Coping With
Multisystem
Complications

Coping With
Multisystem
Complications

Mosby

St. Louis Baltimore Boston Carlsbad Chicago Minneapolis New York Philadelphia Portland
London Milan Sydney Tokyo Toronto

Publisher	Stanley Loeb
Editorial Director	William J. Kelly
Clinical Director	Cindy Tryniszewski, RN, MSN
Associate Editors	Julie Cullen, John L. Harvey
Clinical Project Manager	Maryann Foley, RN, BSN
Editors	Margaret Eckman, Catherine E. Harold, Elizabeth L. Mauro, Laura J. Ninger, Nancy Priff
Clinical Editors	Marlene Ciranowicz, RN, MSN, CDE; Barbara Mankey, RN, MSN; Colleen Seeber, RN, MSN, CCRN
Designer	Lynn Foulk
Composition Specialist	Pamela Merritt
Manufacturing Manager	William A. Winneberger, Jr.

Copyright © 1998 by Mosby, Inc.

Printed in the United States of America
Composition by Mosby Electronic Production, Philadelphia
Printing and binding by R.R. Donnelley & Sons, Inc./CTP

Mosby, Inc.
11830 Westline Industrial Drive
St. Louis, Missouri 63146

Library of Congress Cataloging-in-Publication Data
Coping with multisystem complications.
    p.   cm.
Contributors: Sally A. Brozenec and others.
Includes bibliographical references and index.
ISBN 1-55664-484-1
  1. Multiple organ failure—Pathophysiology. 2. Multiple organ
failure—Nursing. I. Brozenec, Sally A. (Sally Ann), 1943-   .
  [DNLM: 1. Chronic Disease—nursing. 2. Chronic disease—nurses'
instruction. WY 152 C783 1997]
RB150.M84C67 1997
616.07—dc21
DNLM/DLC
for Library of Congress
                                                  97-30022
                                                  CIP

98 99 00 01 02 / 9 8 7 6 5 4 3 2 1

A word about pronouns

You will notice that in *Coping With Multisystem Complications,* as in life, patients come in both sexes. In roughly one half of the chapters, we've used masculine pronouns to refer to patients; in the other half, we've used feminine pronouns.

Contents

1   Diabetes Mellitus   1

2   Hypertension   51

3   Myocardial Infarction   87

Contributors and Consultants

Contributors

Sally A. Brozenec, RN, PhD
Assistant Professor
Rush University College of Nursing
Chicago, Illnois

Heather A. Butler, RN, MSN, CCRN, CNS
Clinical Nurse Educator
St. Joseph's Hospital Health Center
Syracuse, New York

Kay Carpenter, RN, MSN, ARNP, CCRN
Clinical Nurse III, Medical ICU
Saint Luke's Hospital
Kansas City, Missouri

Marilyn A. Folcik, RN, MPH, ONC
Assistant Director, Department of Surgery
Hartford Hospital
Hartford, Connecticut

Marilyn R. Graff, RN, BSN, CDE
Diabetes Care Team, Program Coordinator
Longmont Clinic
Longmont, Colorado

Sharon Kumm, RN, MN, CCRN
Clinical Instructor
University of Kansas School of Nursing
Kansas City, Kansas

Sharon Lehmann, RN, MS, CCRN
Senior Hospital Nurse Clinician
Cardiovascular Interventional Radiology
University of Minnesota Academic Health Center
Minneapolis, Minnesota

Tamara Luedtke, RN, MSN, CCRN
Nurse Manager, Critical Care Unit
Hendrick Health Systems
Abilene, Texas

Andrea R. Mann, RN, MSN
Third Level Chair, Instructor Advanced Medical-
Surgical Nursing
Frankford Hospital School of Nursing
Philadelphia, Pennsylvania

Marci Majors Moreno, RN, MSN
Program Manager, Pulmonary Rehabilitation
Drake Center
Cincinnati, Ohio

Brenda K. Shelton, RN, MS, CCRN, AOCN
Critical Care Clinical Nurse Specialist
The Johns Hopkins Oncology Center
Baltimore, Maryland

Gloria Sonnesso, RN, MSN
Clinical Consultant
Nellcor Puritan Bennett
Pleasanton, California

Deborah Summers, RN, MSN, CCRN
Neuroscience Clinical Nurse Specialist
Saint Luke's Hospital
Kansas City, Missouri

Robyn Tyler, RN, MS, CS, CDE
Clinical Nurse Specialist
Department of Veterans Affairs Medical Center
Sioux Falls, South Dakota

Patti Westrope, RN, MSN, CCRN, CS
Advanced Practice Nurse
Saint Luke's Internal Medicine
Kansas City, Missouri

Consultants

Peggy Bourgeois, RN, MN, APRN, CDE
Director, Diabetes Center
Baton Rouge General Medical Center
Baton Rouge, Louisiana

Mary Jo Gerlach, RN, MSNEd
Assistant Professor, Adult Nursing
Medical College of Georgia, School of Nursing
Athens, Georgia

JoAnne Konick-McMahan, RN, MSN, CCRN
Advanced Practice Nurse
School of Nursing, University of Pennsylvania
Philadelphia, Pennsylvania

Colleen Lucas, RN, MN, CS
Clinical Nurse Specialist
Legacy Good Samaritan Hospital and Medical
Center
Portland, Oregon

Carrie McCoy, RN, MSN, CEN
Associate Professor of Nursing
Northern Kentucky University
Highland Heights, Kentucky

Patricia L. Vaska, RN, MSN, CNP, CNS, CCRN
Cardiovascular Surgery Nurse Practitioner,
Clinical Nurse Specialist
Sioux Valley Hospital
Sioux Falls, South Dakota

Foreword

Today, patients who have more than one major disorder aren't the exception, they're the rule. Take a patient admitted for a myocardial infarction who also has diabetes mellitus, or a home care patient with a cerebrovascular accident who contracts pneumonia. Such patients tend to develop further complications—complications that can be subtle and dangerous.

No matter where you work, caring for these patients presents a complex nursing challenge, perhaps the nursing challenge of today and tomorrow. Yet, of all the nursing books you own, only *Coping With Multisystem Complications* gives you the practical nursing strategies you need to meet this challenge. In langue that's clear and concise, *Coping With Multisystem Complications* explains how major disorders interact and how the interactions affect patients. More important, this book tells you how to modify your patient care and how to anticipate, recognize, and respond to complications triggered by the disorders.

Specifically, *Coping With Multisystem Complications* addresses three distinct types of patients:
- Those who have one disorder that produces a second disorder—for example, *a patient with heart failure who develops pulmonary edema.*
- Those with two related disorders who experience a serious complication triggered by one of them—for example, *a patient with rheumatoid arthritis and a hip fracture who develops fat embolism from the fracture.*
- Those with two unrelated disorders who have a crisis that exacerbates one of them—for example, *a patient with an intestinal obstruction and a myocardial infarction who develops a stress ulcer from gastrointestinal hemorrhaging.*

Organization

As you can imagine, organizing practical information on complex, interrelated disorders and their complications presents an interesting challenge of its own. *Coping With Multisystem Complications* meets the challenge by first focusing on 13 of the most common disorders among hospital patients—diabetes mellitus, hypertension, myocardial infarction, heart failure, rheumatoid arthritis, cerebrovascular accident, emphysema, pneumonia, peripheral vascular disease, asthma, peptic ulcer disease, pancreatitis, and intestinal obstruction. Each of these disorders has its own chapter that starts with a review of relevant anatomy and physiology, pathophysiology, assessment findings, diagnostic tests, medical interventions, and nursing interventions.

Then the major disorder is linked to other disorders patients are most likely to have. For instance, in Chapter 4, heart failure is linked to myocardial infarction, pulmonary edema, and chronic obstructive pulmonary disease. The discussion on each of these pairings covers how the disorders affect each other and how you can best adapt your ongoing nursing care. Next, you'll read about how to recognize and respond to complications that commonly stem from the two disorders. For instance, under the pairing of heart failure and myocardial infarction, you'll find specific discussions of reinfarction, cardiogenic shock, and renal failure. In all, *Coping With Multisystem Complications* covers more than 100 such complications.

Features

As you'll see, *Coping With Multisystem Complications* contains several recurring features that aid your understanding and help you sharpen your skills.

- **Anatomy review** provides a quick memorable refresher with crisp illustrations of relevant anatomy.
- **Pathophysiology** uses illustrations and flowcharts to show you how two disorders progress and interact.
- **Comfort measures** spells out steps you can take to ease your patient's discomfort and provide support.
- **Adapting your care** gives helpful tips on how to modify your care in special situations—for instance, when a patient with more than one disorder is undergoing a diagnostic procedure.

- **Drug alert** warns you of dangerous drug interactions that can develop in patients taking drugs for more than one disorder and of adverse effects that can be exacerbated by a second disorder.
- **Going home** helps you teach your patients how to continue their care at home after discharge.
- **Rapid response** succinctly describes the nursing interventions you must perform when a life-threatening complication develops.

Coping With Multisystem Complications addresses an urgent need in our profession today. It explains how to give skilled, comprehensive nursing care to patients who have more than one major disorder and complications stemming from them. Clearly written and effectively organized, this invaluable resource is packed with practical nursing information. No matter how much nursing experience you have or where you work, my advice is the same: Read this book.

Sally A. Brozenec, RN, PhD
Assistant Professor
Rush University
College of Nursing

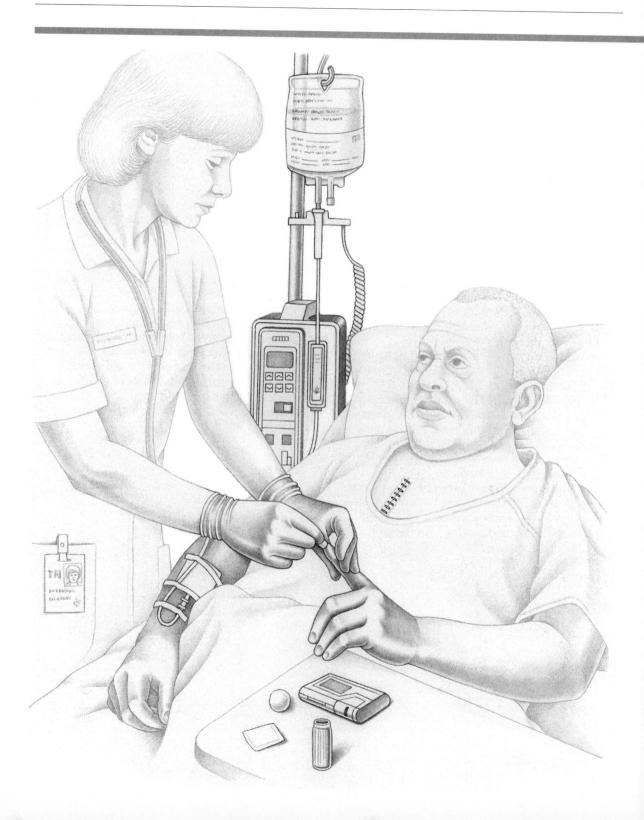

Diabetes Mellitus

The fourth leading cause of death by disease in the United States, diabetes mellitus affects some 16 million Americans. In about half of them, the disease goes undiagnosed. Diabetes strikes males and females of all ages, races, and socioeconomic groups, although the incidence is highest among African-Americans and women over age 60.

A disease of insulin deficiency or resistance, diabetes results when the body's demand for insulin exceeds its supply or when the body can't use insulin. The disease is characterized by altered carbohydrate, fat, and protein metabolism; increased glucose levels; and changes in microcirculation and macrocirculation.

ANATOMY REVIEW

A look at the pancreas

The major organ involved in diabetes, the pancreas functions as both an endocrine and an exocrine gland. The endocrine tissue of the pancreas contains more than a million tiny clusters of alpha, beta, and delta cells, known collectively as the islets of Langerhans. These cells secrete vital hormones, including insulin and glucagon, which play a major role in carbohydrate, fat, and protein metabolism.

The inset below shows a microscopic view of the endocrine tissue of the pancreas.

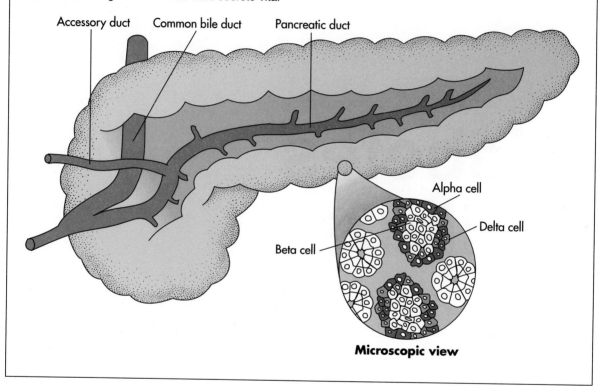

Accessory duct Common bile duct Pancreatic duct

Alpha cell

Delta cell

Beta cell

Microscopic view

Anatomy and physiology review

Located behind the stomach and between the spleen and duodenum, the pancreas contains tiny clusters of hormone-secreting alpha, beta, and delta cells. Known collectively as the islets of Langerhans, these cells are controlled by the sympathetic and parasympathetic nervous systems.

Alpha cells, which account for 20% of the islet cells, secrete glucagon, a hormone that raises blood glucose levels. Beta cells, which make up 75% of the islet cells, secrete insulin, a hormone that lowers blood glucose levels. And delta cells, which account for the remaining 5%, secrete somatostatin, a hormone that regulates alpha and beta cell functions by inhibiting the secretion of insulin, glucagon, and pancreatic polypeptide. Somatostatin also maintains the balance of carbohydrate, fat, and protein metabolism from ingested nutrients (see *A look at the pancreas*).

Insulin

Insulin lowers blood glucose levels by transporting glucose into cells, where it's used immediately for energy or stored as glycogen in the liver and muscles. When insulin levels increase, so do the hepatic uptake of glucose and the conversion of glucose to glycogen. Increased insulin levels also decrease the breakdown of glycogen in the liver and muscles.

Insulin promotes both the conversion of glucose to fat and the storage of fat in adipose tissue. It also promotes the synthesis of triglycerides from glucose within the fat cells and inhibits the breakdown of stored triglycerides. Insulin stimulates protein synthesis by increasing the active transport of amino acids into cells. Plus, insulin inhibits gluconeogenesis (the formation of glucose from fats and protein stored in the liver). When glucose and insulin are present in sufficient amounts, protein is spared because the body is able to use glucose and fats for energy.

Without insulin, the body's tissues can't get the nutrients they need for fuel and storage. Liver, muscle, and adipose tissues require that insulin bind to a receptor on their plasma membrane to metabolize carbohydrates. At the target cell, insulin binds with a receptor to activate tyrosine kinase. In turn, this activates glucose transporters, necessary for the diffusion of glucose into the cells, and protein kinase. Protein kinase then activates or deactivates the target enzymes necessary for glucose metabolism. During this process, potassium, phosphate, and magnesium also enter the cell.

Stimulated by increased blood glucose levels, insulin secretion reaches peak levels about 30 minutes after meals and returns to normal in 2 to 3 hours. Between meals or during a period of fasting, insulin levels remain low, and the body uses its supply of stored glucose and amino acids to provide energy for the tissues (see *Understanding insulin secretion*, page 4).

Glucagon
An insulin antagonist, glucagon helps maintain blood glucose levels between meals and during periods of fasting. Glucagon secretion is stimulated by amino acids and inhibited by insulin. Glucagon works primarily in the liver to increase the blood glucose level by stimulating

glycogenolysis and gluconeogenesis. It enhances the breakdown of fats providing glycerol for gluconeogenesis. It also increases the breakdown of proteins into amino acids for use in gluconeogenesis.

Hormonal regulation of blood glucose levels
Blood glucose levels regulate the secretion of insulin and glucagon. Insulin secretion is stimulated by high blood glucose levels and inhibited by low levels. Conversely, glucagon secretion is stimulated by low blood glucose levels and inhibited by high levels. Both hormones are transported from the pancreas through the portal circulation to the liver, where they exert an almost instantaneous effect on blood glucose levels.

In addition to glucagon, three other hormones help to balance the effect of insulin. These hormones—epinephrine, growth hormone, and cortisol—promote the release of glycogen, thereby raising blood glucose levels. Together with insulin, these hormones help maintain normal blood glucose levels.

A catecholamine, epinephrine helps maintain blood glucose levels during periods of stress. It inhibits the release of insulin, resulting in less movement of glucose into the muscle cells. Epinephrine also stimulates the conversion of glycogen stored in the liver and muscles to glucose and mobilizes fatty acids from adipose tissue. This spares glucose for use in the brain and nervous system.

Growth hormone increases protein synthesis in all body cells. It also mobilizes fatty acids from the adipose tissue and decreases the cellular uptake and use of glucose by the body. This causes blood glucose levels to rise, which, in turn, stimulates the release of insulin and inhibits the secretion of growth hormone. During times of stress—such as prolonged exercise, fasting, or infection—growth hormone secretion increases in response to lower blood glucose levels and insulin secretion.

Glucocorticoid hormones, such as cortisol, regulate blood glucose levels. During times of stress, they stimulate the liver to increase gluconeogenesis. They also decrease tissue use of glucose, thereby sparing glucose for use in the brain and nervous system.

Understanding insulin secretion

The pancreas continuously secretes insulin into the bloodstream at a baseline rate of 1 to 2 units (U) per hour. After a meal, the increased blood glucose stimulates insulin secretion, and 30 to 45 minutes after breakfast, lunch, and dinner, the rate peaks at about 4 to 6 U per hour. Secretion returns to the baseline rate in 2 to 3 hours.

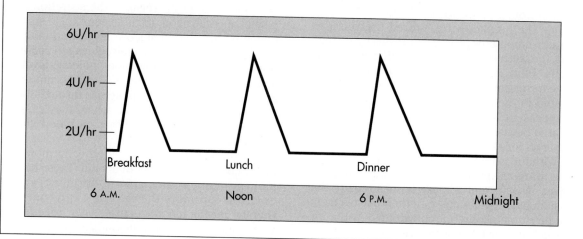

Pathophysiology

In diabetes, the body's insulin supply is either absent or deficient, or target cells resist the action of insulin. This compromises the way the body metabolizes nutrients for energy, leading to hyperglycemia and altered fat metabolism. It also inhibits the conversion of glucose to glycogen. Cells begin to starve, causing the liver to increase its breakdown of glycogen to glucose. This further increases the hyperglycemia.

When peripheral tissues are unable to get the glucose they need, they begin to use their glycogen stores and protein for energy. The liver breaks down lipids for energy, producing ketone bodies from the breakdown of fatty acids. When these ketones accumulate, they can cause ketosis and, eventually, ketonuria.

As blood glucose levels increase, they eventually rise above the renal threshold, and glucose is excreted in the urine. This creates an osmotic diuresis, causing large amounts of water and electrolytes to be excreted from the body, possibly leading to dehydration and electrolyte imbalances.

Types of diabetes mellitus

Diabetes mellitus occurs primarily in two types: Type I, or insulin-dependent diabetes mellitus (IDDM), and Type II, or non–insulin-dependent diabetes mellitus (NIDDM). Two less common types of diabetes also occur. Secondary diabetes develops as a result of another condition, such as pancreatic disease, hormonal disease, or drug or chemical exposure. Gestational diabetes develops during pregnancy.

Type I diabetes mellitus

An autoimmune disorder, Type I diabetes results from the selective destruction of insulin-producing beta cells in the pancreas. With this destruction, the level of circulating insulin is diminished or depleted.

Although the exact mechanism isn't known, the immune system appears to attack and destroy the insulin-producing cells of the pancreas, possibly triggered by genetic and environmental factors. Research findings suggest that genes or groups of genes in the human leukocyte antigen (HLA) region provide susceptibility to Type I diabetes.

Genetic factors associated with antigens on the genes controlling the immune response increase the risk of immune activity against the islet tissues. The autoimmune system also attacks insulin with insulin autoantibodies that result from beta cell destruction.

Viruses may play a role in beta cell destruction. Two such viruses—coxsackie B4 and the mumps virus—have been isolated as possible triggers for Type I diabetes. The incidence of the disease peaks during midwinter and spring, when these viral infections are more prevalent.

Over several years, the beta cells may be completely destroyed. Carbohydrate intolerance results after about 90% of the secretory capacity of a person's beta cell mass has been destroyed.

Type II diabetes mellitus
About 90% of people with diabetes mellitus have Type II diabetes. Of these, 60% to 90% are obese, and about 43% are over age 65. First-degree relatives of patients with Type II diabetes have a 10% to 15% risk of developing diabetes and a 20% to 30% risk of developing impaired glucose tolerance. Type II diabetes is more common in women than in men and in African-Americans than in whites.

Insulin resistance is believed to be the primary cause of hyperglycemia in Type II diabetes. This resistance may result from an alteration of intracellular events involved in glucose metabolism.

Patients with Type II diabetes may have decreased beta cell responsiveness to blood glucose levels and abnormal glucagon secretion. The islet cell dysfunction may result from decreased beta cell mass, abnormal beta cell function, or some combination of the two.

Insulin resistance can also stem from secondary factors that affect target cells. These factors include stress caused by fever or sepsis, pregnancy, and hormonal disorders involving glucocorticoids, growth hormone, catecholamines, glucagon, and thyroid hormones.

A common occurrence with Type II diabetes, syndrome X consists of insulin resistance, hyperinsulinemia, hyperglycemia, upper-body obesity, hypertension, and lipid disorders. This syndrome is associated with abnormalities that increase the risk of other disorders, such as angina, myocardial infarction

(MI), cerebrovascular accident (CVA), and peripheral vascular disease.

Assessment findings

Typically, a patient with Type I diabetes reports a sudden onset of symptoms. Hyperglycemia leads to serum hyperosmolality, which causes water to be drawn out of the cells and into the vascular system. This results in cellular dehydration and increased renal blood flow. Because glucose is also an osmotic diuretic, urine output increases, resulting in polyuria and volume depletion. Excess glucose is excreted in the urine, causing glycosuria. Volume depletion and cellular dehydration lead to thirst and polydipsia.

Because glucose isn't readily available to the cells, energy production decreases, causing malaise and fatigue. Hunger is also stimulated, causing polyphagia. Dehydration and the breakdown of fats and proteins in an attempt to meet the body's energy needs lead to weight loss. Blurred vision may develop because of the osmotic effect on the lenses of the eyes.

As fat stores break down, fatty acids are mobilized and ketosis occurs, resulting in metabolic acidosis. The body compensates by producing respiratory alkalosis, and the patient develops Kussmaul's respiration. At the cellular level, potassium is exchanged for hydrogen ions, resulting in hyperkalemia.

On examination, the eyes may show signs of retinopathy or cataract formation. You may note skin changes resulting from impaired peripheral circulation. The patient also may have muscle wasting and a loss of subcutaneous fat. Skin turgor may be poor, and mucous membranes may appear dry from the osmotic diuresis and resulting dehydration.

Typically, a patient with Type II diabetes reports vague, nonspecific complaints. Signs and symptoms appear more slowly, and the disease may not be diagnosed until the patient seeks health care for another problem. The patient may have polyuria and polydipsia, but usually not polyphagia. Obesity is common; weight loss is uncommon.

Other signs and symptoms of Type II diabetes include blurred vision, fatigue, and paresthesia. Both hyperglycemia and glyco-suria promote the growth of yeast organisms. Many women experience pruritus and vulvo-vaginitis from candidal infections.

Diagnostic tests

Several tests can be used to diagnose diabetes, detect complications, and evaluate the effec-tiveness of treatment. Also, patients can moni-tor their own glucose levels using fingerstick blood samples.

Random blood glucose test

A valuable screening tool for detecting dia-betes mellitus, this test determines a patient's blood glucose level on a random basis. A blood glucose level of 200 mg/dl or more accompa-nied by complaints of polydipsia, polyuria, polyphagia, and weight loss confirms a diagno-sis of diabetes. If the patient hasn't eaten within 2 hours of the test, a blood glucose level greater than 140 mg/dl and less than 200 mg/dl suggests impaired glucose tolerance.

Fasting blood glucose test

Commonly used to screen for diabetes, the fast-ing blood glucose test evaluates the patient's ability to regulate glucose after a fast of at least 4 hours. The normal range for the fasting blood glucose test varies. Generally, normal levels are 70 to 115 mg/dl. Fasting blood glucose levels greater than 140 mg/dl on two or more consec-utive occasions indicate diabetes. Failing to ad-here to the fast or receiving dextrose solution I.V. may affect the test results.

The fasting blood glucose test also can be used to monitor the effects of treatment. Consistent elevations may indicate that the pa-tient's therapy needs to be adjusted.

Glucose tolerance test

When the fasting blood glucose level is nor-mal but signs and symptoms suggest diabetes, a physician may order a glucose tolerance test. This test measures carbohydrate metabo-lism after a patient ingests a challenge dose of glucose. After maintaining a diet that contains at least 150 grams of carbohydrates per day for 3 days, the patient fasts overnight for about 8 hours. Then a blood sample is drawn for a glu-cose level, and a urine sample is obtained and checked for glycosuria. Next, the patient drinks a 75-gram glucose solution. Further blood and urine samples are obtained at 1-hour and 2-hour intervals. During this time, the pa-tient can't eat, but he can drink water.

A physician diagnoses diabetes if two sepa-rate glucose levels exceed 200 mg/dl. Factors such as bed rest, infection, trauma, medica-tions, and stress can alter the test results.

Glycosylated hemoglobin test

Glycosylated hemoglobin levels determine the patient's response to therapy. Normally, when hemoglobin is released from the bone marrow, it doesn't contain glucose. While hemoglobin is in red blood cells, however, glucose attaches itself to it; thus, the hemoglobin becomes gly-cosylated, and substances called glycohemo-globin A_{1a}, A_{1b}, and A_{1c} are formed.

The process of glycosylation is irreversible. Therefore, the level of glycosylated hemoglo-bin in the blood reflects not transient glucose levels, but blood glucose levels over the last 2 months or more. In uncontrolled diabetes, the level of hemoglobin A_{1c} is abnormally high. The normal range for hemoglobin A_{1c} is 4% to 6%. A value of 11% to 15% indicates poor glu-cose control over time.

Related blood tests

Other blood tests can help in evaluating the patient for complications of diabetes. Because diabetes is a risk factor for coronary artery disease and decreased renal function, fasting lipid profiles and blood urea nitrogen (BUN) and creatinine levels can provide valu-able information.

Fasting lipid profile

A fasting lipid profile can detect lipid abnor-malities, which indicate an increased risk of coronary artery disease. After the patient fasts overnight, a blood sample is obtained to mea-sure his total cholesterol, high-density lipo-protein (HDL) cholesterol, low-density lipopro-tein (LDL) cholesterol, and triglyceride levels.

Typically, the patient with Type II diabetes has elevated total cholesterol, LDL cholesterol, and triglyceride levels and decreased HDL cholesterol levels. Elevated total cholesterol, LDL cholesterol, and triglyceride levels increase the risk of coronary artery disease.

BUN and creatinine tests

These tests provide information about a patient's renal function and help detect nephropathy, a complication of diabetes. Because serum creatinine levels aren't affected by dehydration and other problems outside the kidneys, they're a much better indicator of renal function than serum BUN levels. If the serum BUN level is elevated but the serum creatinine level is normal, the cause of the abnormal BUN level may not be renal.

Elevated serum BUN and serum creatinine levels suggest impaired renal function and indicate the need for further testing and follow-up. Impaired renal function and problems with glucose regulation predispose a patient with diabetes to end-stage renal disease and cardiovascular disease.

Urine tests

Urine tests can detect glucose, ketones, and protein in the urine. But today, because blood glucose tests are more accurate than urine glucose tests and because patients routinely use home blood glucose monitoring, urine glucose testing has become obsolete. Glucose appears in the urine only after the renal threshold has been reached, usually when the blood level reaches about 180 mg/dl. Also, the results can be influenced by factors such as fluid intake, urine concentration, and the use of certain drugs. If glucose is detected in the urine during routine urinalysis, the patient should have a blood glucose test to confirm the diagnosis of diabetes.

Testing urine for ketones continues to be an important part of monitoring patients with diabetes, especially those with Type I diabetes who are at risk for developing ketoacidosis. Ketones spill into the urine when the body uses fat instead of glucose for energy. Typically, if blood glucose levels are above 240 mg/dl, ketones appear in the urine. Ketones also can move into the urine when the patient is acutely ill or under stress or when he's developing diabetic ketoacidosis.

Detecting protein in the urine during routine urinalysis may indicate impaired renal function. Because diabetes can severely affect a patient's renal function, a physician should check urine protein levels when the patient is diagnosed and then monitor them periodically. The sudden appearance of protein in the urine indicates the need for further evaluation to determine the cause.

Medical interventions

Currently, diabetes has no cure, but treatment focuses on three major areas: nutrition and diet therapy, drug therapy, and exercise. The goal of diabetes treatment is to keep blood glucose levels as close to normal as possible and therefore minimize the risk of complications. Achieving this goal requires a treatment plan that's tailored to the individual patient's age, lifestyle, nutritional needs, activity level, and self-care ability. Therefore, the patient must be involved in setting goals and creating the treatment plan.

A pancreas transplantation may be an option for treating insulin-dependent diabetic patients. If your patient is between ages 18 and 55 and has diabetic nephropathy, he may undergo a simultaneous kidney transplantation as well. This procedure requires long-term immunosuppression. The use of transplanted pancreatic islet cells is being evaluated as a possible alternative.

Nutrition and diet therapy

An essential part of diabetes treatment, nutrition and diet therapy aims to keep blood glucose and lipid levels within acceptable ranges. It also attempts to meet nutritional needs, prevent wide variations in blood glucose levels, reduce the risks of hypoglycemia and hyperglycemia, and maintain appropriate body weight.

The American Diabetes Association recommends the following distribution of calories daily:
- 55% to 60% from carbohydrates
- 12% to 20% from protein
- less than 30% from fat, primarily polyunsaturated and monounsaturated fats

---

Five approaches to dietary planning

The goal of diet therapy is to provide the diabetic patient with the nutrients he needs to help maintain blood glucose control. This chart compares five common meal-planning methods.

Method	How it works
Exchange lists	• Foods are grouped into categories based on similar calorie, carbohydrate, protein, and fat amounts. • Food selections from each category can be substituted for other, equivalent selections (for example, ½ cup applesauce = ⅓ cup pineapple).
Dietary guidelines for Americans	• Allows a variety of foods. • Features a diet low in fat, saturated fat, and cholesterol. • Encourages use of vegetables, fruits, and grains. • Allows moderate use of sugar, salt, and sodium.
Food guide pyramid	• Foods are divided into six groups. • Encourages use of bread, cereal, rice, and pasta. • Encourages sparing use of fats, oils, and sweets.
Point system	• Points are assigned according to each food's calorie, carbohydrate, protein, and fat content. • The total daily allowance is written as a number of calories and carbohydrates. • Foods are selected according to point distribution.
Sample menus	• Meal plans are devised by a dietitian. • Diet allows for individualized patient needs.

A diabetic person can use nonnutritive sweeteners—such as aspartame, acesulfame K, and saccharin—because they contain few calories and have a negligible effect on blood glucose levels. A diabetic person also can use nutritive sweeteners, such as fructose and sucrose, but they must be substituted for other carbohydrates.

Diet guidelines call for limiting or avoiding alcohol intake because alcohol inhibits gluconeogenesis, thereby interfering with the body's ability to make glucose from noncarbohydrate sources. The result can be hypoglycemia.

An obese patient with Type II diabetes needs to lose weight. Weight reduction slows the release of glucose into the bloodstream and increases the number of insulin receptor cells. With a loss of only 5 to 10 pounds, a person's blood glucose levels begin to improve.

For success, a diabetic patient must follow dietary guidelines consistently and eat meals at regular times. Compliance with diet therapy typically improves when a patient understands the pathophysiology of diabetes and the interrelationships among blood glucose levels, insulin, and food intake. Increased understanding helps the patient control his blood glucose level and minimize the risk of complications (see *Five approaches to dietary planning*).

Drug therapy

All patients with Type I diabetes and some patients with Type II diabetes need drug therapy to control their blood glucose levels. Antidiabetic medications fall into two major categories: insulin and oral hypoglycemic agents. Patients with Type I diabetes need insulin; most patients with Type II diabetes need oral hypoglycemic agents and some need insulin.

Oral hypoglycemic agents

When dietary measures and exercise fail to control blood glucose levels in Type II diabetes, oral hypoglycemic agents are used. For these drugs to be effective, the patient's pancreas must be capable of secreting some insulin.

Oral hypoglycemic agents act primarily by stimulating the pancreas to increase islet cell secretion of insulin. They also appear to make

• less than 10% from saturated fats.

Fiber in a person's diet can delay gastric emptying, increase satiety, and lower total cholesterol and LDL cholesterol levels. Thus, a diabetic person should consume 20 to 35 grams of fiber a day to help promote bowel elimination and lower lipid levels.

tissues more sensitive to insulin by increasing the number of receptor sites available and by enhancing insulin uptake at the postreceptor sites. Some oral hypoglycemic agents also decrease glucose production in the liver.

Most oral hypoglycemic agents are sulfonylureas, which have been used to treat Type II diabetes since the 1950s. Today, two generations of sulfonylureas are available. The second generation drugs are more potent and therefore require smaller doses. They're also less toxic and less likely to interact with other drugs.

Two other common drug categories include biguanides and alpha-glucosidase inhibitors. Biguanides, such as metformin, appear to increase insulin production, increase insulin use in the peripheral tissues, decrease glucose production by the liver, and alter the intestinal absorption of glucose. When taken with the first bite of food, alpha-glucosidase inhibitors, such as acarbose, delay the digestion and absorption of carbohydrates, thereby producing a smaller rise in blood glucose levels following meals (see *Reviewing oral hypoglycemic agents*, page 10).

Insulin

All patients with Type I diabetes must inject insulin daily. Some patients with Type II diabetes also require insulin if diet, exercise, and oral hypoglycemic agents aren't effective. For these patients, insulin is used temporarily during times of stress when blood glucose levels are difficult to control. Like the insulin produced by normally functioning beta cells, injected insulin lowers blood glucose levels by promoting the movement of glucose into cells and by inhibiting the conversion of glycogen and amino acids to glucose.

Several types of insulins are available. Although they have the same mechanism of action, they differ in onset, peak, and duration, thereby affecting the time in which an insulin reaction, such as hypoglycemia, might occur. Insulins are classified as rapid-acting, short-acting, intermediate-acting, and long-acting (see *Reviewing types of insulin*, page 11).

Insulin may be derived from beef, pork, or human sources. Although human insulin causes fewer antigenic reactions, it may have a quicker onset and shorter duration than animal insulins. A patient who changes from an animal insulin to human insulin may need a reduced dosage.

The goal of insulin therapy is to mimic the normal endogenous secretion of insulin. A patient should administer insulin so that it's available when food is consumed, and he should ensure that food is available when insulin is acting. The dosage varies according to the patient's needs and response. It may be increased if a patient is seriously ill, develops an infection, undergoes surgery or trauma, or is experiencing puberty. In some patients, a daily dose of insulin is sufficient. If a patient's blood glucose levels are difficult to control, two different insulins may be combined and administered in a single injection, or different insulins may be administered in separate injections at different times of the day.

Insulin administration: Typically, insulin is administered as a subcutaneous injection, although regular insulin may be given I.V. if a patient needs his blood glucose levels lowered quickly. When insulin is injected subcutaneously, its absorption and duration of action vary depending on the injection site. For example, the quickest absorption and shortest duration occur when insulin is injected into the abdomen. The absorption is slower and the duration is longer when insulin is injected into the arms, legs, or buttocks.

An alternative way to administer insulin, the insulin pump injects regular insulin subcutaneously into the abdomen through an indwelling needle site. Worn externally, the pump can be programmed to infuse insulin continuously at a rate that corresponds to the patient's basal metabolic rate. And a patient can manually activate the pump to deliver a bolus dose before meals. In short, the insulin pump mimics normal endogenous insulin secretion. It also eliminates the need for numerous subcutaneous injections and allows flexibility in meal size and timing. However, a patient must still monitor blood glucose levels closely and comply with other treatments, such as diet therapy and exercise. Many patients receiving insulin pump therapy must check their blood glucose levels up to six times a day and may need to adjust their insulin

Reviewing oral hypoglycemic agents

For patients with Type II diabetes, oral hypoglycemic agents form an important part of therapy.

Agent	Dosage range (mg/day)	Onset (hr)	Peak (hr)	Duration (hr)
Sulfonylureas				
Tolbutamide	250 to 3,000	1	4 to 6	6 to 12
Tolazamide	100 to 1,000	Variable	4 to 6	12 to 24
Acetohexamide	250 to 1,500	1	2 to 4	12 to 24
Chlorpropamide	250 to 500	1	3 to 4	60
Glipizide	5 to 15	1 to 1.5	1 to 3	10 to 16
Glyburide	2.5 to 5	1	4	16 to 24
Glimepiride	1 to 4	1	2 to 3	Not known
Other agents				
Metformin	500 to 2,500	Not known	Not known	10 to 16
Acarbose	75 to 300	Very rapid	1	Not known

dosages according to the results (see *Using an insulin pump,* page 12).

An implantable pump, about the size of a bar of soap, can be surgically placed under the skin and programmed to release insulin into the peritoneal cavity. Like the external pump, this device is programmed to deliver a low, steady flow of insulin throughout the day. At mealtimes, the patient uses a remote control device to deliver a bolus dose. Every 4 to 12 weeks, the physician refills the reservoir with insulin. The advantages of the implantable pump include good control of blood glucose levels, closer imitation of endogenous insulin secretion, and fewer episodes of hypoglycemia. The only disadvantage is that the pump tends to clog and therefore must be rinsed out periodically.

Complications: Patients receiving insulin therapy commonly develop hypoglycemia. This complication may stem from receiving too much insulin, eating late, skipping meals, or exercising too strenuously. Typically, the patient experiences signs and symptoms when blood glucose levels drop to 60 mg/dl or less.

Other possible complications include atrophy or tissue hypertrophy at the injection site, erratic insulin action, insulin allergy, and insulin resistance. Atrophy results from the breakdown of adipose tissue and may be caused by an immune response or an injection of impure insulin. Tissue hypertrophy involves thickening of the subcutaneous tissue and usually results from repeated injections into the same site. Continued use of hypertrophied sites can cause erratic insulin action. Other causes of erratic insulin action include the following:
• excessive eating
• irregular mealtimes
• inaccurate dose measurement
• inadequate mixing of two types of insulin
• irregular exercise
• use of drugs such as aspirin, alcohol, cough syrups, and thiazide diuretics.

Insulin allergy usually results from a hypersensitivity to the animal proteins in animal

Reviewing types of insulin

Depending on its onset, peak, and duration, insulin may be rapid-acting, short-acting, intermediate-acting, or long-acting. When teaching your diabetic patient about insulin therapy, inform him when the insulin will start to take effect, when it will reach its peak level, and how long its effects will last. This information will help him learn when the risk of hypoglycemia is greatest. The chart below summarizes the onset, peak, and duration of the four major types of insulin.

Type	Onset	Peak (hr)	Duration (hr)
Rapid-acting (Lispro)	5 to 15 min	0.5 to 1.5	2 to 4
Short-acting (Regular)	30 to 60 min	2 to 3	6 to 8
Intermediate-acting (NPH, Lente)	1 to 2.5 hr	4 to 15	24
Long-acting (Ultralente)	4 to 8 hr	10 to 30	>36

insulins, although some patients are allergic to insulin or the preservatives in the solution. However, systemic allergic reactions to insulin are rare. Insulin resistance may result from specific insulin antagonists within the blood or from circulating antibodies that bind to insulin, rendering it inactive and unavailable for use by the target tissues. An insulin-resistant patient needs higher than usual doses of insulin. Many such patients need 200 or more units of insulin each day.

Exercise

In patients with Type II diabetes, exercise helps to decrease the occurrence of insulin resistance, decrease weight, and lower triglyceride and LDL cholesterol levels, thus reducing the risk of cardiovascular disease. In patients with Type I diabetes, moderate exercise is worthwhile, but too much exercise can increase the risk of hypoglycemia. A balanced program of insulin therapy, diet therapy, and exercise maximizes the benefits while minimizing the risks.

Before starting an exercise program, a patient should have a thorough physical examination to determine blood glucose levels and detect or evaluate any long-term complications that might contraindicate exercise. For example, a diabetic patient should never start an exercise program until he achieves good blood glucose control. Also, a patient with progressive retinopathy should avoid intense exercise because it may cause blood pressure changes that can increase retinal vessel damage and hemorrhage. And a patient with peripheral neuropathy needs close monitoring during exercise for possible foot injuries. Patients who are age 30 and older, those who have had diabetes for more than 20 years, and those with cardiovascular symptoms must undergo exercise stress testing before starting an exercise program.

As with diet therapy, an exercise program must be individualized. Sedentary patients may require a less intensive program than active patients. The following are general guidelines:
• 5 minutes of warm-up activity
• 5 to 7 minutes of stretching
• 20 to 30 minutes of aerobic activity
• 10 to 15 minutes of cool-down activity.

All exercise programs should identify which exercises the patient should perform, how strenuously he should perform them, how long he should perform them, and how often he should perform them. A patient should start slowly and increase the intensity and duration gradually.

One of the most common risks associated with exercise and diabetes, hypoglycemia strikes more patients with Type I diabetes than patients with Type II diabetes. The following steps can help reduce the risk:

Using an insulin pump

The insulin pump, an alternative to several daily injections of insulin, produces near-normal glucose levels by providing a continuous subcutaneous infusion of insulin. The battery-powered pump contains a syringe and a computer chip that stores information for insulin administration.

To administer insulin, the patient attaches an infusion set with a small catheter to the pump. He then inserts the catheter into his abdomen, arm, or thigh. He can wear the pump 24 hours a day, but he should change the insertion site every 72 hours. He should also change the site if it becomes inflamed or painful or if the system leaks or becomes occluded.

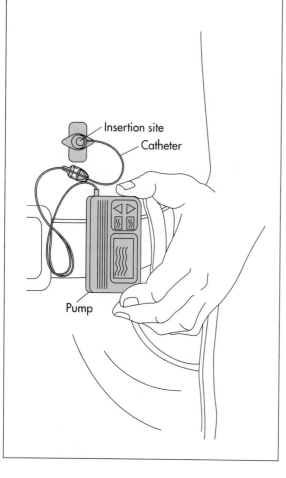

Insertion site

Catheter

Pump

- Learn how your patient responds to different types and intensities of exercise.
- Teach your patient to monitor blood glucose levels before, during, and after exercise.
- Tell your patient to eat a carbohydrate snack if his blood glucose level is less than 100 mg/dl.
- Instruct him to eat 15 to 30 grams of carbohydrates every 30 minutes when engaged in prolonged exercise. Explain that he may need to increase his intake for up to 24 hours after exercising.
- Caution your patient to avoid exercise during peak insulin times.
- Tell your patient to avoid exercise involving the muscles used for insulin injection.
- Inform your patient that hypoglycemia can develop as long as 24 hours after exercising.

Remember, patients with Type II diabetes may not need to increase their intake of carbohydrates because they're less likely to develop hypoglycemia. Increasing their intake increases the chances of overeating and counteracts the benefits of exercise and weight control.

Nursing interventions

You should focus on implementing the measures your patient needs to regain and maintain control over his blood glucose levels. This begins with a thorough assessment, including a patient health history and a physical examination. It also includes obtaining the results of diagnostic tests, such as a fasting blood glucose test, a glucose tolerance test, and a lipid profile.

In the health history, include information about your patient's current complaints, medical history, family history, diet, medication history, lifestyle, health beliefs, and knowledge level. The information you gather will help you formulate an effective, individualized plan of care.

In the physical examination, include a review of systems, focusing on any acute or chronic complications of diabetes. Be alert for possible barriers to the patient's ability to manage his diabetes. For example, a patient with diminished visual acuity may have difficulty reading the numbers on an insulin syringe or medication container. A patient with muscle atrophy or decreased manual dexterity or strength may have difficulty using a certain site for insulin injection. Simple modifications can help ensure that the patient manages his condition adequately.

If your patient is elderly, consider how age-related changes, such as incontinence, may mask diabetes symptoms, such as polyuria. Also, remember that many older adults have several chronic illnesses and take numerous medications, which can disguise or counteract the signs and symptoms of diabetes. For example, certain medications can decrease a person's appetite, leading to weight loss that counteracts the weight gain associated with Type II diabetes.

When caring for a diabetic patient, your primary roles are to facilitate and to teach. Focus your interventions on helping your patient learn to manage his diabetes effectively. This includes controlling blood glucose levels, maintaining adequate nutrition and hydration, preventing complications, and providing emotional support. If possible, include your patient's family in the plan of care and in your teaching.

Controlling blood glucose levels
Blood glucose control is the foundation of diabetes management. Before starting therapy, review baseline laboratory findings, including fasting blood glucose and glucose tolerance test results. Use subsequent test results to help evaluate the effectiveness of the treatment plan.

Check blood glucose levels
Hospitalized diabetic patients have fasting blood glucose levels checked daily, using a blood sample obtained by venipuncture or fingerstick. Report any abnormal findings to the physician as soon as possible because a dosage adjustment may be necessary. To continually monitor the patient's condition, obtain fingerstick blood samples for glucose levels several times a day, such as before meals and at bedtime. Also, check urine specimens for ketones, especially if blood glucose levels are high or the patient is experiencing unusual stress.

Ensure regular meals
Monitor the patient's food intake and make sure he receives his meals on time. If a meal is delayed, give the patient a snack. If the patient

must have nothing by mouth because of a diagnostic test, a procedure, or a problem such as nausea or vomiting, inform the physician, so that any medication adjustments can be made.

Administer insulin
For a patient with Type I diabetes, administer insulin according to the established regimen. Keep in mind that regimens vary and often require adjustments. When administering insulin, check the dosage and the type of insulin. Consider its time of onset, peak, and duration and be prepared to offer a snack if hypoglycemia occurs. Remember that the rate of absorption varies with the injection site. Abdominal injections are absorbed the quickest.

Administer insulin subcutaneously, with the needle at a 45-degree to 90-degree angle. The greater the amount of subcutaneous tissue, the closer the needle should be to a 90-degree angle. When using the abdomen as an injection site, avoid the area within 2 inches of the umbilicus. Rotate injection sites within one area before moving to another area to prevent irregularities in absorption rates.

Administer oral hypoglycemic agents
For a patient with Type II diabetes who's receiving oral hypoglycemic agents, administer the medications as prescribed. Give a sulfonylurea 30 minutes before meals or with meals to prevent gastrointestinal (GI) upset. If more than one daily dose is prescribed, expect to give the second dose with the evening meal. If the patient is receiving metformin, administer it before meals or with the meal to prevent GI irritation. Metformin may be combined with a sulfonylurea to achieve better glucose control. If a patient is receiving an alpha-glucosidase inhibitor, administer it three times a day with the first bite of the main meals. It may be given with a sulfonylurea or insulin for better glucose control.

Manage hypoglycemia
Throughout therapy, monitor your patient for signs and symptoms of hypoglycemia, such as nervousness, tremors, palpitations, pallor, anxiety, diaphoresis, and tachycardia. If you detect these findings, obtain a blood glucose level. Blood glucose levels below 70 mg/dl indicate mild hypoglycemia; levels below 60 mg/dl

indicate moderate to severe hypoglycemia. If your patient is alert, awake, and able to swallow, give him 15 grams of a rapidly absorbed carbohydrate, such as 8 ounces of fruit juice, 6 to 8 ounces of regular soda, three 5-mg glucose tablets, or a small tube of glucose gel. If he's taking an alpha-glucosidase inhibitor, be sure to use glucose, not sucrose, to counteract the effects of hypoglycemia.

If the patient's symptoms aren't relieved after 15 minutes, give another 15 grams of a rapidly absorbed carbohydrate. If the symptoms worsen or the patient is unconscious, notify the physician immediately and prepare to give an I.V. bolus injection of 25 to 50 grams of 50% dextrose solution. If the patient doesn't have an I.V. catheter in place, administer 0.5 to 1 mg of glucagon subcutaneously or intramuscularly.

After the patient responds, give him a liquid carbohydrate and then a snack. After the patient's signs and symptoms resolve completely, give him a meal of complex carbohydrates and proteins. Continue to monitor his blood glucose levels frequently until his condition stabilizes.

When the patient's condition is stable, try to determine the cause of the hypoglycemic episode. Check to see that he received his medications on time and that he has had his meals and snacks. If he receives combination drug therapy, consider the possibility of an additive effect. Also, consider the possibility of interactions with other medications the patient is receiving.

Maintaining adequate nutrition and hydration

A balanced diet plan is crucial for the diabetic patient. Enlist the aid of a nutritionist or dietitian to develop a realistic, individualized program. Assess the patient's nutritional needs, as determined by his height, weight, and laboratory studies. Review his current nutritional intake and habits, likes and dislikes, and cultural or ethnic influences. Evaluate his lifestyle, schedules, activities, and economic status. Use this information to develop a diet plan that includes the appropriate amounts and types of calories, nutrients, carbohydrates, proteins, and fats. And be sure to work with the patient to establish mutual goals.

For a patient with Type I diabetes, the nutritional plan stresses eating a consistent amount of food each day, maintaining a desirable weight, and integrating insulin therapy with the type and amount of food eaten. For a patient with Type II diabetes, the nutritional plan focuses on the composition of the diet, the timing of meals, and the distribution of the day's calories among meals and snacks. If the patient is obese, the diet plan also aims to reduce weight.

Throughout therapy, monitor the patient's intake. Check his meal trays for what and how much he's eating. Note any changes in appetite or refusal to eat certain foods. Help the patient complete his daily menu selection, enlisting the dietitian's aid, if necessary.

Make sure the patient's fluid intake is adequate, especially if his blood glucose level is high, because increased blood glucose promotes osmotic diuresis. Encourage fluid intake of 2,500 to 3,000 ml/day. Monitor his intake and output and watch for signs of dehydration. Assess the patient's skin turgor and check his mucous membranes. Monitor the results of serum electrolyte levels and report any abnormal values to the physician.

Preventing complications

Because of disease-related changes, diabetic patients risk developing acute and chronic complications. Therefore, measures to promote safety and prevent injury are crucial. Diabetic patients who suffer a loss of muscle mass and deconditioning may benefit from a balanced schedule of activity and rest. Gradually increase the patient's activity, as his condition permits. Assist him with activities of daily living and ambulation, as needed. Caution him to avoid overexertion. If he participates in an exercise program, stress the need to allow time for warming up, stretching, and cooling down. Also, monitor him for signs and symptoms of hypoglycemia, especially if he has Type I diabetes.

Look for the Somogyi and dawn phenomena

If your patient has Type I diabetes, be alert for the Somogyi phenomenon, a reaction characterized by alternating periods of hypoglycemia and hyperglycemia. In this phenomenon, abnormally low blood glucose levels caused by excessive insulin therapy trigger the release of counterregulatory hormones—including glucagon, epinephrine, growth hormone, and cortisol—which leads to hyperglycemia. Commonly seen as nocturnal hypoglycemia and subsequent early morning hyperglycemia, the Somogyi phenomenon can occur at any time of day. Typically, the blood glucose level drops at around 3:00 A.M., causing nightmares, restlessness, and increased perspiration. If the patient wakes up, he'll notice signs and symptoms of hypoglycemia, such as clammy skin, shakiness, weakness, and confusion. If he sleeps through the night, he'll complain of a headache in the morning. If hormonal stimulation causes the blood glucose level to rise high enough, ketones may spill into the urine. Without realizing that the underlying cause is excessive insulin therapy, a physician may order more insulin to counteract the hyperglycemia, instead of reducing the dose.

Also, be alert for the dawn phenomenon, early morning hyperglycemia that doesn't occur in response to hypoglycemia. This phenomenon can affect all diabetic patients, although it's most common in those with Type I diabetes. Research suggests that it results from the release of growth hormone, which causes the tissues to become insulin resistant, thereby raising blood glucose levels.

To determine whether your patient is experiencing either phenomenon, check his blood glucose levels at bedtime, 3:00 A.M., and 7:00 A.M. Blood glucose levels less than 60 mg/dl at 3:00 A.M. and greater than 120 mg/dl at 7:00 A.M. indicate the Somogyi phenomenon. Anticipate giving a patient with this phenomenon a lower dose of intermediate-acting insulin in the evening. Make sure you give him a bedtime snack and continue to check his blood glucose levels at 3:00 A.M. and 7:00 A.M. until they've stabilized. Blood glucose levels that remain within normal limits until about 3:00 A.M. and then begin to rise suggest the dawn phenomenon. Anticipate increasing the patient's intermediate-acting insulin dose at bedtime and possibly reducing or eliminating the patient's evening snack.

Check for DKA and HHNK syndrome

Elevated blood glucose levels also can cause two life-threatening acute complications: diabetic ketoacidosis (DKA) and hyperglycemic hyperosmolar nonketotic (HHNK) syndrome. If your patient develops either of these conditions, you'll need to maintain a patent airway, provide sufficient oxygenation, maintain his circulation, and protect him from injury (see *Comparing DKA and HHNK syndrome*, page 16).

Check for infection

Diabetic patients are susceptible to infection because the skin's effectiveness as the first line of defense is altered by the loss of fat stores and the breakdown of glycogen and protein. Protein loss interferes with the inflammatory response and wound healing. It can also affect the action of the leukocytes in combating infection. Vascular changes can result in decreased circulation to a body part, thereby interfering with nutrient transport to the cell. As a result, healing is delayed and the risk of infection increases even more.

Assess the patient's skin carefully. Be especially alert when assessing warm, moist areas, such as between the toes, under the breasts, and in the axillae and groin. Assess the patient's feet for color, temperature, sensory function, and pulses, comparing one side to the other. Examine the feet for corns, calluses, cuts, bruises, cracks, and infection. Consult a podiatrist, if necessary.

Help the patient perform meticulous hygiene to keep his skin supple yet dry. Emphasize the need to dry thoroughly any body cracks and crevices. Because diabetic patients may experience sensory loss from peripheral neuropathy, make sure that bath water is 84° to 90° F (29° to 32° C) to prevent burning.

Take precautions to help the patient avoid illness and possible complications. Advise him to avoid people with upper respiratory tract infections. If he develops an infection or illness, evaluate him immediately. Monitor his blood glucose levels and check his urine for ketones every 2 to 4 hours. Continue administering insulin or oral medications, even if he can't eat. Omitting insulin can cause ketosis, especially in patients with Type I diabetes. Anticipate

Comparing DKA and HHNK syndrome

Diabetic ketoacidosis (DKA) and hyperglycemic hyperosmolar nonketotic (HHNK) syndrome are acute complications of diabetes mellitus. Although both are triggered by hyperglycemic crisis, they're treated differently. Without proper treatment, either may result in coma and death.

	DKA	HHNK syndrome
Patients primarily affected	Patients with Type I diabetes	Elderly patients with Type II diabetes
Onset	Relatively rapid	Gradual
Signs and symptoms	• Increased thirst • Nausea, vomiting, anorexia • Abdominal cramping • Lethargy and weakness • Polyuria leading to oliguria • Kussmaul's respiration • Fruity acetone breath odor • Blood glucose levels 300 mg/dl to 800 mg/dl • Urine ketones	• Poor fluid intake • Dehydration • Hypotension, circulatory collapse • Lethargy, confusion leading to coma • Polyuria leading to oliguria • Focal neurologic deficits, seizures • Blood glucose levels greater than 800 mg/dl • Absent or slight urine ketones
Nursing management	• Administer isotonic saline solution for fluid and electrolyte replacement. • Administer low-dose continuous infusion of regular insulin at 0.1 to 0.2 U/kg/hr. • Administer potassium replacement based on serum levels and urine output. • Insert indwelling urinary catheter, nasogastric tube, and invasive monitoring lines, depending on severity of patient's condition. • Monitor vital signs and intake and output. • Assess level of consciousness. • Evaluate arterial blood gas results. • Monitor blood glucose levels. • Comfort and support patient and family.	• Administer 0.9% normal saline solution at 1 L/hr for fluid replacement or (if patient has hypernatremia or heart failure) 0.45% normal saline solution at 1 L/hr. • Administer low-dose continuous insulin infusion at 0.1 to 0.2 U/kg/hr. • Administer potassium replacement based on serum levels. • Monitor vital signs and intake and output. • Assess neurologic status; reorient patient as necessary. • Institute seizure precautions. • Monitor hemodynamic status. • Institute cardiac monitoring. • Comfort and support patient and family.

adding a short-acting insulin to control hyperglycemia and ketosis. Encourage the patient to drink at least 8 ounces of fluids every hour to prevent dehydration.

Providing emotional support

The fact that diabetes has no cure and requires numerous lifestyle changes can be devastating to your patient and his family. Allow them to work through any feelings of loss, shock, disbelief, identity change, or anger. Be understanding with your patient and allow him to grieve for actual and potential losses.

Avoid overwhelming your patient with information and instructions. Give him time to learn and master a skill by working at his own pace, particularly as you teach him about insulin administration and fingerstick blood glucose testing. Include family members as appropriate to give them a better understanding of what the patient is experiencing. Refer the patient and his family to agencies, such as the local chapter of the American Diabetes Association, and community support groups. As patients cope with chronic illness, they may become noncompliant with part or all of their treatment plan, perhaps as a way of testing its importance. If this happens, accept the patient's behavior without labeling him. Don't assume that noncompliance only results from knowledge deficits. Complying with a diabetes regimen takes time, energy, and money. Try to find out why your patient isn't complying and help him overcome the cause. If appropriate, refer him to social services.

Patient teaching

Focus your teaching on helping your patient gain the knowledge and skills he needs to manage his diabetes. He'll be much less likely to experience complications if he keeps his blood glucose under tight control with frequent monitoring, regular medication, an exercise program, and a healthy diet.

Before you begin teaching, assess the patient's level of knowledge and readiness to learn. Make sure he understands basic information about his condition and its treatment. Then teach him how to integrate the treatment regimen into his lifestyle. Even if he isn't newly diagnosed, review previously taught information to help correct any misconceptions that could lead to poor compliance and complications.

Your primary goal is to teach your patient how to maintain an optimal blood glucose level, ranging from 90 mg/dl to 140 mg/dl. Begin by teaching him how to monitor his blood glucose levels. Watch him perform the procedure to ensure that he's doing it correctly. Tell him to make sure he has adequate supplies available and to check the expiration dates. Give him guidelines for target blood glucose values, and teach him what to do if the values are abnormally high or low. Inform him when he should call his physician. Also, teach your patient with Type I diabetes how to monitor his urine for ketones. Explain that if he finds ketones in the urine, he should notify his physician because an adjustment in his insulin may be required.

If your patient uses insulin, teach him how to prepare the injection, select and prepare the injection site, and inject the insulin. Instruct him to inject the insulin in a different site every time but in the same body part, for example, the abdomen or thigh. Instruct him to store the bottle he's using at room temperature and to refrigerate any additional bottles. Suggest that he use a chart to record the injection site and keep a log of insulin doses and blood glucose levels.

If your patient takes an oral hypoglycemic agent, make sure he understands how and when to take it. Explain the action, dosage, possible side effects, interactions, and any precautions. If your patient takes more than one medication, help him remember when to take them by using a chart or checklist. Inform him about possible interactions and how to avoid them. For example, antacids can interfere with the absorption of some medications. If your patient needs to take a medication for a minor illness along with his diabetes medication, teach him about the action, dosage, possible side effects, interactions, and any precautions needed for the other medication as well. Also, teach him how to plan his meals and snacks, so he continues to receive adequate nutrition, even if the illness decreases his appetite.

Explain the role and purpose of diet therapy. Teach your patient how to choose nutritious foods that minimize fluctuations in blood glucose levels. Also, instruct him to schedule meals and snacks carefully, including before and after exercise, to avoid hypoglycemia.

Finally, document your teaching in the patient's chart. Reinforce any verbal instructions and demonstrations with written instructions and handouts (see *Diabetes: Patient teaching checklist*, page 18).

Diabetes mellitus and hypertension

Adults with diabetes are at risk for hypertension and hyperlipidemia. Risk factors for hypertension in diabetic patients include genetic predisposition; conditions that affect cardiac output, such as increased heart rate and fluid volume; and neural stimulation, which may activate the counterregulatory process. Hypertension also

GOING HOME

Diabetes: Patient teaching checklist

Before your diabetic patient is discharged from the hospital, make sure you've taught him what he needs to know about his condition and its treatment. This checklist identifies the major topics to cover.

Diabetes as a disease
- Pathophysiology
- Type of diabetes
- Blood glucose levels and diabetes
- Effect of activity on blood glucose levels
- Effect of illness and stress on blood glucose levels
- Available community resources

Nutrition
- Prescribed diet plan, including snacks
- Appropriate food choices
- Food restrictions
- Consistency of meals and snacks
- Effect of food on blood glucose levels

Exercise
- Exercise plan
- Effect of exercise on blood glucose levels
- Precautions and risks
- Benefits

Insulin therapy
- Types of insulin (including onset, peak, and duration)
- Schedule
- Preparation
- Injection technique
- Site rotation
- Storage
- Care of equipment
- Signs and symptoms to report to physician

Oral hypoglycemic agents
- Name of prescribed drug
- Action
- Dosage
- Side effects
- Interactions
- Signs and symptoms to report to physician

Blood glucose monitoring
- Rationale for monitoring
- Target range for blood glucose levels
- Procedure, including fingerstick, sample collection, proper care and use of meter
- Signs and symptoms to report to physician

Prevention of complications
- Signs and symptoms of hypoglycemia and hyperglycemia
- Signs and symptoms of infection
- Care measures during minor illness
- Foot care measures

---

may be caused by increased insulin concentrations, which stimulate sodium reabsorption and fluid retention. Diabetes itself may be a risk factor, along with male gender, age, and obesity. In a diabetic patient, hypertension increases the risk of a CVA and nephropathy, factors that can change hormonal balance and aggravate hypertension.

Pathophysiology

In diabetic patients, macrovascular changes from atherosclerosis develop at an earlier age, progress faster, and usually are more severe and extensive. This results in decreased vessel lumen size, compromised blood flow, and decreased oxygen delivery to the tissues—conditions that set the stage for hypertension. Atherosclerotic lesions appear to stem from several causes, including endothelial injury. Endothelial lesions occur when smooth-muscle cells proliferate, lipids accumulate, and an extracellular matrix forms. These events are accelerated by abnormal lipid levels, tissue hypoxia, platelet changes, hormonal changes, and possibly hyperglycemia. Because insulin plays a major role in lipid metabolism, lipid disorders

Understanding vascular changes in diabetes mellitus and hypertension

Patients with diabetes mellitus and hypertension experience vascular changes that can compromise the entire vascular system. In diabetes, vascular injury begins with damage to the intimal vessel layer from high levels of glucose, free fatty acids, and cholesterol. Fatty streaks and fibrous plaques form, causing damage and obstructing blood flow. In hypertension, vascular injury stems from sustained elevation of blood pressure, which leads to medial necrosis and possibly occlusion, aneurysm, or rupture.

High blood glucose levels in diabetes and elevated blood pressure in hypertension lead to endothelial injury. Lipids and platelets then accumulate in the injured area, and macrophages are drawn to the area.

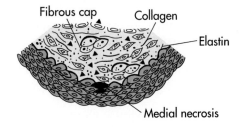

The injured endothelium becomes more permeable to circulating lipids and plasma proteins. Platelets aggregate and adhere to the injured area. Smooth-muscle cells and macrophages migrate into the intima and engulf the lipids, forming a fatty streak. As the fatty streak enlarges, the endothelial cells are pulled apart, and the underlying connective tissue is exposed, providing an additional area for platelet aggregation and adherence and, possibly, thrombus formation.

Smooth-muscle cells, which now contain lipids, continue to proliferate. A fibrous cap forms on the smooth-muscle cells. Intimal thickening occurs, increasing the amount of elastin and collagen in this area and leading to the formation of fibrous plaques. Plaque may occlude the arterial lumen, impeding blood flow. Meanwhile, damage from the leakage of plasma components, such as platelets, fibrinogen, and fibrin-containing proteins, may cause medial necrosis.

Hemorrhage, calcification, medial necrosis, and mural thrombosis may cause the lipid-filled core of the plaque to enlarge. The surface may develop cracks, disintegrate, or ulcerate, attracting the cellular elements that form clots. Thrombi form, increasing plaque size and further occluding the arterial lumen. Sustained elevation of blood pressure further stresses the arterial wall and can cause the plaque to rupture.

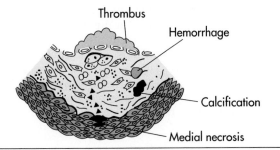

are common among diabetic patients.

Of course, blood pressure regulation is directly related to changes in cardiac output and peripheral vascular resistance. Cardiac output is affected by blood volume, which is influenced by sodium levels. Peripheral vascular resistance is affected by the arterial vessel lumen diameter, which is controlled by hormones. Diabetic patients may develop sodium retention because of elevated insulin levels resulting from the insulin therapy needed to achieve blood glucose control. In patients with Type II diabetes, insulin levels are elevated because high levels are secreted to combat insulin resistance. Even mild insulin elevations increase the tubular reabsorption of sodium because kidney cells don't experience insulin resistance as do other cells and tissues. Insulin also alters the movement of electrolytes in and out of the cells and increases intracellular levels of sodium and calcium. This makes the vessels more responsive to endogenous vasopressors, thereby increasing peripheral vascular resistance and blood pressure.

Another factor that contributes to hypertension is an elevated intracellular pH, which is believed to stimulate a response to growth factors. This, in turn, leads to cellular proliferation, thickening of the vascular media, and narrowing of the vessel lumen, thus increasing peripheral vascular resistance. Also, insulin stimulates the sympathetic nervous system, causing arteriolar vasoconstriction, increasing cardiac output, and increasing renal sodium retention. This overstimulation of the sympathetic nervous system may alter glucose metabolism, resulting in excess catecholamine levels that can lead to insulin resistance and hyperinsulinemia.

Prolonged blood pressure elevation causes vessel changes. The large vessels become sclerosed and tortuous. The lumens narrow, and blood flow is decreased. In the small vessels, the intima become damaged, fibrin accumulates, local edema develops, and intravascular clotting may ensue. This results in a decreased blood supply to the tissues (see *Understanding vascular changes in diabetes mellitus and hypertension*, page 19).

Adapting nursing care

Nursing care focuses on controlling hypertension with nonpharmacologic therapy, including lifestyle modifications, such as weight reduction, sodium restriction, alcohol avoidance, risk factor modification, and stress management. If necessary, drug therapy is prescribed. Antihypertensives include diuretics, angiotensin-converting enzyme (ACE) inhibitors, adrenergic inhibitors, and calcium channel blockers.

ACE inhibitors and calcium channel blockers serve as first-line antihypertensive drugs because they enhance insulin sensitivity. To avoid drug interactions, administer antihypertensive and blood glucose control medications cautiously (see *Diabetes drugs and antihypertensives: Dangerous interactions*).

Be alert for orthostatic hypotension and resting tachycardia, complications that may result if autonomic neuropathy affects the cardiovascular system. Many antihypertensive drugs also produce orthostatic hypotension. Check the patient's blood pressure in both arms while he lies down, sits, and stands, comparing the right and left sides. A blood pressure drop of more than 10 mm Hg with position changes indicates orthostatic hypotension. Encourage the patient to change positions slowly. Advise him to sit on the edge of the bed before rising and to stand up slowly. Suggest that he wear elastic stockings to improve venous return and that he elevate the head of the bed to minimize position changes. If the patient feels dizzy or lightheaded, institute safety measures to prevent injury.

The physician may order a low-dose thiazide diuretic to reduce the patient's total exchangeable sodium levels. If your patient is receiving a diuretic, monitor his serum potassium levels. Loop and thiazide diuretics promote potassium excretion, which may require replacement to prevent a deficit. Monitor your patient's intake, output, and daily body weight. Watch for signs and symptoms of dehydration, such as poor skin turgor.

Monitor blood glucose levels and blood pressure to determine the effectiveness of treatment, and be prepared to change the treatment regimen, if indicated.

Emphasize the patient's need to modify his lifestyle. Teach him how to plan meals that include the appropriate amounts of calories, fat,

DRUG ALERT

Diabetes drugs and antihypertensives: Dangerous interactions

Diabetes drugs	Antihypertensives	Adverse effects	Nursing actions
• Insulin and sulfonylureas	• Beta blockers	• Beta blockers may prolong hypoglycemic effect, delay recovery from hypoglycemia, and mask signs and symptoms of hypoglycemia.	• Monitor patient for signs and symptoms of hypoglycemia, such as diaphoresis and tremors. • Check blood glucose levels at least four times a day. • If hypoglycemia occurs, check blood glucose levels to evaluate response to therapy. • Anticipate need for increased amounts of glucagon or dextrose to treat hypoglycemia. • Expect dosage adjustments of both drugs if hypoglycemia occurs.
	• Vascular smooth-muscle relaxants	• Vascular smooth-muscle relaxants may increase hypoglycemic effect.	
	• Potent vasodilators	• Potent vasodilators may inhibit endogenous insulin secretion, causing hypoglycemia.	
	• Thiazide diuretics	• Thiazide diuretics antagonize effects of insulin and sulfonylureas, resulting in hyperglycemia.	• Check for signs and symptoms of hyperglycemia, such as weakness, fatigue, nausea, and vomiting. • Check blood glucose levels frequently. • Anticipate need for increased dosage of insulin or sulfonylurea.
• Sulfonylureas	• Centrally acting alpha$_2$ blockers	• Alpha$_2$ blockers may prolong hypoglycemic effect and mask signs and symptoms of hypoglycemia.	• Monitor patient for signs and symptoms of hypoglycemia, such as diaphoresis and tremors. • Check blood glucose levels at least four times a day. • If hypoglycemia occurs, check blood glucose levels to evaluate response to therapy. • Anticipate need for increased amounts of glucagon or dextrose to treat hypoglycemia. • Expect dosage adjustments of both drugs if hypoglycemia occurs.
	• Loop diuretics	• Loop diuretics may cause hyperglycemia.	• Check blood glucose levels frequently. • Check for signs and symptoms of hyperglycemia, such as weakness, fatigue, nausea, and vomiting. • Anticipate need for increased dosage of sulfonylurea.
• Biguanides	• Calcium channel blockers • Thiazide diuretics	• Calcium channel blockers and thiazide diuretics may cause hyperglycemia.	• Monitor blood glucose levels frequently. • Check for signs and symptoms of hyperglycemia, such as weakness, fatigue, nausea, and vomiting. • Anticipate need for increased dosage of biguanide.

and sodium. Review with him which foods are high and low in sodium and potassium. If appropriate, instruct him to reduce or eliminate his use of tobacco and alcohol. Describe how exercise effectively controls blood glucose levels, reduces blood pressure, and helps maintain or achieve normal body weight. Encourage the patient to exercise for at least 20 minutes a day, three times a week. Help him choose an exercise and an appropriate level of intensity. Then help him develop an exercise plan. Teach him stress-management techniques, such as progressive relaxation and imagery, if indicated.

Before the patient is discharged from the hospital, make sure he understands his medication regimen. Review all medications with him, including what he should take and when he should take it. Make sure he knows the dosage for each drug and the timing of its action. Teach him how to recognize side effects, respond appropriately, and take steps to prevent them. Make sure he knows when he should call his physician. If necessary, use a chart to help him organize his medication schedule.

If appropriate, have the patient demonstrate the technique for insulin administration. Also, review with him self-monitoring techniques for blood glucose testing and urine testing. Teach him how and when to monitor his blood pressure and pulse rate. Explain the need for him to weigh himself daily. Help him establish a system to record the dates, times, and results of all self-monitoring, and make sure he knows when to notify his physician.

Teach your patient how to care for himself during minor illnesses. Emphasize the need to eat regular meals and snacks, even if his appetite is diminished. If he smokes, discuss the need to stop and help him develop a smoking cessation plan.

Complications

For a diabetic patient with hypertension, possible complications include CVA, retinopathy, thromboembolism, and peripheral neuropathy.

Cerebrovascular accident

Because of associated vascular changes and injury, diabetes and hypertension are risk factors for CVA. The risk is heightened by the macrovascular changes caused by atherosclerosis. Vascular changes in the cerebral arteries lead to cerebral ischemia. Short-term ischemia produces temporary deficits, and prolonged ischemia produces cerebral infarction and permanent deficits.

The most common cause of CVA, cerebral thrombosis results from cerebrovascular atheromatosis, which makes the blood more coagulable and viscous. Atherogenesis is enhanced in diabetic patients because of lipid metabolism abnormalities associated with the glycemic control of diabetes.

Confirming the complication

A patient experiencing temporary ischemia will have transient ischemic attacks (TIAs). Typically, the patient complains of weakness in the lower portion of the face, fingers, hands, arms, and legs. Transient dysphagia and sensory impairment also may occur. These deficits resolve, and the results of neurologic examinations between episodes are normal.

The signs and symptoms of a CVA depend on the area of the brain affected. They may include a sudden feeling of weakness and unsteadiness, possibly resulting in a momentary loss of consciousness. These findings may be accompanied by a loss of arm or leg movement, numbness or tingling in any part of the body, an excruciating headache, confusion, difficulty speaking, and blurred or double vision or a loss of vision in one eye. Unconsciousness and seizures may occur because both are related to generalized ischemia and the brain's response to abrupt hypoxia.

A lumbar puncture will usually reveal increased cerebrospinal fluid pressure. A computed tomography scan will show the area of infarction. A cerebral angiogram or digital subtraction angiography may be used for a patient with a TIA to identify any blocked or occluded arteries.

Nursing interventions

The key to care is prevention through adequate blood pressure and blood glucose control. Nursing care during the acute phase of a CVA involves helping the patient survive and preventing further brain injury. A CVA places additional stress on the body, thereby affecting the body's ability to control blood pressure and blood glucose levels.

Frequently monitor the patient's vital signs and blood glucose levels and compare them to his baseline values. Be alert for blood pressure changes. An increased blood pressure and a widening pulse pressure, followed by a drop in blood pressure, indicate continuing elevated intracranial pressure and a deterioration of the patient's condition.

If the added stress of the CVA causes hyperglycemia, the dosage of the patient's diabetes medication may need to be adjusted. If the patient is unconscious, be prepared to administer medications I.V., as prescribed.

After the patient's condition stabilizes, focus on preventing complications or a recurrence. Continue to monitor blood glucose levels and blood pressure frequently. Adjust medications, as ordered. Plan for appropriate exercise as soon as his condition permits to help increase his HDL cholesterol levels and to promote rehabilitation.

Arrange for a dietitian to talk with your patient about diet modifications to decrease triglyceride levels and reduce weight, if indicated. Discuss community weight-loss programs with him, if appropriate.

Modify care to accommodate any residual deficits, such as diminished awareness, visual-field deficits, decreased mental status, weakness, or paralysis. These deficits may affect the patient's ability to manage his hypertension and diabetes. For example, a patient with a visual-field deficit may have trouble reading the numbers on an insulin syringe or the label of a medication container or locating an injection site. A patient with paralysis of his dominant side may have difficulty opening a medication container, administering an insulin injection, or performing a fingerstick for glucose monitoring. Evaluate your patient for any deficits and modify his regimen or help him adapt, as appropriate. For example, having him use a magnifier may help him overcome visual deficits. Enlist the help of your patient's family members, friends, or caregiver, if necessary.

Before your patient is discharged from the hospital, review his home care needs with him. Make sure he understands all instructions and self-care procedures. Arrange for a home care nurse to meet with the patient to discuss follow-up care.

Retinopathy

The leading cause of new cases of legal blindness in the United States, diabetic retinopathy stems from microvascular changes in the eye. In hypertension, sustained blood pressure elevation causes papilledema, hemorrhage, and exudates in the retina. This contributes to the progression of retinopathy, placing diabetic patients with hypertension at high risk.

Retinopathy occurs in three stages: nonproliferative, preproliferative, and proliferative retinopathy. Patients with Type I diabetes are at greater risk for proliferative diabetic retinopathy; patients with Type II diabetes are at greater risk for macular edema (retinal thickening or hard exudates adjacent to the thickened retina near the center of the macula). Prompt photocoagulation therapy can reduce vision loss by 50%.

Confirming the complication

Patients with retinopathy may complain of spots floating in the visual field, rapid visual changes, fogged vision, or loss of vision. Blurred central vision leading to a loss of central vision indicates macular edema. Ophthalmoscopic examination may reveal blood vessel damage, yellow lipid deposits, small intraretinal hemorrhages, and macular edema.

The earliest sign, a retinal capillary microaneurysm, can be detected by ophthalmoscopic examination. Fluorescein angiography can detect retinal capillary abnormalities from leakage or from capillary nonperfusion, possibly revealing retinal hemorrhages or hard exudates. If the patient has macular edema, he may have a loss of visual acuity. As retinopathy progresses, large patches of acellular capillaries develop and terminal arterioles become occluded, producing a soft exudate called cotton-wool spots.

In proliferative diabetic retinopathy, new blood vessels appear on the surface of the retina, possibly obscuring vision. These new vessels may multiply over weeks or months. Contraction of the vitreous humor may lead to retinal detachment and bleeding of the retina into the vitreous humor. Visual symptoms may include a few floating spots that last only an hour or a loss of vision except for light perception and hand-movement perception (see *Understanding diabetic retinopathy*).

Nursing interventions

The key to nursing care is prevention. Emphasize the need to control blood glucose levels and blood pressure to minimize the risk of vascular changes, which can lead to retinopathy. Encourage the patient to visit an ophthalmologist at least once a year, or more often if visual problems develop.

If your patient already has visual impairment, provide support. Describe the room, remove clutter, and place the call light and personal objects within his reach. Speak to him before touching him. If his visual deficits don't improve, modify his self-care regimen. Investigate self-help devices designed for visually impaired patients. And refer him to appropriate community agencies and support groups.

Thromboembolism

Thromboembolism results from venous stasis, endothelial damage to the vessel lining, and hypercoagulability. It commonly affects patients with diabetes and hypertension because of the vascular changes associated with the two disorders. Thromboembolic complications may occur with DKA because of the elevation of several clotting factors. The risk of thromboembolism is also high during HHNK syndrome because of the patient's hyperglycemia, hyperosmolarity, dehydrated state, and possibly his comatose condition.

Confirming the complication

Signs and symptoms of thromboembolism depend on the location of the affected vessel, the size of the thrombus, and the presence of collateral circulation. Commonly, a thrombus forms at the bifurcation of a deep vessel of the leg. Calf pain, edema, and increased calf circumference may develop. If the thrombus is at the level of the iliac or femoral vessels, pain and extensive limb swelling result. If the thrombus is large enough to occlude the vessel completely, signs and symptoms of decreased circulation—such as pallor, coolness,

and absent pulses—will occur. An embolus can break off from a thrombus and enter the bloodstream, migrating to the lungs and causing a pulmonary embolism.

Nursing interventions

Focus your interventions on preventing thromboembolism. Encourage your patient to maintain good blood pressure and blood glucose control, in part by adhering to his diet and exercise plan. Emphasize the need for continued follow-up care. Periodically monitor hematocrit and hemoglobin levels and coagulation studies, such as activated partial thromboplastin time (APTT) and prothrombin time (PT).

RAPID RESPONSE ▶ If your patient develops a pulmonary embolism, you'll need to act quickly to prevent serious complications, such as heart failure. Place him in a position that promotes chest expansion and eases breathing. Rapidly assess his respiratory status, including the rate and depth of his respirations. Auscultate his breath sounds and administer oxygen, as prescribed. Expect to give a bolus of 5,000 to 10,000 units of heparin, followed by a continuous infusion of 1,000 units per hour. Carefully monitor his APTT and adjust the infusion, as prescribed. Continuously monitor oxygen saturation levels with pulse oximetry. Also, obtain blood for arterial blood gas (ABG) studies to evaluate his oxygenation status. Monitor his electrocardiogram (ECG) for arrhythmias. As you care for your patient, be alert for embolisms in other parts of the body.

If the patient is receiving anticoagulants, advise him to watch for petechiae, bleeding gums, and signs of GI bleeding. Maintain adequate fluid intake. ◀

Peripheral neuropathy

The most common complication of diabetes, diabetic peripheral neuropathy involves three pathologic changes. First, the walls of the blood vessels that supply nerves thicken, causing a decrease in nutrients to the nerve tissue. Second, Schwann cells that surround and insulate the nerves demyelinate, slowing nerve conduction. And third, sorbitol accumulates within the Schwann cells, impairing nerve conduction. Vascular changes associated with hypertension

Understanding diabetic retinopathy

Most diabetic retinopathy begins as nonproliferative retinopathy. The patient's vision may not be affected, but on examination the physician finds microaneurysms, small hemorrhages, cotton-wool spots, hard exudates, and capillary closure. Nonproliferative retinopathy can then lead to preproliferative or proliferative retinopathy. With preproliferative retinopathy, the capillaries continue to deteriorate and become obstructed, leading to retinal ischemia and infarction. Proliferative retinopathy involves the retina and the vitreous humor. As capillaries become blocked, new blood vessels form in a process called neovascularization. Eventually, these new vessels become fibrous and rupture, causing hemorrhage and vitreous humor contraction. If the capillaries hemorrhage while the vitreous humor contracts, the patient is at risk for developing tractional retinal detachment. If the macula is involved, he's at high risk for losing his vision.

These illustrations show what you may see when you look at your patient's eye through an ophthalmoscope.

Normal retina

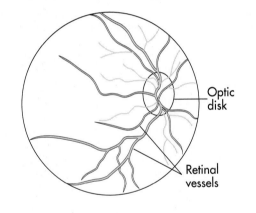

Nonproliferative retinopathy

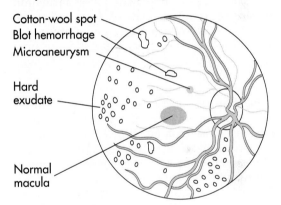

Preproliferative retinopathy

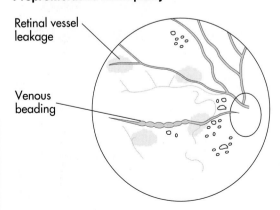

Proliferative retinopathy

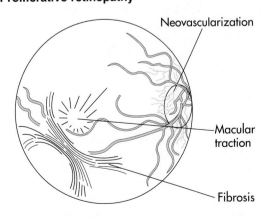

further impair the blood supply to the tissues, causing an even larger decrease in the nutrients available.

Confirming the complication

Peripheral neuropathy results from tissue changes that cause either painful symptoms, such as a burning sensation in the legs, or an inability to sense touch and pain. Typically, the signs and symptoms depend on the location of the lesion; generally, they appear first in the toes and feet and then progress upward. Insensate tissues break down because of unnatural stress on the limb. With nerve impairment and continuous trauma, ulcers develop and infection sets in.

Signs and symptoms of peripheral neuropathy include paresthesia, hyperesthesia, hypoesthesia, anhidrosis, heavy callus formation over pressure points, loss of deep tendon reflexes, and loss of vibratory, temperature, and position sense. The patient is at risk for trophic ulcers, footdrop, changes of foot shape, muscle atrophy, changes in the bones, and joint and neuropathic fractures.

Diabetic patients are prone to foot infections caused by gram-positive and gram-negative organisms. More than one type of organism can be present in the same wound. A fungal organism may infect the nails. Osteomyelitis can develop following a chronic perforating ulcer. Abscess of the plantar spaces can cause swelling and redness in the sole of the foot.

Nursing interventions

Nursing care focuses on reducing the risk of peripheral neuropathy by controlling blood pressure and blood glucose, maintaining adequate tissue perfusion, and preventing injury.

Explain to your patient that exercise improves circulation to the limbs. Encourage him to walk slowly with frequent rest periods. Advise him to avoid sitting or standing for a prolonged time, crossing his legs, and wearing constrictive clothing. Caution the patient to avoid exposure to the cold, which can cause vasoconstriction, further impairing his circulation.

Assess the color, temperature, and pulses of the limbs, comparing the results bilaterally. Report any significant changes immediately.

Assess the patient's skin, paying particular attention to the hands and feet. Teach him how to inspect his feet daily for blisters, skin tears, open wounds, redness, cracks, swelling, and tenderness. Advise him to wash his feet daily with soap and water, to pat them dry, and to wear properly fitting shoes.

Caution the patient to protect his hands and feet from injury. Explain that he may have diminished reflexes, muscle weakness, and atrophy. He also may be unable to perceive the movement or position of his limbs. Thus, he could injure himself and not feel the injury.

To prevent burns, caution him to check bath water with his elbow or inner wrist before submerging his feet. Instruct him not to use a hot-water bottle or heating pad on his feet because decreased sensation can result in burns. Advise the patient against soaking his feet, which could lead to tissue maceration.

Frequently monitor the patient's blood pressure and blood glucose levels and adjust his medication dosages, as prescribed. Also, monitor him closely for hypoglycemia or hyperglycemia.

If the patient has a wound infection, obtain a specimen for culture and sensitivity testing to identify the causative organism. Initiate antibiotic therapy immediately, as ordered.

If peripheral neuropathy interferes with the patient's manual dexterity, help him modify his self-care management regimen. Suggest the use of assistive devices and equipment, such as syringe holders and nonchildproof caps.

Diabetes mellitus and coronary artery disease

Among diabetic patients, coronary artery disease (CAD) accounts for 40% to 60% of all deaths. In these patients, the left coronary artery is affected more often than the right.

The cause of CAD differs, depending on the type of diabetes a patient has. The high rate of kidney disease in Type I diabetes can lead to hypertension and probably contributes to atherosclerosis and cardiovascular disease. In patients with Type II diabetes, however, the causes of CAD appear to be the same as those in nondiabetic patients: autoregulatory dysfunction, renal sodium retention, abnormal cellular transport, and increased intracellular calcium. Genetic conditions that cause abnormalities of the sympathetic and parasympathetic systems also may lead to CAD in patients with either Type I or Type II diabetes.

Pathophysiology

In CAD, the endothelial layer of the arteries becomes damaged. This damage worsens with high levels of glucose, free fatty acids, and cholesterol. Elevated lipoprotein and triglyceride levels, seen in patients with insulin resistance, also increase damage to the endothelial lining. Monocytes adhere to the damaged area and macrophages migrate there, contributing to lipid accumulation and the development of an atherosclerotic plaque. The macrophages release growth factor, causing the smooth-muscle cells to enlarge, multiply, and migrate through the layers of the vessel, further narrowing the vessel lumen. Meanwhile, platelets also adhere to the damaged area, especially in hyperglycemic patients, causing a thrombus to form. The combination of endothelial damage and increased platelet aggregation accelerates the thickening of the arteries, leading to vasoconstriction.

Progressive atherosclerosis results in reduced coronary artery blood flow, placing the patient at risk for myocardial ischemia and MI. In a diabetic patient, CAD often leads to GI upset, a silent MI, and heart failure.

Adapting nursing care

Focus your care on preventing CAD, detecting it early, and reducing risk factors. Teach your patient how to modify his diet, so that saturated fats account for less than 10% of his total daily caloric intake and all fats account for less than 30%. Teach him to reduce his cholesterol intake to 250 to 300 mg per day. Obtain baseline blood lipid levels, and monitor these levels to detect changes and evaluate the effectiveness of treatment.

Keep in mind that drug therapy can reduce cholesterol and other lipid levels, but it's not the first line of treatment. If diet, weight loss, antihypertensive therapy, and exercise aren't

effective, then antilipemic drugs may be prescribed. Commonly used drugs include bile-sequestering agents (cholestyramine and colestipol), fibric acid derivatives (clofibrate and gemfibrozil), cholesterol synthesis inhibitors (fluvastatin, lovastatin, pravastatin, and simvastatin), and nicotinic acid. If your patient is receiving an antilipemic drug, monitor his blood glucose levels closely (see *Sulfonylureas and antilipemic agents: Dangerous interactions*, page 28).

Exercise and weight control also help maintain blood glucose and blood pressure control and reduce the risk of CAD. Help the patient develop an effective exercise program, if necessary. Emphasize the need to monitor blood glucose levels before, during, and after exercise to prevent hypoglycemia.

If your patient smokes, encourage him to stop. Explain that cigarette smoking increases his risk of developing CAD because it reduces oxygen delivery to the heart and increases his heart rate and blood pressure. Also, advise your patient to avoid second-hand smoke. Explain that even 2 hours of passive smoke exposure can decrease oxygen delivery to the heart, decrease exercise time, and increase heart rate and blood pressure. Refer him to a smoking-cessation program, if necessary. If appropriate, discuss with the physician the use of a dermal nicotine delivery system, such as a nicotine patch, or a chewing gum containing nicotine.

Before the patient is discharged from the hospital, make sure he understands the risk factors for CAD and knows how to modify them. Also, reinforce the need for good blood glucose and blood pressure control through adherence to his treatment plan.

Complications

Diabetic patients with CAD are at risk for several complications, including angina, MI, and cardiac arrest.

Angina
Progressive atherosclerosis results in decreased coronary artery blood flow, which places the patient at risk for myocardial ischemia. Myocardial cells become ischemic within

DRUG ALERT

Sulfonylureas and antilipemic agents: Dangerous interactions

Sulfonylureas	Antilipemic agents	Adverse effects	Nursing actions
• First and second generation sulfonyl-ureas	• Fibric acid derivatives	• Fibric acid derivatives may increase hypoglycemic effect.	• Check for signs and symptoms of hypoglycemia, such as diaphoresis and tremors. • Monitor blood glucose levels. • Anticipate lowering dosage of sulfonylurea based on blood glucose levels. • Warn patient of possible drug interaction. • Stress the need to watch for signs of hypoglycemia and to notify physician if any occur.
	• Nicotinic acid	• Nicotinic acid antagonizes the effect of sulfonylureas, leading to development of insulin resistance.	• Check for signs and symptoms of hyperglycemia, such as weakness, fatigue, nausea, and vomiting. • Monitor blood glucose levels. • Anticipate increasing dosage of sulfonylurea.

10 seconds of coronary artery occlusion. After several minutes of ischemia, the cells convert to anaerobic metabolism because they've been deprived of needed glucose and oxygen, thus producing lactic acid as a by-product. As lactic acid accumulates, pain develops.

Confirming the complication

A lack of oxygen to the myocardial muscles precipitates pain, which may be in the chest and may radiate to the jaw or arm. Typically, pain strikes in the early morning and lasts less than 5 minutes. It may occur in cold weather or with physical exertion, emotional or psychosocial stress, or eating. In some cases, the pain abates after the patient stops the activity. In others, the pain doesn't subside until the patient has taken up to three sublingual nitroglycerin tablets. Instead of pain, a patient may complain of chest heaviness, shortness of breath, and nausea and vomiting. He also may be diaphoretic.

ECG tracings may be normal or may show ST-segment elevation. Radioisotope imaging reveals areas of poor perfusion as cold spots. Coronary angiography confirms the presence of a partial or complete blockage of the coronary artery.

Nursing interventions

A patient with diabetes and CAD may not experience typical signs and symptoms of angina, especially if he has autonomic neuropathy. Therefore, you should teach him to be alert for and to report chest heaviness, shortness of breath, fatigue, nausea, vomiting, and palpitations.

Administer medications, as prescribed. If your patient is receiving insulin along with a beta blocker, such as propranolol, remember that it can impair epinephrine secretion and mask the signs and symptoms of hypoglycemia. A patient receiving insulin may be able to tolerate low doses of a cardioselective beta$_1$ blocker, such as atenolol, metoprolol, or acebutolol. However, you still need to monitor blood glucose levels closely for changes.

Also, monitor the patient's heart rate, ECG tracing, and vital signs for changes indicating a progression of the ischemia. If appropriate, obtain serum enzyme levels to rule out an MI. If your patient is receiving nitrate therapy for angina, keep in mind that nitrates don't interfere with blood glucose control but may cause severe hypotension. Monitor his blood pressure closely.

Institute safety measures to protect the patient from injury and help him identify activities that precipitate an attack. Teach him what to do if chest pain develops:

- Stop the activity.
- Sit down and rest.
- Take nitroglycerin if prescribed, repeating the dose every 5 minutes if necessary for a maximum of three doses.
- Notify his physician and seek emergency treatment if the pain doesn't subside.

Explain to your patient that he might not be able to distinguish angina symptoms from hypoglycemic symptoms, especially if he doesn't experience typical chest pain. If this happens, advise him to check his blood glucose level and treat hypoglycemia if he detects it. If the symptoms persist, tell him to take sublingual nitroglycerin. If the symptoms persist after three doses, advise him to seek emergency medical attention.

Some diabetic patients with angina can benefit from percutaneous transluminal coronary angioplasty, which restores blood flow in blocked coronary arteries. Coronary artery bypass graft surgery also may be performed, but diabetic patients are at high risk for postoperative complications, such as mediastinitis. After either procedure, the patient requires close monitoring of blood glucose levels and, possibly, medication adjustments. Patients with Type II diabetes may require short-term insulin therapy.

Review with your patient the causes of angina and the need for lifestyle changes to avoid complications of CAD and diabetes. Explain that CAD and angina can be controlled, although they can't be cured. Talk with your patient about starting a cardiac rehabilitation program, if his physician has recommended one. Emphasize the need to monitor his heart rate and blood glucose levels before and after exercise. And suggest that he eat frequent small snacks to reduce the likelihood of hypoglycemia.

Before your patient is discharged, reinforce all home care instructions with him. Provide information about lifestyle changes, diet, medications, and signs and symptoms that require follow-up care.

Myocardial infarction

If myocardial ischemia progresses, blood and oxygen supply to the myocardium is drastically reduced, causing necrosis and an MI. Patients with diabetes are more likely to suffer a silent MI if they have autonomic neuropathy, which masks the typical warning signs and symptoms.

In general, women have smaller coronary arteries than men. And patients with diabetes have a higher incidence of disease in their small blood vessels. Consequently, diabetic patients, especially women, have more complications and a higher rate of mortality from MI. Complications in diabetic patients with an MI include recurrent infarction, cardiogenic shock, conduction abnormalities, heart failure, and myocardial rupture.

Confirming the complication

If your diabetic patient has autonomic neuropathy, he may be asymptomatic or may not recognize the signs and symptoms of an MI. Such a patient may report atypical signs and symptoms, such as confusion, dyspnea, fatigue, nausea, and vomiting. Because these findings mimic those of hyperglycemia and hypoglycemia, he may delay seeking treatment. Typically, a diabetic patient with autonomic neuropathy who experiences angina becomes aware of his symptoms later in the course of the ischemia than a patient without autonomic neuropathy.

An ECG is useful in detecting myocardial injury and MI. However, ECG monitoring may not give a true picture of the infarction in diabetic patients because many such patients have non–Q wave MIs, which don't show up on an ECG. Coronary angiography may be ordered to diagnose coronary artery occlusion. Angioplasty or atherectomy may be performed to relieve the occlusion. These procedures usually are restricted to diabetic patients who are acutely ill because the contrast medium can cause renal impairment, especially if the patient also has nephropathy. Radionuclide imaging can be used to distinguish between normal and abnormal tissue and to indicate the size and extent of the infarction. Elevations in serum cardiac enzyme levels confirm the diagnosis of MI.

Nursing interventions

If the diabetic patient is in the acute phase of an MI, nursing care focuses on promoting oxygenation, tissue perfusion, and adequate cardiac output. Administer oxygen and monitor oxygen saturation levels, using pulse oximetry and ABG studies. Also, monitor vital signs for changes. Institute cardiac monitoring to detect ECG changes that indicate a progression of the MI or the development of arrhythmias. Place the patient in the semi-Fowler position to promote diaphragmatic expansion.

You may be asked to assist with thrombolytic therapy using streptokinase, urokinase, tissue plasminogen activator, or anisoylated plasminogen streptokinase activator complex. For greatest effectiveness, thrombolytic therapy should be given within 6 hours of the onset of chest pain. This may not be possible for diabetic patients who don't experience chest pain.

If your patient does have chest pain, institute pain-control measures, as appropriate. Typically, morphine is administered I.V. in small doses. Nitrates are given for their vasodilatory effect.

The physician may use reperfusion therapy to limit the size of the infarction or angioplasty to relieve ischemia. The physician may order coronary artery bypass surgery, although the long-term survival rate appears to be lower in diabetic patients.

Monitor blood glucose levels closely, especially after administering insulin. If the patient becomes hypoglycemic, arrhythmias can develop as catecholamines are released. Remember that in ischemia, the heart shifts from aerobic metabolism, with fatty acids as the primary fuel source, to anaerobic metabolism, with glucose as the primary fuel source. This makes glucose transport into the myocardial cells crucial. Insulin promotes glucose uptake; ketones and high levels of free fatty acids found in insulinopenia inhibit glucose transport. The excess of catecholamines often associated with an MI may further worsen myocardial metabolism in the diabetic patient, decreasing the insulin secretory reserve and promoting lipolysis and myocardial uptake of free fatty acids.

Diabetic patients with poorly controlled glucose levels during an MI have a much poorer prognosis. A patient who experiences severe hyperglycemia is at risk for DKA or HHNK syndrome, which leads to further myocardial damage because less oxygen is available for the myocardial tissue.

Make sure your patient gets adequate rest to help decrease the heart's workload. Keep in mind, however, that bed rest can contribute to a reduced need for insulin. Continue to monitor blood glucose levels closely, especially as the patient's activity level increases. Adjust the insulin dosage, as indicated.

Provide support and comfort to help alleviate the patient's anxiety. Remember that anxiety increases myocardial oxygen demands, further stressing the heart. It may also increase blood glucose levels, requiring additional glycemic control.

After your patient's condition has stabilized, focus your interventions on medication therapy, lifestyle modifications, diet, exercise rehabilitation, and patient teaching. Continue to monitor blood glucose levels and adjust medication therapy accordingly. Be especially alert for subtle signs that might indicate reinfarction.

Before your patient is discharged, make sure he clearly understands his prescribed medication regimen and any possible drug interactions. Reinforce the physician's instructions about lifestyle modifications, diet, and exercise. Make sure your patient knows which signs and symptoms to watch for and report to his physician. Review all aspects of diabetes self-management with the patient.

Cardiac arrest

After an acute MI, diabetic patients have a higher risk of death because of factors such as underlying cardiomyopathy and an accelerated atherosclerotic process. Your patient's ability to adapt to hemodynamic stress from autonomic dysfunction, hypertension, small-vessel CAD, a silent MI, or underlying ventricular dysfunction also may be impaired.

In diabetic patients with an MI, ketoacidosis greatly increases the likelihood of death. Insulin deficiency may impair the myocardial uptake of glucose. Plus, the increased output of adrenal steroids and catecholamines may inhibit the action of insulin.

Confirming the complication

A diabetic patient who suffers a cardiac arrest will experience the same signs and symptoms as a nondiabetic patient. The patient will be unresponsive, pale, and cyanotic, without spontaneous respirations, without heart sounds, and without a pulse or blood pressure.

Nursing interventions

Focus your nursing care on preventing a cardiac arrest and responding quickly and appropriately if one does occur. Keep emergency resuscitation equipment and medications available for immediate use.

If your patient suffers a cardiac arrest, you'll need to establish a patent airway and begin rescue breathing and circulation. Call for help and begin cardiopulmonary resuscitation. When equipment and help arrive, resuscitate the patient according to current advanced cardiac life-support guidelines. Monitor the patient's ventilations, the effectiveness of resuscitative measures, his electrolyte levels, ABG studies, and blood glucose levels. Anticipate the need to administer drugs, including I.V. insulin to treat hyperglycemia.

After your patient's condition has stabilized, continue to monitor him for changes indicating deterioration. Also, continue to monitor his blood glucose levels, which may fluctuate.

Diabetes mellitus and nephropathy

Diabetic nephropathy is the most common cause of new cases of end-stage renal disease in the United States, especially among men. A microvascular complication of diabetes, diabetic nephropathy causes a persistent leakage of protein into the urine (more than 0.5 gram of protein per 24 hours). Diabetic nephropathy is diagnosed only after other causes of proteinuria, such as infection or heart failure, have been ruled out. Most patients with diabetic nephropathy also experience diabetic retinopathy and hypertension.

The prevalence of nephropathy in patients with Type I diabetes increases with time. About 21% of people who've had Type I diabetes for 20 to 25 years have this complication.

Patients with Type II diabetes who develop nephropathy also have a high incidence of hypertension, high arterial pressure, and inadequate blood glucose control.

When nephropathy leads to a decline in renal function and a glomerular filtration rate that is about 25% of normal, renal insufficiency ensues. Enough nephrons remain to allow the kidney to function. However, any additional physiologic stress—such as illness, dietary changes, or nephrotoxic drugs—can lead to renal failure.

Pathophysiology

The exact cause of renal destruction in diabetic nephropathy isn't known. Damage to the glomerulus causes scar tissue to replace normal tissue, resulting in glomerulosclerosis. This process leads to complete obliteration of the glomerulus, thereby impairing renal function.

When renal function is impaired, the number of nephrons able to excrete solutes progressively declines. In response, the remaining nephrons hypertrophy to compensate. This adaptive mechanism can maintain fluid and electrolyte balance until 75% of the nephrons are destroyed. When this occurs, the filtration rate and the number of solutes for each nephron are so high that the kidneys can no longer maintain the balance between filtration and reabsorption. The kidneys lose their ability and flexibility to excrete and conserve electrolytes and water. Even modest changes can further upset this balance.

Adapting nursing care

Nursing care aims to prevent or slow the progress of diabetic nephropathy and minimize the effects of renal insufficiency, thus preserving as much renal function as possible (see *Diabetic nephropathy: Preventing further damage,* page 32).

Additional renal damage and renal insufficiency can result from the diabetic patient's exposure to other conditions. For example, a urinary tract infection (UTI) can further impair renal function. Use of nephrotoxic drugs to treat the infection can compound the problem.

Diabetic nephropathy: Preventing further damage

Certain circumstances—including infections, treatments, and procedures—can worsen your patient's diabetic nephropathy. To help prevent further renal damage, you should be aware of the following four circumstances and take appropriate action.

- Urinary tract infections can further impair renal function in patients who have nephropathy. And many of the antibiotics used to treat these infections can cause additional impairment. To address the problem, suggest that the physician prescribe a less nephrotoxic drug such as norfloxacin.
- Many radiographic studies are nephrotoxic. If such studies are necessary, anticipate administering mannitol I.V. to induce diuresis.
- Poorly controlled blood glucose levels contribute to the onset and rapid progression of nephropathy. Monitor your patient's blood glucose levels frequently and encourage him to do the same when he returns home.
- A high-protein diet increases the rate of urine albumin secretion, leading to proteinuria. Encourage your patient to restrict his protein intake to 0.8 g/kg/day.

If the patient has a UTI, expect to administer an antibiotic that's less nephrotoxic, such as norfloxacin. If necessary, other antibiotics may be used in reduced dosages to minimize their nephrotoxic effects.

Carefully review the patient's medications, especially those that are excreted in the urine. If the patient has renal impairment, his physician may reduce the dosage or prescribe a different drug. For example, a patient with decreased kidney function who uses insulin may need a reduced dosage because about one-third of the dose is metabolized and excreted by the kidneys. Also, a patient who takes oral sulfonylureas may need a reduced dosage because the active metabolites of some of these drugs are excreted in the urine. Certain sulfonylureas, such as glipizide, may be used because they have a shorter half-life and break down to inactive metabolites that are excreted in the urine. If

your patient is receiving metformin, monitor him for lactic acidosis, a complication that results when plasma levels of metformin are greater than 5 mg/ml. If lactic acidosis occurs, immediately stop administering metformin and anticipate the need for hemodialysis.

Remember that certain dyes used in radiographic studies can be nephrotoxic. If a contrast medium is used, anticipate giving mannitol I.V. 1 hour before the test to induce diuresis and minimize the nephrotoxic effects. Encourage the patient to drink fluids after the test to help dilute the dye and eliminate it from the kidneys.

Monitor blood glucose levels frequently and adjust therapy as indicated by the results. Remember that optimal blood glucose control is crucial in helping to delay the onset and progression of nephropathy. It also can help reduce the frequency and severity of hypoglycemic episodes, thereby minimizing the risk of physiologic stress that can lead to further deterioration and possible renal failure.

If needed, restrict the patient's dietary protein intake to reduce the rate of urine albumin excretion and to slow the rate of kidney deterioration. You may need to restrict protein to 0.8 g/kg/day or less. Help the patient adhere to the restriction, which is substantially less than the typical intake of 1.2 to 1.4 g/kg/day. Ask the dietitian to help with meal planning to ensure that the patient maintains the recommended allowances for glucose control.

Aggressive treatment for hypertension may slow the progression of diabetic nephropathy. For example, diabetic patients with microalbuminuria and possible hypertension may benefit from ACE inhibitors. If administering captopril, remember that it may cause hyperkalemia. Monitor serum potassium levels to detect increases promptly. Also, administer thiazide diuretics cautiously because they may worsen hyperlipidemia and hyperglycemia. If the patient receives beta blockers, be aware that they may mask or alter the signs and symptoms of hypoglycemia. If he has hypertension, explain the need for additional lifestyle modifications.

Monitor the patient's renal function. Obtain a urine specimen for baseline urinalysis to detect glucose, ketones, and protein and do a 24-hour urine test to evaluate protein, serum creatinine, and BUN levels and creatinine clearance.

Assess electrolyte levels for imbalances, possibly caused by decreased renal function. As appropriate, institute measures to increase or decrease electrolyte levels, keeping in mind that treatment for one imbalance may ultimately result in the opposite imbalance. For example, if you administer potassium supplements to treat hypokalemia, you may induce hyperkalemia.

Dialysis and transplantation

If the patient's renal function continues to deteriorate, anticipate the need for hemodialysis, peritoneal dialysis, or possibly kidney transplantation. Because patients with diabetes are prone to developing sclerotic blood vessels, they may have limited access for hemodialysis. For this reason, many patients with diabetes who require hemodialysis are candidates for kidney transplantation. If your patient is receiving dialysis, stress the need to comply with diet and fluid restrictions. A patient receiving peritoneal dialysis will absorb extra calories from the dialysate as it dwells in the peritoneum. Therefore, he may be required to take in fewer calories during the day. Monitor weight and blood glucose levels closely. Also, monitor the patient's access site frequently for signs of infection. Keep in mind that peritonitis is a common complication of peritoneal dialysis. Watch for an elevation in serum leukocytes as well as fever and rebound abdominal tenderness. Check the arteriovenous (AV) shunt or fistula for adequate perfusion. It should be warm with an audible bruit and palpable thrill. To prevent occlusion of the AV access site, don't take blood pressure readings from the arm with the shunt or fistula. Remember that patients receiving dialysis may be more prone to depression, anxiety, and stress, so provide emotional support.

Prepare your patient for surgery, if indicated. Some patients with Type I diabetes may benefit from a kidney and pancreas transplantation or a kidney and islet cell transplantation. Both procedures aim to eliminate the need for exogenous insulin and dietary restrictions, improve renal function, and stabilize microvascular and macrovascular complications. If your patient receives an organ transplant, you'll need to prepare him for lifelong immunosuppressive therapy. Keep in mind that immunosuppressive

drugs can have serious adverse effects and may increase blood glucose levels. Expect to adjust your patient's insulin dosage because his insulin requirement will change after surgery.

Remember that treatment options may involve making difficult decisions that affect not only the patient but also his family. What's more, the patient's options may be limited by financial demands, insurance restrictions, and an inability to find a matching donor. Provide current, accurate information to enable the patient and his family to make informed decisions. If the patient's ability to concentrate and think clearly is affected by uremia, delay important discussions and decisions about treatment options until his condition improves with dialysis treatment. Offer emotional support, and allow the patient and his family to express their feelings and concerns. Enlist the help of a mental health professional, if necessary. Refer the patient and his family to support groups where they can share their feelings and experiences.

Self-care

Before the patient is discharged from the hospital, make sure that he understands his medication and treatment regimens and the need for follow-up care. Reinforce all aspects of glucose control, hypertension management, diet, and renal care. Have him repeat your demonstrations of self-care procedures, such as fingerstick blood glucose monitoring, urine testing, and blood pressure monitoring. Confirm that he can identify the signs and symptoms of complications, including decreased renal function, and that he knows when to notify his physician. Refer him to a home care nurse for evaluation, reinstruction, and follow-up care.

Complications

Diabetic patients with nephropathy are prone to renal complications, including proteinuria, nephrotic syndrome, and renal failure.

Proteinuria

Protein in the urine indicates increasing renal function deterioration. Among patients with persistent proteinuria, 25% develop end-stage renal disease within 6 years of onset, and 75% develop it within 15 years. Diabetic patients with proteinuria are 15 times more likely to develop CAD.

Confirming the complication

In a diabetic patient, proteinuria may be accompanied by signs of retinopathy, such as visual changes; increased serum creatinine and BUN levels; and decreased creatinine clearance. If renal function drops below 25% of normal, anemia occurs because the increase in retained nitrogenous wastes inhibits the kidneys' ability to produce erythropoietin, which normally stimulates red blood cell (RBC) production in the bone marrow.

Nursing interventions

Nursing care aims to prevent further renal function deterioration while maintaining diabetic control. Focus your interventions on controlling blood glucose levels and hypertension, restricting dietary protein, and administering medication therapy.

Expect to administer an ACE inhibitor, such as captopril. Captopril effectively treats diabetic nephropathy in patients with Type I diabetes, retinopathy, serum creatinine levels less than 2.5 mg/dl, and proteinuria greater than 500 mg/day. Captopril slows the rate of progression of renal insufficiency, thus decreasing the need for renal transplantation or dialysis. It also delays the progression to proteinuria and reduces the albumin excretion rate when given to patients with Type I diabetes, retinopathy, and microalbuminuria.

Currently, captopril is approved for use in treating diabetic nephropathy in patients with or without hypertension. When administering this drug, monitor the patient carefully for hyperkalemia. Obtain serum electrolyte levels and note any changes. Be especially alert for hyperkalemia if the patient is also receiving a potassium sparing diuretic, such as spironolactone, triamterene, or amiloride, because these drugs may significantly increase serum potassium levels.

Teach the patient about diabetes and renal insufficiency, including information about diagnosis and treatment. Review with him information about captopril, including the dosage (usually 25 mg orally three times a day). Also, discuss the possibility of side effects, such as hypotension, especially if he's receiving a diuretic or another drug for hypertension. Arrange for follow-up laboratory tests, including urinalysis, a 24-hour urine test, serum creatinine and BUN levels, and creatinine clearance, to evaluate renal function and serum electrolyte levels.

Nephrotic syndrome

A common complication in diabetic patients with renal insufficiency, nephrotic syndrome refers to a set of symptoms caused by protein wasting that results from diffuse glomerular damage. In this disorder, the glomerular basement membrane is abnormally permeable to proteins, particularly albumin, resulting in excessive protein filtration and excretion into the urine. Pressure changes occur in the kidney, causing edema.

Confirming the complication

A patient with nephrotic syndrome typically has proteinuria, hypoalbuminemia, and generalized edema. The edema usually begins slowly but eventually becomes extensive and severe. Other signs and symptoms include waxy skin pallor, anemia, anorexia, malaise, irritability, and abnormal menses. Proteinuria may account for losses of 4 to 30 grams of albumin daily. Serum albumin concentrations may be as low as 1 to 2.5 g/dl. Urinalysis typically reveals granular and epithelial cell casts and fat bodies. The patient also may have hematuria.

Nursing interventions

Focus on decreasing the patient's edema. Closely monitor his fluid balance, intake and output, and daily weight measurements. Obtain a baseline measurement of his abdominal girth and compare it to subsequent measurements. As prescribed, administer loop diuretics, such as furosemide, and plasma volume expanders, such as salt-poor albumin, plasma, and dextran, to pull fluid from the extracellular spaces for filtration by the kidney. Administer these medications carefully because diabetic patients with renal insufficiency have a reduced capacity to tolerate sudden shifts in intravascular volume. Assess the patient for signs and symptoms of electrolyte imbalance because loop diuretics predispose patients to hypokalemia.

If your patient is receiving corticosteroid therapy, monitor him closely for signs of infection, which may be masked. Also, monitor blood glucose levels because corticosteroids can disrupt glucose control.

Teach the patient about dietary management, including how to follow a sodium-restricted diet, if prescribed. The amount of dietary protein allowed depends on the amount lost in the urine over 24 hours. Typically, the patient with nephrotic syndrome has a diminished appetite. Offer small, frequent meals. Work with the dietitian to develop a diet plan that provides the calories, protein, fat, and carbohydrates needed to maintain glycemic control and minimize the effects on renal function. Monitor the patient's blood glucose levels for changes and adjust medications accordingly.

Because of microvascular changes and large protein losses, a diabetic patient with nephrotic syndrome is at risk for infection. Monitor vital signs closely. If you suspect an infection, obtain a specimen for culture and sensitivity testing. Administer antibiotics, as prescribed. Keep in mind that many antibiotics are nephrotoxic, so the dose may need to be reduced or the drug replaced. Because infection increases the risk for hyperglycemia, you may also need to increase the patient's insulin dose.

Remember that edematous tissue is prone to cellulitis and infection, especially when the legs are affected. If a diabetic patient has neuropathy, he may not be aware of the pain, swelling, or skin breakdown that could signal infection. Position him carefully and encourage him to change positions often. Inspect pressure areas, especially the sacrum, heels, and elbows, for signs of breakdown. Have the patient use an air or water mattress.

Avoid injecting insulin into edematous tissue; doing so may interfere with insulin absorption. During the acute phase of edema, you may need to administer insulin I.V. until the patient's condition stabilizes.

After the patient's condition stabilizes, prepare a teaching plan that encompasses all aspects of his care and begin planning for discharge. Anticipate the need for follow-up home care, and refer the patient to community agencies for support.

Renal failure

Before renal transplants and dialysis became common, renal failure was the primary cause of death in diabetic patients with renal insufficiency. Renal failure occurs when the kidneys can no longer maintain homeostasis because they're irreversibly damaged. In diabetic patients with nephropathy and renal insufficiency, renal failure results from progressive damage to the glomerulus and the deterioration of renal function.

Confirming the complication

Signs and symptoms of renal failure result from fluid and electrolyte imbalances, such as hyperkalemia, and altered regulatory function, such as in the synthesis of erythropoietin. Although the course of renal failure varies among patients, common characteristics include fluid retention, anemia, and heart failure. The patient also may develop cardiac insufficiency, peripheral vascular disease, and peripheral neuropathy. Chronic renal failure affects many body systems (see *Effects of renal failure on patients with diabetes*, page 36).

Nursing interventions

Renal failure ultimately results in uremia and death unless the patient undergoes dialysis or renal transplantation. Treatment doesn't cure renal failure, but it may slow its progression. Focus your nursing care on preserving the remaining renal function, improving the patient's physiologic status, alleviating any associated symptoms, and helping improve quality of life.

Discuss treatment options with the patient and his family, including kidney transplantation, kidney and pancreas transplantation, and dialysis. If the patient chooses not to receive treatment, he'll still need home or hospice care. Reinforce the physician's explanation of treatment options. Provide support and answer any questions about the risks and benefits of each treatment to help the patient make an informed decision.

Effects of renal failure on patients with diabetes

In patients with diabetes, renal failure is devastating. This chart summarizes its effects on major body systems.

Body system	Effects
Cardiovascular	• Hypervolemia • Hypertension • Tachycardia • Arrhythmias • Heart failure • Pericarditis
Hematopoietic	• Anemia • Leukocytosis • Platelet dysfunction • Thrombocytopenia
Neurologic	• Lethargy, confusion, stupor, coma • Seizures • Sleep disturbances • Asterixis • Muscle irritability • Unusual behavior
Gastrointestinal	• Anorexia • Nausea and vomiting • Constipation or diarrhea • Abdominal distention • Uremic fetor (halitosis)
Skin	• Pallor • Pigmentation • Pruritus • Ecchymosis • Excoriation
Genitourinary	• Uremic frost • Decreased urine output and specific gravity • Proteinuria • Casts and cells in urine • Decreased urine sodium
Skeletal	• Osteodystrophy • Renal rickets • Joint pain • Retarded growth
Reproductive	• Infertility • Decreased libido • Impotence • Amenorrhea

Take appropriate measures to relieve pruritus, and discourage the patient from scratching his skin. Explain that scratching can cause excoriation, which places a diabetic patient at high risk for infection. Treatment may include the use of topical lotions and emollients, antihistamines, I.V. lidocaine, and ultraviolet B light therapy. Dialysis also may relieve pruritus. Use comfort measures and try to prevent further skin breakdown.

Emphasize the need for personal safety precautions, especially if the patient has peripheral neuropathy or visual problems related to retinopathy, because decreased sensation can mask injuries. When the patient is in bed, keep the side rails up and encourage him to use the call light for assistance. Keep necessary items within his reach.

If the patient's mental alertness is diminished, reorient him as necessary and take the time to explain information thoroughly. Remember, changes in mental status can result not only from renal failure, but also from hypoglycemia and hyperglycemia. Therefore, monitor the patient's blood glucose levels frequently.

Assess the patient's learning needs. Inform him and his family about renal failure, including its outcome and treatment. If the patient will be receiving home dialysis, provide thorough teaching and a referral for home care. Discuss the need for lifestyle modifications. Offer support and stress the need to comply with the prescribed treatment program.

Diabetes mellitus and pneumonia

An infectious and inflammatory process, pneumonia usually occurs when normal defense mechanisms are weakened or overcome by the virulence, quality, or number of microorganisms in the lungs. Diabetes is a risk factor for developing pneumonia because increased blood glucose levels and impaired white blood cell (WBC) function make the patient more vulnerable to infection. In a patient with Type I diabetes, pneumonia may lead to

DKA. The infection can increase the level of hormones, such as glucagon. And this, in turn, leads to the breakdown of fats and proteins that causes hyperglycemia. A patient with DKA will have elevated blood glucose and urine ketone levels.

Pathophysiology

Normally, the presence of microorganisms in the lungs activates the body's defense mechanisms, such as the cough reflex, ciliary clearance, phagocytosis, and the inflammatory response. In susceptible patients, the invading microorganisms multiply, releasing toxins and stimulating a full-scale inflammatory and immune response that causes damaging side effects. Also, the antigen-antibody reactions and the endotoxins released by some organisms can damage the bronchial mucous and alveolar membranes. In diabetic patients, pathogens may proliferate more rapidly because of the increased glucose in body fluid. WBC function in diabetic patients is also impaired.

Most cases of pneumonia start with a viral upper respiratory tract infection. The viral infection progressively worsens, or a secondary bacterial infection occurs. The patient may develop a fever, chills, cough, malaise, pleural pain, and sometimes dyspnea and hemoptysis. Usually, the WBC count is elevated. Chest X-rays show infiltrates. A sputum culture identifies the causative organism.

Adapting nursing care

Aggressive treatment of the pneumonia infection is essential in diabetic patients because of the high incidence of serious complications and death. Keep in mind that the counterregulatory hormones—cortisol, epinephrine, growth hormone, and glucagon—will increase blood glucose levels, thus increasing the patient's insulin requirements. Plus, lipolysis and ketogenesis may cause ketonuria.

When your diabetic patient develops pneumonia, you should focus not only on treating the pneumonia but also on dealing with its effects on the patient's diabetes. Like any infection, pneumonia can cause a diabetic patient to develop dangerous complications, such as hyperglycemia, hypoglycemia, and dehydration. As part of your patient's immediate care, you'll need to control blood glucose levels, maintain a patent airway, provide sufficient oxygenation, and maintain fluid and electrolyte balance (see *Providing support, easing discomfort,* page 38). Also, as the patient undergoes diagnostic tests for pneumonia, such as bronchoscopy, you'll need to tailor your care (see *When your patient with diabetes and pneumonia needs bronchoscopy,* page 39).

Blood glucose levels

For a diabetic patient with pneumonia, you'll need to monitor blood glucose and urine ketone levels at least four times a day and adjust the insulin dosage accordingly. If your patient develops DKA, you'll need to increase his insulin dosage. A patient with Type II diabetes may develop HHNK syndrome, a complication that may be caused by infections such as pneumonia. A patient with HHNK syndrome will have extremely high blood glucose levels (greater than 800 mg/dl) but no ketones in his urine. Because this dangerous syndrome creates profound dehydration, you'll need to infuse large amounts of fluids I.V., usually a hypotonic solution, such as 0.45% normal saline solution. Then, give the prescribed insulin I.V. until the patient's blood glucose levels return to normal.

Many patients with pneumonia lose their appetite, and some develop nausea and vomiting. Therefore, hypoglycemia can develop unless the patient's oral hypoglycemic agent or insulin is withheld or the dose is reduced. Be alert for symptoms of hypoglycemia, such as clammy skin, shakiness, weakness, and confusion. If vomiting persists, an antiemetic may be prescribed. However, certain antiemetics, such as chlorpromazine, may be contraindicated for diabetic patients.

Vomiting, DKA, or HHNK syndrome can lead to fluid and electrolyte imbalances. To correct the imbalances, you'll probably first administer hypotonic solutions I.V., then replace electrolytes, such as potassium and phosphate.

COMFORT MEASURES

Providing support, easing discomfort

- Before performing any procedure or treatment, tell the patient who you are and explain what you're about to do, even if he's unconscious or confused.
- When your patient's blood glucose levels stabilize, reassess how often they need to be monitored. Reducing the number of fingersticks and venipunctures will help prevent skin breakdown of the finger pads and protect the integrity of the veins.
- During chest physiotherapy, be sure to cup your hands so your patient doesn't feel pain or discomfort and his skin remains intact.
- When you perform nasotracheal suctioning, lubricate the catheter generously and apply suction only as you withdraw it, not as you insert it. Taking these steps helps prevent hypoxia, mucosal irritation, and discomfort. Also, avoid using suction pressure greater than 120 mm Hg and don't suction for more than 15 seconds at a time. If bronchospasm occurs during suctioning, gently pull back on the catheter. Before and after suctioning, give the patient supplemental oxygen.
- If your patient has an endotracheal tube or a tracheostomy, inspect the skin under the security ties for signs of irritation or breakdown.
- When using continuous pulse oximetry, alternate the monitoring sites every 8 to 12 hours to ensure comfort and to prevent skin breakdown or rashes beneath the probe sensor.

Airway and oxygenation

You also need to establish and maintain a patent airway and ensure adequate oxygenation. Depending on the severity of the pneumonia and your patient's overall health, he may need supplemental oxygen or even mechanical ventilation.

Monitor the effectiveness of treatment using pulse oximetry and ABG studies. To loosen mucus and facilitate expectoration or suctioning, use humidified oxygen, perform chest physiotherapy, and reposition the patient often. Bronchodilators also may be prescribed; if albuterol is used, be alert for signs of hyperglycemia, which may result from the drug's beta-adrenergic effects. If the patient has chronic obstructive pulmonary disease or asthma and is receiving glucocorticoid treatment, his blood glucose levels may increase.

Fluid and electrolyte balance

Increased blood glucose levels increase urine output and, in turn, fluid requirements. To maintain fluid balance, you'll need to monitor your patient's intake and output and daily weight measurements and replace lost fluids accordingly. You'll also need to monitor serum BUN, creatinine, and electrolyte levels to detect nephropathy. Plus, you should monitor renal studies closely, because many antibiotics are nephrotoxic and can further impair renal function.

Self-care

Make sure your patient knows how to manage his diabetes when he has a minor illness, such as a cold, flu, or upset stomach. If he's weak, he may need help with his self-care regimen.

Before your patient is discharged from the hospital, review his diabetic treatment regimen and explain how his pneumonia has affected it. Also, explain and demonstrate any respiratory care measures, such as coughing, deep breathing, incentive spirometry, or bronchodilator inhalation therapy. And teach him to recognize and report signs and symptoms of respiratory problems.

As you care for your patient, stress the importance of preventing pneumonia. Advise him to avoid exposure to crowds or to people with active respiratory infections and to use proper hygiene measures to reduce the risk of droplet transmission. Also, recommend that he receive a polyvalent pneumococcal vaccine and a yearly influenza immunization.

Complications

A diabetic patient with pneumonia risks developing complications, such as hyperglycemia and respiratory failure.

ADAPTING YOUR CARE

When your patient with diabetes and pneumonia needs bronchoscopy

The stress of an illness such as pneumonia or a procedure such as bronchoscopy, which requires an 8-hour fast, can alter your diabetic patient's insulin requirements. To minimize the disruption to his normal meal regimen, schedule the procedure early in the day. Also, to prevent serious complications—such as hypoxemia, hypoglycemia (or marked hyperglycemia), ketoacidosis, and fluid and electrolyte imbalance—take the following steps.

Before bronchoscopy
- Give the prescribed oral hypoglycemic drug. The patient's physician may withhold this drug the day before and the day of the procedure.
- Give the prescribed insulin. The physician may lower the doses of short-acting (regular) and intermediate-acting (NPH or Lente) insulin the day before the procedure and may lower the dose of long-acting (Ultralente) insulin 1 to 2 days before the procedure. To control hyperglycemia, administer regular insulin as needed.
- Make sure your patient takes nothing by mouth for 8 hours before the procedure. If appropriate, insert an I.V. line and administer fluids I.V. to maintain hydration.
- Several hours before the procedure, check the patient's blood glucose and plasma ketone levels. If he has ketosis, the bronchoscopy may be postponed.
- The morning of the procedure, administer the prescribed insulin. Typically, this will be a reduced dose of intermediate-acting insulin (one-half to two-thirds of the usual morning dose of NPH or Lente).
- Elevate the head of the bed between 45 and 90 degrees until the procedure begins. This mea-

sure promotes comfort and helps the patient breathe more easily.
- Assess the patient for signs and symptoms of hypoxemia (such as restlessness and tachycardia) and hypoventilation (such as cyanosis and Cheyne-Stokes respirations). Administer oxygen by nasal cannula or mask, if necessary.

During bronchoscopy
- Monitor the patient's heart rate and respiratory rate. Use continuous pulse oximetry to monitor his oxygenation status.
- Administer fluids I.V. as prescribed to maintain fluid and electrolyte balance.
- Administer the prescribed conscious sedation medication, such as meperidine or midazolam.
- Monitor the blood glucose level, which should remain between 150 and 200 mg/dl. If it rises above 200 mg/dl, administer regular insulin as prescribed.

After bronchoscopy
- Place the patient in the semi-Fowler position or on his side to help remove secretions. Use nasotracheal suctioning, if necessary.
- Monitor the patient's vital signs. Assess his breath sounds and respiratory rate frequently. Encourage him to cough and breathe deeply.
- Administer oxygen by nasal cannula or mask, if indicated. Monitor the patient's oxygenation status, using continuous pulse oximetry.
- Check blood glucose levels and, if necessary, administer regular insulin as prescribed.
- When the local anesthetic wears off and the patient's gag and swallow reflexes return, encourage him to eat.

Hyperglycemia
Diabetic patients with pneumonia may develop acute hyperglycemia because the physiologic stress of the pneumonia increases the secretion of counterregulatory hormones. Epinephrine decreases the uptake of glucose by the muscle tissue, inhibits the release of endogenous insulin, and stimulates the breakdown of glycogen in the liver. Cortisol increases glucose production in the liver and inhibits the uptake of insulin by the muscle cells. And growth hormone and glucagon raise blood glucose levels.

Confirming the complication
Initially, the patient with hyperglycemia may be asymptomatic. As blood glucose levels rise, polyuria, polydipsia, polyphagia, and weight loss (especially in patients with Type I diabetes)

occur. Blood glucose levels higher than 200 mg/dl before eating confirm the diagnosis. If left untreated, hyperglycemia can progress to DKA or HHNK syndrome.

Nursing interventions

Your immediate goal is to reduce the patient's blood glucose level. If he has Type I diabetes, you may need to administer supplemental doses of regular insulin. If he has Type II diabetes, you may need to administer insulin to control blood glucose levels until the pneumonia resolves; if he's already receiving insulin therapy, you may need to increase his insulin dosage.

For a patient with DKA or HHNK syndrome, your primary goals are to maintain his airway, breathing, and circulation and to protect him from injury. Therefore, check his vital signs and assess his level of consciousness. If the level of consciousness is altered, protect him from injury. Look for signs of dehydration, including dry mucous membranes, poor skin turgor, tachycardia, and blood pressure changes. Expect to begin cardiac monitoring and, if your patient is dehydrated, replace fluids with hypotonic normal saline solution.

Monitor your patient's blood glucose levels closely. Draw blood for baseline glucose, ketone, and electrolyte measurements. Keep in mind that blood glucose levels may be affected by dehydration and shock.

Administer regular insulin I.V., as prescribed. Then administer a continuous infusion at the prescribed rate, which will be adjusted according to the patient's blood glucose levels. Continue to check blood glucose levels every 1 to 2 hours.

Monitor your patient's intake and output; insert an indwelling urinary catheter, if necessary, to monitor output every hour. If his level of consciousness is altered, you may need to insert a nasogastric tube to prevent aspiration. Monitor vital signs, cardiac rhythm, and electrolyte levels frequently. In a patient with DKA, the potassium level will drop as the acidosis resolves.

After your patient's condition has stabilized, review with him all aspects of his diabetic regimen. Stress the importance of managing his diabetes when he has a minor illness. Teach him to take his temperature properly and to report a fever to his physician. Make sure he knows how to recognize the signs and symptoms of respiratory infections. Advise him to check with his physician before taking any over-the-counter cough or cold medications because they may contain glucose and alcohol, which can affect blood glucose levels.

Respiratory failure

In a diabetic patient with pneumonia, respiratory failure can result from worsening of the pneumonia or a failure to treat it. Also, respiratory failure may occur as a complication of acute emergencies, such as DKA or HHNK syndrome.

Confirming the complication

Signs and symptoms of respiratory failure include apprehension, confusion, headache, respiratory distress, slowed respiratory rate, paradoxical respirations, and somnolence that can progress to coma. ABG studies confirm the diagnosis. Typically, the partial pressure of arterial oxygen (Pao_2) is 60 mm Hg or less, the partial pressure of arterial carbon dioxide ($Paco_2$) is 50 mm Hg or more, and, if the patient has acidosis, the pH is 7.35 or less.

Nursing interventions

As needed, initiate oxygen therapy to maintain the patient's Pao_2 between 60 and 90 mm Hg. Maintain a patent airway and encourage coughing, deep breathing, and frequent position changes. Elevate the head of the bed to facilitate breathing. And suction the airway as necessary to remove secretions. Provide fluids to mobilize secretions. Anticipate the need for mechanical ventilation if the patient's pulmonary status deteriorates.

If respiratory failure results from DKA or HHNK syndrome, the patient will be dehydrated. As prescribed, administer fluids I.V. and monitor intake and output. Assess renal function studies carefully because diabetic nephropathy may not produce symptoms.

Monitor blood glucose levels frequently—every hour, if indicated. As prescribed, administer insulin I.V. based on the blood glucose levels.

After your patient's condition stabilizes, review with him the events that precipitated respiratory failure. Reinforce the need to control blood glucose levels, to notify the physician of adverse signs and symptoms, and to manage diabetes during minor illnesses. If your patient with Type II diabetes needs insulin therapy for a short time, teach him as you would a newly diagnosed patient with Type I diabetes. Arrange for a home care nurse to consult with him about the need for follow-up care.

Diabetes mellitus and peripheral vascular disease

Peripheral vascular disease (PVD) occurs sooner and more commonly in diabetic patients. Typically, a diabetic patient with PVD develops occlusions and poor collateral circulation in both legs. By contrast, a nondiabetic patient with PVD may develop a problem in only one leg and still have adequate collateral circulation.

PVD can cause muscle atrophy and lower leg and foot ulcers. It also accounts for more than one-half of all nontraumatic leg amputations, which are up to 20 times more likely to occur in diabetic patients.

Pathophysiology

In PVD, blood and oxygen flow through the peripheral vessels is reduced. Usually, this results from atherosclerotic changes in the peripheral arteries that lead to thrombus formation and arterial occlusion, thereby diminishing the supply of oxygen and nutrients to the tissues. Other causes include increased coagulability of the blood, blood pressure changes, and inflammation. As the tissues' oxygen needs exceed the supply, areas of ischemia develop, ultimately resulting in necrosis. To compensate for the decreased blood supply, collateral circulation usually develops. However, diabetic patients may not be able to develop adequate collateral circulation to bypass the occlusion because of microvascular changes associated with diabetes.

Venous system problems occur when the transport of blood from the capillary beds to the heart is altered. Changes in the smooth muscle and connective tissue impair the veins' ability to expand and contract. The valves may not function, resulting in a backflow of blood and, ultimately, tissue ischemia and necrosis.

If the arteries are affected, pulses are diminished or absent. Muscle atrophy; thin, hairless, cool skin; thick, ridged toenails; and a bruit over the affected arteries may occur. When the leg is elevated above the heart, the skin is pale gray; when it's dependent, the skin is dusky red.

If the venous system is affected, superficial veins are dilated, tortuous, and cordlike. The patient may experience pain when the legs are dependent. Edema, dependent cyanosis, brown skin discoloration, pruritus, and paresthesia can occur. Temperature remains normal, and pulses are usually present, although they may be difficult to palpate through the edema.

Adapting nursing care

Nursing care focuses on reducing risk factors and promoting tissue perfusion. You'll also need to help maintain the patient's skin integrity, promote activity, and prevent injury. Even minor trauma to the legs can lead to infection, ulceration, and, ultimately, loss of function.

Monitor your patient for pain, paresthesia, paralysis, pallor, and pulselessness. If necessary, use a Doppler stethoscope to locate the pulses and mark the areas with a permanent felt-tip pen, so you can relocate them.

Thoroughly assess your patient's skin for pressure areas or tears. If he has peripheral or autonomic neuropathy, he may be less sensitive to touch, pain, or temperature. He also may experience paresthesia and be unaware of changes or injury. Also, assess capillary refill and check for any changes in feeling, such as numbness or tingling.

Foot ulceration can be a serious complication for a diabetic patient with PVD. If infection develops, further ischemia and possibly gangrene can develop, ultimately requiring an amputation. Provide meticulous foot care along with optimal blood glucose control to decrease the risk of complications. Reposition your patient at least every 2 hours and have him perform range of motion exercises, as tolerated. Wash his feet with warm water and mild soap. Make sure that his feet, especially the areas between the toes, are completely dried. Inspect the feet and apply moisturizing lotion daily. Use protective padding, foot cradles, and an air or water mattress to reduce the risk of pressure injuries. To prevent constriction, avoid using elastic antiembolism stockings. Make sure the patient wears shoes or slippers that fit properly to avoid further breakdown.

If your patient has an ulcer that may be infected, obtain a wound culture and begin antibiotic therapy. Maintain adequate hydration and monitor renal function closely. Depending on its extent, the wound may require an incision, drainage, or debridement, and dressing changes. Use aseptic technique for wound care to reduce the risk of further infection. Be alert for increased redness, swelling, and foul-smelling, purulent drainage.

Administer the prescribed pain medications. Pentoxifylline may help improve intermittent claudication by increasing the RBC flexibility and decreasing blood viscosity, plasma fibrinogen, and platelet aggregation. This, in turn, improves blood flow and enhances tissue oxygenation. Monitor the patient for headache, dizziness, nausea, and vomiting. Also, check his WBC count for neutropenia.

Platelet inhibitors, such as aspirin or ticlopidine, may be given to slow the progression of atherosclerosis. If your patient is receiving ticlopidine, monitor his complete blood count and WBC differential for neutropenia. Assess his liver function tests for elevations that indicate liver dysfunction.

Invasive and surgical procedures

Invasive treatments include laser angioplasty and percutaneous transluminal angioplasty of the femoral, iliac, or popliteal artery. Usually, surgery is considered if pain interferes with the patient's ability to function, if foot ulcers or infection don't respond to treatment, or if the patient has gangrene. The decision to perform arterial bypass grafting depends on the location and severity of the occlusion and the patient's overall medical condition. The aim of this surgery is to restore circulation to the affected limb and reduce the risk of amputation.

Closely monitor your patient's blood glucose levels before and after surgery. The physiologic demands of surgery, lack of food intake, and emotional stress will affect blood glucose control.

After surgery, take steps to promote and maintain circulation. Monitor the neurovascular status of the legs, and assess the patient for severe pain, loss of pulses, cold limbs, and new complaints of numbness or tingling. To reduce edema, elevate the affected leg and caution the patient not to cross his legs or sit for long periods of time.

Self-care

Focus your patient teaching on reducing risk factors, providing proper foot care, and preventing complications. Review with the patient his medication regimen and make sure he understands any modifications needed for glucose management. Also, stress the importance of exercise to control blood glucose levels and help increase circulation.

If your patient has diabetic retinopathy, keep in mind that impaired vision may affect his ability to inspect and care for his feet. And if he has diabetic neuropathy, decreased sensation may mask changes or injuries. Assess his ability to care for his feet. Provide written care instructions and enlist the aid of family members. Urge the patient to report any changes to his physician. Refer him to a podiatrist, if necessary (see *Foot care guidelines*).

Complications

A diabetic patient with PVD risks developing complications, such as arterial occlusion, deep vein thrombosis (DVT), chronic venous insufficiency, and gangrene.

Arterial occlusion

Progressive narrowing of the vessel lumen may result in arterial occlusion. The onset is usually gradual, although microvascular changes place diabetic patients with PVD at increased risk for acute arterial occlusion, with arteriosclerosis and atheromatous occlusion commonly developing below the knee. Peripheral vascular bypass surgery has been successful with these types of occlusions.

Confirming the complication

Typically, the patient complains of intermittent claudication, which he may describe as a tightening pressure in the calves, thighs, or gluteal muscles or as a sharp, cramplike sensation that occurs during walking and disappears 1 to 2 minutes after resting. Eventually, exercise tolerance decreases, and symptoms occur more often with less exertion. The patient also may feel pain at rest, usually at night when he's lying down. Pain increases when the legs are elevated because of decreased blood flow. Nerve ischemia may occur, causing a dull, aching sensation in the toes or forefoot that's relieved by hanging the foot over the side of the bed or by walking.

If the occlusion is acute, your patient may have pain, pallor, pulselessness, paresthesia, or paralysis. Muscle necrosis may occur as early as 2 to 3 hours after the occlusion. Complete paralysis, with stiffness of muscles and joints, indicates irreversible damage.

Nursing interventions

Care measures focus on improving tissue perfusion, promoting skin integrity, preventing infection, relieving pain, and reducing the risk of injury. Close monitoring of blood glucose levels is essential to minimize the risk of hypoglycemia and hyperglycemia.

If the patient requires diagnostic testing, tell him what to expect before, during, and after the procedure. Remember that in diabetic patients who have PVD, angiography can increase the risk of precipitating renal insufficiency or renal failure because the contrast medium is nephrotoxic. Intervene to reduce this risk by promoting diuresis with adequate hydration and I.V. mannitol before the test. Use nonionic contrast agents, as prescribed.

Explain to the patient the role that exercise plays in increasing circulation. Before he starts an exercise program, teach him to check his pulse rate. Suggest exercises such as interval training, stationary biking, swimming, walking on a slow treadmill, or chair exercises involving upper-body movements. Reinforce that the patient should check blood glucose

 GOING HOME

Foot care guidelines

For a patient with diabetes and peripheral vascular disease, proper foot care can help prevent the loss of a limb. Before your patient is discharged, teach him these routine care measures:
- Inspect your feet every day at the same time.
- Wash your feet with mild soap and water. Avoid soaking them and using harsh chemicals.
- Check the temperature of bath water to make sure it's not too hot before you step into the tub.
- Use good lighting and a mirror to inspect the soles of your feet.
- Apply lotion containing lanolin to the soles of your feet, but not between your toes.
- If your feet perspire, apply powder to them.
- Cut your toenails straight across with clippers or rounded-edge scissors after you bathe or shower.
- See a podiatrist for corns, calluses, and other foot problems.
- Wear properly fitting shoes or slippers and cotton socks. Change your socks daily.
- Don't walk barefoot or wear shoes without socks.
- Choose leather shoes with thick rubber soles and soft tops. Don't wear rubber or plastic shoes or high heels with pointed toes.
- Guard against injury and burns. Keep your feet warm, but don't use hot-water bottles, heating pads, or electric blankets.
- Notify your physician immediately if redness, tenderness, swelling, or other signs or symptoms of infection appear.

levels before, during, and after exercise because he can become hypoglycemic while exercising. Assess his tolerance of the exercise plan. Keep in mind that if he has a leg or foot ulcer, exercise is contraindicated because it can cause further ischemia.

Because of poor circulation, a patient with chronic arterial occlusion is prone to ulceration and infection. Lesions tend to heal poorly, if at all. Keep the affected area clean and free from pressure and irritation. Assess the surrounding tissue for edema, capillary refill, pallor, dependent rubor, and skin temperature. Encourage bed rest to reduce the oxygen demands of the impaired tissue. If the wound is debrided, change the dressing, as needed; doing so further debrides the wound. Carefully assess the patient's femoral, popliteal, and dorsalis pedis pulses.

If the patient has an acute arterial occlusion, place him on bed rest and protect the affected limb from pressure and other trauma. Closely assess the leg for signs of further deterioration, such as paralysis with stiffening muscles and joints.

Typically, the patient's anticoagulant therapy will begin with a heparin infusion; later, he'll receive an oral anticoagulant. During therapy, monitor his APTT and PT. Watch for signs of hemorrhage, including hematuria, epistaxis, bruising, petechiae, hematoma formation, hematemesis, and bleeding from the gums and rectum.

If your patient will continue anticoagulant therapy at home, teach him about the medication regimen, including how and when to take the medication and which signs and symptoms to watch for and report. Encourage him to use a soft toothbrush instead of a hard one and an electric razor instead of razor blades to minimize the risk of injury and bleeding. If he's taking warfarin, caution him to avoid foods that are high in vitamin K, which can interfere with the drug's intended action. If your patient injects insulin, advise him to rotate injection sites on his abdomen to minimize the risk of hematoma formation that may occur with anticoagulant therapy. Also, warn him not to use bruised injection sites because insulin is poorly absorbed in these areas.

Before the patient is discharged from the hospital, be sure he understands instructions for medication therapy, exercise, and foot care. Review with him how to manage his blood glucose level and help him modify his regimen, if necessary.

Deep vein thrombosis

This complication stems from venous stasis, vessel wall injury, and hypercoagulability of the blood. Stasis can occur with incompetent valves or inactive muscles. The risk is especially great among diabetic patients with PVD who are on prolonged bed rest.

Thrombus formation in the veins is similar to that in the arteries. As RBCs, platelets, and fibrin accumulate and attach to the vein wall, a thrombus forms. The proximal end of the thrombus freely floats in the lumen, ready to break apart and migrate into the circulation, causing an embolus.

Confirming the complication

Signs and symptoms depend on the level of the affected vein, the size of the thrombus, and the presence of collateral circulation. For example, a thrombus at the level of the iliac and femoral veins may cause pain and extensive swelling of the entire limb.

Other signs and symptoms may include tenderness along the iliac vessels and the femoral canal, in the popliteal space, and over the deep calf veins. Also, a patient may have ankle edema, a low grade fever, or tachycardia. However, some patients have no symptoms unless they develop a pulmonary embolus.

Nursing interventions

The key to nursing care is prevention by teaching patients how to reduce risk factors. If DVT occurs, expect to begin treatment with anticoagulant therapy, usually I.V. heparin followed by an oral anticoagulant agent, such as warfarin. The physician also may prescribe thrombolytic agents. Monitor the patient's PT and APTT to evaluate the effectiveness of therapy. Watch for signs of hemorrhage, such as hematuria, epistaxis, bruising, petechiae, hematemesis, and bleeding from the gums and rectum. If your patient will continue anticoagulant therapy at home, teach him about the medication regimen, including how and when to take the medication and which signs and symptoms to watch for and report. Also, teach him appropriate safety precautions.

Keep the patient on bed rest during the acute stage to prevent emboli and pressure fluctuations in the venous system that occur with walking or sitting. Remember, however, that inactivity can contribute to a reduced need for insulin. Monitor blood glucose levels closely because inactivity may cause his normal insulin regimen to heighten the risk of hypoglycemia.

Institute measures to protect the skin, such as using a bed cradle, heel protectors, and an air or water mattress, especially if your patient has diabetic neuropathy, which increases the risk of skin breakdown. After the threat of emboliza-tion is over, encourage your patient to walk and to exercise in bed to decrease venous pressure and promote blood flow. Monitor his blood glu-cose levels closely as his activity level increases and adjust his insulin dosage, if necessary.

Elevate your patient's legs above the level of the heart to relieve edema and pain and to fa-cilitate blood flow, thereby helping to prevent venous stasis and the formation of new thrombi. As directed, apply warm, moist soaks to the affected leg. If your patient has diabetic neuropathy, monitor the affected leg because decreased sensation can result in burns if the soaks are too hot.

Before your patient is discharged from the hospital, teach him about his medication ther-apy, activity restrictions, and signs and symp-toms to watch for and report. Reinforce instruc-tions about how to manage his blood glucose level.

Chronic venous insufficiency

Chronic venous insufficiency stems from dys-functional valves that reduce venous return. The resulting increase in venous pressure causes venous stasis. Diabetic patients with PVD are at high risk for this problem because of the vascular changes that occur in both dis-orders, each compounding the other.

Confirming the complication

Chronic venous insufficiency often progresses to obstruction. The patient may be asympto-matic, or he may experience swelling from edema, leading to tissue fibrosis, redness over the muscle, engorgement of superficial veins, and cyanosis. He may complain of tenderness, aching, or severe pain in the affected arm or leg. Chronic venous insufficiency can lead to necrosis of distal tissue, causing stasis ulcers, which make the patient vulnerable to sec-ondary infections. He may experience fever, chills, or malaise because of the infection.

Nursing interventions

Try to prevent chronic venous insufficiency by teaching your patient about the disease and by reducing risk factors. Encourage strict adher-ence to his treatment regimens for PVD and di-abetes. Explain that adequate blood glucose

control helps to minimize the risk associated with macrovascular complications. Stress the importance of meticulous skin care and hy-giene measures for preventing skin breakdown and infection. Tell him to take any antibiotics prescribed for infection.

Gangrene

Because of the increased risk of tissue isch-emia, skin breakdown, and infection from the vascular changes associated with diabetes and PVD, patients with these diseases are at high risk for gangrene. If the patient also has neu-ropathy, he's less likely to notice a problem or change in the affected area, placing him at an even higher risk.

Gangrene can be dry or moist. Dry gangrene usually results from coagulative necrosis that occurs without subsequent bacterial decompo-sition. Moist gangrene results from necrosis of tissues when proteins are broken down by bac-terial action. This usually occurs in the internal organs.

A special type of gangrene, gas gangrene re-sults when wounds become infected with a species of *Clostridium*. These anaerobic bacte-ria produce enzymes that cause a gas and a serosanguineous exudate, which fill the muscles and subcutaneous tissue and destroy cellular membranes. This can be fatal if the enzymes lyse the RBC membranes and destroy their ability to carry oxygen.

Gangrenous tissue must be completely re-moved before healing can occur. Gangrene is a leading cause of amputation.

Confirming the complication

If your patient has dry gangrene, the skin over the affected area will appear very dry, shrunken, and wrinkled. The color will change to dark brown or black. If he has moist gan-grene, the affected area will be swollen, cold, and black and have a foul odor. If your patient has gas gangrene, you'll detect localized swelling and dusky brown or reddish discol-oration. Bullae form over the wound and rup-ture, revealing a dark red or black necrotic muscle. A foul-smelling, watery or frothy dis-charge may appear. The patient may be pale and

---

Recognizing the types of gangrene

Patients with diabetes and peripheral vascular disease are at risk for developing gangrene. This table helps you distinguish the three types of gangrene at a glance.

Type of gangrene	Signs and symptoms
Dry gangrene	• Dry, shrunken, and wrinkled skin. • Skin color dark brown or black.
Moist gangrene	• Swollen, cold, and black skin. • Foul odor.
Gas gangrene	• Swollen and dusky brown or reddish skin. • Bullae rupture, revealing dark red or black necrotic muscle. • Foul-smelling, watery, or frothy discharge. • Patient may be pale and motionless.

---

motionless because of systemic toxicity. Subcutaneous emphysema is a hallmark sign (see *Recognizing the types of gangrene*).

Nursing interventions

RAPID RESPONSE ▶ To prevent further tissue necrosis, provide emergency care. Obtain a culture of the wound and institute antibiotic therapy immediately. If the patient has diabetic nephropathy, you may need to administer a reduced dose of the antibiotic. Because infection is likely to cause hyperglycemia, expect to give insulin or increase the dose the patient is already receiving. Monitor blood glucose levels as often as every hour, depending on the patient's condition.

Meticulous wound care is essential to control infection. Use strict aseptic technique to prevent further contamination. Typically, if the patient has dry gangrene, you'll need to keep the wound dry. If he has moist gangrene, you'll need to clean the wound. If the patient has gas gangrene, the wound should be opened, so that

air can enter and the wound can drain. The wound then is debrided and irrigated. If gangrene is massive, amputation may be necessary.

Monitor the wound closely for appearance, size, and drainage. Notify the physician if the wound worsens, drainage increases, or the odor changes. Also, monitor the patient's vital signs to help detect sepsis. ◀

To promote the patient's comfort, deodorize the room to control any foul odors. If appropriate, prepare him for surgical intervention and treatments, such as debridement. Remember, your patient is acutely ill and may be anxious about the prospect of losing a limb to amputation. A below-the-knee amputation may be necessary if arterial reconstruction is impossible or if the patient has a serious infection or intractable pain at rest. Help the patient adjust to the possibilities of amputation and prosthesis use.

Diabetes mellitus and wound infection

Wound infection commonly occurs in diabetic patients, sometimes with life-threatening results. In poorly controlled diabetes, wound healing is delayed because of protein catabolism, impaired nutritional status, and diminished peripheral circulation.

Pathophysiology

Compromised skin integrity makes a diabetic patient more susceptible to infection. In diabetes, glycosylated hemoglobin in the RBCs impedes the release of oxygen to the tissues. Elevated blood glucose levels also make some pathogens thrive and proliferate rapidly. Vascular changes decrease blood, oxygen, and nutrient supply to the tissues and affect the supply of WBCs in the area. Because the WBCs don't function properly, phagocytosis is defective.

Adapting nursing care

For a diabetic patient, care of a wound infection focuses on preventing complications, including further infection. Be prepared to perform aggressive and immediate debridement and excision of any necrotic tissue to prevent further infection. You'll also need to provide rapid fluid resuscitation to correct any fluid or electrolyte imbalance and insulin therapy to control blood glucose levels. Obtain blood and wound cultures and administer the prescribed broad-spectrum antibiotic I.V., possibly at a reduced dosage to avoid nephrotoxicity.

During antibiotic therapy, monitor the patient's renal status closely. Check serum creatinine, BUN, and creatinine clearance levels for changes indicating a deterioration in renal function. Also, monitor his vital signs for fever and decreased blood pressure, which may indicate bacteremia and septic shock. If septic shock goes untreated, multiple organ dysfunction may result.

Complications

A diabetic patient with a wound infection risks developing complications, such as DKA, delayed wound healing, and superinfection.

Diabetic ketoacidosis

An acute emergency, DKA requires rapid intervention. Without insulin, cells can't use glucose, and the body starts using fats instead of carbohydrates for energy. Glucose levels rise, and the fat metabolism produces excessive ketones as a by-product. These ketones make the body's pH acidic. Also, as the body tries to eliminate the excessive ketones, excessive urination and profound dehydration develop. Uncontrolled wound infection can trigger DKA because it increases the metabolic rate and results in hyperglycemia.

Confirming the complication

The signs and symptoms of DKA usually begin within 12 to 24 hours of insulin deficiency and may extend over several days. The patient may experience a decreased level of consciousness, weight loss, polyuria, polydipsia, and lethargy.

Associated findings include signs and symptoms of infection, such as fever, purulent drainage from the wound, tenderness, and localized erythema.

Because DKA causes excessive diuresis, your patient may show signs of dehydration, such as tachycardia, orthostatic hypotension, dry mucous membranes, and poor skin turgor. As the condition progresses, he may become confused, stuporous, and eventually comatose. The diuresis causes electrolyte imbalances, such as hypokalemia and hypomagnesemia. As DKA progresses, the patient develops Kussmaul's respirations with a fruity, acetone breath. His urine is positive for ketones. Typically, blood glucose levels range from 300 to 800 mg/dl. ABG measurements reveal metabolic acidosis.

Nursing interventions

RAPID RESPONSE ▶ Immediate care focuses on correcting fluid imbalance, controlling blood glucose levels, and preventing complications. Quickly evaluate the patient's hydration status. Assess his vital signs, weight, intake and output, urine specific gravity, and serum osmolality. Check skin turgor and mucous membranes.

Administer fluids to correct dehydration. During fluid replacement, watch for signs of fluid overload, such as pulmonary crackles, labored respirations, tachycardia, and dependent edema. Continue to monitor the patient's electrolyte levels for improvement. Also, monitor his ECG for changes that may indicate electrolyte imbalances.

If necessary, provide glucose control by administering I.V. insulin. Begin with an infusion of regular insulin in 0.9% normal saline solution, making sure to flush the tubing with about 50 ml of the insulin solution, so the tubing is saturated. Insulin binds to the plastic in the I.V. tubing, and if the flush isn't performed, the patient won't get the correct dose. Use a pump to regulate the infusion.

Monitor glucose levels hourly. When levels decrease to 250 to 300 mg/dl, anticipate switching the I.V. solution to 5% dextrose with 0.45% normal saline solution to prevent hypoglycemia. Continue to monitor the patient's blood glucose levels, and adjust the insulin dosage accordingly. After his condition stabilizes, switch to subcutaneous injections. ◀

Provide comfort measures. Moisten the patient's lips and mucous membranes and provide frequent oral care to alleviate thirst. Turn and position him every 2 hours to prevent skin breakdown, and avoid disturbing the wound.

Provide wound care, as ordered. Frequently check the I.V. insertion site for signs and symptoms of infiltration or infection, such as redness, swelling, and tenderness.

When your patient's condition permits, explain what occurred and why. Reinforce all aspects of his glucose control regimen, especially if it has changed because of his wound infection and the development of DKA. Explain the rationale for any changes and help him incorporate them into his self-care routine.

Delayed wound healing

Proper wound healing requires protein. But a diabetic patient with a wound infection may not have enough protein available to heal the wound in the normal time. In diabetes, a wound infection generates a hyperglycemic state, which increases the catabolism of protein for use as energy. Also, macrovascular and microvascular changes that occur in diabetes can interfere with circulation to the tissues, thus decreasing the amount of oxygen and nutrients available for tissue repair.

Confirming the complication

Typically, the patient will have a pale-colored wound that takes longer to heal than expected. He also may have signs and symptoms of infection, such as redness, warmth, and drainage.

Nursing interventions

Treat the wound infection with the prescribed antibiotic therapy. Closely monitor the patient's renal function for possible renal impairment from the combination of diabetic nephropathy and use of nephrotoxic antibiotics. Perform wound care, as prescribed, using strict aseptic technique.

Because infection increases the patient's insulin requirements, blood glucose control is essential to promote healing. Monitor blood glucose levels frequently, adjusting insulin dosages according to the results. If your patient has Type II diabetes, he may need insulin to maintain glycemic control until the infection heals, at which time he can resume oral therapy.

Before your patient is discharged from the hospital, teach him about all aspects of his self-care regimen. If he'll continue wound care at home, have him repeat your demonstration of the procedure. Enlist the aid of a family member, especially if your patient has diabetic neuropathy or retinopathy. Stress the importance of good hand washing to minimize the risk of additional infection. Also, review with the patient the signs and symptoms of infection. Advise him to check his temperature at least once a day and to notify the physician of a fever or a change in the wound. Refer the patient to a home care nurse for follow-up care and evaluation of wound healing.

Superinfection

In superinfection, the patient develops a second infection in the same wound or in another body area, but this time with a new organism. The new organism—*Staphylococcus aureus*, for example—is generally more virulent or drug resistant than the first. If the infection progresses, bacteremia may develop.

Often, antibiotics used to treat a bacterial infection destroy normal flora. This allows organisms, such as the yeast-like fungus *Candida albicans*, to proliferate and create a second infection in another body area, such as the mouth or vagina. Because antibiotics aren't effective against fungi, the yeast organisms continue to grow unchecked.

Confirming the complication

A diabetic patient with a superinfection typically shows signs of infection, such as fever, tenderness, swelling, and redness. A wound culture identifies the causative organism and confirms the diagnosis. A blood culture detects bacteremia.

Nursing interventions

Carefully monitor the use of antibiotics to avoid the development of drug-resistant organisms that may result from overuse. Be alert for signs of superinfection. If you note such signs, reculture the wound to identify any additional organism.

Be especially alert for yeast infections. Watch for signs of oral thrush and vaginal candidiasis. And administer antifungal agents, as prescribed.

Control the patient's exposure to possible sources of infection from visitors and staff members. Everyone should thoroughly wash his hands before and after contact with the patient, and any contaminated articles and equipment must be properly disposed of or disinfected. Minimize invasive procedures as much as possible to reduce the risk of exposure.

Help the patient to maintain good nutrition and personal hygiene. Work with the dietitian to plan a healthy diet with sufficient nutrients to combat infection, promote healing, and maintain glucose control. Reinforce the need for frequent monitoring of blood glucose levels and adjust the patient's therapy accordingly.

Review the appropriate aspects of drug therapy with the patient. Teach him appropriate measures to prevent infection. Also, teach him to recognize signs and symptoms of infection and to notify the physician immediately if any occur.

Suggested readings

Bressler P, Defronzo R. Drugs and diabetes. *Diabetes Rev.* 1994;2(1).

Cirone N. Unmasking a hidden disorder: diabetes in the elderly, part I. *Nursing.* March 1996;34-39.

Cirone N, Schwartz N. Finding the balance for drug therapy: diabetes in the elderly, part II. *Nursing.* March 1996;40-45.

Diabetes in America. 2nd ed. Bethesda, Md: National Institutes of Health, National Institute of Diabetes and Digestive and Kidney Diseases publication NIH 95-1468; 1995.

FAX STAT on drugs. *Facts and Comparisons.* Dec 20, 1996;Vm #5.

Fishman T, Freedline AD, Kahn D. Putting the best foot forward. *Nursing.* Jan 1996;58-60.

Haire-Joshu D. *Management of diabetes mellitus: perspectives of care across the life span.* 2nd ed. St Louis, Mo: Mosby–Year Book, Inc; 1996.

Huether SE, McCance KL. *Understanding pathophysiology.* St Louis, Mo: Mosby–Year Book, Inc; 1996.

Lewis S, Collier I, Heitkemper M. *Medical-surgical nursing: assessment and management of clinical problems.* 4th ed. St Louis, Mo: Mosby–Year Book, Inc; 1996.

McKenry LM, Salerno E. *Mosby's pharmacology in nursing.* 19th ed. St Louis, Mo: Mosby–Year Book, Inc; 1995.

Mosby's 1998 Nursing drug reference. St Louis, Mo: Mosby–Year Book, Inc; 1998.

Phipps WJ, Sands J, Lehman MK, Cassmeyer V. *Medical-surgical nursing: concepts and clinical practice.* 5th ed. St Louis, Mo: Mosby–Year Book, Inc; 1995.

Polaski AL, Tatro SE. *Luckmann's core principles and practice of medical-surgical nursing.* Philadelphia, Pa: WB Saunders Co; 1996.

Price SA, Wilson LM. *Pathophysiology: clinical concepts of disease processes.* 5th ed. St Louis, Mo: Mosby–Year Book, Inc; 1996.

Seidel HM, Dains JE, Ball JW, Benedict GW. *Mosby's guide to physical examination.* 3rd ed. St Louis, Mo: Mosby–Year Book, Inc; 1995.

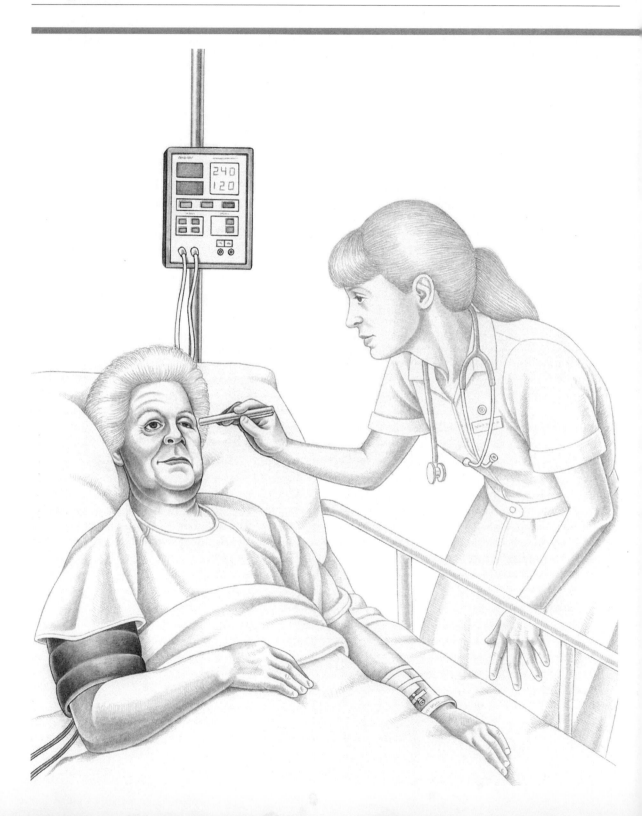

Hypertension

Called the silent killer by many health
care professionals, high blood pressure (hypertension) affects nearly 60 million people in the
United States—about one in four Americans. It
rarely causes telltale symptoms; in fact, up to
half of hypertensive people don't even know
they're in danger.

But they are in danger. Hypertension raises
the risk for and complicates a number of life-
threatening disorders, including aortic aneurysm, cerebrovascular disease, coronary artery
disease, and renal insufficiency.

As a nurse, you're responsible not only for understanding the far-reaching effects of hypertension but also for preventing them—and

ANATOMY REVIEW

Inside the arteries

Arteries are composed of several tissue layers adapted to accommodate blood flowing at high speeds and forceful pressures. Large elastic arteries, such as the aorta, have a thick layer of connective tissue that expands with each ventricular contraction (tunica adventitia). Smaller muscular arteries have a thick layer of smooth muscle that allows constriction and dilation (tunica media). The illustrations below highlight the major layers of typical arteries.

Elastic artery

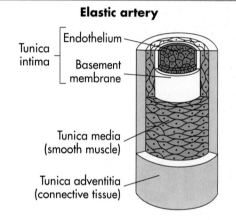

Tunica intima
- Endothelium
- Basement membrane

Tunica media (smooth muscle)

Tunica adventitia (connective tissue)

Muscular artery

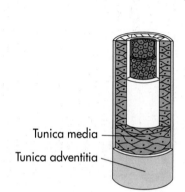

Tunica media

Tunica adventitia

---

teaching patients how to prevent them—whenever possible.

Anatomy and physiology review

Blood pressure is a term used to describe the force exerted by blood against the interior walls of the body's blood vessels. Accordingly, there are three categories of blood pressure that correspond to the three types of blood vessels: arterial, capillary, and venous.

Where hypertension is concerned, arterial pressure is the measurement to watch because it reaches the highest levels. As you know, arterial blood pressure is recorded as two numbers. One reflects the higher pressure exerted during ventricular contraction (systolic pressure) and the other reflects the lower pressure exerted during ventricular relaxation (diastolic pressure).

Arterial adaptations

Because of their relative proximity to blood flowing forcefully from the heart, arteries must withstand the highest pressures of all the body's blood vessels. Fortunately, their thick, muscular walls are adapted to withstand the added pounding (see *Inside the arteries*).

Arteries are classified as either elastic or muscular by their size, location, and relative amounts of elastic connective tissue and smooth-muscle fibers. Elastic arteries have a thick tunica media and more elastic fibers than smooth-muscle fibers, which allows them to stretch as blood pressure rises during systole. They recoil during diastole, helping to maintain diastolic pressure between ventricular contractions. Elastic arteries include the aorta and its major branches.

Muscular arteries include medium and small vessels that carry blood to the arterioles. These smaller vessels are farther away from the heart than the elastic arteries, and they contain a greater proportion of smooth-muscle fibers. Because of their smooth-muscle content, muscular arteries can be stimulated to contract and relax, resulting in vasoconstriction and vasodilation.

Arteries branch into arterioles, tiny vessels that regulate the flow of blood into capillaries. They contain primarily smooth muscle. They too can constrict and relax.

Understanding blood pressure regulation

The body requires a relatively constant blood pressure level to ensure adequate perfusion of its organs and tissues. To maintain that steady level, it must balance and react to a number of factors, including:
- the volume of blood in the circulatory system
- blood viscosity
- arterial elasticity
- stroke volume (the amount of blood ejected by the heart)
- heart rate
- peripheral vascular resistance.

Blood pressure varies with the volume of blood in the circulatory system. If blood volume increases, blood pressure increases, and vice versa.

The more viscous the blood, the more slowly it moves through arteries, especially narrow ones. This restricted flow causes increased blood pressure.

Normally, arterial elasticity absorbs some of the force of blood being ejected from the heart. If the arteries become more rigid, however, they can't distend as readily to absorb the force—and blood pressure rises.

The resistance of peripheral blood vessels can affect blood pressure in either direction. If the arterioles constrict, peripheral vascular resistance increases and impedes blood flow from the arterioles to capillaries. As a result, blood pressure rises. If the arterioles relax, peripheral vascular resistance decreases and blood flows more rapidly and easily through the capillaries. Thus, blood pressure falls.

The body employs several mechanisms—neural, hormonal, and physical—to influence these factors, thereby maintaining blood pressure at a relatively steady level and channeling adequate blood throughout the body.

Neural mechanisms

Specialized nerve endings in the walls of some arteries help to regulate blood pressure by sensing pressure and resistance inside the vessel, then transmitting that information to the brain. These specialized nerve endings are called baroreceptors and chemoreceptors.

Also known as stretch receptors, baroreceptors are embedded primarily in the walls of the internal carotid arteries and aortic arch. When increased blood pressure causes arterial walls to stretch, baroreceptors detect the lengthening of smooth-muscle fibers. They then discharge more rapidly, sending increased neural impulses to the medulla's cardiovascular control center by way of cranial nerve IX and the vagus nerve. The result? Increased parasympathetic activity and decreased sympathetic activity, which leads to peripheral vasodilation, a decreased heart rate, and decreased cardiac contractility. Arterial blood pressure decreases.

Conversely, when blood pressure decreases, baroreceptors detect the shortening of smooth-muscle fibers. Baroreceptors then trigger peripheral vasoconstriction, an increased heart rate, and increased contractility.

Remember, however, that baroreceptors function only in response to changes from the established pressure level. In a person with sustained high blood pressure, baroreceptors become accustomed to the higher level and lose their ability to reduce blood pressure back to a truly normal range.

Like baroreceptors, chemoreceptors are embedded in the walls of the carotid arteries and aorta. They're also found in the medullary area of the brain stem. Chemoreceptors are sensitive to oxygen and carbon dioxide concentrations and to the blood's pH. In response to low levels of oxygen and increased levels of carbon dioxide in the blood, they stimulate sympathetic activity and inhibit parasympathetic activity, increasing arterial pressure.

Hormonal mechanisms

Several hormones work in concert to help control blood pressure levels:
- epinephrine, secreted by the adrenal glands
- norepinephrine, secreted by the presynaptic nerve terminals
- renin, secreted by the juxtaglomerular cells of the kidneys

How renin raises blood pressure

When blood pressure drops excessively, the kidneys react to bring it back up. They do so by releasing an enzyme called renin, which accelerates the conversion of the plasma protein angiotensinogen to the hormone angiotensin I.

When blood containing angiotensin I reaches the lungs, angiotensin-converting enzyme in small lung vessels converts it to angiotensin II, a potent vasoconstrictor. Angiotensin II cues the kidneys to decrease the excretion of sodium and water. And it prompts the adrenal cortex to secrete aldosterone, which further decreases sodium and water excretion.

Vasoconstriction and increased fluid volume help to increase blood pressure. Increased blood pressure provides negative feedback to halt renin production, as shown in the flowchart below.

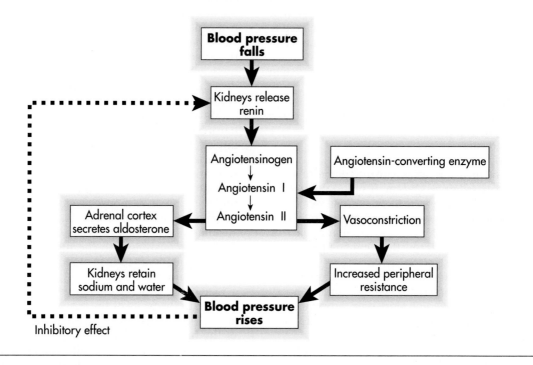

- antidiuretic hormone (ADH), secreted by the hypothalamus
- atrial natriuretic peptide (ANP), secreted by the right atrium
- prostaglandins, secreted by numerous body tissues.

Epinephrine and norepinephrine increase heart rate, blood pressure, automaticity, and contractility. They stimulate alpha and beta receptors in the sympathetic nervous system throughout the vasculature. Alpha stimulation causes vasoconstriction; beta stimulation causes vasodilation.

When blood pressure drops, the kidneys release an enzyme called renin, which begins a chain reaction designed to bring blood pressure back up (see *How renin raises blood pressure*). The multistep reaction results in vasoconstriction and decreased excretion of sodium and water, which work together to raise blood pressure.

Also in response to decreasing blood pressure, the hypothalamus secretes ADH. It acts on renal tubules to promote water retention, which increases plasma volume, peripheral resistance, and blood pressure.

Cells of the right atrium secrete ANP when right atrial pressure increases. ANP acts to inhibit ADH by increasing the amount of sodium lost in urine. As a result, the body excretes a large volume of dilute urine, thus decreasing blood volume and, consequently, blood pressure.

Several prostaglandins are involved in blood pressure regulation as well. In general, prostaglandins A and E dilate arteries and veins. Prostaglandin F constricts veins.

Physical mechanisms

Blood vessels can constrict and dilate temporarily in response to short-term changes in blood pressure, which provides a physical mechanism for regulating blood pressure. Fluid also shifts in and out of capillaries to compensate for changes in blood pressure. When arterial pressure rises sharply, for example, capillary hydrostatic pressure increases, causing fluid to shift into the interstitial space. Thus, the volume of circulating fluid declines and blood pressure drops. The reverse is also true.

Pathophysiology

Hypertension occurs in two main forms: primary and secondary. Although they each produce similar long-term damage, they differ in that secondary hypertension can be attributed to an identifiable underlying disorder. A less common form of the disease, malignant hypertension is a severe, rapidly progressing disorder that quickly leads to death if left untreated.

Primary hypertension

Commonly known as essential hypertension, primary hypertension has no specific, identifiable cause. About 95% of hypertensive patients have this form of the disorder. Although the cause isn't known, certain risk factors are known.

For example, under age 55, the incidence of hypertension is higher in men than in women. African-Americans tend to develop more significant hypertension, and at an earlier age, than whites. Hypertension also crops up more commonly among lower-income, less-educated people. A host of other physiologic and psychosocial factors influence its development as well.

Psychosocial influences

Anything that enhances vasoconstriction and peripheral vascular resistance can influence the development of primary hypertension or worsen an existing condition. Such lifestyle factors include:
- excessive alcohol consumption
- stress and emotional upset
- tobacco use
- overstimulation with caffeine and other stimulant drugs
- obesity.

Genetic makeup

Genetic makeup also seems to play a prominent role in primary hypertension. Abnormal intracellular sodium concentration is one likely genetic factor. A child who inherits this abnormality will likely have increased intracellular calcium as well. Increased calcium, in turn, contributes to increased vascular tone, which can lead to hypertension.

Decreased sodium excretion is another probable genetic factor, possibly caused by impaired ANP secretion. Decreased sodium excretion leads to increased vascular volume, thus increasing blood pressure. ANP also has direct vasodilatory properties.

Whether a person has a genetic defect in sodium transport, sodium excretion, or both, experts speculate that the result is the same. If the patient consumes too much salt, the underlying genetic problem could accelerate the development of hypertension.

Role of insulin

Insulin affects blood pressure in several ways, all of which may influence the development or degree of hypertension. For starters, insulin promotes renal sodium resorption. Hyperinsulinemia (a hallmark of insulin resistance) may increase extracellular volume and impair sodium excretion. Although insulin resistance and hyperinsulinemia typically are associated with obesity, they also show up in hypertensive patients who aren't obese. Insulin also may increase vascular smooth-muscle tone by directly affecting the exchange of sodium and hydrogen in tissues.

In addition, insulin has significant effects on the sympathetic nervous system. Specifically, it spurs the release of epinephrine from the adrenal medulla and norepinephrine from pre-synaptic nerve terminals. As a result, cardiac output increases (mediated mainly by epineph-rine) and vascular resistance increases (medi-ated mainly by norepinephrine). In fact, insulin may well be the chief factor responsible for sympathetic nervous system activation after food ingestion.

Renin-angiotensin connection

A defective renin-angiotensin-aldosterone sys-tem may be one of the main mechanisms by which hypertension develops. It also may ac-count for why many hypertensive patients have normal or increased renin levels.

But up to a third of people with primary hy-pertension, especially elderly and African-American people, have low renin levels. These people probably don't have a renin-angiotensin defect. Instead, their hypertension may result from a reduced number of nephrons in the kid-neys' filtration surface. Fewer nephrons means the kidneys can't excrete as much sodium, and the resulting increase in sodium leads to ex-cess volume, which results in hypertension.

Because angiotensin II acts as a growth factor in vascular smooth muscle, it too may influence the development of hypertension. Increased lev-els produce structural hypertrophy in the ves-sels, which may create or enhance peripheral resistance that contributes to hypertension. Once hypertension develops, it tends to con-tinue even if levels of angiotensin II decline.

Secondary hypertension

Secondary hypertension results from one of sev-eral specific conditions, including renal paren-chymal disease, aldosteronism, pheochromocy-toma, renal stenosis, and Cushing's syndrome.

Renal parenchymal disease

The most common cause of secondary hyper-tension, renal parenchymal disease develops in patients who have diabetic nephropathy, hy-pertensive nephrosclerosis, polycystic kidney disease, chronic pyelonephritis, or one of many other acute renal diseases, including glo-merulonephritis and oliguric renal failure. If the patient has renal parenchymal disease but no renal insufficiency, hypertension develops through activation of the renin-angiotensin-aldosterone system. If the patient has renal in-sufficiency, defective sodium excretion leads to excess volume, which raises blood pressure.

Aldosteronism

Aldosterone is a type of hormone (a mineralo-corticoid) produced by the zona glomerulosa of the adrenal gland. In excess, aldosterone causes the body to retain sodium, thus increasing vol-ume and creating or worsening hypertension.

Excess aldosterone may result from primary or secondary aldosteronism. In primary aldos-teronism, excess hormone stems either from a solitary adrenocortical adenoma or from bilat-eral hyperplasia of the zona glomerulosa. Secondary aldosteronism results from in-creased renin activity, typically from nephrotic syndrome, cirrhosis, idiopathic edema, heart failure, trauma, burns, or other types of stress.

Aldosterone-related hypertension also may result from excessive use of substances that contain glycyrrhetenic acid, a mineralocorti-coid. They include chewing tobacco, certain liquors, and licorice candy.

Pheochromocytoma

A rare neoplasm of the adrenal medulla, pheo-chromocytoma causes excess production of norepinephrine and epinephrine in a sympa-thetic ganglion. The result is increased cardiac output, vasoconstriction, and hypertension.

Renal stenosis

Renovascular hypertension results when ische-mia reduces glomerular perfusion pressure and activates the renin-angiotensin-aldosterone system. Atherosclerosis is the most common cause of renal ischemia, followed by fibro-muscular dysplasia, blockage by an embolus, and compression of an artery by a nearby tumor.

Cushing's syndrome

Cushing's syndrome results either from excess cortisol production by the adrenal cortex or from prolonged treatment with glucocorticoids. Either way, blood pressure rises from sodium retention and volume expansion.

What's more, glucocorticoids cause patients to gain weight in abdominal subcutaneous and visceral tissues, resulting in abnormalities of free fatty acid metabolism and possibly contributing to insulin resistance and hyperinsulinemia.

Glucocorticoids also enhance blood vessel reactivity to pressor substances, such as norepinephrine, which increases vascular tone.

Effects of long-standing hypertension

Early in its course, hypertension produces no obvious changes in blood vessels or organs. Over time, however, widespread damage surfaces in large and small blood vessels, especially those in the eyes, heart, kidney, and brain. Accordingly, common results of uncontrolled hypertension include failing vision, coronary artery occlusion, renal failure, and cerebrovascular accident (CVA).

In long-standing hypertension, large vessels become sclerosed and tortuous. Lumens narrow, decreasing or perhaps blocking blood flow to the organs and limbs. Small vessels sustain damage to the intimal layer, causing fibrin to accumulate and local edema to form. Intravascular clotting may develop, also reducing blood supply to the tissues and organs.

Meanwhile, the heart must contract more vigorously to force blood through the narrowed arterioles and maintain cardiac output. Over time, this increased demand leads to left ventricular hypertrophy, which can then lead to coronary insufficiency, myocardial ischemia, and infarction. If the left ventricle can't sustain sufficient cardiac output, the left and possibly the right ventricle may fail, reducing blood flow to the kidneys and decreasing renal perfusion. Kidney failure further aggravates hypertension.

Damage to the arteries' intimal lining, coupled with the increased pressure of cardiac contractions, can cause the vessel walls to weaken and possibly to rupture.

Assessment findings

Normally, the body's compensatory mechanisms restrict blood pressure to a fairly narrow range, in the vicinity of 120/80 mm Hg. However,

Classifying your patient's hypertension

Use this table to categorize your patient's arterial blood pressure. If a patient's systolic and diastolic pressures are in different categories, assign the higher one. If systolic pressure is 140 or above and diastolic pressure is 90 or below, document the patient's condition as isolated systolic hypertension and assign it the appropriate stage based on the systolic pressure.

This table is based on the Fifth Report of the Joint National Committee on Detection, Evaluation, and Treatment of High Blood Pressure from the National Institutes of Health.

Category	Systolic pressure (mm Hg)	Diastolic pressure (mm Hg)
Normal blood pressure	<130	<85
High normal blood pressure	130–139	85–89
Stage 1 (mild) hypertension	140–159	90–99
Stage 2 (moderate) hypertension	160–179	100–109
Stage 3 (severe) hypertension	180–209	110–119
Stage 4 (very severe) hypertension	≥210	≥120

blood pressure varies from person to person. It also varies normally throughout the day, with the highest pressures in the morning and the lowest in the evening. Blood pressure also varies in response to meals and exercise.

Consequently, an isolated above-normal blood pressure reading doesn't mean your patient has hypertension. By definition, your adult patient has hypertension if you obtain resting readings on three separate occasions of 140/90 mm Hg or above—160/95 mm Hg or above in a person age 50 or older (see *Classifying your patient's hypertension*).

Keep in mind that some patients become overly anxious in a medical office and may appear to be hypertensive when, in all other settings, they aren't. Blood pressure that rises only during medical visits is called white-coat hypertension. If a patient with mild or moderate hypertension appears anxious in the office, you may want to consider having additional blood pressure readings taken in other locations, especially at the patient's home. Doing so may give you a more accurate picture of your patient's typical pressure. Performing a careful health history will complete the picture by giving you a good idea of the patient's risk profile.

Health history

Unless your patient has severe or long-standing hypertension, she'll probably have few or no symptoms of the problem. Even if your patient does have symptoms, they may not be pronounced or consistent enough for her to think them worth mentioning. That's why so many cases of hypertension surface during screening tests, routine check-ups, and treatments for other disorders. And that's why a detailed history is so important. It can help you not only uncover risk factors for hypertension but also catalog the patient's current condition and plan measures to counteract the effects of increased pressure.

During the health history interview, be sure to investigate your patient's family history. Hypertension, heart disease, hyperlipidemia, and diabetes mellitus in the family history are all associated with hypertension. Also, ask about medication use. Use of such medications as diet pills, decongestants, cold remedies, and especially oral contraceptives and corticosteroids have been linked to hypertension.

Note personal and lifestyle characteristics that could raise the patient's risk of hypertension, and ask the patient about possible contributing factors. A review of the patient's personal habits may reveal a diet high in salt, caffeine, and fat. Remember, obesity is associated with primary hypertension, and a recent unintentional weight loss may be linked to pheochromocytoma. Use of alcohol, tobacco, and recreational drugs (especially cocaine) are associated with elevated blood pressure.

Ask the patient if she's experiencing any of these signs and symptoms: chest pain, palpitations, difficulty breathing, light-headedness, unsteadiness, headache, blurred vision, flushing, sweating, nighttime urination, or frequent urination. All may result from the effects of hypertension on the patient's organ systems. Also, note if the patient has or has ever had a myocardial infarction (MI), heart failure, hyperlipidemia, hypothyroidism, diabetes, pyelonephritis, eclampsia, a transient ischemic attack (TIA), asthma, or emotional stress. Ask if she's ever been treated for hypertension.

During your initial evaluation, also watch for certain groups of symptoms that could point to possible causes of secondary hypertension. For example, if your patient reports episodes of chest pain, palpitations, headache, sweating, and light-headedness, she could have pheochromocytoma. If she complains of frequent urination, awakening at night to urinate, and muscle weakness, she may have primary aldosteronism. Hyperactivity of the sympathetic nervous system may appear as dilated pupils, excessive sweating, and a rapid pulse.

Physical examination

The most important aspect of examining a potentially hypertensive patient is obtaining the most accurate blood pressure readings possible. If the patient's arm is relatively large, use a larger-than-normal cuff to avoid falsely elevated readings. If you suspect hypertension, measure the pressure in both arms, with the patient in both the supine and upright positions. If your first reading indicates possible hypertension, you'll need to confirm the increased level with at least two more readings at later times.

During your examination, pay attention to possible warning signs of hypertension or related conditions. For example, blood pressure readings above 200/120 mm Hg may suggest that the patient has pheochromocytoma, primary aldosteronism, or renal artery stenosis. Orthostatic hypotension (pressure that drops 10 mm Hg or more when the patient rises) is common in patients with pheochromocytoma, a condition in which hypertension may be either sustained or intermittent. An abdominal or flank bruit may warn of possible renal artery stenosis, aortic coarctation, or aneurysm. Unequal pressures between arms may suggest coarctation of the aorta. Palpable, enlarged kidneys may reflect a renal basis for hypertension. And truncal obesity and purple striae are associated with Cushing's syndrome.

To obtain information about the duration and severity of hypertension, you can examine the fundus of the patient's eye with an ophthalmoscope. Moderately severe to severe hypertension may be evident as narrowed retinal arteries, retinal hemorrhage, retinal exudates, and papilledema. Patients with these changes may complain of vision problems.

Careful cardiopulmonary examination may reveal the effects of hypertension on the patient's heart. For example, if you detect a lift or heave, or if the point of maximal impulse is displaced laterally, the patient may have left ventricular hypertrophy. If you hear an S_3 or S_4 heart sound or if you find an increased heart rate, the patient could be developing heart failure, especially if she also has pedal edema. Listen for crackles and wheezes because pulmonary congestion is also associated with heart failure.

Diagnostic tests

Diagnostic testing aims to define possible predisposing factors, possible causes of hypertension, and the presence and extent of related organ damage.

Routine tests

Routine tests for your patient may include blood chemistries, such as sodium and potassium levels; blood glucose, calcium, uric acid, blood urea nitrogen (BUN), creatinine, and cholesterol level measurements; a complete blood count (CBC); microscopic examination of urine; a chest X-ray; and an electrocardiogram (ECG). Results of these tests can give clues to possible causes of the hypertension and the presence of organ damage (see *Finding the cause of hypertension*, page 60).

Hypokalemia suggests aldosteronism, renal artery stenosis, or Cushing's syndrome. High serum sodium values suggest aldosteronism and high renin states. Elevated serum glucose may be related to Cushing's syndrome or pheochromocytoma. Hypercalcemia may suggest primary hyperparathyroidism, which may be associated with primary hypertension or multiple endocrine neoplasia, a group of syndromes in which Cushing's syndrome or pheochromocytoma can occur. Hyperuricemia may indicate renal impairment, a possible result of untreated primary hypertension. Elevated BUN and creatinine levels confirm renal insufficiency. Hyperlipidemia increases the risk of atherosclerotic and cardiovascular complications. Anemia commonly accompanies renal insufficiency. Polycythemia may reveal hemoconcentration in a patient with pheochromocytoma. And urinalysis may reveal glycosuria, proteinuria, or microscopic evidence of such chronic renal diseases as pyelonephritis or glomerulonephritis.

The chest X-ray can provide a clue to aortic coarctation by showing either the coarctation itself or rib notching. It also may reveal the cardiomegaly that commonly indicates left ventricular hypertrophy. Characteristic ECG changes indicate left ventricular hypertrophy or dilation. Evidence of hypokalemia or hypercalcemia also appears on the ECG.

Further tests

Typically, hypertensive patients undergo additional testing if their moderate or severe hypertension doesn't respond to antihypertensive medications. Also, certain unusual circumstances may warrant more extensive testing. For example, significant hypertension in a person under age 30 may result from a curable cause. Likewise, a patient with a flank bruit or hypokalemia may have an underlying cause.

Any patient with a strong possibility of secondary hypertension probably will undergo some special tests, commonly starting with 24-hour urine collection. For example, measuring free cortisol levels can rule out endogenous Cushing's syndrome. Comparing urine potassium levels with serum potassium levels, especially in response to a salt load, can confirm aldosteronism. Checking aldosterone excretion

Finding the cause of hypertension

Diagnostic testing can provide clues to conditions that may be contributing to a patient's hypertension. Below are some of the tests the physician may order for your patient.

Diagnostic test	Abnormal findings	Possible causes
Serum sodium measurement	>145 mEq/L	• Renal artery stenosis • Aldosteronism
Serum potassium measurement	<3.5 mEq/L	• Aldosteronism • Renal artery stenosis • Cushing's syndrome
Uric acid measurement	>7.8 mg/dL	• Essential hypertension • Gout
Hemoglobin measurement	<11.0 or >15.0 g/dL (women) <13.0 or >17.0 g/dL (men)	• Renal insufficiency (low value) • Pheochromocytoma (high value)
Hematocrit measurement	<33% or >46% (women) <40% or >50% (men)	• Renal insufficiency (low value) • Pheochromocytoma (high value)
Fasting blood glucose measurement	>100 mg/dL	• Cushing's syndrome • Pheochromocytoma
Blood urea nitrogen measurement	>20 mg/dL	• Renal insufficiency
Creatinine measurement	>1.2 mg/dL	• Renal insufficiency
Blood calcium measurement	>10.5 mg/dL	• Primary hyperparathyroidism
Chest X-ray	• Cardiomegaly • Rib notching	• Aortic coarctation

during salt loading can confirm primary aldosteronism. Measuring metanephrines or fractionated catecholamines can rule out pheochromocytoma.

If biochemical tests confirm primary aldosteronism or pheochromocytoma, the patient most likely will undergo computed tomography (CT) scanning of the adrenal glands to localize the tumor. About 70% of patients with primary aldosteronism have a single adrenal adenoma. About 90% of pheochromocytomas are located in the adrenal glands. If CT scanning fails to identify the adrenal pheochromocytoma, the physician may order whole-body ^{131}I metaiodobenzylguanidine scintiscanning.

Screening for renal artery stenosis may involve an I.V. pyelogram, a renal scan with technetium-99m diethylenetriamine pentaacetic acid (alone or with the angiotensin-converting enzyme inhibitor captopril), or ultrasonography.

Medical interventions

Interventions appropriate for the hypertensive patient depend on the severity of the condition and should reflect accepted follow-up guidelines (see *Follow-up care for hypertensive patients*).

For most hypertensive patients, interventions involve lifestyle changes, antihypertensive medications, or both. For many, lifestyle changes alone can restore normal blood pressure. If not, the physician may begin prescribing medications according to the step-care approach recommended by the Joint National Committee on Detection, Evaluation, and Treatment of High Blood Pressure from the National Institutes of Health (see *Step-care approach*, page 62).

For patients with primary hypertension, treatment aims to reach and maintain an arterial blood pressure below 140/90 mm Hg. For patients with secondary hypertension, treatment aims to control or correct the underlying disease, reduce blood pressure quickly and safely, and minimize hypertension's long-term effects.

Lifestyle modifications

Modifications that help reduce blood pressure include controlling or reducing weight, moderating intake of alcohol and dietary stimulants, participating in regular exercise, reducing sodium intake, and staying away from tobacco products.

Controlling or reducing body weight helps to normalize blood pressure by decreasing the strain on the left ventricle, thus slowing or preventing hypertrophy. Reducing body weight also lowers levels of fats and lipids circulating in the bloodstream. Consequently, fewer fats and lipids adhere to the inner walls of blood vessels and, over time, the vessels sustain less damage than they would have if the patient remained overweight. For most patients, the best way to reduce body weight is by learning to select low-fat foods, avoiding high-fat snacks, reducing daily calorie intake, and avoiding fad and crash diets that reduce weight only temporarily. Decreased alcohol and sodium consumption also help to reduce weight.

By constricting peripheral blood vessels, caffeine and nicotine decrease blood flow and increase heart rate and blood pressure. That's why hypertensive patients should avoid all products containing caffeine or nicotine.

Exercise offers another effective lifestyle modification to the hypertensive patient. Regular, moderate exercise (such as walking or swimming) helps control blood pressure by

---

Follow-up care for hypertensive patients

These guidelines list appropriate follow-up actions for patients with hypertension. The guidelines are based on the Fifth Report of the Joint National Committee on Detection, Evaluation, and Treatment of High Blood Pressure from the National Institutes of Health.

Category	Follow-up action
Normal blood pressure	Recheck blood pressure in 2 years.
High normal blood pressure	Recheck blood pressure in 1 year.
Stage 1 hypertension	Confirm hypertension within 2 months.
Stage 2 hypertension	Evaluate patient or refer for care within 1 month.
Stage 3 hypertension	Evaluate patient or refer for care within 1 week.
Stage 4 hypertension	Evaluate patient or refer for care immediately.

---

promoting blood flow, increasing oxygen consumption, and strengthening cardiac muscle so the heart can beat at a slower rate. In the meantime, it also reduces stress and appetite levels. Most patients achieve the best results by starting slowly and then gradually increasing the exercise intensity as tolerance develops.

In addition to lifestyle modifications, relaxation techniques may help reduce blood pressure, especially in patients who have excessive sympathetic activity. Meditation, yoga, and biofeedback all have the potential to reduce blood pressure.

Drug therapy

If lifestyle modifications alone fail to bring blood pressure within normal limits, the physician

Step-care approach

This table shows the steps recommended by the National Institutes of Health for treating hypertension. If following the guidelines presented in step 1 doesn't bring the patient's blood pressure down adequately, then a physician will move to step 2. If the first attempt at medication doesn't reduce blood pressure enough, the patient will have to move on to step 3, and finally, if necessary, to step 4.

Step	Treatment action
Step 1	• Modify lifestyle: control weight, reduce alcohol consumption, exercise regularly, reduce sodium consumption, and avoid tobacco.
Step 2	• Continue lifestyle modifications. • Begin taking an antihypertensive, usually a diuretic or beta blocker.
Step 3	• Continue lifestyle modifications. • Increase dose of current drug OR Substitute another drug OR Add a second drug from a different class.
Step 4	• Continue lifestyle modifications. • Add a second or third drug or a diuretic, if not already prescribed.

may prescribe one or more antihypertensive drugs. A wide variety of drugs can be used to control hypertension, including diuretics, beta blockers, angiotensin-converting enzyme (ACE) inhibitors, angiotensin II inhibitors, calcium channel blockers, alpha antagonists, and vasodilators (see *Classes of antihypertensive drugs*).

According to the step-care approach, a physician prescribes drugs one at a time. A combination of potent drugs with differing mechanisms of action makes for an effective treatment approach as long as dosages are titrated carefully and the patient is assessed regularly for adverse effects.

Diuretics

Diuretics are recommended for first-line therapy in treating hypertension. In general, diuretics are safe and inexpensive, especially when used in doses low enough to avoid potential problems for patients with diabetes, cardiac abnormalities, or lipid abnormalities.

Thiazide diuretics are especially beneficial in African-American patients and elderly patients. Loop diuretics (such as furosemide and bumetanide) are a good choice for patients with compromised renal function. And potassium-sparing diuretics are commonly given to patients susceptible to hypokalemia.

Beta blockers

Beta blockers provide another mainstay of hypertension therapy. They've proven particularly beneficial in white patients under age 40. Beta blockers also tend to work well in patients who have angina, in patients recovering from MI, and in patients with anxiety or resting tachycardia.

Beta blockers should be given cautiously to patients with diabetes because these drugs adversely affect insulin action and triglyceride metabolism. They also may mask the signs and symptoms of hypoglycemia and prolong recovery from a hypolgycemic episode. Beta blockers are contraindicated for patients who have asthma, heart block, impotence, or depression, although beta$_2$ blockers may be used cautiously in these patients.

ACE inhibitors

ACE inhibitors, such as captopril and enalapril, have several benefits. Patients with heart failure who use these drugs have lower mortality rates. Also, left ventricular function improves. Arterial compliance increases as well. These drugs have a neutral or beneficial effect on lipid levels and insulin sensitivity. And they have anti-ischemic and antiarrhythmic effects.

Angiotensin II inhibitors

A newer class of drugs, angiotensin II inhibitors interfere with the binding of angiotensin II to specific receptor sites in the vascular smooth muscle and adrenal glands. This action stops angiotensin II from triggering vasoconstriction

Classes of antihypertensive drugs

This table highlights major antihypertensive drug classes, their mechanisms of action, and some commonly prescribed examples.

Drug class	Actions	Selected examples
Thiazide and thiazide-like diuretics	• Block sodium reabsorption in the tubules • Increase water and sodium excretion, thereby decreasing blood volume	• chlorothiazide • chlorthalidone • hydrochlorothiazide • metolazone
Loop diuretics	• Block sodium reabsorption in the tubule • Promote rapid diuresis	• bumetamide • furosemide
Potassium-sparing diuretics	• Inhibit aldosterone • Cause sodium rather than potassium to be excreted in urine	• spironolactone • triamterene
Beta blockers	• Block beta receptors in sympathetic nervous system, causing decreased heart rate and blood pressure	• atenolol • metoprolol • nadolol • pindolol • propranolol
Angiotensin-converting enzyme inhibitors	• Inhibit conversion of angiotensin I to angiotensin II, ultimately blocking aldosterone release	• captopril • enalapril • lisinopril
Angiotensin II inhibitors	• Block binding of angiotensin II, preventing renin-angiotensin-aldosterone system from causing vasoconstriction and stopping aldosterone release	• losartan
Calcium channel blockers	• Inhibit movement of calcium into cells • Reduce spasms and promote vasodilation	• nifedipine • verapamil
Peripherally acting adrenergic blockers	• Deplete catecholamines in peripheral sympathetic fibers • Block release of norepinephrine	• guanethidine • reserpine
Centrally acting alpha agonists	• Activate central receptors, suppressing vasomotor and cardiac centers • Decrease peripheral vascular resistance	• clonidine • guanfacine • methyldopa
Alpha$_1$ blockers	• Block synaptic receptors, causing vasodilation	• prazosin • terazosin
Combined alpha and beta blockers	• Block beta receptors of sympathetic nervous system, decreasing heart rate and blood pressure	• labetalol
Vasodilators	• Directly relax vascular smooth muscle	• hydralazine • minoxidil

and the release of aldosterone. As a result, blood pressure decreases. Angiotensin II inhibitors seem to be at least as effective as ACE inhibitors and better tolerated by some patients.

Calcium channel blockers

Calcium channel blockers, such as nifedipine, produce cardiac effects similar to those produced by ACE inhibitors. These drugs are beneficial in elderly and African-American patients.

Alpha agonists and blockers

Alpha agonists and blockers interact with central or peripheral alpha receptors. Clonidine, for example, is a central alpha agonist that also acts on presynaptic alpha receptors to inhibit the release of norepinephrine. It can produce a dry mouth and sedation. It also may result in fluid retention, which requires the patient to take a diuretic as well.

Prazosin, terazosin, and doxazosin are peripheral alpha blockers that reduce peripheral vascular resistance. They may help patients who have trouble taking other drugs, such as patients unable to take beta blockers because of asthma. Alpha blockers have a neutral or positive effect on lipid levels and may improve insulin sensitivity. These drugs may cause fatigue and orthostatic hypotension.

Vasodilators

Vasodilators, such as hydralazine and minoxidil, act directly on vascular smooth muscle to dilate the vessel and thus lower blood pressure. Side effects include light-headedness, headache, and tachycardia.

Nursing interventions

Because hypertension causes few symptoms and the treatment regimen may be unpleasant or costly, many patients don't comply with it. Therefore, you may need to encourage your hypertensive patient to comply with her regimen and help her manage it successfully. You also may play the leading role in coordinating the patient's care team, which commonly includes a physician, a pharmacist, and a dietitian.

Emphasize to the patient with mild or moderate hypertension that, even though she feels no symptoms, her hypertension is serious and has the potential to cause real, possibly life-threatening, problems later on. Urge her to adopt sound nutritional principles, make important lifestyle adjustments, begin an exercise program, and follow her medication regimen as meticulously as possible. Through detailed teaching and assistance, you can help your patient do just that.

Improving nutrition

Urge your hypertensive patient to restrict her dietary sodium intake to 2 grams per day. One way to drop sodium intake dramatically is to avoid processed or fast foods and replace them with fresh, natural foods. This change can be especially challenging if the patient eats out routinely. In fact, she may need special help from a dietitian to learn how to make healthy selections from restaurant menus.

Also, discourage your patient from adding salt to food while cooking. Reassure her that, although unsalted foods may taste bland initially, the body becomes accustomed to the change, and taste perception typically improves over time. If it doesn't, suggest that she try a non-sodium substitute. Recommend only sparing use of half-potassium, half-sodium salt substitutes because the added potassium can create problems for patients at risk for heart failure.

Encourage your patient to limit her intake of calories from dietary fat to no more than 30% of total calories. This step alone may help her lose weight, even if she doesn't try to consume less food. Teach the patient to eat high-fat foods (such as meats, cheeses, nuts, and fried foods) only occasionally. Snack foods are a major hidden source of fat, so take special care to help your patient make low-fat selections, such as fresh fruits and vegetables. Many low-fat and fat-free snack options now appear on grocery store shelves, but remind the patient to check serving sizes carefully on the label.

Modifying lifestyle

Explain to your patient that she must be willing to drop harmful behaviors and adopt healthy ones that she can follow for the rest of her life. For most people, regular exercise tops the list.

The ideal exercise program to control weight and reduce hypertension includes 20 to 30 minutes of continuous aerobic activity nearly every day of the week. But rather than urging your patient to make a dramatic change, encourage her to make a steady, gradual change from getting no exercise to getting moderate exercise 3 to 4 times a week. Warn her to avoid exercises that raise her blood pressure without yielding an aerobic benefit—weight lifting, for example.

Both alcohol and nicotine raise blood pressure. If your patient drinks or smokes, explain the effect on her blood pressure and encourage her to stop. As appropriate, help your patient devise a plan to stop drinking or smoking.

Taking medications

Clearly, your patient carries the responsibility for taking her medications correctly. But you can do much to help her succeed. First, be sure you know which drugs she's taking and at which dosages. Discuss the patient's medications with her to be sure she knows as well.

Also, be sure the patient knows how to take her medications in relation to meals. For example, ACE inhibitors should be taken on an empty stomach, 1 hour before or 2 hours after meals, to ensure proper absorption. If the patient takes a diuretic and complains of stomach upset, tell her that she can take the medication with food.

Antihypertensive drugs tend to cause orthostatic hypotension, especially when given in combination. You'll need to monitor your patient's blood pressure frequently. Check it while she's lying down, sitting, and standing up. Note any decrease in pressure after she changes position. Also, note any complaints of dizziness or light-headedness. If she develops orthostatic hypotension, take steps to protect her from injury. And encourage her to avoid sudden position changes and to sit at the edge of the bed before standing up.

If your patient takes a diuretic, monitor her carefully because it may cause fluid and electrolyte problems. Loop and thiazide diuretics can lead to hypokalemia. Potassium-sparing diuretics can lead to hyperkalemia. These changes in electrolyte levels can predispose the patient to further problems, especially if she has other underlying conditions, such as heart disease. Also, assess your patient's hydration status by tracking her intake and output and recording her weight daily. Check her skin turgor and mucous membranes for signs of fluid volume deficit. Keep in mind that, although reduced fluid volume helps decrease blood pressure, if fluid volume declines too much, cardiac output becomes impaired, leading to further problems with tissue perfusion.

Note any factors that may interfere with the patient's ability or willingness to comply with drug therapy. Discuss these factors with her, and stress the need to take medications exactly as prescribed. Help the patient design a dosing schedule that she can remember and that works for her. For example, if she takes a diuretic twice daily, suggest that she take the second dose late in the afternoon to minimize the need to urinate at night.

Patient teaching

Unfortunately, many hypertensive patients receive little or no education about their disease and the importance of proper treatment. As a result, a large proportion of these patients fail to bring their blood pressure into the normal range. Many stop taking their medications and fail to appear for follow-up appointments. Through increased patient and family involvement, you can help to reverse this trend.

The lifestyle changes required to control hypertension affect not just the patient but her entire family. That's why you should involve the whole family in the patient's treatment regimen. Make sure family members know that uncontrolled hypertension increases the risk of heart disease, kidney disease, vision problems, and CVA.

During follow-up visits, ask the patient whether she has any problems with her medications. If so, involve the physician in helping her switch to a more acceptable alternative.

For many hypertensive patients, home blood-pressure monitoring provides a means of tracking the success of therapy. It also involves the patient in managing her disease and gives you an opportunity to evaluate the patient's blood pressure in her normal daily environment.

If you think your patient can benefit from home blood-pressure monitoring, explain its purpose and procedures to her. Provide information about home blood-pressure monitors, and help the patient select a reliable one. In general, an aneroid sphygmomanometer with a stethoscope attached to a microphone beneath the cuff provides the most reliable option.

After the patient has purchased her monitor, teach her to use it and then ask her to try it, so you can watch. Agree on a monitoring schedule and urge the patient to record her measurements and bring her records to all follow-up appointments.

Hypertension and aortic aneurysm

An aortic aneurysm is an abnormal outpouching of the aorta. Most result from atherosclerosis, hypertension, or both. Especially in patients with hypertension, an aortic aneurysm raises the risk of vascular rupture, a potentially life-threatening event.

Pathophysiology

Aortic aneurysms come in several types, all of which result from a weakness in the aorta's medial layer (see *Types of aneurysms*). This layer contains collagen, elastin, and vascular smooth muscle, which provide strength, elasticity, and tone. When a weakness develops in the vessel wall, the wall dilates gradually. As it does, tension increases. The wall becomes progressively thinner and weaker, more unstable, and more apt to rupture. By increasing arterial pressure, hypertension increases stress on the aortic wall, raises the risk of aneurysm, and accelerates the dilation process after an aneurysm develops.

Adapting nursing care

Nursing care for a hypertensive patient at risk for an aortic aneurysm focuses on reducing the risk by controlling blood pressure levels. It also involves maintaining a keen sensitivity to subtle signs and symptoms that could point to a possible aortic aneurysm. And it involves adaptations designed to reduce the risk of a rupture and maximize the success of surgical repair.

Aortic aneurysms typically produce no symptoms. When they do, the symptoms usually relate to how large the aneurysm is, where it is, and whether it's exerting pressure on nearby anatomic structures. If your hypertensive patient becomes hoarse for no apparent reason, an aneurysm on the aortic arch may be pressing on her larynx. If she has trouble swallowing, it may be pressing on her esophagus. If you palpate just above the suprasternal notch, you may be able to feel an aneurysm on the aortic arch.

If a hypertensive patient develops a cough, dyspnea, wheezing, stridor, or recurrent pneumonitis, the problem could stem from an aneurysm on the thoracic aorta that's pressing on the tracheobronchial tree. As the aneurysm dilates, it may obstruct venous return from the patient's head and arms, eventually causing superior vena cava syndrome. If a hypertensive patient develops hemoptysis and sudden excruciating pain, suspect that she has a ruptured thoracic aneurysm and act immediately.

If your hypertensive patient complains of boring, gnawing midabdominal or lumbar pain unaffected by movement, recognize that she may have an abdominal aortic aneurysm. Sudden severe pain may warn of an expansion of an aneurysm or an impending rupture. Check for a bruit or pulsating, possibly tender, abdominal mass, and notify the physician right away.

In all cases of aortic aneurysms, the risk of rupture is greatest when vessel diameter reaches about 6 cm (especially if the patient also has symptoms). If the diameter is under 5 cm and a hypertensive patient has no symptoms, your nursing care will focus on educating her about the need for regular follow-up to detect any changes in the size of the aneurysm. Emphasize the importance of sticking to the antihypertensive regimen and controlling blood pressure to reduce the risk of an expansion or rupture.

If the aneurysm exceeds 5 cm, you may be involved in preparing the patient physically and emotionally for surgery. Anticipate the need for preoperative testing, including pulmonary function tests to minimize the risks of complications.

Types of aneurysms

Most aneurysms are either fusiform or saccular. A fusiform aneurysm is a circumferential dilation, usually caused by atherosclerosis of the descending aorta. A saccular aneurysm looks more like a balloon attached to the side of the aorta. It commonly contains a blood clot. Saccular aneurysms tend to arise in the thoracic aorta; fusiform aneurysms tend to arise in the abdominal aorta distal to the renal arteries.

A dissecting aneurysm develops when an inner arterial layer tears and blood forces its way between the layers, creating an unstable pocket or cavity. It may span the artery's circumference or produce a unilateral pouching.

The term *false aneurysm*, or *pseudoaneurysm*, applies when all layers of the arterial wall are torn. Blood or a blood clot then escapes and becomes trapped by a thin layer of tissue or by surrounding organs and tissues.

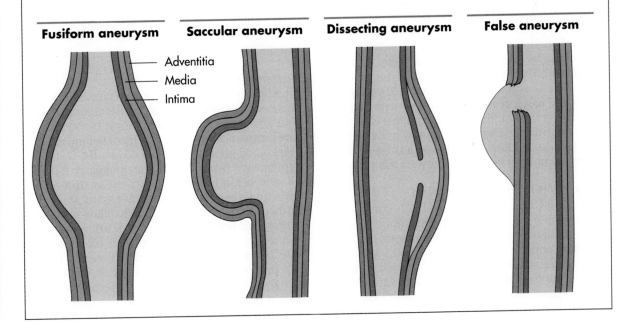

Fusiform aneurysm — Adventitia — Media — Intima

Saccular aneurysm

Dissecting aneurysm

False aneurysm

Stress the need for coughing and deep breathing after surgery. Teach the patient how to splint the incision, perform incentive spirometry, and do isometric leg exercises. And stress the benefits of early ambulation.

Ask the physician how to handle the patient's prescribed antihypertensive therapy before surgery. She may receive it I.V. on the day of surgery, or she may be allowed to take it orally with a sip of water. If the patient takes an ACE or angiotensin II inhibitor, make sure the surgeon knows about it. ACE inhibitors block angiotensin II formation that would otherwise result from the release of renin during surgery, and angiotensin II inhibitors interfere with the binding of angiotensin II. So the surgical team will need to monitor the patient's blood pressure closely.

Before discharge, inform the patient of any activity limitations imposed by the surgery. Reinforce the importance of controlling her blood pressure.

Complications

Hypertension and abdominal aortic aneurysm can result in a number of complications. For instance, the enlarging aneurysm can interfere with arterial blood flow, causing abdominal ischemia. The aneurysm can also obstruct venous blood flow back to the heart, resulting in superior vena cava syndrome. Paraplegia from compression of the anterior spinal artery, CVA, and cardiac tamponade can also occur. But the most common complication for a patient with hypertension and abdominal aortic aneurysm is dissection.

Dissection

A patient with hypertension and an aortic aneurysm has an increased risk for dissection of the aneurysm because of the thin vessel wall and increased pressure inside the vessel. It happens like this: The loss of structural integrity in the medial layer eventually leads to a tear in the intimal layer. Then, pressure exerted during systole (especially increased pressure caused by hypertension) can force blood into the medial layer, enlarging the tear and creating a false channel. Although aortic aneurysms usually occur in the arch or descending aorta, dissecting aneurysms most commonly develop in the ascending aorta.

Confirming the complication

A patient with a dissection invariably complains of pain in the chest, between the scapulae, or in the abdomen. Be especially suspicious of a dissecting aortic aneurysm if the patient says the pain is the worst she's ever experienced or rates it a 10 on the pain scale. She may describe it as stabbing or tearing pain. As the dissection continues, the pain may migrate or expand to both the thoracic and abdominal regions.

Neurologic symptoms and even syncope may occur with proximal dissection; syncope typically indicates a poor prognosis. Proximal dissection can produce aortic valvular incompetence and occasionally cardiac tamponade. Cardiac tamponade may then result in heart failure.

Physical findings alone may confirm the complication. Common findings include pulse abnormalities (an asymmetric reduction in or loss of a pulse), a murmur of aortic regurgitation, and neurologic deficits. Other physical findings may include Horner's syndrome (unilateral ptosis, miosis, and decreased facial sweating), a pulsating neck mass, and such respiratory signs as coughing, wheezing, and stridor that result from compression of the tracheobronchial tree.

Most patients also have diastolic pressures as high as 160 mm Hg. However, some may develop hypotension from decreased cardiac output related to cardiac tamponade or aortic insufficiency.

Laboratory findings typically don't help much. Chest X-rays almost always show a widened aortic shadow, but this finding isn't diagnostic. Two-dimensional and especially transesophageal echocardiography can help identify an aortic dissection. A CT scan using contrast media or a magnetic resonance imaging (MRI) scan also may help. However, the most valuable test is aortic angiography. The angiogram will confirm the dissection, establish the site of origin, and indicate the extent.

Nursing interventions

A patient suspected of having an aortic dissection needs emergency surgery. Before surgery, your goal is to maintain her systolic blood pressure between 100 and 120 mm Hg or her mean arterial blood pressure at about 60 mm Hg. If she's hypotensive from blood loss, administer fluids I.V. and begin blood replacement as ordered. Give analgesics to control her pain as prescribed. Expect to insert an indwelling urinary catheter to monitor the patient's urine output and an arterial line to monitor her blood pressure and response to treatment. If possible, provide preoperative teaching to help ease her fears.

If the patient is hypertensive despite blood loss, a potent vasodilator, most commonly nitroprusside, is the drug of choice for reducing blood pressure. Also, anticipate giving a beta blocker, which reduces the force of left ventricular contraction and thus aortic pressure during systole. Labetalol, a combined alpha and beta blocker, may be particularly useful in managing aortic dissection. Patients with refractory hypertension from renal artery ischemia may receive parenteral enalapril or a calcium channel blocker.

Keep in mind that oliguria may signal impending renal artery occlusion. A change in level of consciousness and other neurologic signs warn of cerebral perfusion compromised by the progressing dissection. Hypotension or cardiac arrhythmias may indicate the development of cardiac tamponade.

COMFORT MEASURES

Controlling anxiety during aortic dissection

By worsening hypertension, anxiety has the potential to complicate the course of an aortic dissection. And because the patient with aortic dissection has a life-threatening condition that requires intensive care, anxiety is a common but counterproductive reaction. Your actions can help calm the patient and possibly improve the outcome.

- When the patient is moved from her room to intensive care, make sure she knows when, where, and why she's going. If possible, go with her during the transfer. If not, have someone else go along for support.
- In the intensive care unit, introduce yourself to the patient. Ask her to tell you if she feels any pain, unusual discomfort, or worsening symptoms.
- During your introduction, assess the patient for signs and symptoms of anxiety, such as restlessness, tachycardia, pallor, and diaphoresis. Rule out other possible causes before deciding whether these problems reflect the patient's anxiety level or a worsening of her condition.
- Maintain a quiet, calm environment. If possible, partially close the door or pull the curtain. Try to minimize traffic in and out of the room. When speaking to the patient, use a calm, reassuring tone. Use therapeutic touch as appropriate.

- Tell the patient what to expect. Explain all treatments and procedures. Prepare her for the insertion of a pulmonary artery catheter to monitor her status. Reassure her that the devices used to monitor her condition can prevent any further problems.
- Stay with the patient and provide reassurance during procedures and treatments. Explain why the procedure is being done and what is happening.
- Tell the patient that her blood pressure will be monitored continuously for changes and that she may need additional medications to control it.
- Give a sedative as prescribed, and assess the patient frequently for adverse reactions, such as oversedation or depressed respiratory function.
- Administer supplemental oxygen as necessary. Monitor the patient's oxygen saturation with pulse oximetry as appropriate. Watch for signs of hypoxemia, such as decreased oxygen saturation levels, cyanosis, and a decreased level of consciousness.
- Involve the family in the patient's care. If family members calm the patient, allow them to stay with her as much as possible. Otherwise, allow the family members to visit the patient briefly and give them frequent updates in the family waiting room.

Cardiac tamponade, a life-threatening complication, results when fluid accumulates in the pericardial cavity, restricting ventricular filling during diastole and thus limiting venous return. As a result, venous pressure rises, and cardiac output and arterial pressure decline.

RAPID RESPONSE ▶ If your patient develops cardiac tamponade, take the following steps to prevent shock and death:

- Begin cardiac monitoring and evaluate the patient's ECG for arrhythmias and ischemic changes.
- Monitor the patient's blood pressure every 15 minutes—continuously if she has an arterial line in place. Watch for a paradoxical pulse.
- Help insert a pulmonary artery catheter to monitor hemodynamic status. Assess hemodynamic pressures according to your facility's policy.
- Provide supplemental oxygen as prescribed.

- Start two I.V. lines using large-bore needles.
- Give isoproterenol as prescribed to enhance myocardial contractility and decrease peripheral vascular resistance. Start the infusion at a rate of 1 μg/minute as prescribed. Be alert for cardiac arrhythmias.
- Prepare your patient for pericardiocentesis. ◀

After surgery for aortic dissection, the patient will need close monitoring. Your main goals are to maintain her systolic blood pressure between 100 and 120 mm Hg, promote optimal hemodynamic and respiratory status, and reduce her pain and anxiety.

If your patient is hypertensive, expect to continue such medications as nitroprusside and alpha and beta blockers. If she's hypotensive, expect to continue fluids and blood to maintain her blood pressure. Watch closely for signs of bleeding—hypotension, tachycardia, and tachypnea—at the aneurysm graft site. Also, be alert for sudden, excruciating back pain, a signal that the graft site may be tearing.

Expect that the patient will need mechanical ventilation. Frequently check her arterial blood gas (ABG) levels—an indication of her oxygenation status—and monitor her oxygen saturation. Assess her breath sounds frequently.

Give your patient medications for pain and anxiety as prescribed, and teach her what she needs to know to help her understand her condition. Keep in mind that controlling her fears and anxiety level may present one of your most challenging assignments. Remember that your reactions and responses to her may greatly help or hinder her ability to cope with this frightening, life-threatening problem (see *Controlling anxiety during aortic dissection,* page 69).

Hypertension and cerebrovascular disease

Cerebrovascular disease is a broad term that refers to problems created by an inadequate blood supply to the brain. The supply may be restricted by lesions in blood vessel walls, thrombotic or embolic occlusion of the lumen, rupture of the vessel, or altered blood characteristics (such as altered platelet function). CVA is the most common example of cerebrovascular disease. Other examples include aneurysms and arteriovenous malformations. Patients who have hypertension and cerebrovascular disease face an increased risk for thrombosis, embolism, and hemorrhage.

Pathophysiology

The brain receives a constant supply of nutrients and oxygen from blood carried by the internal carotid arteries and cerebral arteries (see *Sources of cerebral blood supply*). Normally, if one of these arteries becomes blocked, collateral circulation develops to shunt blood to the affected area. Autoregulatory mechanisms also maintain cerebral circulation at a constant rate despite changes in arterial pressure. Specifically, they prompt vasoconstriction and vasodilation in response to the serum oxygen level, carbon dioxide level, and arterial blood pressure. When blood pressure decreases or the carbon dioxide level increases, cerebral arteries dilate to increase the blood flow. When blood pressure increases, cerebral arteries constrict to maintain the flow and pressure. If the patient has hypertension, however, these compensatory mechanisms can become overworked, possibly leading to impaired cerebral blood flow and ischemia. If the impairment lasts for more than a few minutes, the deprived area can become a zone of infarction.

Hypertension aggravates this potentially serious situation in several ways. For one, it raises the risk of developing atherosclerosis, the most common factor linked to cerebral ischemia and infarction. Prolonged hypertension also causes vascular changes that raise the risk of thrombi and emboli. Over time, hypertension causes the artery's intimal layer to thicken. Lipids and fibrin accumulate, lining the artery with plaques that project into the lumen and eventually restrict blood flow through the vessel. Plaques also raise the risk of ulceration, which attracts platelets and fibrin and may lead to the formation of a thrombus that partially or completely occludes the vessel lumen, interrupting blood flow to part of the brain. If a fragment of the thrombus breaks off and travels in the bloodstream, it may eventually lodge in a small cerebral artery, causing occlusion, ischemia, and possibly infarction.

Hypertensive patients also face an increased risk of a cerebral aneurysm because of the increased wall tension and the accelerated decline of the medial layer. Although more common in the aorta, aneurysms also can develop in the vessels of the brain, commonly near or at the bifurcation of the circle of Willis, in the vertebrobasilar arteries, or in the carotid arteries. As with an aortic aneurysm, hypertension raises the risk of a rupture.

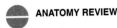

Sources of cerebral blood supply

To function normally, the brain must receive a steady supply of oxygenated blood. The illustration below shows you the arteries that supply the brain.

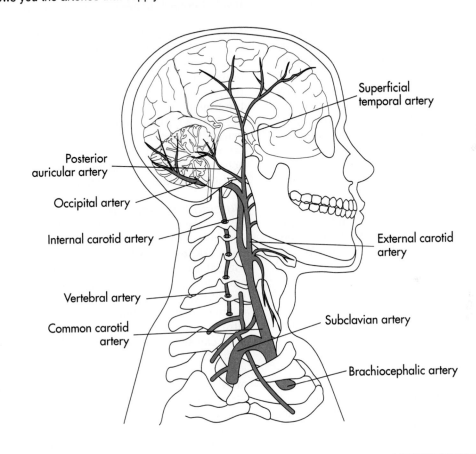

It also raises the risk of a rupture for patients who have arteriovenous malformations, which are tangled masses of blood vessels that have abnormally thin walls. If an arteriovenous malformation is large enough, blood shunts to the malformation, decreasing cerebral perfusion. Hypertension can worsen the problem by predisposing the patient to cerebral hemorrhage.

Adapting nursing care

For patients with hypertension and cerebrovascular disease, your care will focus on preventing cerebral occlusion by reducing or eliminating risk factors. For example, stress the dangers of smoking. Explain that nicotine raises blood pressure. Mention that inhaled carbon monoxide displaces oxygen, reducing blood supply to the tissues. And explain that tobacco use shortens clotting time and increases the risk of blood clots.

Also, teach your patient and her family members about the role of diet, exercise, and weight reduction in controlling blood pressure and reducing the risk of cerebrovascular and cardiovascular disease. Emphasize that hypertension is a major risk factor for cerebrovascular disease and that patients and families should make every effort to keep blood pressure under control.

Explain that combining risk factors can produce risk levels considerably higher than the sum of individual problems. For example, patients with hypertension and cerebrovascular disease who also smoke tobacco and take oral contraceptives have a high risk of a CVA. Patients with hypertension and cerebrovascular disease who also have impaired glucose tolerance and elevated blood lipid levels should be monitored closely and receive intense education about lifestyle modifications and medical treatment to reduce the risk of a CVA.

Complications

Common complications for patients with hypertension and cerebrovascular disease include a TIA, CVA, and subarachnoid hemorrhage.

Transient ischemic attack

A TIA results from a microembolus that breaks free from an atherosclerotic plaque in the cerebral arterial system, usually the carotid arteries. The embolus lodges in a smaller vessel downstream, temporarily interrupting blood flow to an area of the brain. The signs and symptoms of a TIA depend on which area of the brain is deprived of blood flow. Although, by definition, a TIA resolves within 24 hours, it may herald a future CVA. This is especially true if the patient has hypertension, which damages the vessels and raises the risk of plaques and emboli.

Confirming the complication

A TIA can be confirmed from its course of signs and symptoms. The patient may report numbness or tingling on one or both sides of the body and disturbances in vision, speech, or balance. Commonly, these symptoms may already have resolved by the time the patient can see a physician about them.

Nonetheless, the patient should receive a thorough neurologic examination that covers level of consciousness, balance and coordination, speech, and motor and sensory function. Laboratory tests should include a CBC with differential (to check for polycythemia or leukocytosis), sedimentation rate and antinuclear antibody test (to screen for vasculitis), and activated partial thromboplastin time and prothrombin time (to guide anticoagulation therapy, if needed). A CT or MRI scan may be obtained but usually is normal. Ultrasound of the carotid arteries may reveal atherosclerotic disease. An echocardiogram can exclude valvular disease. An ECG may indicate atrial fibrillation.

Nursing interventions

If you care for a patient who has hypertension, cerebrovascular disease, and a history of a recent TIA, evaluate her vital signs and neurologic status frequently. Monitor her blood pressure closely. The patient's family may be able to help you identify neurologic deficits. Remember that a sudden increase in blood pressure, a rapid and bounding pulse, and a headache can signal an impending CVA.

Educate the TIA patient about the warning signs and symptoms of a CVA. Urge her to seek medical care immediately if they develop. Stress the importance of blood pressure control in reducing the risk of further neurologic events. Help the patient define and implement needed changes in diet and lifestyle. Make sure she knows the importance of complying with her medication regimen. Also, make sure she knows that people with hypertension and cerebrovascular disease who take antihypertensives are at increased risk for adverse reactions (see *Antihypertensives and aspirin: Dangerous interactions*).

If the patient is receiving anticoagulation therapy, teach her about foods and medications that can alter warfarin requirements by influencing drug absorption or affecting how warfarin binds to plasma proteins. Tell her

DRUG ALERT

Antihypertensives and aspirin: Dangerous interactions

If your patient takes aspirin regularly, adding an antihypertensive drug to her regimen could cause unwanted effects. The table below outlines some of those effects and lists appropriate nursing actions.

Antihypertensives	Effect of antihypertensive and aspirin	Nursing actions
• Loop diuretics	• Increased risk of salicylate toxicity • Decreased diuretic effect	• Monitor patient for signs and symptoms of aspirin toxicity, such as tinnitus, headache, hearing loss, nausea, vomiting, diarrhea, and thirst. • Monitor serum salicylate levels. • Monitor fluid intake and output and weigh patient daily. • Monitor blood pressure frequently for changes that could indicate fluid-volume overload. • Watch for additional signs of fluid-volume excess, such as increased weight and edema. • Anticipate changing to another antiplatelet drug, lowering aspirin dosage, increasing diuretic dosage, or adding a diuretic, depending on the adverse effect.
• Potassium-sparing diuretics	• Decreased diuretic effect	• Monitor fluid intake and output and weigh patient daily. • Monitor blood pressure frequently for changes that could indicate fluid-volume overload. • Watch for additional signs of fluid-volume excess, such as increased weight and edema. • Monitor serum potassium levels for hyperkalemia. • Anticipate changing to another antiplatelet drug, increasing diuretic dosage, or adding another diuretic.
• Angiotensin-converting enzyme inhibitors • Beta blockers	• Decreased antihypertensive effect	• Monitor blood pressure closely and note any changes in blood-pressure control. • Anticipate changing to another antiplatelet drug, increasing antihypertensive dosage, or switching to another antihypertensive. • If antihypertensive dosage is increased or another antihypertensive is added, watch for adverse reactions and potentiation.

that foods rich in vitamin K may increase warfarin requirements, and advise her to eat small but consistent amounts of foods that contain vitamin K, such as cabbage, cauliflower, broccoli, and asparagus.

Cerebrovascular accident

A CVA, also called stroke, stems from interrupted arterial blood supply to the brain. It results in a cerebral infarction that may leave the patient with permanent neurologic deficits that correspond to the affected area. CVA is the third leading cause of death in the United States. Hypertension is its most important risk factor (especially isolated systolic hypertension), although it's not the only risk factor. In general, hypertension increases the risk of a CVA by about three to four times. The incidence of CVAs increases proportionately with increasing blood pressure.

The most common cause of a CVA is thrombosis of a cerebral artery resulting from cerebrovascular atherosclerosis. If the patient has hypertension, thrombosis is likely to develop in small penetrating arteries deep in the white matter of the brain. The resulting disorder, called a lacunar CVA, usually involves the basal ganglia, internal capsule, or brain stem.

Cerebral thrombosis disproportionally affects the elderly (who commonly have cardiac disease, atherosclerotic disease, or both) and African-Americans (who are more prone to hypertension). Embolism also may result from an endocardial clot; this is common in patients with atrial fibrillation, endocarditis, or a recent MI.

Risk factors for a CVA include:
- a history of cardiovascular problems, such as an MI, hypertension, atrial fibrillation, valvular disease, and hyperlipidemia
- a history of polycythemia, trauma, or obesity
- a family history of CVA
- unhealthy behaviors, such as smoking and a sedentary lifestyle
- use of oral contraceptives.

Confirming the complication

Depending on the size and location of the infarcted area, signs and symptoms may include loss of consciousness, mental disturbances, hemiplegia, weakness, aphasia, dysphasia, dysarthria, apraxia, loss of voluntary muscle control, seizures, flaccid paralysis, loss of deep tendon reflexes, and sensory losses.

Laboratory tests—such as an erythrocyte sedimentation rate, clotting and lipid profiles, and electrolyte levels—are usually normal. A CT or MRI scan can usually indicate the location and extent of cerebral thrombosis, although an abnormality may not be apparent until 24 to 48 hours after the event. An electroencephalogram may be used, especially if the patient has seizures or is comatose. An echocardiogram and ECG should be performed to exclude a cardiac embolic source, as can occur with atrial fibrillation.

Nursing interventions

During the acute phase of a CVA, your nursing care for a patient with hypertension will be the same as if the patient didn't have hypertension. You'll be working to help the patient survive and to avoid further brain injury. Specifically, you'll need to support the patient's vital functions, assess for and prevent complications, and initiate rehabilitation. Monitor the patient's blood pressure closely to reduce the risk of further infarction. If you detect increased blood pressure and a widening pulse pressure, followed by declining blood pressure, the patient may have increasing intracranial pressure (ICP).

Severely elevated blood pressure can cause cerebral edema and increased ICP and may require increased antihypertensive therapy. The trick is to achieve a delicate balance between reducing blood pressure far enough to minimize the risk of cerebral edema and increased ICP, but not far enough to impair cerebral perfusion and risk further ischemia.

Depending on the size and area of the brain involved, your patient may require endotracheal intubation and mechanical ventilation for oxygenation and management of respiratory secretions. Assess the patient's breathing patterns, oxygen saturation, and ABG levels to evaluate ventilation and respiratory function. Raise the head of the bed 30 degrees to promote drainage of oral secretions and also to prevent increased ICP. For the mechanically ventilated patient, aggressive pulmonary management—including hyperinflation with 100% oxygen before and after suctioning, chest percussion, and incentive spirometry—helps mobilize secretions, maximize oxygenation and ventilation, and prevent complications.

Frequent, thorough neurologic examination is essential to assess cerebral perfusion and evaluate the patient for signs of increased ICP. If the patient becomes agitated or has seizures, she may need special interventions to protect her from injury. These may include an oral airway, supplemental oxygen, suctioning, padded side rails, restraints, and a prescribed anticonvulsant.

Long-term therapy: After the patient's condition stabilizes, focus on preventing complications and minimizing the chance of a recurrence. Your goals include maintaining nutrition; helping the patient compensate for perceptual difficulties; promoting activity, communication, and rehabilitation; and providing emotional support and education. Continue to monitor the patient's blood pressure frequently. Adjust medication dosages as prescribed and plan for appropriate exercise.

You'll also need to provide support to the patient's family. Recognize that they're almost certainly under tremendous emotional stress, and give them frequent but simple explanations of the patient's condition. Be honest, consistent, and compassionate. It may be helpful to hold a patient care conference, in which all the patient's caregivers meet and talk with the family.

Early rehabilitation is important and appropriate for most CVA patients to minimize functional loss. Focus on preventing further impairment, maintaining and optimizing existing abilities, and helping the patient attain as much independence as possible. For most patients, the pace is slow and frustrating. Try to maintain a consistently supportive approach.

Remember that residual perceptual problems (such as visual-field deficits or mental status problems) and impairments (such as weakness, paralysis, and difficulty swallowing) may affect the patient's ability to manage her hypertension regimen. She may have trouble reading the medication label, for example. Or she may have trouble opening the container. If she has trouble swallowing, she may not be able to take her drugs. Nevertheless, you'll need to stress the importance of continuing the hypertension regimen and help the patient identify and compensate for new obstacles to compliance. If necessary, make sure the patient's medication comes with a nonsafety cap. Obtain a hand grip if it will help her open the container. If she has trouble swallowing, find out if she can crush her pills and take them with applesauce or other foods. If not, find out if the drug comes in liquid form.

Before discharge, review all aspects of the patient's care and make sure she and her family understand all your instructions. Anticipate the need for a home care referral (see *Teaching the hypertensive patient after a CVA*, page 76).

Subarachnoid hemorrhage

If arteries in the brain begin to bleed into the subarachnoid space or the parenchyma, the increasing volume of blood presses on surrounding brain tissue. Eventually, it presses strongly enough to produce ischemia and cause a catastrophic cerebrovascular event.

Subarachnoid hemorrhage occurs most commonly among people with a berry aneurysm or arteriovenous malformation, especially people under age 50. Although the cause of the rupture isn't always known, hypertension is a leading risk factor. Hypertension-related hemorrhage can arise anywhere in the brain, but it tends to develop in the brain stem, cerebellum, or basal ganglia.

Confirming the complication
A headache may be a prominent prodromal symptom of a neurologic deficit. The patient also may suffer confusion, vertigo, and fainting. In most cases, however, the onset is sudden and characterized by:
• excruciating headache
• photophobia
• neck rigidity
• nausea and vomiting
• loss of consciousness
• seizures
• signs and symptoms of increased ICP
• respiratory distress
• shock.

A CT or MRI scan may show intracerebral bleeding. Angiography can confirm the size, shape, and location of the aneurysm. A lumbar puncture may reveal blood, protein, or both in the cerebrospinal fluid. However, this procedure is contraindicated if the patient has increased ICP.

Nursing interventions
First, focus on the patient's airway, breathing, and circulation. Assess her neurologic status frequently and report any signs of deterioration.

Controlling the patient's hypertension may be crucial in preventing further bleeding. Assess her blood pressure frequently to make sure systolic pressure stays below 160 mm Hg. A recurrence of bleeding commonly develops within 24 hours or between 7 and 10 days after the initial hemorrhage. Because vasospasm may occur (usually 3 to 4 days after the initial bleeding), you may need to give the calcium channel blocker nimodipine as a preventive measure, as prescribed. Patients with intraparenchymal bleeding risk increased ICP, so be sure to monitor them regularly.

Teaching the hypertensive patient after a CVA

As much as any other disorder, a cerebrovascular accident (CVA) affects the spirit, motivation, and ability of the patient and her family. CVA patients tend to be elderly. They may be confused. They may feel helpless and out of control. And they may have physical limitations they've never experienced. They need a great deal of teaching and sometimes a great deal of help. It may seem a daunting task. But if you can teach your patient and her caregivers thoroughly and methodically, you can set your patient up for success at home.

Managing medications

In all likelihood, your patient will continue to take an antihypertensive when discharged after her CVA. But even though she may have taken the very same drug before her CVA, you'll need to review the regimen with her and her caregivers.

Emphasize that she still must control her blood pressure. Doing so could prevent another CVA. With the patient and her caregiver, review her antihypertensive drugs, their dosages, and their possible adverse effects. Warn them of the possibility of interactions with other drugs or foods. Finally, help them set up a dosing schedule that fits their daily routine.

Many patients are left with motor deficits, sensory deficits, or both after a CVA. If your patient has such deficits, you'll want to take steps to solve any problems that could lead to noncompliance.

For example, if the patient can't swallow normally, check with the pharmacist to see if the patient can crush her drugs before taking them. If so, suggest that she take them with a bit of applesauce, pudding, or another thickened liquid. If not, see whether the medication is available in liquid form and show the patient's caregiver how to administer it. Some patients prefer to place the medication between the cheek and gum to the rear of the unaffected side of the mouth. Others prefer a medication spoon or a syringe to place the medication.

If the patient has trouble opening her mouth, suggest that the caregiver stroke the muscle under her chin or touch her lips with the tip of the medication device to stimulate mouth opening.

If the patient can't swallow at all and needs enteral nutrition, show her, her caregiver, or both how to administer medication through the tube. Ask them to give you a return demonstration before discharge. Remind them to flush the tube after each dose to prevent clogging and ensure a full dose.

Success at home

Many people have trouble communicating after having a CVA. To help reduce the patient's frustration and encourage interaction, try to work out a system of verbal and nonverbal cues, so the patient can let you or a caregiver know how and what she's feeling. Some patients prefer using a pen and paper. Others prefer using a talking board or magnetic alphabet letters. Whenever possible, let the patient choose a communication system that feels comfortable for her.

Also, be sure to work out a system for obtaining blood pressure measurements at home. If the patient can't take her own pressure, teach a caregiver how to do it and ask for a return demonstration. Ask the physician to define a blood pressure range that's acceptable for the patient and write it down for them to take home. Establish a schedule they should follow for taking the patient's blood pressure, and encourage them to write the readings down in a daily record book.

Let the patient and caregiver know that a single blood pressure reading outside the accepted range is acceptable. Two such readings, however, may indicate a problem, and the patient or caregiver should notify the physician. Urge them to bring their daily record book to their follow-up appointments.

Clearly, having a CVA changes a person's lifestyle and abilities forever. Taking time to address these changes with the hypertensive patient and her caregiver helps promote feelings of self-esteem and independence. In the long run, those feelings will provide a firm foundation for compliance.

If necessary, prepare the patient for surgical intervention to clip the aneurysm or to place a coil that embolizes it. The latter procedure is usually performed by a neuroradiologist.

Also, protect the patient from injury, maintain her nutrition, and support her fluid and electrolyte balance. Usually, the earlier rehabilitation starts, the more completely a patient will recover.

Hypertension and coronary artery disease

Coronary artery disease (CAD) causes more deaths in the United States than any other single disorder. Hypertension not only acts synergistically with hyperlipidemia in causing CAD, but it also raises the risk of adverse effects from CAD.

Pathophysiology

Uncontrolled hypertension speeds the development of atherosclerosis, leading to premature CAD, endothelial damage, and smooth-muscle hypertrophy. Endothelial damage may be linked to the development of smooth-muscle hypertrophy because endothelial cells normally produce vasoactive substances that act on underlying smooth-muscle cells. These substances—nitric oxide, endothelial-derived relaxant factor, and endothelins—may play a role both in the pathogenesis of hypertension and the vascular damage that results from it. Lipoproteins influence the production of these vasoactive substances, which may partly explain the link between hyperlipidemia, hypertension, and coronary atherosclerosis. The proliferation of smooth muscle thickens vascular walls, thus perpetuating the hypertension.

The major cause of left ventricular hypertrophy is hypertension, which increases cardiac work by increasing peripheral vascular resistance. Although hypertrophy provides an effective compensatory mechanism temporarily, over time, the ventricle fails. The combination of increased demand and decreased supply results in ischemia, which in turn increases the risk of arrhythmia, heart failure, and sudden death.

Adapting nursing care

When caring for a patient with hypertension and CAD, focus on preventing the complications of both disorders by teaching her to modify certain risk factors. Tell your hypertensive patient that measures she takes to control blood pressure will also help control the development of CAD.

Obviously, controlling blood pressure—especially systolic pressure and especially in older patients—is crucial in reducing the risks of CAD complications. Thus, you need to ensure that your patient knows the importance of taking her hypertensive drugs as prescribed.

Also, try to reduce the patient's other CAD risk factors. Chief among them is hyperlipidemia, which magnifies the effects of hypertension. As with hypertension, patients can reduce the risk with lifestyle modifications, such as adopting a low-fat, low-sodium, low-alcohol diet. Only 30% or less of calories should come from dietary fat, and the patient should strictly limit the intake of saturated fat and cholesterol. Also, the patient should reduce sodium intake to 2 grams a day. Some patients may need antilipemic medications as well. But they should still follow recommended lifestyle modifications closely.

Urge your patient to stop smoking because it's an independent risk factor for CAD, separate from its effect on blood pressure. Remember that women age 35 and over who use oral contraceptives are at increased risk for CAD; concurrent smoking and use of oral contraceptives magnifies the risk at any age. Oral contraceptives also affect blood coagulation, platelet function, and fibrinolytic activity and may alter the integrity of the vascular endothelium, placing the patient at risk for additional complications.

Help your patient arrange an exercise plan and a method for controlling her weight, if necessary. And be sure the patient understands all the risk factors for hypertension and CAD.

Complications

Common complications for patients with hypertension and CAD include angina pectoris, arrhythmias, and heart failure.

Angina pectoris
Angina pectoris is a term used to describe the set of signs and symptoms that result from myocardial ischemia. It affects more than 5 million people in the United States. And it almost

always results from coronary atherosclerosis, a condition accelerated by hypertension.

Confirming the complication

The signs and symptoms of angina occur most commonly during exertion, exposure to cold, or ingestion of a large meal, but they may occur even when the patient is resting. Substernal chest pain is the chief symptom. In most cases, it lasts only a short time, typically less than 5 minutes. It may radiate to the arms, neck, or jaw and can be accompanied by dyspnea, diaphoresis, and nausea. Some patients complain of chest heaviness, shortness of breath, and vomiting rather than chest pain.

The patient's ECG may show signs of ST-segment elevation. If myocardial injury develops, ST-segment changes—such as elevation or a horizontal depression at least 2 mm deep and more than 80 milliseconds in duration—may appear. If an MI occurs, the ECG will most likely reveal abnormalities, such as symmetric T-wave inversion or elevation. Pathologic Q waves indicate myocardial necrosis or irreversible myocardial damage.

Levels of serum enzymes—including lactic dehydrogenase, aspartate transaminase, and creatine kinase—are normal in a patient with angina but increase as a result of myocardial damage.

If an ECG and laboratory tests don't indicate myocardial damage, a physician may order a treadmill exercise test or an echocardiogram (with or without exercise) to detect the presence of myocardial ischemia. A thallium scan with exercise is very sensitive for ischemia. Ultimately, coronary angiography confirms the presence of a partially or completely blocked coronary artery.

Nursing interventions

Initially, focus on helping the patient control pain and maintain hemodynamic stability. Pain commonly causes blood pressure to rise, which can worsen ischemia by increasing the myocardial workload. Consequently, relieving the patient's pain may reduce blood pressure and relieve ischemia.

Some medications used to reduce ischemia and relieve pain, such as nitroglycerin and calcium channel blockers, also decrease blood pressure. Remember to monitor the patient's blood pressure closely if she receives these drugs because she may develop severe hypotension. The goal is a blood pressure high enough to maintain perfusion but not high enough to increase cardiac afterload.

Depending on your patient's condition and risk factors, she may require thrombolytic therapy, angioplasty, coronary artery stent placement, or coronary artery bypass surgery. Meanwhile, monitor the patient's heart rate, ECG, and vital signs for changes that could indicate worsening ischemia. Obtain serum enzyme levels to rule out MI.

When you have the opportunity, help the patient identify activities that precipitate an attack. And teach her that if an attack occurs, she should stop what she's doing, sit down and rest, and take the prescribed dose of nitroglycerin.

If the pain doesn't subside, she should repeat the dose every 5 minutes for a maximum of three doses. If the pain still doesn't subside, she should notify the physician and seek emergency medical treatment.

Review the cause of angina with the patient and the need for lifestyle changes to decrease the risks of CAD and hypertension. Explain that CAD and angina can be controlled. Before discharge, reinforce all your instructions with the patient. Provide information about lifestyle changes, diet, medications, and signs and symptoms of problems that require follow-up. If the physician has recommended a cardiac rehabilitation exercise program, be sure to provide the appropriate referral and answer the patient's questions about the program.

Arrhythmias

As a result of myocardial ischemia, a patient with hypertension and CAD may develop arrhythmias, including atrioventricular conduction defects and ventricular ectopy. Acute, severe ischemia may cause ventricular tachycardia, ventricular fibrillation, and sudden death. Arrhythmias may increase ischemia by decreasing myocardial oxygen supply or increasing myocardial workload. In a hypertensive patient, the hypertrophic ventricle raises the risk of arrhythmias because of the increased possibility of ischemia.

The type of arrhythmia that develops depends largely on which part of the conduction system is affected by ischemia. For example, ischemia that results from an occlusion in the left anterior descending or circumflex coronary arteries, which supply the atrioventricular node, the bundle of His, and the bundle branches, may cause premature ventricular contractions and ventricular tachycardia or supraventricular tachyarrhythmias.

Confirming the complication
You'll probably discover an arrhythmia by noticing irregular peripheral pulses or hearing irregular heart sounds. Continuous cardiac monitoring determines the exact arrhythmia. A 12-lead ECG can help distinguish between a supraventricular and ventricular tachyarrhythmia.

Nursing interventions
For the patient who develops an arrhythmia, nursing care focuses on controlling it, controlling cardiac output, and promoting cardiac function. Cardiac arrhythmias typically are treated according to advanced cardiac life support (ACLS) guidelines. Depending on the particular arrhythmia, you may administer such drugs as atropine, lidocaine, or esmolol. For an arrhythmia in a hypertensive patient, a calcium channel blocker may be the drug of choice. Also, anticipate the need for external pacing, cardioversion, or defibrillation.

In the hypertensive patient with CAD who develops an arrhythmia, you'll want to lower blood pressure to reduce cardiac ischemia. Monitor the patient's blood pressure and ECG tracings continuously to evaluate the effectiveness of therapy. Administer supplemental oxygen as needed and monitor oxygen saturation and ABG values as indicated.

Heart failure
In heart failure, impaired cardiac function decreases cardiac output so much that it fails to meet the body's metabolic needs. Hypertension and CAD create more work for the heart, raising the risk of heart failure, which eventually leads to left ventricular hypertrophy.

The sympathetic nervous system tries to compensate for heart failure by causing the arterioles to constrict in an effort to decrease the body's metabolic needs. But instead, this further increases peripheral vascular resistance

and myocardial workload. The sympathetic nervous system also reduces renal blood flow. In response, the renin-angiotensin-aldosterone system is activated, which promotes water and sodium retention and leads to increased blood volume. This further stresses an already overly stressed heart and blood vessels.

In severe heart failure, systolic blood pressure may decrease because of reduced stroke volume. However, vasoconstriction may increase diastolic pressure.

Confirming the complication
In heart failure, increased sympathetic activity and hypervolemia may lead to acutely elevated blood pressure. Tachycardia is common. The patient may be anxious, confused, tachypneic, diaphoretic, and cyanotic. Other findings may include crackles or wheezes, venous jugular distention, an S_3 or S_4 heart sound, hepatojugular reflux, weight gain, and peripheral edema.

The patient's chest X-ray may reveal cardiomegaly, pulmonary vascular congestion, pleural effusion, or all three. The ECG may show an arrhythmia. ABG analysis may indicate hypoxemia and respiratory acidosis. Bedside hemodynamic monitoring helps to confirm the degree of failure and guide therapy. Usually, patients with heart failure have increased central venous pressure, pulmonary artery pressure, and pulmonary artery wedge pressure. Cardiac output and cardiac index typically are reduced, and systemic vascular resistance typically is increased.

Nursing interventions
For the hypertensive patient with heart failure, lowering the blood pressure may be enough to relieve the signs and symptoms of heart failure. Any of several drugs may be prescribed. For example, ACE inhibitors are highly effective. Diuretics, such as furosemide, help reduce extracellular fluid volume. Inotropic drugs, such as dopamine and dobutamine, may be given to improve myocardial contractility and cardiac output. Occasionally, an afterload reducer, such as nitroprusside, can help, especially if the patient has markedly increased systemic vascular resistance.

For most patients, these drugs are titrated upward to achieve the optimal cardiac index. Therefore, you'll need to assess your patient's hemodynamic status frequently to evaluate her response to the medications.

Other supportive measures include providing supplemental oxygen. Some patients may need mechanical ventilation. Either way, monitor the patient's oxygen saturation and ABG values to evaluate her ventilation and respiratory function. Each day, check the patient's weight and intake and output to monitor her response to treatment. Notify the physician if the patient develops complications, such as hypokalemia, hyponatremia, or prerenal azotemia.

Patients with heart failure tend to be anxious. Helping the patient control her anxiety not only helps her emotional state, but also reduces her oxygen demand. To ease her anxiety, do your best to establish a calm, quiet environment. Reassure the patient and give her routine reports about her condition. Tell her the reasons for any invasive interventions. Anticipate the need for analgesics. Morphine I.V., for example, may not only help to decrease anxiety, but may also reduce preload.

Before discharge, reinforce all your instructions for controlling blood pressure and modifying risk factors to prevent complications. Discuss any instructions related to her treatment for heart failure. In particular, make sure she understands the dosages and adverse effects of any newly prescribed drugs.

Hypertension and renal insufficiency

Functioning normally, the kidneys maintain the quality of extracellular fluid. They remove water, urea, creatinine, and other waste products from the body. They form urine, maintain electrolyte balance (such as sodium-potassium balance), and maintain acid-base balance. Together with the circulatory and endocrine systems, they help regulate blood pressure.

In renal insufficiency, the kidneys partially fail: They form a reduced amount of urine and can't maintain homeostasis. Hypertension can be both a cause and a consequence of renal insufficiency. In fact, hypertension is the leading cause of renal disease in the United States.

Pathophysiology

The mechanism by which hypertension leads to impaired renal function isn't clear. Normally, increased perfusion pressure increases urine output and renal sodium excretion. But primary hypertension seems to alter this relationship, preventing increased blood pressure from prompting increased excretion. Instead, the body maintains intravascular volume despite the elevated blood pressure. Renal blood flow decreases and renal vascular resistance increases, at least in part because renal vascular resistance develops along with the systemic vascular resistance that accompanies hypertension.

In uncomplicated primary hypertension, the kidney protects itself from increased systemic arterial pressure through autoregulation of afferent and efferent arteriolar tone. Thus, it maintains normal glomerular pressure and a normal filtration rate. This may explain why primary hypertension usually doesn't cause renal failure. In severe hypertension and prolonged, uncontrolled hypertension, however, this protective mechanism fails, exposing the glomerulus to excessive pressure and resulting in glomerular damage. As hypertension-induced nephron damage progresses, the patient develops a gradual decrease in creatinine clearance, an increase in serum creatinine and urea, and a loss of the kidneys' urine-concentrating ability.

Renal disease also may precede hypertension. For example, in patients with Type I diabetes, hypertension may develop after the glomerular filtration rate increases and microalbuminuria appears.

Adapting nursing care

Controlling blood pressure in hypertensive patients can slow the progress of renal insufficiency and reduce the risk of renal failure. Be sure to discuss the benefits of controlled blood pressure, not just with patients but also with their families. Early diagnosis, lifestyle changes, and drug therapy all can help reduce the overall risk of renal damage.

Teach hypertensive patients or those at risk for hypertension to control blood pressure by losing weight, limiting sodium and alcohol intake, and exercising. Home blood-pressure monitoring can help promote compliance. But make sure your patient has a reliable blood-pressure monitor and knows how to use it properly.

Identify and share with the patient the specific goals of therapy. In patients with primary hypertension, blood pressure should be lowered to at least 140/90 mm Hg when possible.

Patients with hypertension and renal insufficiency also should have baseline renal function tests. Expect to obtain baseline urinalysis for glucose, ketones, and protein as well as a 24-hour urine collection for initial and ongoing changes in protein, serum creatinine, and BUN levels and creatinine clearance. Assess the patient's electrolyte levels for changes that suggest an imbalance. Remember that decreased renal function may disrupt the patient's electrolyte balance. Institute measures to replace or remove electrolytes as necessary, keeping in mind that treatment for one imbalance may result in another.

Complications

The most common complication for patients with hypertension and renal insufficiency is chronic renal failure. Other complications that develop are actually indications of the patient's progression toward chronic renal failure.

Chronic renal failure

Chronic renal failure occurs when the glomerular filtration rate decreases below 25% of normal. The process occurs over a period of years, and the damage results in uremia. Chronic renal failure differs from acute renal failure in that it involves progressive, irreversible damage to one or both kidneys.

Renal failure develops in patients who have hypertension and renal insufficiency because of the progressive damage to the glomeruli and the resulting deterioration of renal function (see *How hypertension and renal insufficiency lead to chronic renal failure,* pages 82 and 83). The kidneys continue to function until 75% of the nephrons have been destroyed. Then the solute load exceeds the kidneys' remaining ability to absorb it, and osmotic diuresis occurs. Nephrons continue to be damaged, which leads to retention of waste products and eventually to oliguria.

Confirming the complication

The signs of renal failure include anemia, azotemia, and an impaired ability to concentrate and dilute urine. The patient with chronic renal failure typically complains of fatigue, itching, weakness, anorexia, a tendency to bleed, nausea, and insomnia. She may or may not be oliguric. In fact, many patients with chronic renal failure have polyuria and nocturia because of the kidneys' impaired concentrating ability. Physical findings include dry skin, bruising, abdominal distention, Kussmaul's respirations, tachycardia, pericardial friction rub, signs of pulmonary edema, confusion, and lethargy.

Laboratory findings include elevated BUN and serum creatinine levels, hyperkalemia, hyperphosphatemia, hypocalcemia, and metabolic acidosis. Serum creatinine typically exceeds 3.0 mg/dL, and creatinine clearance is 10 to 50 ml/min. When creatinine clearance reaches 15 ml/min or less, the patient has end-stage renal disease. Uric acid typically is elevated. The patient may have hypertriglyceridemia and usually has mild to moderate anemia with normocytic or microcytic red blood cell (RBC) indices. The anemia probably results from a suppression of erythropoietin, which is produced by the kidneys. A renal ultrasound scan may reveal small, symmetric kidneys. Excretory urography will identify any urinary obstruction.

Nursing interventions

For a patient with hypertension, renal insufficiency, and chronic renal failure, controlling blood pressure should be high on your list of priorities. If successful, you'll slow the decline in renal function.

ACE inhibitors and other antihypertensives can help reduce the rate of declining renal function. However, most patients with renal insufficiency need two, three, or even four drugs to control blood pressure adequately. Be especially alert for increased adverse reactions resulting from the use of several drugs.

Also, monitor the patient for signs and symptoms of drug toxicity. The patient may need
(Text continues on page 84.)

How hypertension and renal insufficiency lead to chronic renal failure

1. Normally, blood flows to each glomerulus through an afferent arteriole. Blood then flows through a glomerular capillary tuft and out of the glomerulus through an efferent arteriole. The juxtaglomerular cells, which store renin, line the glomerular end of the afferent arteriole and help regulate blood pressure. Glomerular filtration occurs as fluid moves out of the glomerular capillary tuft, into Bowman's capsule, and then out through the proximal convoluted tubule. Filtrate then passes through the distal convoluted tubule for eventual excretion from the body as urine.

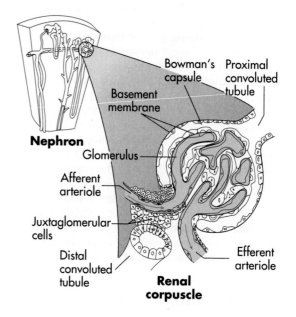

2. In hypertension, high-pressure renal blood flow causes hyaline thickening of the walls of the renal afferent arteriole. This thickening strengthens the walls and prevents their rupture from the increased pressure. However, as the walls thicken they become stiff and sclerosed. This narrows the lumen of the arterioles, causing decreased blood flow, which prompts the juxtaglomerular cells to release renin, an enzyme used by the kidneys to increase blood pressure further.

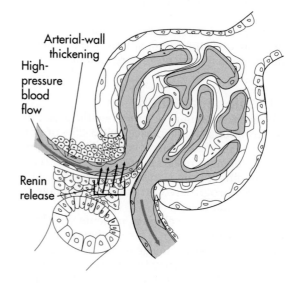

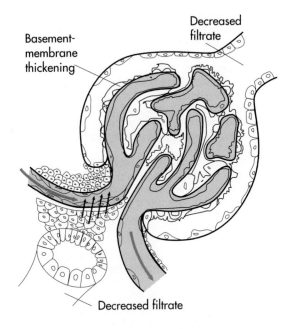

Basement-membrane thickening

Decreased filtrate

Decreased filtrate

3. Over a long period of time, high-pressure blood flow injures glomerular cells, resulting in basement-membrane thickening and scarring. Scarring reduces the amount of filtrate surface available in the glomerulus, which in turn decreases the functional ability of affected nephrons. If hypertension is not brought under control, renal insufficiency eventually occurs as the damaged nephrons fail to function.

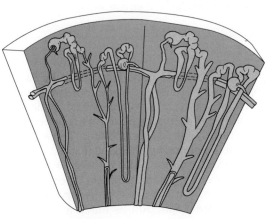

Nonfunctioning nephron **Hypertrophied nephron**

4. As more and more nephrons become damaged from long-standing, uncontrolled hypertension, renal insufficiency gradually progresses to chronic renal failure. The remaining nephrons hypertrophy and are unable to keep up with the increased workload created by the nonfunctioning nephrons. Chronic renal failure develops when more than 75% of nephrons lose their filtering ability.

ADAPTING YOUR CARE

Helping the hypertensive patient who needs dialysis

If your hypertensive patient needs dialysis, you'll have to adapt your nursing care appropriately to minimize an already significant risk of fluid imbalance.

Before dialysis
• Monitor the patient's fluid balance closely. Body weight provides an important indicator of how much fluid should be removed during dialysis. Weigh the patient at the same time each day, on the same scale, with the patient wearing the same amount of clothing. Steady weight gain indicates fluid retention.
• Monitor the patient for signs and symptoms of heart failure, including tachycardia, distended neck veins, increased central venous pressure, edema, crackles, and shortness of breath. If you note these signs and symptoms, notify a physician right away.
• Keep in mind that antihypertensive medications are usually withheld before and during dialysis to help prevent hypotension.

During dialysis
• Watch for fluid volume deficit caused by the hypertonicity of the dialysate or bleeding from the vascular access puncture. Signs and symptoms include poor skin turgor, decreased central venous pressure, and tachycardia.
• During peritoneal dialysis, watch for fluid overload. Catheter complications can block the exchange fluid in the peritoneal cavity, or a severely scarred peritoneum can prevent an adequate exchange.
• During hemodialysis, watch for fluid overload resulting from compromised regulatory mechanisms. Signs and symptoms include an increase in blood pressure, difficulty breathing, and crackles. Excess fluid volume aggravates hypertension.
• Monitor the hemodialysis patient for hemorrhage because heparin is used to prevent clotting as blood flows through the dialyzer.
• Check the patient's blood pressure and pulse every 30 to 60 minutes.

After dialysis
• Apply pressure to the puncture site and avoid venipunctures and intramuscular injections for at least 60 minutes.
• Tell the patient to notify you or her physician right away if she develops any bleeding.
• Check with a physician about restarting the patient's medications when she returns from dialysis.

---

lower-than-usual doses because impaired renal function interferes with drug clearance. Antihypertensive treatment presents an even greater challenge for patients who must submit to the dramatic volume changes caused by dialysis (see *Helping the hypertensive patient who needs dialysis*).

Because a patient with renal failure typically retains sodium, the physician may prescribe a diuretic, usually a loop diuretic, to reduce fluid volume while controlling blood pressure. Provide the patient with a moderately sodium-restricted diet and check her weight daily. Also, watch for electrolyte imbalance, typically hyperkalemia, and the cardiac arrhythmias that may result from it.

If the patient is anemic, the physician may order RBC transfusion. Transfusion can reduce the risk of hyperkalemia, possibly through improved oxygenation and less acidemia. Erythropoietin can reduce the need for transfusion and improve exercise tolerance and tissue oxygenation by raising the patient's hematocrit.

Ultimately, chronic renal failure leads to uremia and death unless the patient starts dialysis or receives a donor kidney. Either way, treatment doesn't cure the problem, it only slows its progress. Care focuses on preserving the remaining renal function as much as possible, improving the patient's physiologic status, alleviating associated symptoms, and maintaining her quality of life.

To some degree, the patient's quality of life depends on your teaching. Teach your patient and her family about the disease, its outcome, and its treatment. Be sure to talk with them about the relative risks and benefits of treatment. Provide emotional support to the patient and her family and encourage them to bring their questions and concerns to you. If the patient will receive home dialysis, she and her family will need thorough teaching and a home care referral. Remember that even in the face of a devastating disease, the physiological and psychosocial support you provide can make a dramatic difference in a patient's quality of life.

Suggested readings

Abe K, Iwanaga H, Inada E. Effect of nicardipine and diltiazem on internal carotid artery blood flow velocity and local cerebral blood flow during cerebral aneurysm surgery for subarachnoid hemorrhage. *J Clin Anesth.* 1994;6:99-105.

American Heart Association. *Heart and stroke facts.* Dallas, Tx: American Heart Association; 1994.

American Heart Association. *Heart and stroke facts, 1996 statistical supplement.* Dallas, Tx: American Heart Association; 1995.

Anonymous. 1993 guidelines for the management of mild hypertension. Memorandum from a World Health Organization/International Society of Hypertension meeting. Guidelines subcommittee of the WHO/ISH mild hypertension liaison committee. *Hypertension.* 1993;22:392-403.

Anonymous. The fifth report of the Joint National Committee on Detection, Evaluation and Treatment of High Blood Pressure (JNC V). *Arch Intern Med.* 1993;153:154-183.

Boden G. Fatty acids and insulin resistance. *Diabetes Care.* 1996;19:394-395.

Brown RD, Whisnant JP, Sicks JD, Fallon WM, Wiebers DO. Stroke incidence, prevalence, and survival: secular trends in Rochester, Minnesota through 1989. *Stroke.* 1996;27:373-380.

Chait A, Brunzell JD, Denke MA, et al. Rationale of the diet-heart statement of the American Heart Association. Report of the Nutrition Committee. *Circulation.* 1993;88:3008-3029.

Davies MK. Effects of ACE inhibitors or coronary haemodynamics and angina pectoris. *Heart* 1994;72(3 Suppl):S52-S56.

Falkenhahn M, Gohlke P, Paul M, Stoll M, Unger T. The renin-angiotensin system in the heart and vascular wall: new therapeutic aspects. *J Cardiovasc Pharmacol.* 1994;24(Suppl 2):S6-S13.

Fuster V, Gotto AM, Libby P, Loscalzo J, McGill HC. 27th Bethesda Conference: matching the intensity of risk factor management with the hazard for coronary disease events. Task Force 1. Pathogenesis of coronary disease: the biologic role of risk factors. *J Am Coll Cardiol.* 1996; 27:964-976.

Gifford RW Jr, Manger WM, Bravo EL. Pheochromocytoma. *Endocrinal Metab Clin North Am.* 1994;23:387-404.

Gudbjörnsdottir S, Lönnroth P, Sverrisdóttir YB, Wallin BG, Elam M. Sympathetic nerve activity and insulin in obese normotensive and hypertensive men. *Hypertension.* 1996;27:276-280.

Harper R, Ennis CN, Heaney AP, et al. A comparison of the effects of low- and conventional-dose thiazide diuretic on insulin action in hypertensive patients with NIDDM. *Diabetologia.* 1995;38:853-859.

King BF Jr. Diagnostic imaging evaluation of renovascular hypertension. *Abd Imaging.* 1995; 20:395-405.

Levine DM, Cohen JD, Dustan HP, et al. Behavior changes and the prevention of high blood pressure. Workshop II. AHA Prevention Conference III. Behavior change and compliance: keys to improving cardiovascular health. *Circulation.* 1993;88:1387-1390.

Lewis EJ, Hunsicker LG, Bain RP, Rohde RD. The effect of angiotensin-converting-enzyme inhibition on diabetic nephropathy. The Collaborative Study Group. *N Engl J Med.* 1993;329:1456-1462.

Lithell H. Metabolic aspects of the treatment of hypertension. *J Hypertension.* 1995;13(Suppl 2): S77-S80.

Pohl MA. The ischemic kidney and hypertension. *Am J Kidney Dis.* 1993;21(Suppl 2):22-28.

Raine AE. Hypertension and the kidney. *Br Med Bull.* 1994;50:322-341.

Saito I, Saruta T. Hypertension in thyroid disorders. *Endocrinal Metab Clin North Am.* 1994; 23:379-386.

Saruta T. Mechanism of glucocorticoid-induced hypertension. *Hypertension Res.* 1996;19:1-8.

Sheps SG, Canzanello VJ. Current role of automated ambulatory blood pressure and self-measured blood pressure determinations in clinical practice. *Mayo Clin Proc.* 1994;69:1000-1005.

Subcommittee on Advanced Cardiac Life Support. *Textbook of advanced cardiac life support.* Dallas, Tx: American Heart Association; 1994.

Welle S. Sympathetic nervous system response to intake. *Am J Clin Nutr.* 1995;62(Suppl 5):1118S-1122S.

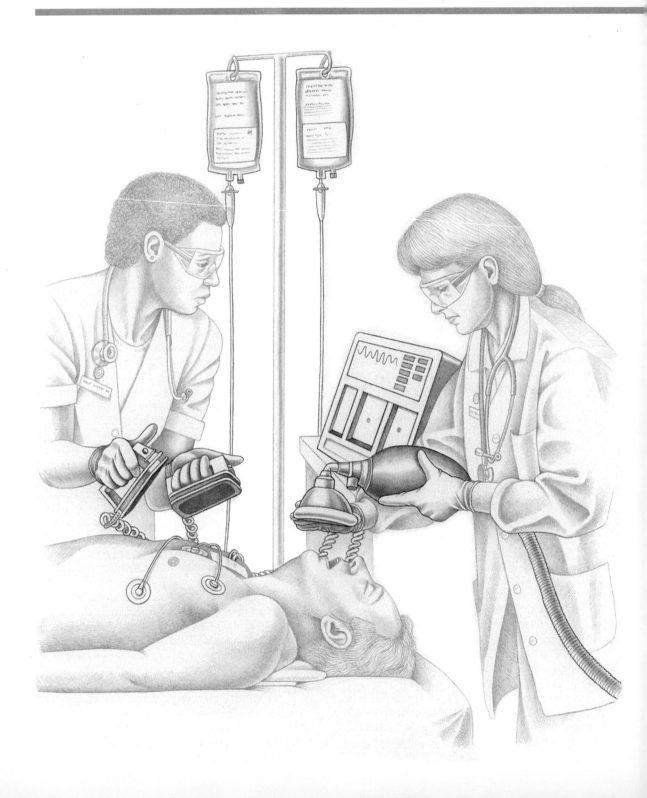

3

Myocardial Infarction

Myocardial infarction (MI), a common and typically life-threatening result of coronary artery disease (CAD), strikes about 300,000 people each year in the United States. About 25% of them die, half within the first hour after symptoms begin.

Unfortunately, many disorders can raise the risk of MI or complicate its course. They include coagulation defects, hypertension, diabetes mellitus, and thyroid disease. In combination with MI, these disorders can cause complications as serious as life-threatening hemorrhage, cardiogenic shock, cardiac arrhythmias, aneurysm, and dramatic changes in blood glucose and fluid volume levels.

ANATOMY REVIEW

Locating the coronary arteries

These illustrations show the locations of the coronary arteries on the surface of the heart. Naturally, the location at which coronary circulation is compromised has a direct effect on the type of myocardial infarction (MI) your patient experiences.

- Occlusion of the right coronary artery or one of its branches usually results in a posterior or right ventricular MI.

- Occlusion of the left anterior descending artery causes an infarction of the septum or the anterior, anterolateral, or inferior wall of the left ventricle.
- Occlusion of the left circumflex artery may result in a lateral or posterior infarction.
- Occlusion of the left coronary artery before it branches usually is fatal because the infarction affects most of the left ventricle.

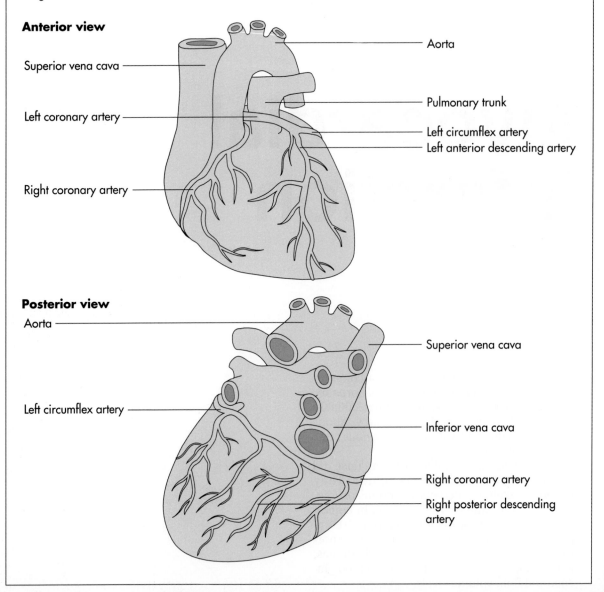

Anterior view

Superior vena cava

Left coronary artery

Right coronary artery

Aorta

Pulmonary trunk

Left circumflex artery

Left anterior descending artery

Posterior view

Aorta

Left circumflex artery

Superior vena cava

Inferior vena cava

Right coronary artery

Right posterior descending artery

Anatomy and physiology review

The heart, seat of the body's circulatory system, is a hollow muscular organ that delivers blood and oxygen to tissues in all parts of the body. It does so by contracting rhythmically, forcing blood to circulate through its chambers at a resting rate of about 5 liters per minute.

The heart has four chambers that work in concert: two atria that function partly as holding tanks and two heavily muscled ventricles that contract with great pressure, forcing oxygen-depleted blood to the lungs and oxygen-rich blood to the rest of the body.

Blood moves steadily through the heart's chambers because of a series of four valves that open as blood moves forward and close against backward pressure, thus preventing backward flow. The tricuspid valve lies between the right atrium and right ventricle, and the mitral (or bicuspid) valve lies between the left atrium and left ventricle. The pulmonary valve lies between the right ventricle and the pulmonary artery, and the aortic valve lies between the left ventricle and aorta.

Coronary circulation

As blood flows from the left ventricle into the ascending aorta, some of it leaves the aorta and enters two coronary arteries. These arteries emanate from the root of the aorta and supply oxygenated blood to the heart muscle (see *Locating the coronary arteries*).

The position and function of the coronary arteries varies somewhat from person to person. Usually, however, the right coronary artery and its branch, the posterior descending artery, supply the right atrium, right ventricle, posterior wall of the left ventricle, apical half of the septum, sinoatrial (SA) node, and atrioventricular (AV) node. The left coronary artery divides into two branches: the left anterior descending (LAD) and the circumflex. The LAD branch supplies the anterior and inferior walls of the left ventricle, the basal half of the septum, the right and left bundle branches, and, occasionally, the anterior wall of the right ventricle. The circumflex branch supplies the left atrium and the lateral and, occasionally, the posterior walls of the left ventricle.

To perfuse the thick myocardium, coronary arteries branch at right angles and penetrate into the heart wall. Even so, the endocardial layer has the poorest blood supply. Consequently, it usually sustains the worst damage if ischemia develops (see *Layers of the heart wall*, page 90).

Because the myocardium is perfused only during diastole, any condition that shortens diastole—tachycardia, for example—may decrease myocardial perfusion and compromise myocardial oxygenation, possibly leading to ischemia or infarction.

Cardiac conduction

The heart contracts regularly because electrical signals spread predictably and repeatedly across the heart muscle through the cardiac conduction system. Unlike other muscles in the body, the normal heart muscle possesses certain electrophysiologic properties that allow it—indeed, force it—to contract over and over, at a steady rate and with a regular rhythm. These properties include automaticity, excitability, conductivity, and refractoriness.

- Automaticity is the ability of the myocardial cells to initiate a regular and spontaneous impulse. Under normal circumstances, this property is most prominent in the SA node.
- Excitability refers to the ability of the myocardial cells to respond to a stimulus. As a result of stimulation, the electrical charge of the resting myocardial cells changes, creating an action potential. Functioning as a unit, once stimulated, the entire heart muscle contracts.
- Conductivity refers to the ability of the myocardial cells not only to respond to an impulse but also to transmit that impulse along a cell membrane.
- Refractoriness is the inability of the myocardial cells to respond to a new stimulus while still contracting from an earlier stimulus. This property prevents rapid, uncontrolled contractions, thus preserving heart rhythm.

Paths of cardiac conduction

In the normal heart, conduction begins in the SA node—the heart's pacemaker. Each impulse produced by the SA node results in depolarization, or a rapid reversal of the cell membrane's resting potential. Normally, cells have a negative

ANATOMY REVIEW

Layers of the heart wall

The heart wall consists of three layers: an outer epicardium, a thick myocardium composed of interlacing bundles of cardiac muscle fibers, and a thin innermost endocardium. The epicardium is also one of the layers of the serous pericardium; the other is the parietal pericardium. Between these layers is the pericardial space, which normally contains a small amount of lubricating fluid.

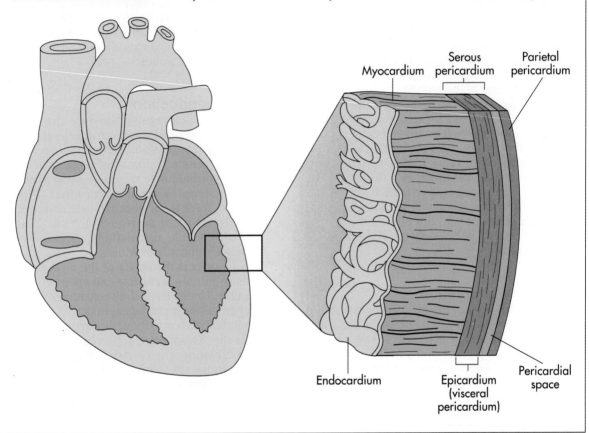

internal charge and a positive external charge. However, the electrical impulse causes the cell membrane to become more permeable to sodium ions, producing a rapid influx. As a result, potassium moves out of the cell. This movement of ions across the cell membrane creates an electrical current. When sodium ions inside the cell reach a critical level, an electrical impulse—a wave of depolarization—moves from cell to cell until all of the heart's cells have fired. At the end of depolarization, the cell membrane becomes less permeable to sodium.

Sodium moves out of the cell, and potassium moves back in, resulting in repolarization.

Beginning at the SA node, the wave of depolarization spreads through the right and left atria by way of the anterior, middle, and posterior intranodal tracts and Bachmann's bundle. This results in atrial contraction (see *Path of cardiac conduction*).

The AV node then takes up impulse conduction. Normally, the AV node forms the only electrical connection between the atria and ventricles. Initially slowing the impulse, this

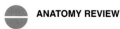

Path of cardiac conduction

The sinoatrial (SA) node emits 60 to 100 electrical impulses per minute. The impulses travel over the atria to the atrioventricular (AV) node, and then over the ventricles.

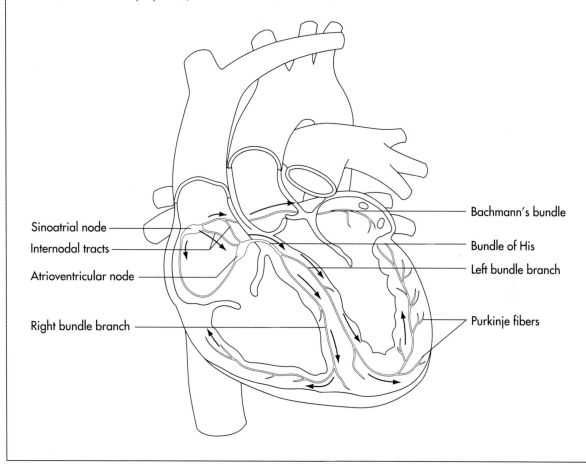

connection delays ventricular activity and allows blood to move from the atria to the ventricles. Conduction then progresses quickly through the AV node to the bundle of His.

The bundle of His is a network of fibers that arises in the AV node and extends along the right interventricular septum. It divides in the ventricular septum to form the right bundle branch and left bundle branch. The right bundle branch innervates the right ventricle. The left bundle branch divides into two fascicles or bundles (anterior and posterior) to supply the larger left

ventricle. The impulse rapidly spreads through these fibers to both ventricles.

Purkinje's fibers, the distal portions of the left and right bundle branches, fan across the subendocardial surface of the ventricles, from the endocardium through the myocardium. As the electrical impulse spreads through Purkinje's fibers, it prompts ventricular contraction.

Control of cardiac conduction

When a person is at rest, the parasympathetic nervous system controls heart function through branches of the vagus nerve. During activity or stress, the sympathetic nervous system takes over, stimulating the heart's nerves to fire more rapidly and the ventricles to contract more forcefully. The sympathetic nervous system stimulates the heart and blood vessels via branches of the cervical and thoracic nerves. It also stimulates the heart through the effects of circulating catecholamines: norepinephrine and epinephrine.

The actions of the sympathetic nervous system can be grouped according to the responses produced. Stimulation of alpha receptors in vascular smooth muscle causes arterial and venous constriction. Stimulation of $beta_1$ receptors in the heart increase heart rate, atrioventricular conduction, and contractility. $Beta_1$ stimulation also enhances automaticity.

The vagus nerve decreases heart rate and slows impulse transmission through the AV node and the ventricular conduction system. Baroreceptors, specialized nerve tissues located in the internal carotid arteries and the aorta, respond when they're stretched, activating the vagus nerve to decrease heart rate and AV conduction.

Cardiac output

Cardiac output is the amount of blood pumped by the heart in one minute. It reflects the number of heart beats per minute multiplied by the amount of blood ejected with each beat (stroke volume). Three factors affect stroke volume: preload, afterload, and contractility.

Preload refers to the passive stretching force exerted by blood in the ventricle on the ventricular muscle at the end of diastole. The more the muscle fibers are stretched during diastole, the more forcefully they'll contract in systole.

Afterload refers to the pressure required for ventricular muscles to force the aortic valve open and eject blood into the aorta by overcoming its greater pressure.

Contractility refers to the myocardium's ability to contract normally.

Pathophysiology

When the heart muscle doesn't receive enough oxygen to support its function, an MI may

result. Usually, an MI results from coronary artery occlusion severe enough and long-lasting enough to cause prolonged ischemia. If ischemia lasts long enough, cardiac muscle normally supplied by the blocked artery dies, permanently losing its ability to contract. Coronary artery obstruction typically results from CAD, an embolus or thrombus, or vasospasm.

The most common cause of an MI, CAD results from a diffuse buildup of plaque in the intimal layer of the coronary arteries. Experts believe that plaque buildup begins in response to chronic injury of the arteries' endothelial lining.

Injury to the endothelial lining causes platelets, white blood cells, fibrin, and lipids to converge at the injured site. Macrophages collect under the damaged intima, gradually thickening the intimal layer and narrowing the lumen of the coronary artery. If plaque builds up gradually, the body may respond by creating collateral circulation, thus reducing the heart's reliance on a narrowed artery. If the artery becomes occluded, collateral circulation may prevent extensive damage. However, the lumen may close abruptly from atherosclerotic thickening, hemorrhage into the intimal wall, thrombus formation, or an embolus.

A rupture of coronary plaque can trigger sudden coronary occlusion. The risk of a rupture may depend more on plaque composition than on size, with plaques of soft extracellular lipids and macrophages more likely to rupture. Macrophages are the primary inflammatory cells in atherosclerotic plaques. They release lytic enzymes that can weaken the fibrous cap and allow the plaque to rupture. Repeated rupture and healing narrows the intimal lumen. Plus, plaque rupture may cause thrombus formation, resulting in a complete occlusion.

Thrombi—composed of platelets, fibrin, erythrocytes, and leukocytes—play a role in most MIs. Platelets within the thrombi release potent vasoconstrictors, including thromboxane A_2, serotonin, and thrombin. No one knows exactly what causes these thrombi to form, but plaque fissure and hemorrhage are predisposing factors.

The exact cause of coronary artery vasospasm is also unknown. Thromboxane A_2, released by the sympathetic nervous system during physical or emotional stress, is a precipitating factor. Other factors include cigarette smoking, alcohol ingestion, and cocaine use (see *Identifying MI risk factors*).

Classifying MIs

Myocardial infarctions can be classified as anterior, inferior, lateral, or posterior based on the area of heart muscle involved. They also can be classified by the depth of injury or the muscle layer involved. Infarctions usually occur in the left ventricular wall (called left ventricular MIs) and the interventricular septum because of the increased muscle mass and workload of the left ventricle. The particular coronary arteries involved also help determine the type of MI.

A subendocardial infarction involves the endocardium and the myocardium. A subepicardial infarction involves the epicardium and the myocardium. Because the endocardium has a higher oxygen demand than the epicardium, subendocardial infarctions are more common.

A transmural infarction involves all three muscle layers in the heart wall and produces a higher incidence of ventricular dysfunction. Transmural infarction affects both myocardial depolarization and repolarization.

Progression of an MI

When myocardial oxygen demand exceeds supply, anaerobic metabolism results. Lactic acid builds up in the heart muscle, stimulating nerve endings and producing a sensation of pain. If reversible, this sensation is called angina pectoris. If prolonged cellular hypoxia kills myocardial cells, however, the result is an MI.

Necrotic myocardial cells can lead to a decrease in contractility, stroke volume, and blood pressure. Hypotension stimulates baroreceptors in the aortic arch and carotid bodies, which in turn stimulate the sympathetic nervous system to release epinephrine and norepinephrine. These catecholamines increase the heart rate and cause peripheral vasoconstriction, which further increases myocardial oxygen demand.

In an MI, the area of dead cells is known as the zone of infarction. Surrounding the zone of infarction are zones of injury and ischemia. Both of these zones contain viable tissue. That's

---

Identifying MI risk factors

Myocardial infarction (MI) is most common in men over age 50 and postmenopausal women. Risk factors for MI mirror those for coronary artery disease:
- family history of MI
- cigarette smoking
- hyperlipidemia
- hypertension
- diabetes mellitus
- obesity
- sedentary lifestyle
- stress
- use of illicit drugs, especially cocaine and amphetamines.

---

why you need to recognize and respond to an MI quickly; prompt treatment can help preserve tissues in these potentially functional zones.

Characteristic changes in the patient's electrocardiogram (ECG) can help locate the zones of infarction, injury, and ischemia. In a zone of infarction, the lack of impulse conduction causes a pathologic Q wave. In the zone of injury, hypoxic cells don't fully repolarize, producing an elevated ST segment. The zone of ischemia has delayed repolarization, resulting in T-wave inversion on the ECG. In fact, impaired repolarization associated with the zone of ischemia produces many of the arrhythmias associated with MI.

The myocardium begins to heal within 24 hours after an infarction. Leukocytes infiltrate the area of infarction to degrade and remove necrotic tissue. Within 3 weeks, scar tissue begins to form. During this period, the patient faces the highest risk of ventricular wall rupture because absorption of necrotic tissue results in a thin ventricular wall. Within 6 weeks, scar formation is complete. Depending on the extent of the scar tissue, the heart's performance may be hampered by decreased myocardial contractility, altered ventricular wall movement, reduced stroke volume, reduced ejection fraction, and increased ventricular end-diastolic volume.

Assessment findings

Typically, an MI produces chest pain unrelieved by rest or nitroglycerin that lasts 30 minutes or more. Other typical findings include nausea, diaphoresis, shortness of breath, and a feeling of impending doom. The patient may be extremely anxious and restless.

Most patients describe the pain of MI as an overwhelming squeezing, pressing, or crushing sensation. Usually the pain is substernal, but it may radiate to the shoulder, neck, jaw, arm, or back. In some patients, the pain may be mild and mistaken for indigestion. In others—for example, diabetic patients—an MI may produce no pain at all.

If you care for a patient who complains of chest pain, perform a focused, thorough assessment addressing the history, onset, duration, and location of the pain and methods the patient has used to try to relieve it. In many cases, a patient with a history of CAD may report an increase in the frequency, severity, or duration of angina.

If the patient's right ventricle is involved, you may note jugular vein distention. Tachycardia and hypertension may result from sympathetic nervous system stimulation. You also may detect abnormal heart sounds (S_3, S_4, or a paradoxical splitting of S_2), a new systolic murmur (if papillary muscles are involved), and a low-grade fever. If the patient is experiencing a transmural MI or has developed pericarditis, auscultation may reveal a pericardial friction rub.

Diagnostic tests

The diagnosis of an MI is based on the patient's symptoms, cardiac enzyme measurements, ECG, echocardiogram, and scanning and imaging studies.

Cardiac enzyme levels

Cardiac enzyme level measurement is the most effective diagnostic test for MI. Cardiac enzymes are released from irreversibly damaged or infarcted myocardial cells. The enzymes released include creatine kinase (CK), lactic dehydrogenase (LD), and troponin (see *Tracking cardiac enzyme levels*).

CK, the most commonly assessed biochemical marker, has three isoenzymes that indicate muscle (MM), brain (BB), and cardiac (MB) origin. CK-MB is currently the most specific and sensitive indicator for diagnosing MI. CK-MB serum levels begin to rise 2 to 4 hours after an infarction, peak in 12 to 24 hours, and return to normal levels in 48 hours. Serial serum levels are drawn at admission and every 4 to 6 hours for 24 hours to monitor their rise and peak.

LD is composed of five isoenzymes. When myocardial cells sustain damage, the levels of isoenzymes LD_1 and LD_2 rise, with LD_1 rising higher than LD_2. The normal ratio of LD_1 to LD_2 is less than 1. With an MI, the ratio becomes greater than 1 and is said to be flipped.

Levels of LD rise 12 to 48 hours after an MI and peak in 72 to 144 hours. An LD_1 level that exceeds LD_2 suggests that an MI occurred at least 24 hours earlier. Analysis of LD provides a useful tool when caring for a patient who has delayed treatment for 24 hours or more after developing chest pain.

Cardiac troponin T and cardiac troponin I are proteins unique to the myocardium. They provide sensitive and specific tools to help detect an MI. Cardiac troponin appears 6 to 10 hours after the onset of an MI, and levels may remain elevated for days or even weeks. Cardiac troponin I has no skeletal muscle component and has been useful in detecting MIs in patients with cardiac contusions or perioperative infarctions.

Electrocardiogram

The second most effective diagnostic test is the ECG. If it shows T-wave inversion, ST-segment elevation or depression, and pathologic Q waves, the patient may have had an infarction. In most cases, a pathologic Q wave alone is diagnostic of an MI.

Evidence of ischemia may appear in a single monitored lead, but accurate diagnosis requires a series of 12-lead ECGs. Ischemia impairs repolarization and appears on the 12-lead ECG as inverted T waves. Prolonged ischemia results in myocardial injury, which produces ST-segment elevation or depression (depending on the lead

Tracking cardiac enzyme levels

Changes in cardiac enzyme levels can help determine the presence of a myocardial infarction (MI). This graph depicts the typical rise in the levels of three key enzymes after an MI: creatine kinase, troponin, and lactic dehydrogenase.

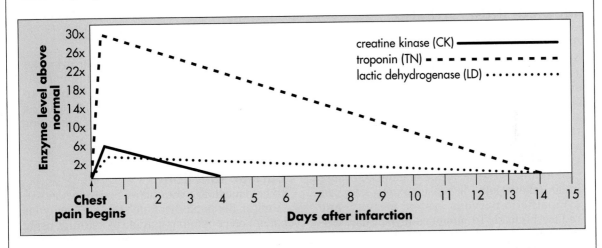

monitored). As injury progresses to infarction, cells die and conduct no electrical activity, producing a deep, wide Q wave. Typically, this pathologic Q wave is 0.04 second in duration and at least 25% the height of the R wave.

Echocardiogram

An echocardiogram can help assess abnormal ventricular wall motion and wall thinning, which correlate with ischemia and infarction. An echocardiogram also may reveal global systolic dysfunction. Transesophageal echocardiography offers superior visual images and more direct visualization of the atrium and great vessels; however, it has the disadvantage of being invasive.

Scanning and imaging studies

Radionuclide imaging may be used when the patient's history, ECG, and laboratory findings can't confirm an infarction.

Cardiac nuclear scanning with technetium 99m pyrophosphate has a sensitivity of 90%

when used 24 hours after an infarction. It's less sensitive when used within 24 hours or after 7 days. Thallium imaging can help detect an infarction 8 to 10 hours after the onset of symptoms, but it's less sensitive after 24 hours. However, both tests may not be able to distinguish a recent infarction from an old one. Cardiac nuclear imaging with antimyosine antibody can more accurately differentiate a recent infarction from an old one.

Magnetic resonance imaging can help diagnose an MI by revealing nonfunctional infarcted zones. And multiple-gated acquisition scans can be used to assess ventricular performance after an MI and to evaluate ventricular volumes, abnormalities in wall motion, and ejection fractions.

Additional tests

Additional diagnostic tests include chest X-rays and hematologic, coagulation, and serum lipid studies. A chest X-ray can determine the size and shape of the heart and may reveal excess fluid in the pulmonary vasculature. Hematologic studies can determine the blood's oxygen-carrying capacity. Coagulation studies determine serum clotting effectiveness and the risk of developing thrombi. And serum lipid studies help determine the risk of progressive CAD.

Medical interventions

The goals of medical intervention include preserving myocardial function, relieving pain, and controlling dangerous arrhythmias. The first 6 hours after an MI are the most crucial time for accomplishing these goals. During this time, the physician may attempt to reperfuse the myocardium through thrombolysis, percutaneous transluminal coronary angioplasty, or emergency coronary artery bypass surgery.

Morphine is the analgesic of choice because it can relieve pain, decrease anxiety, decrease sympathetic nervous system activity, and reduce preload. To minimize myocardial oxygen demand by reducing preload or afterload, the physician may give patients nitrates, beta blockers, and calcium channel blockers I.V. Or the physician may dilate the coronary arteries. Supplemental oxygen, rest, and a liquid or soft diet also help reduce tissue hypoxia.

Because most patients have ventricular arrhythmias early in the infarction period, the patient will need continuous monitoring of his heart rate and rhythm. A hemodynamically unstable patient may be monitored using a pulmonary artery catheter.

Because most MIs involve thrombosis, the patient may receive thrombolytic therapy with streptokinase, urokinase, tissue plasminogen activator, or anistreplase. These drugs convert plasminogen to plasmin, which dissolves fibrin clots. For thrombolytic therapy to be beneficial, the drug should be administered within 4 to 6 hours after the onset of symptoms. In fact, the earlier thrombolytic therapy starts, the better the result.

In addition to thrombolytic therapy, an anticoagulant, such as heparin, may be administered to decrease the risk of clotting complications. An antiplatelet drug (such as aspirin, sulfinpyrazone, or dipyridamole) may be given to decrease platelet release of thromboxane A_2, thereby decreasing vasopasms and platelet aggregation.

Additional diagnostic studies can help assess the patient's continuing risk and important components of short-term and long-term management. These studies include echocardiography and angiography to assess ventricular function and exercise stress testing to assess the heart's electrical activity.

Nursing interventions

If your patient has had an MI, your priorities include assessing and maintaining cardiac function, controlling pain, balancing myocardial oxygen supply and demand, recognizing and preventing complications, and educating the patient and his family.

Cardiac function

To help maximize your patient's cardiac output, monitor his hemodynamic status. Place your patient on continuous cardiac monitoring, using a lead that allows you to detect arrhythmias and ischemic changes. Monitor your patient's ECG tracing closely for changes. Also, assess his heart rate and rhythm and pulse.

If your patient has left ventricular failure, he'll probably need a pulmonary artery catheter to provide continuous hemodynamic monitoring. A pulmonary artery catheter will tell you the patient's pulmonary artery pressure and pulmonary artery wedge pressure (PAWP) and will help you determine his cardiac output (CO), cardiac index (CI), and systemic vascular resistance. Record these values every 2 to 4 hours or more frequently, as indicated. Report PAWP above 18 mm Hg, CO less than 4 liters per minute, and CI less than 2.5 liters per minute. Some hemodynamic monitors track cardiac output continuously. You also may need to monitor mixed venous oxygen saturation to assess oxygen supply and demand balance.

Also, monitor your patient's hemodynamic status by checking his vital signs, urine output, and peripheral circulation. Promptly report a heart rate at or over 100 beats per minute or under 60 beats per minute, a urine output under 30 ml per hour, pallor, cyanosis, and decreased peripheral pulses.

Assess your patient's level of consciousness (LOC). Note any restlessness or changes in responsiveness or heart and breath sounds.

Give medications as prescribed. Nitrates, beta blockers, and calcium channel blockers help reduce myocardial oxygen demand. Vasodilators and inotropic drugs improve cardiac output. Make sure your patient has at least two I.V. sites available: one for a thrombolytic followed by an anticoagulant and one for drawing blood. If he'll receive a nitrate, make sure he has three I.V. sites available.

If your patient is receiving thrombolytic therapy, monitor him throughout the infusion for signs of bleeding, including occult bleeding. Continuously assess his neurologic status for changes. Put pressure on any needle puncture sites, and protect the patient from bleeding or bruising. If you see any signs of bleeding, report them immediately. Expect to stop the infusion to reverse anticoagulation. Also, the patient may need such blood products as fresh frozen plasma to prevent possibly life-threatening complications (see *When a patient with an MI receives thrombolytic therapy*, page 98).

During and after thrombolytic therapy, monitor your patient's serum electrolyte levels, cardiac enzyme levels, and coagulation studies for changes.

Also, watch for complications, including:
• a hyperdynamic state, which produces tachycardia and hypertension
• hypotension from hypovolemia or decreased cardiac output
• reocclusion if the artery has been recannulized
• reperfusion injury and arrhythmias
• bleeding after cardiac procedures (such as cardiac catheterization or percutaneous transluminal coronary angioplasty).

Pain relief
Monitor your patient's pain carefully. Look for nonverbal indicators as well as changes in heart rate, respiratory rate, and blood pressure. Ask the patient to tell you immediately if he feels any chest pain. Emphasize that an early response to pain may reduce its intensity and duration and may reduce any further damage to his heart.

If an MI patient has pain, it usually means that myocardial ischemia is continuing. Relieving the pain decreases sympathetic nervous system activity as well as anxiety, which promotes balanced myocardial oxygen supply and demand.

Oxygen, nitrates, and morphine are first-line interventions for the pain of MI. After establishing I.V. access, administer morphine as prescribed. Morphine relieves pain—which, in turn, may lessen apprehension—and promotes vasodilation. After administering the morphine, monitor your patient's respiratory status carefully. Notify a physician if your patient's respirations fall below 12 breaths per minute.

Oxygenation and tissue perfusion
Diminished tissue perfusion causes cellular hypoxia and subsequent ischemia, cellular swelling, and cellular death. To combat these potential problems, you'll probably administer oxygen by nasal cannula at 2 to 4 liters per minute for the first 24 to 48 hours after an MI. Raise the head of your patient's bed to maximize lung expansion and increase oxygen supply.

If pain persists or if hypotension, dyspnea, or arrhythmias develop, continue administering oxygen as ordered. Use a pulse oximeter and monitor the patient's oxygen saturation levels continuously. Obtain and monitor arterial blood gas (ABG) measurements, as indicated.

Comfort, rest, and activity
Initially, your patient will be confined to bed rest to limit the size of the infarction and prevent complications. Emphasize the importance of complete rest for the first 24 hours; urge your patient to use a bedside commode. Also, help him with activities of daily living to minimize energy expenditures and thereby decrease myocardial oxygen demands. Provide frequent rest periods between activities, procedures, and treatments.

After the initial rest period, encourage your patient to increase his activity level gradually, depending on the extent of his infarction. Begin by having him sit in a chair for increasing periods of time, then progress gradually to walking. Suggest that your patient attend a cardiac rehabilitation class. Continually monitor

When a patient with an MI receives thrombolytic therapy

As you know, thrombolytic drugs can successfully dissolve artery-blocking blood clots. However, they also increase the risk of hemorrhage.

If you'll be caring for a patient who's receiving thrombolytic therapy, take the following measures before administering the drug:
- Establish at least two I.V. sites. To decrease the risk of reocclusion, your patient will receive heparin after receiving the thrombolytic. The second site allows for blood sampling without repeated venipunctures. If your patient will also be receiving nitroglycerin, establish a third I.V. site.
- Have antidotes to thrombolytic drugs readily available.
- Make sure your patient's blood has been typed and crossmatched and that blood is available for transfusion. Anticipate the need for coagulation factors in case of severe hemorrhage.
- Obtain laboratory samples for coagulation factors and hematocrit.
- Administer oxygen to increase tissue oxygenation.
- Explain all routines, procedures, and equipment to your patient. Tell your patient that some bruising at the administration site is normal.
- Administer the thrombolytic according to manufacturer directions, using an infusion pump.

Preventing complications
After giving the thrombolytic, take these measures to prevent complications:
- Administer heparin as prescribed to prevent reocclusion. The therapeutic goal of heparin therapy is to keep the activated partial thromboplastin time (APTT) at 2 to 2.5 times the control.
- Monitor your patient frequently for hypotension and tachycardia, which may indicate hemorrhage.
- Assess your patient frequently for ecchymosis, oozing, or bleeding from I.V. and arterial sites, previous puncture sites, and mucous membranes.
- Assess your patient at least every 4 hours for signs of change in his neurologic status that

may indicate intracranial hemorrhage. For example, watch for headache, altered level of consciousness, pupillary changes, paralysis, nausea, and vomiting.
- Administer an antacid or H_2 blocker to decrease acidity and prevent gastric bleeding. Assess your patient for gastrointestinal bleeding by auscultating bowel sounds, measuring abdominal girth, and checking for frank or occult blood in vomitus and feces.
- Administer stool softeners to prevent straining.
- Avoid giving your patient intramuscular injections or performing arterial blood sampling for 24 hours if possible.

Teaching precautions
If your patient needs long-term anticoagulant therapy, instruct him to take extra precautions:
- Review with your patient the actions, dosage, and potential side effects of the anticoagulant. Make sure he understands that he must take the drug at the same time each day.
- Stress the importance of keeping appointments to monitor the effectiveness of the anticoagulant.
- Instruct your patient to consult his physician before taking any over-the-counter medication because it may alter anticoagulant effectiveness.
- Tell your patient not to take medication that contains aspirin, ibuprofen, or naproxen. These medications alter platelet adhesiveness and promote bleeding.
- Instruct your patient to check his skin, mucous membranes, urine, and stool daily for bleeding.
- Teach your patient to use a soft toothbrush and an electric razor, to avoid contact sports, and to wear slippers or shoes when he's not in bed.
- Advise your patient to wear a medical identification tag.
- Tell him who to contact if bleeding occurs. Explain when and how to apply pressure to the site.

him for changes in vital signs, for complaints of pain, and for arrhythmias.

Don't forget that fear and anxiety initiate the stress response, releasing catecholamines that boost myocardial oxygen demand. Try to reduce your patient's anxiety level whenever possible. Provide a calm, nonthreatening atmosphere. Anticipate administering anxiolytic drugs or sedatives as needed to help reduce his anxiety.

Help your patient and his family express their fears and concerns. Explain the events happening around them and the rationale for needed treatments and procedures. Offer support and guidance.

Nutrition

Usually, only fluids and soft foods are permitted during the first 24 hours after an MI. This decreases the risk of aspiration if cardiac arrest should occur. And because fluids and soft foods are easily digested, myocardial oxygen consumption and basal metabolic rate decrease. As your patient's condition improves, he may begin to eat a low-fat, low-cholesterol, low-salt diet. Small, frequent meals may be better tolerated and also help to conserve your patient's energy.

Decreased activity and narcotic analgesics may cause constipation, so the physician may prescribe a stool softener to prevent your patient from straining. Remember, straining can change the blood pressure and heart rate, increasing myocardial oxygen demand and possibly triggering ischemia, arrhythmias, pulmonary embolism, or even cardiac arrest.

Patient teaching

During the acute phase of an MI, your teaching should focus on simple, concrete explanations and directions about the events going on around the patient. Provide explanations of the equipment being used, procedures being performed, and medications being given.

After your patient's condition stabilizes, focus on the disease process and needed lifestyle changes. Make sure your patient and his family understand the rationale for activity restrictions, dietary restrictions, and medications. Key areas to address include the following:
- underlying changes associated with an MI
- the extent of myocardial damage
- management of chest pain
- activity restrictions
- medication regimen
- risk factor modifications
- dietary modifications
- danger signs to report to a physician
- follow-up care.

Myocardial infarction and coagulation defects

Coagulation disorders come in two forms: coagulopathies, which involve inadequate clotting, and thrombotic diseases, which involve excessive clotting. Either form can exert a profound effect on the care of a patient who has had an MI. Coagulopathies, either inherited or acquired, increase the risk of hemorrhage when an MI patient receives an anticoagulant, an antiplatelet drug, or a thrombolytic. Thrombotic diseases increase the risk of MI and may increase the size of the infarcted area.

Pathophysiology

Under normal conditions, the hematologic system is in constant balance between coagulation and fibrinolysis. In patients with coagulation disorders, this balance is disrupted, complicating the treatment of an MI.

Coagulopathies

Coagulopathies result from a defect in the vascular reaction to an injury, in platelet plug reaction, in fibrin clot formation, or in clot lysis. The small blood vessels are most vulnerable in coagulopathy. Bleeding may appear as ecchymotic areas, petechiae, occult blood in feces, or oozing from mucous membranes. Persistent bleeding depletes the patient's coagulation factors and may worsen the clotting disorder.

Patients who have had MIs receive many medications that interfere with clotting and platelet function, the most common being heparin, aspirin, procainamide, nitroprusside, dipyridamole, propranolol, epinephrine, furosemide, anticoagulants, and thrombolytic drugs. Patients who receive vasodilators have decreased arterial constriction as well as reduced platelet aggregation and clot production.

Thrombolytic drugs are given to dissolve a clot. These drugs are used in conjunction with anticoagulants and antiplatelet drugs to decrease the risk of reocclusion. Thrombolytic drugs are usually contraindicated in patients with known coagulopathies.

Thrombotic diseases

Thrombotic diseases arise from excessively active platelets or clotting factors. Cigarette smoking, hyperlipidemia, hypercholesterolemia, atherosclerosis, high estrogen levels, and diabetes mellitus contribute to the problem. Clotting activity also is increased by factors that promote blood stasis, such as bed rest, immobility, dehydration, obstructed blood flow, edema, and heart failure. Clotting factors are also elevated by corticosteroids and oral contraceptives.

Thromboses of the arterial or venous system reduce blood flow distal to the site. If a vessel is completely occluded, tissue becomes necrotic distal to the site. Venous thromboses produce a localized inflammatory reaction that includes pain, warmth, and swelling. Arterial thromboses create acute circulatory symptoms of pain, pallor, coolness, and diminished pulses.

A patient who has had an MI is in a hypercoagulable state, raising the risk that his infarction will expand. Thrombosis may also develop in his peripheral veins, especially with prolonged bed rest, hypotension, or hypovolemia. Typically, antiplatelet drugs and anticoagulants are administered to counteract the patient's hypercoagulable state.

Adapting nursing care

Nursing care of the patient with an MI and a coagulation defect requires maintaining a delicate balance of blood clotting mechanisms to prevent hemorrhage while minimizing the risk of thrombosis. To accomplish this balance, monitor your patient closely for signs and symptoms of bleeding. Cautiously administer anticoagulants I.V., using an infusion pump to prevent overdosage. Remember that thrombolytic therapy is usually contraindicated in patients with a history of coagulopathies.

Obtain baseline coagulation studies, such as prothrombin time, activated partial thromboplastin time, platelet counts, and activated coagulation times. Then monitor these studies to determine the effectiveness of therapy and to maintain values within the therapeutic range. If your patient requires cardiac catheterization to determine the extent of damage or the need for angioplasty, explain the procedure to him fully (see *When a patient with an MI and a coagulation defect needs cardiac catheterization*).

Inspect the patient's skin closely for signs of petechiae, bruising, and ecchymoses. Check his urine and stool for occult blood. If bleeding occurs, notify a physician because it may be necessary to reverse the anticoagulation and administer blood products.

Perform safety measures to minimize the risk of trauma to the patient. For example, avoid intramuscular injections, not only to reduce the risk of bleeding but also to prevent an elevation of muscle enzymes that may interfere with serial enzyme monitoring. Apply pressure to all venipuncture sites for at least 5 minutes and all arterial puncture sites for at least 10 minutes or until bleeding stops. Inspect any venipuncture or catheter sites for oozing or bleeding.

Of course, a patient with an MI and a coagulation defect is also at risk for thrombosis. And the bed rest required in the initial phase of MI therapy can predispose the patient to stasis. Also, hypercholesterolemia, hyperlipidemia, and atherosclerosis—common in MI patients—increases the risk of thrombosis.

To promote circulation, encourage your patient to perform isometric exercises while he's on bed rest. Gradually increase his activity level as his condition permits. Encourage your patient to walk as soon as possible. Note any complaints of chest pain or ECG changes that occur when he increases his activity, and thus his myocardial oxygen demands. The key is to increase activity gradually, without causing ischemia.

Check your patient's arms for a positive Homans' sign, which may indicate thrombophlebitis. Evaluate pedal pulses and monitor your patient for pedal edema. If you note a decrease in color or pulses or if your patient complains of pain or paresthesia, notify the physician. To prevent stasis, tell your patient to avoid crossing his legs. Use alternating sequential compression devices as indicated to promote venous return.

If your patient is at risk for thrombosis, he's also at risk for emboli. Monitor his neurologic,

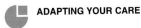
ADAPTING YOUR CARE

When a patient with an MI and a coagulation defect needs cardiac catheterization

Cardiac catheterization poses risks for any patient with a myocardial infarction (MI). But if the patient also has a coagulation defect, the risk of bleeding increases. If you're caring for such a patient, take the following measures before and after the procedure.

Before the procedure

• Fully explain cardiac catheterization to the patient and his family, both the reason for it and what to expect during and after the procedure. This will not only help the patient feel more comfortable about what will happen to him but may also help lower his myocardial oxygen demand by lessening his anxiety. Your explanation will also help the patient recognize and tell you if something seems to be different from your explanation, allowing you to intervene more quickly. Plus, he's more likely to comply with any restrictions after the procedure if he understands the reasons for them.

• Obtain baseline coagulation studies, including prothrombin time, activated partial thromboplastin time, and platelet counts. Make sure that the results appear on the patient's chart before the procedure. Point out to the physician any abnormalities or changes from the patient's baseline.

After the procedure

• Monitor the patient closely. Because of the coagulation defect, he has a higher risk for bleeding, so keep especially close tabs on his vital signs, electrocardiogram (ECG), and hemodynamic measurements.

• Watch for changes in pulse and blood pressure, which may point to bleeding.

• Assess the pulse on the operative side every 15 minutes for at least 1 hour, then every 30 minutes for 2 to 3 hours, according to hospital policy.

• If the physician inserted the catheter in the brachial site, take the patient's blood pressure in the unaffected arm.

• Monitor the patient's ECG for signs of increasing myocardial ischemia. Also, monitor coagulation studies for changes from the patient's baseline.

• Report decreased or absent pulses, extremity coolness, mottling, decreased capillary refill time, and cyanosis.

• Pay close attention to any complaints the patient might have. If he tells you he feels numbness, pain, or tingling at the insertion site, he may have an occlusion. Complaints of pain in the thigh, groin, or back could point to bleeding in the retroperitoneal area. Reports of increased pain or tenderness at the insertion site could be early signs of bleeding.

• To minimize the risk of bleeding, keep the patient's arm (for brachial artery insertion) or leg (for femoral artery insertion) straight. Tell him not to flex his elbow or hip for at least 6 hours. If the femoral artery was used, don't elevate the head of the bed more than 30 degrees or the risk of bleeding and hematoma formation will increase.

• Inspect the insertion site for hematoma, oozing, and bleeding. Report any such findings at once, and apply a pressure dressing or maintain pressure at the site with a sandbag that's 2.5 pounds to 5 pounds.

pulmonary, and renal status to detect this complication. Note any restlessness, anxiousness, or disorientation. Also, watch for decreasing oxygen saturation levels, pallor, cyanosis, and decreased urine output. Deterioration in these body systems may result from other causes as well, such as decreased cardiac output or hemorrhage.

Also, provide adequate hydration, but prevent fluid overload, which can further stress the already compromised heart. Monitor intake, output, and daily weights. Frequently assess your patient's lungs for adventitious breath sounds and his heart for abnormal heart sounds.

Complications

Common complications for patients with an MI and a coagulation defect include hemorrhage and cardiogenic shock.

Hemorrhage

Most MI patients receive heparin and aspirin, which increase the risk of hemorrhage. Thrombolytic therapy increases it even more. If your patient already has coagulopathy, these medications further increase his risk of hemorrhage. If hemorrhage occurs, cardiac output and tissue perfusion decrease, further compromising heart function.

Confirming the complication

The most obvious confirmation of hemorrhage is frank bleeding from puncture sites and mucous membranes and blood in vomitus, urine, or stool. Bleeding into the cranium, abdomen, or soft tissue may be more difficult to detect. Bleeding into the cranium may produce neurologic changes, such as changes in LOC or signs that warn of a cerebrovascular accident. Bleeding into the abdomen will produce an increasing abdominal girth and a rigid, boardlike abdomen. Bleeding into soft tissue will cause ecchymoses and, in an extremity, an increase in the extremity's diameter.

Decreases in the hemoglobin level and hematocrit may indicate bleeding or hemodilution. If you know that fluid overload isn't the cause of the decreases, investigate the possibility of blood loss. Chest or abdominal X-rays may reveal areas of hemorrhage. Computed tomography, magnetic resonance imaging, and arteriograms are more definitive in locating a source of bleeding.

Nursing interventions

All MI patients who receive antiplatelet drugs, anticoagulants, or thrombolytic drugs should be assessed for bleeding.

If your patient has received antiplatelet drugs, anticoagulants, or thrombolytic therapy, take the following measures to prevent or detect bleeding:

- Check for bleeding from all puncture sites.
- Check for the development of petechiae, purpura, ecchymoses, and hemorrhagic gingivitis.
- Check LOC and pupil reaction at least every 4 hours.
- Monitor urine, sputum, vomitus, and stool for frank and occult blood.
- Assess the patient's abdomen, arms, and legs and note tenderness, pain, or increasing girth.

- Monitor oxygenation status, including pulse oximetry and ABG values. Assess lung sounds. Instruct the patient to notify you if he becomes short of breath.
- Teach the patient to wear slippers or shoes when he's out of bed, to use a soft toothbrush, and to use an electric shaver rather than a straight razor. Also teach the patient to watch for blood in his urine and stool and to look for bleeding after brushing his teeth.

Hemorrhage is a medical emergency. If your patient begins to hemorrhage, he'll need prompt intervention to prevent hypotension, increased myocardial ischemia, and death.

RAPID RESPONSE ▶ If your patient starts to hemorrhage, notify the physician at once. Then take these measures:

- Place the patient in the supine position, with his legs slightly elevated to increase venous return.
- Apply direct pressure to sites where you see bleeding.
- Prepare to administer blood products and volume expanders, such as dextran.
- Administer normal saline solution or lactated Ringer's solution, as indicated, to increase vascular volume. If intravascular volume is inadequate, inotropic drugs such as dopamine won't increase blood pressure.
- Give supplemental oxygen if the patient isn't already receiving it. Monitor his oxygen levels using pulse oximetry or ABG levels.
- Monitor the patient's hemoglobin level and hematocrit closely. A drop of 1 gm/dl of hemoglobin points to a blood loss of 500 ml; an increase of 1 gm/dl should result from the infusion of 1 unit of blood. ◀

Cardiogenic shock

Cardiogenic shock refers to the heart's failure to effectively pump blood forward. This emergency occurs most commonly when more than 40% of the myocardium becomes dysfunctional as a result of ischemia or infarction. Cardiogenic shock occurs in about 15% of patients with acute MI. Other causes of cardiogenic shock include arrhythmias, papillary muscle rupture, and septal rupture.

The ventricles' impaired ability to pump an adequate volume of blood results in decreased

Compensatory mechanisms of cardiogenic shock

A common complication of myocardial infarction (MI), cardiogenic shock develops when ventricular function, primarily left ventricular function, decreases by more than 40% and the heart fails to pump blood efficiently into the circulatory system, causing a drop in cardiac output. To maintain adequate tissue perfusion, the body compensates by triggering a series of compensatory mechanisms, which are controlled by the sympathetic nervous system and the release of chemical substances.

Baroreceptors
The sympathetic nervous system triggers baroreceptors in the aortic arch and carotid sinus to release epinephrine and norepinephrine, which improve cardiac output by increasing peripheral vascular resistance, heart rate, and myocardial contractility. But the increased heart rate also increases myocardial oxygen demand, and results in further ischemia.

Eventually, oxygen delivery to the cells becomes inadequate. Aerobic metabolism shifts to anaerobic metabolism, producing less adenosine triphosphate and more lactic acid, which further decreases myocardial function. Poor blood flow prevents the removal of carbon dioxide, which then combines with water to form high levels of carbonic acid. These accumulating acids and other waste products act as powerful vasodilators, decreasing venous return and cardiac output.

As cardiac output continues to decrease, the sympathetic nervous system is continually stimulated, causing blood vessels to constrict. This constriction further reduces blood flow to the cells, causing hypoxia and acidosis. As they become worse, more myocardial cells are destroyed, which depresses contractility even more.

Fluid shifts
Sympathetic nervous system activity is aided when the hypothalamus releases catecholamines and vasopressin, which promote the movement of fluid from interstitial spaces into the blood vessels to restore blood volume. But as hypoxia and acidosis continue, destructive enzymes increase capillary and cell membrane permeability, causing fluid to move from the blood vessels into the cells.

Renin-angiotensin-aldosterone system
When renal ischemia occurs, the renin-angiotensin-aldosterone system releases renin, which is converted to a strong vasoconstrictor called angiotensin II. This conversion stimulates the release of aldosterone, which increases sodium and water resorption by the renal tubules to help maintain intravascular volume. Also, the posterior pituitary gland releases antidiuretic hormone to assist with this resorption of sodium and water. As cardiogenic shock continues, sodium ions begin to move into the cells and potassium ions begin to move out of the cells, causing hyperkalemia.

stroke volume and increased ventricular preload. The increased preload results in backed-up blood. If the right ventricle is impaired, blood backs up into the systemic circulation. If the left ventricle is impaired, blood backs up into the pulmonary system. The decrease in stroke volume results in decreased cardiac output, which leads to impaired tissue perfusion and decreased cellular oxygenation. A coagulation defect hastens the process (see *Compensatory mechanisms of cardiogenic shock*).

Confirming the complication
The initial signs and symptoms of cardiogenic shock—such as hypotension, decreased LOC, oliguria, tachycardia, tachypnea, and cool, pale,

moist skin—result from decreased cardiac output. The patient will be anxious and restless.

As the body loses its ability to compensate, the skin becomes cold, mottled, and cyanotic, and peripheral pulses disappear. Tachycardia and tachypnea worsen, and eventually bradycardia develops.

When compensatory mechanisms fail, myocardial ischemia worsens, and the patient develops angina and arrhythmias. Respiratory and metabolic acidosis and hypoxemia develop as the pulmonary system fails. As cerebral blood flow and oxygenation diminish, the response to stimuli decreases, and eventually neurologic deficits develop. The mortality rate for cardiogenic shock is 75% to 95%.

Nursing interventions

Because cardiogenic shock can cause rapid deterioration and death, you must intervene immediately and then monitor the patient closely.

RAPID RESPONSE ▶ Focus on enhancing myocardial oxygen supply, limiting myocardial oxygen consumption, and improving cardiac output. To enhance myocardial oxygen supply:

- Maintain a patent airway.
- Administer supplemental oxygen, and monitor oxygen saturation using pulse oximetry. If supplemental oxygen isn't adequate, the patient may need endotracheal intubation and mechanical ventilation.
- Monitor breath sounds, ABG values, capillary refill time, and skin color.
- Administer sodium bicarbonate and increase the ventilation rate and depth to correct acidosis.
- Give low-dose morphine as prescribed to promote venous pooling and decrease dyspnea as well as anxiety and pain.
- Continuously monitor your patient's ECG because hypoxia raises the risk of arrhythmias.

To limit myocardial oxygen consumption:

- Position the patient comfortably.
- Keep the environment as calm and quiet as possible.
- Administer nitroglycerin or other prescribed nitrate to reduce preload and afterload, improve stroke volume, and reduce myocardial oxygen consumption.
- Administer anxiolytics as prescribed.

To maximize cardiac output:

- Administer an inotropic drug, such as dopamine, as ordered to increase contractility, increase stroke volume, and raise cardiac output.
- Monitor the patient for hemodynamic instability. Monitor pulmonary artery pressures and central venous pressures at least hourly to evaluate your patient's response to therapy.
- Monitor blood pressure and mean arterial pressure. A mean arterial pressure under 60 mm Hg adversely affects cerebral perfusion.
- Titrate fluids and inotropic drugs to maintain a systolic blood pressure of at least 80 mm Hg. ◀

Be alert for complications. Monitor the patient for decreased urine output, abnormal renal function tests, falling arterial oxygen concentration, and a deteriorating LOC. Patients who need an intra-aortic balloon pump to improve the effectiveness of the heart's pumping action require special monitoring for complications, which include emboli, infection, aortic rupture, thrombocytopenia, improper balloon placement, balloon rupture, and circulatory occlusion of the cannulated extremity.

To decrease the risk of worsening heart failure, take these measures before discharge:

- Review the actions, dosages, and potential side effects of all medications. Your patient may be receiving several types of cardiac medications—angiotensin-converting enzyme (ACE) inhibitors to decrease myocardial wall thinning, vasodilators to decrease preload and afterload, inotropic drugs to improve contractility, and diuretics to decrease preload.
- Instruct your patient to report indications of peripheral edema, such as shoes or rings feeling tighter, and any increasing shortness of breath.
- Instruct your patient about a low-fat, low-salt diet. Teach him to read food labels to determine fat and sodium content. Initiate nutritional counseling if needed.
- Encourage your patient to enroll in a cardiac rehabilitation class.

Myocardial infarction and hypertension

A patient with hypertension has an increased risk of MI because of increased myocardial oxygen consumption and the accelerated atherosclerosis that results from damage to the intimal layer of the arteries. Mechanical stress on vessels from hypertension activates angiotensin II and promotes the growth of smooth-muscle cells, which decreases the arterial lumen. Also, a patient with an MI and hypertension faces an increased risk of an extended infarction because of increased myocardial oxygen demand. The risk is even greater if a hypertensive crisis caused the patient's MI.

Pathophysiology

Hypertension causes an increased resistance, or afterload, that the ventricles must work against—particularly the left ventricle. To develop more pressure to meet the increased afterload, the ventricular muscle hypertrophies. The increased muscle mass increases the myocardial need for oxygen and usually reduces ventricular compliance. Consequently, the myocardium has a decreased oxygen supply and an increased demand.

Nonhemodynamic factors that contribute to the development of left ventricular hypertrophy include high sodium intake, growth-promoting hormones (such as insulin and thyroxine), sympathetic nerve activity, the renin-angiotensin-aldosterone system, blood viscosity, glucose levels, and genetics.

As left ventricular mass increases in hypertensive patients, contractility decreases. These patients have decreased diastolic ventricular relaxation because of the increased wall thickness, which interferes with filling. Hypertensive patients with left ventricular hypertrophy risk sudden death from ventricular arrhythmias.

Adapting nursing care

If your patient has an MI and hypertension, you'll need to focus on decreasing his blood pressure without decreasing his cardiac output, thus maintaining adequate tissue perfusion. You'll also need to teach your patient what he needs to do to keep his blood pressure under control.

To accomplish this, first review your patient's history. Note which antihypertensive measures were prescribed in the past. Then, assess your patient's understanding of and compliance with those measures. If hypertension is a new diagnosis, your patient will need more extensive teaching, including teaching about treatment measures as they're implemented.

Make sure your patient understands that he'll need to restrict sodium and alcohol consumption. Teach him how to recognize foods and seasonings that contain sodium. Explain that he'll have to avoid adding salt to his food, even during cooking. Total daily sodium intake shouldn't exceed 2.3 grams a day. Explain, too,

that alcohol can elevate arterial blood pressure; he'll need to restrict his intake to no more than 1 ounce of alcohol a day.

If your patient weighs more than 10% above his ideal weight, you'll need to teach him about weight reduction. Teach him the kinds of exercises he can perform that won't exacerbate his MI. Use the exercise program outlined in his cardiac rehabilitation program as your guide. Explain to the patient that, even after his heart muscle has healed, he'll need to avoid such muscle-building exercises as weight lifting and wrestling; these can increase blood pressure to dangerous levels. Also, suggest relaxation techniques to further reduce blood pressure.

If your patient smokes, he'll need to give up tobacco completely. Provide encouragement to help him take this difficult step. Tell him to enroll in a program to help him quit as soon as he's discharged. Explain that his physician may tell him not to use any type of nicotine patch because the nicotine could strain his already-compromised cardiovascular system.

The physician may also order medications to keep the patient's blood pressure under control. Typically, drug therapy consists of a thiazide diuretic or a beta blocker. But if the patient has congestive heart failure from the MI, he may need a calcium channel blocker or an ACE inhibitor instead of a beta blocker. Explain the drug regimen to your patient and tell him that, if the prescribed drugs don't bring his blood pressure under control within 3 months, his physician will likely change his prescription.

Your patient will need close monitoring to determine his response to the measures taken to lower his blood pressure. If his blood pressure suddenly rises to dangerous levels, he may be experiencing a hypertensive crisis, which can cause further myocardial damage. If you observe such an increase in blood pressure, notify the physician and prepare to administer a potent antihypertensive drug, as ordered.

RAPID RESPONSE ▶ Medications commonly used to treat a hypertensive crisis include furosemide, nitroprusside, nitroglycerin, phentolamine, and labetalol. Your nursing care for a patient in hypertensive crisis should include the following measures:

• Titrate the antihypertensive drug according to the target blood pressure set by the physician.

DRUG ALERT

Antianginals and antihypertensives: Dangerous interactions

Antianginals	Antihypertensives	Adverse effects	Nursing actions
• Calcium channel blocker (diltiazem, nifedipine, verapamil)	• Beta blocker (metoprolol, propranolol)	• Calcium channel blocker decreases heart rate and reduces blood pressure, causing profound bradycardia and hypotension. • Combination of beta blocker and diltiazem is most common cause of bradycardia.	• Monitor heart rate and blood pressure frequently. • Administer atropine for symptomatic bradycardia. • Administer a vasopressor for hypotension. • Administer 200 to 500 ml of volume expanders for hypotension and assess response. • Watch closely for signs and symptoms of heart failure.
• Nitrate (isosorbide, nitroglycerin)	• Calcium channel blocker (diltiazem, nifedipine, verapamil)	• Vasodilatory effects of nitrate may produce profound hypotension.	• Monitor blood pressure frequently. • Position patient supine with legs elevated if hypotension develops. • Administer 200 to 500 ml of volume expanders and assess response. • Watch closely for signs and symptoms of heart failure. • Decrease I.V. nitrate dosage to increase blood pressure. • Administer vasopressor cautiously to prevent increased myocardial oxygen demand.
	• Beta blocker (metoprolol, propranolol)	• Both drugs may cause hypotension. • Beta blocker prevents reflex tachycardia.	• Monitor blood pressure frequently. • Position patient supine with legs elevated if hypotension develops. • Administer 200 to 500 ml of volume expanders and assess response. • Watch closely for signs and symptoms of heart failure. • Decrease I.V. nitrate dosage to increase blood pressure.
• Any vasodilator (calcium channel blocker, nitrate)	• Diazoxide or hydralazine	• Vasodilator causes reflex tachycardia and hypotension, which increase myocardial oxygen demand at time of decreased oxygen supply.	• Monitor heart rate and blood pressure. • Request a prescription for a beta blocker to prevent reflex tachycardia. • Position patient supine with legs elevated if hypotension develops. • Administer 200 to 500 ml of volume expanders and assess response. • Watch closely for signs and symptoms of heart failure. • Administer vasopressor cautiously to prevent increasing cardiac workload and ischemia.

• Monitor your patient's blood pressure every 5 to 15 minutes during antihypertensive titration and every 15 to 30 minutes after his blood pressure stabilizes.

• Assess your patient for such complications as shock, myocardial ischemia, and arrhythmias.
• Watch for signs and symptoms of cerebral bleeding (confusion, stupor, seizures, coma);

a rapidly decreasing blood pressure may cause cerebral ischemia.

- Monitor your patient's fluid intake and output hourly; a hypertensive crisis can trigger acute renal failure.
- Watch for drug interactions that adversely affect cardiac output (see *Antianginals and antihypertensives: Dangerous interactions*).
- If your patient is also receiving nitroprusside, monitor him for thiocyanate toxicity. (Thiocyanate is a metabolite of nitroprusside.) Check his blood levels for thiocyanate, and look for signs and symptoms of toxicity, including fatigue, nausea, disorientation, psychosis, seizures, and tachycardia. ◀

Complications

Common complications for patients with an MI and hypertension include arrhythmias and aortic aneurysm.

Arrhythmias

About 95% of patients who have an MI develop arrhythmias afterward. The most common cause of arrhythmias after an MI is ischemia of the pacemaker cells. Such ischemia may alter the discharge of the SA node, enhance its automaticity, or cause circus reentry. In patients with hypertension, the hypertrophic ventricle increases the risk of arrhythmias because of its resistance to microvascular perfusion, which results in ischemia.

Myocardial ischemia may cause all types of arrhythmias, including atrioventricular conduction defects and ventricular ectopy. Acute, severe ischemia may lead to ventricular tachycardia, ventricular fibrillation, and sudden death. Arrhythmias may further increase ischemia by decreasing myocardial oxygen supply or increasing myocardial demand.

Besides ischemia, arrhythmias also may result from reperfusion after thrombolytic therapy, electrolyte imbalances, acid-base imbalances, hemodynamic instability, digoxin toxicity, and chamber dilation.

Confirming the complication

Irregular peripheral pulses and heart sounds indicate arrhythmias. A diagnosis of the exact arrhythmia is determined by cardiac monitoring and 12-lead ECG (see *Characteristics of cardiac arrhythmias*, pages 108 and 109).

Nursing interventions

Key nursing interventions for hypertensive patients who develop arrhythmias after an MI are similar to those for any patient who develops arrhythmias after an MI. Interventions include controlling the arrhythmia, maintaining cardiac output, and promoting cardiac perfusion. You'll use cardiac monitoring to detect the arrhythmia and help evaluate the effectiveness of therapy.

RAPID RESPONSE ▶ Any arrhythmia that might result in cardiac compromise calls for immediate action. Whenever you detect an arrhythmia, take these measures:

- Check the patient's LOC, and check for a pulse. If the patient is pulseless, call for help and begin cardiopulmonary resuscitation (CPR).
- If the patient has a pulse, assess him for evidence of hemodynamic compromise, such as hypotension; an irregular, rapid, or slow pulse; dyspnea; tachypnea; chest discomfort; decreased LOC; dizziness; and pallor.
- If he's hypotensive, position him on his back with his legs elevated, remove any transdermal nitrate patches, and administer fluids I.V. to expand blood volume. If the patient is receiving a vasodilator I.V., the administration rate should be slowed or the drug discontinued.
- Follow advanced cardiac life support (ACLS) guidelines for the specific arrhythmia the patient has.
- Be prepared to use an external pacemaker, cardioversion, or defibrillation, if needed.
- Monitor and correct any imbalances in the patient's oxygen status, acid-base balance, and electrolytes (especially potassium and magnesium). ◀

Aortic aneurysm

About 90% of patients who have an aortic aneurysm, which is a localized dilation of the aortic wall, also have hypertension. The most common cause of aneurysms is a degeneration of the medial wall of the aorta, and hypertension increases the risk of medial degeneration.

Characteristics of cardiac arrhythmias

Arrhythmia	Description	Symptoms
Sinus arrhythmias		
Sinus tachycardia	• P waves followed by QRS complex • Heart rate 100–150 beats/minute	• Possible palpitations • If prolonged, may lead to decreased cardiac output
Sinus bradycardia	• P waves followed by QRS complex • Heart rate <60 beats/minute	• May cause decreased cardiac output • Light-headedness, faintness • Chest pain
Atrial arrhythmias		
Atrial tachycardia	• P wave present; may merge with previous T wave • QRS complex normal • Heart rate >150 beats/minute	• Palpitations • Anxiety
Atrial fibrillation	• Rapid, irregular P waves (>350 beats/minute) • Irregular ventricular rhythm • Varying ventricular rate, possibly increasing to 150 beats/minute if untreated	• Pulse deficit • Decreased cardiac output (if rate is rapid) • Possible thrombus formation in atria
Ventricular arrhythmias		
Premature ventricular contractions (PVCs)	• Early, wide, bizarre QRS complex; not associated with P wave • Irregular rhythm	• Possible palpitations • If frequent, may decrease cardiac output
Ventricular tachycardia	• No P wave before QRS complex • QRS complex wide and bizarre • Ventricular rate >100 beats/minute	• Decreased cardiac output • Hypotension • Loss of consciousness • Respiratory arrest
Ventricular fibrillation	• Chaotic electrical activity • No recognizable QRS complex	• No cardiac output • Absent pulse and respiration • Cardiac arrest
Ventricular asystole	• P waves possibly present • No QRS complex • Straight line	• No cardiac output • Absent pulse and respiration • Cardiac arrest

(continued)

The ascending aorta and the aortic arch are the most common sites of dissection.

Many patients with MIs have underlying atherosclerosis that decreases the lumen size of major arteries and increases the stress on the vessels. Coupled with the vascular changes associated with hypertension, these changes place the patient at high risk for developing an aortic aneurysm.

Confirming the complication

If an aortic aneurysm is increasing in size or if a dissection is developing, the patient may have signs and symptoms similar to those of an MI. Typically, he'll experience a sudden onset of intense, severe, tearing pain that may be localized at the site of the aneurysm or may radiate. An ascending aortic aneurysm produces central chest pain; a descending aortic

Characteristics of cardiac arrhythmias (continued)

Arrhythmia	Description	Symptoms
Impulse conduction deficits		
First-degree atrioventricular (AV) block	• PR interval prolonged over 0.20 second	• Warning of possible increased conduction problems
Bundle-branch block	• Normal sinus rhythm with QRS complex duration >0.10 second	• Warning of increased conduction problems, such as second-degree and third-degree AV block
Second-degree AV block	• P waves occurring regularly at rates consistent with SA initiation • Not all P waves followed by QRS complexes • PR interval may lengthen before nonconducted P wave • QRS complex possibly widened	• Decreased heart rate and cardiac output
Complete third-degree AV block	• Atria and ventricles beat independently • P waves occur without relation to QRS complexes • Ventricular rate possibly low, at 20 to 40 beats/minute	• Decreased cardiac output (with low rates) • Light-headedness, faintness • Chest pain

aneurysm produces pain radiating to the back, abdomen, or legs. The pain may move if the aneurysm dissects. Other signs may include severe hypertension, shock, acute neurologic deficits, absent peripheral pulses, a new murmur (caused by aortic regurgitation), and such GI signs and symptoms as acute abdominal pain and hyperactive bowel sounds.

To distinguish an MI from a dissecting aneurysm, a physician relies on cardiac enzyme measurements and an ECG. An MI complicated by a thoracic aortic aneurysm is usually confirmed by a chest X-ray that shows the aneurysm. For patients with suspected aneurysms, such diagnostic procedures as aortogram, magnetic resonance imaging, and computed tomographic scanning may confirm the diagnosis.

Nursing interventions

RAPID RESPONSE ▶ If a patient's aneurysm is dissecting or it's larger than 4 mm in diameter, prepare him for immediate surgery. Otherwise, take the following measures to control his blood pressure and pain:

• Insert two large-bore I.V. catheters in case he needs fluid resuscitation.
• If the patient is hypertensive, administer a potent vasodilator, such as labetalol or nitroprusside. Monitor his blood pressure continuously.
• Assess his cardiovascular and neurovascular status hourly. Hypotension, pallor, cool and clammy skin, and a decreased LOC may indicate an aortic rupture. Be prepared to administer a vasopressor and fluids.
• Continuously monitor his ECG. An aneurysm in the ascending aorta may dissect into the aortic valve, resulting in ST-wave and T-wave changes.
• Maintain a quiet environment.
• Assess and treat the patient's pain. Be aware that analgesics should be used sparingly because they may mask symptoms of dissection. Immediately report any complaints of new or worsening pain; such complaints may signal a progression of the dissection. ◀

Before your patient goes home, discuss activity restrictions, dietary restrictions, medications, and smoking cessation. Tell your patient to notify his physician if he has difficulty breathing, the surgical incision becomes infected, circulatory changes occur in his arms or legs, or he has increased abdominal or incisional pain.

Myocardial infarction and diabetes mellitus

Diabetes mellitus increases the risk of and worsens the prognosis for MI. In fact, diabetes is an independent risk factor for death after an MI, especially in patients under age 65. An MI, in turn, can elevate the diabetic patient's glucose levels, which may require treatment changes and worsen other conditions related to his diabetes. Together, these two disorders present a formidable pair—a pair that demands special attention and skilled application of your nursing expertise.

Pathophysiology

Over time, diabetes mellitus causes structural and functional cardiac changes that raise the patient's risk of ischemic heart disease, cardiomyopathy, and congestive heart failure. Poor glucose control, hyperinsulinemia, and lipid disorders speed the development of atherosclerosis. And diabetes raises the risk of thrombosis by altering platelet function, coagulation, fibrinolysis, and endothelial function.

As a result, patients with diabetes tend to develop atherosclerotic disease early. And they're more likely to have two or three diseased vessels. Their increased catecholamine sensitivity may constrict small arteries, worsening myocardial ischemia. And because of the neuropathies associated with diabetes, these patients may have atypical cardiac pain. If this lack of typical symptoms delays treatment for ischemic disease, the patient's condition becomes more complicated.

Initially, diabetic autonomic neuropathy affects parasympathetic neurons, leading to increased sympathetic tone, resting tachycardia, and vasoconstriction. Later, sympathetic neurons become affected, and the patient develops postural hypotension. Ventricular arrhythmias may develop, raising the patient's risk of sudden death.

Treatments used to prevent or treat an MI, such as percutaneous transluminal coronary angioplasty and coronary artery bypass surgery, tend not to work as well in diabetic patients because of their diffuse coronary disease.

Adapting nursing care

Because your patient may develop ischemia or an extension of his infarction without experiencing pain, you'll need to monitor his cardiac rhythm carefully for changes that reveal ischemia and infarction. Also, monitor his hemodynamic status to help detect the onset of heart failure. Check for signs of fluid overload by listening frequently for crackles at his lung bases and the presence of an S_3 heart sound (see *Preventing ischemia in a diabetic patient*).

If your diabetic patient is scheduled for percutaneous transluminal angioplasty to restore blood flow in the blocked coronary artery, remember that he may receive a contrast agent during the procedure. These agents can be toxic to the kidneys, especially if the patient already has some nephropathy. To reduce his risk, be prepared to administer mannitol I.V. 1 hour before the procedure. You'll also want to increase his oral or I.V. fluids after the procedure to help his kidneys excrete the dye. Monitor the patient's renal function after the procedure by checking his serum creatinine and blood urea nitrogen levels carefully for changes.

One of your most important goals for a diabetic patient who has had an MI is to help him control his blood glucose levels. You'll need to monitor his glucose levels at least four times daily.

Remember that patients not dependent on insulin to control their glucose levels may need insulin for a time after an MI. The bed rest required after an MI severely decreases the patient's activity. Because exercise helps lower blood glucose levels, the lack of exercise that results from bed rest may increase the patient's need for exogenous insulin. Also, keep in mind that patients usually able to manage a diabetic

COMFORT MEASURES

Preventing ischemia in a diabetic patient

If your patient with a myocardial infarction (MI) also has diabetes, try to keep him comfortable and calm. Why? Because if myocardial oxygen demand exceeds supply, patients with long-standing diabetes and autonomic neuropathy may develop undetectable—but life-threatening—complications.

Silent danger

In general, health care professionals are taught to recognize cardiac ischemia and infarction by a certain set of signs and symptoms, including chest pain, nausea, and diaphoresis. However, a diabetic patient may not have any of these warning signs.

So, if you're caring for a diabetic patient who has had an MI, be on the lookout for even the most subtle signs of continuing trouble. For example, watch for fatigue, vague shortness of breath, or reports of palpitations. If these problems develop, or if your patient experiences chest pain, remember that he may become very frightened, worsening his condition. Your swift interventions may not only restore comfort and calm but also prevent life-threatening complications.

Nursing interventions

Use the following guidelines as you care for a diabetic patient after an MI:
- When you introduce yourself and orient your patient to his room, ask him to tell you right away if he experiences any feelings of discomfort. Specifically mention feelings of chest pain, tightness, or pressure. Also mention sweating or nausea. Emphasize that, for him, signs of continued heart trouble may be more subtle than for patients who don't have diabetes.
- Tell your patient to report even atypical discomfort, such as fatigue, shortness of breath, palpitations, toothaches, or discomfort in the neck, back, or right arm. Use the term *discomfort* instead of *pain* to help him understand the meaning of atypical symptoms of angina.
- If your patient is on continuous cardiac monitoring, explain that the electrocardiogram (ECG) tracing on the cardiac monitor doesn't always tell you when the heart isn't getting enough oxygen. So you may have no way of knowing that something is wrong unless he tells you about any feelings of discomfort. Emphasize that, even if the discomfort turns out to be nothing,

you'd rather know about it. Assure him that he won't be bothering you.
- If your patient complains of discomfort or pain, assess it for intensity, quality, precipitating symptoms, location, and radiation.
- If your patient isn't already being oxygenated, provide supplemental oxygen. Give 2 liters of oxygen per minute by nasal cannula. Because patients with diabetes are susceptible to skin breakdown and delayed healing, check the nares for signs of impaired skin integrity from the nasal cannula. If your patient has skin irritation or breakdown, talk with his physician or respiratory therapist about switching to a face mask.
- If appropriate, monitor your patient's oxygenation with a pulse oximeter. To prevent skin breakdown, change the oximeter's location every 8 hours. If your patient checks his blood glucose levels with a fingerstick, avoid using the same finger for the oximeter and the fingersticks to reduce discomfort and trauma to the skin.
- If ordered, obtain a 12-lead ECG to help diagnose the area of ischemia. Monitor precordial lead placement sites for signs of skin irritation or an allergic reaction to the electrodes or conductive gel or paste. Change the electrodes every 24 hours to decrease skin irritation. If your patient develops a localized skin reaction, talk with his physician about prescribing a topical agent, such as hydrocortisone cream, to alleviate itching or burning. If your patient has an allergic reaction, replace the skin electrodes with a hypoallergenic brand.
- Administer antianginal and pain medications as prescribed and evaluate your patient's response.
- Make sure your patient follows his activity limitations. To help reduce his myocardial oxygen demand, provide him with frequent rest periods. Your patient will probably be on bed rest with bathroom privileges, but be sure to reposition him at least every 2 hours. Assess his skin for signs of pressure or breakdown.
- To reduce anxiety, explain routines, activity limitations, and equipment. Before each procedure, tell your patient what you're going to do. Maintain a calm, quiet atmosphere. If your patient is restless or overly anxious, administer anxiolytics (such as alprazolam) to decrease his myocardial oxygen demand.

regimen on their own may need help after an MI because of changes in their routine, their energy level, or both.

As your patient gradually increases his activity level, his insulin dosages may need to be adjusted to prevent hypoglycemia. Remind him to monitor his blood glucose levels frequently as he begins to participate in a cardiac rehabilitation program. Tell him that his physician will monitor his ECG regularly for ischemic changes as he increases his activity level.

Diabetic MI patients also require in-depth teaching about lifestyle changes needed to reduce the risk of another infarction (see *Teaching a diabetic patient after an MI*).

Complications

Common complications for patients with an MI and diabetes mellitus include hyperglycemia, hypoglycemia, and acute arterial occlusion.

Hyperglycemia

An MI induces the stress response, which increases endogenous glucose production by stimulating the sympathetic nervous system. If the hyperglycemia that results is severe, it can lead to diabetic ketoacidosis (DKA) or hyperglycemic hyperosmolar nonketotic (HHNK) syndrome. Both conditions lead to severe dehydration and electrolyte imbalances. Dehydration promotes microcoagulation, increasing the risk for further infarction. An electrolyte imbalance—especially hypokalemia—increases the risk of lethal arrhythmias.

Confirming the complication

Confirm hyperglycemia by checking your patient's blood glucose levels at least every 4 hours and correlating your findings with his signs and symptoms. Keep in mind that some patients may not have the signs and symptoms of hyperglycemia—polyuria, polydipsia, polyphagia, and fatigue—even though their blood glucose levels are high.

If the patient's hyperglycemia is severe, look for confirmation of DKA or HHNK syndrome. Indications of DKA include a fruity breath odor, restlessness, confusion, signs of dehydration, and Kussmaul's respirations. The patient's

blood glucose levels will range from 300 to 800 mg/dl, and his urine will test positive for ketones.

If the patient develops HHNK syndrome, he'll appear severely dehydrated, with multiple neurologic abnormalities that may be mistaken for signs of stroke. His blood glucose level may reach 2,000 mg/dl.

If your patient has DKA or HHNK syndrome, monitor his ABG studies for signs of acidosis and decreased oxygenation and his serum electrolyte levels for changes that could affect his heart. Also monitor his ECG for early signs of ischemia—the result of microcoagulation.

Nursing interventions

Your primary goal for a diabetic patient recovering from an MI is to prevent hyperglycemia. Hyperglycemic patients have an increased risk of arrhythmias and extension of the infarction.

Frequently monitor your patient's blood glucose levels, ABG studies, serum potassium levels, vital signs, and urine output. If your patient develops hyperglycemia, focus on changing his diabetic treatment to bring his blood glucose levels down, as prescribed. For the patient whose diabetes was previously controlled without insulin, this may mean starting insulin therapy; for the patient already using insulin, this may mean increasing his dosage or changing the insulin regimen.

If your patient develops DKA or HHNK syndrome, monitor him as frequently as every hour. Also, take immediate steps to reduce his blood glucose level, including starting fluid, insulin, and electrolyte therapy.

Fluid replacement: A crucial treatment, fluid replacement must be done quickly and carefully. RAPID RESPONSE ▶ Be sure to include the following steps when providing fluid replacement for a diabetic patient with an MI:
• Administer fluids as prescribed. Expect to give more fluid than you would to a patient with an MI alone, but less than you would to a diabetic patient with DKA. For a diabetic patient with DKA or HHNK syndrome, you'd normally expect to administer normal saline solution at a rate of 1 L per hour for an hour or more and then 500 ml per hour for the

Teaching a diabetic patient after an MI

A diabetic patient faces special risks after experiencing a myocardial infarction (MI). Before your diabetic patient goes home, provide him with complete instructions to prevent complications and help ensure a complete recovery. Emphasize an exercise program, a healthy diet, and smoking cessation.

Keep in mind that any patient would find it difficult to make all these changes at once. Work with your patient to help him decide which issues to focus on first, then help him devise a plan for success.

Exercise

Immediately after an MI, your patient will have to decrease his activity level to allow his heart time to heal. Explain to him and his family how important it is to adhere to these activity restrictions.

After 4 to 6 weeks, your patient will resume normal activities and begin an exercise program. To reduce myocardial oxygen demand, suggest that he avoid exercising in extreme temperatures. To prevent hypoglycemia, encourage him to check his blood glucose level before beginning to exercise and any time during exercise if he experiences unusual symptoms, such as extreme fatigue or dizziness. Suggest he keep snacks available, and tell him to eat a snack during prolonged exercise. (For example, after 30 minutes of exercise, he may need a snack that contains about 15 grams of carbohydrates, the equivalent of one starch or fruit serving.) Give your patient information about cardiac rehabilitation, or refer him to an exercise program.

Talk with your patient and his partner about when he can resume sexual activity. Inform him that nitroglycerin taken 5 to 10 minutes before sex may help prevent angina.

Diet

In addition to the diabetic diet your patient already follows, he will need to monitor his fat, sodium, and caffeine intake. Find out whether your patient and his family know how to read food labels to determine the fat, sodium, and carbohydrate content of foods. For patients and families that seem overwhelmed, consider making a referral for nutritional counseling.

Smoking cessation

If your patient smokes, urge him to quit. Ask if he has ever tried to quit before. Talk about why previous attempts failed, and offer advice for overcoming these problems. Also tell the patient that previous failures have no bearing on future success. In fact, some researchers believe that previous attempts to quit only make a smoker more likely to succeed. Tell your patient about smoking cessation programs in his area.

Discharge instructions

Review all postdischarge medications with your patient, including their actions, dosages, and potential side effects. If your patient will be using sublingual nitrates, reinforce correct storage and usage as follows:

- Instruct your patient to store the tablets in the original bottle.
- Advise him to keep the medication with him at all times but not to carry it next to his body.
- Instruct your patient to buy a new supply of tablets every 6 to 9 months and to throw out any tablets older than 9 months.

Provide a written copy of all discharge teaching for your patient and his family to review after they get home. Include the name of a person to contact if they have questions.

Because your diabetic patient may have autonomic neuropathy, instruct him and his family to watch for atypical symptoms of a cardiac problem, such as fatigue, dizziness, or shortness of breath. Tell him and his family what to do if signs and symptoms of cardiac problems appear and how to summon the local emergency service. To help reduce their anxiety, encourage the family to enroll in a cardiopulmonary resuscitation class.

next hour or more, with the amount given slowly tapered off as the patient's hydration status improves. But because your patient also has an MI, he may not be able to tolerate such a rapid infusion. Adjust the flow rate frequently, based on his tolerance.

- Watch closely for pulmonary edema, a telltale sign that the patient's weakened heart can't keep up with the fluid replacement. Also monitor his heart rate and rhythm.

- Assess your patient's lungs every hour, reporting crackles, dyspnea, cough, and frothy sputum immediately. Also report decreased pulse oximetry values. If you note such signs, slow the infusion rate at once unless instructed to do otherwise.
- Evaluate the effectiveness of fluid replacement hourly. Check your patient's vital signs, skin turgor, peripheral pulses, capillary refill time, urine output, and LOC. Also check serum osmolality every hour. A sudden decrease may trigger cerebral edema, a life-threatening complication.
- When your patient's blood glucose level approaches 250 mg/dl, change his I.V. solution to one containing 5% dextrose to prevent hypoglycemia. If hypoglycemia occurs, notify a physician and provide treatment as ordered. ◄

Insulin therapy: A key component in the treatment of DKA and HHNK syndrome, insulin therapy is most effective when fluid replacement therapy begins first. Take the following steps when administering insulin therapy:
- Expect to administer regular insulin because it works the fastest.
- Although insulin can be given I.V. or intramuscularly, administer it I.V., as prescribed, to prevent altering your patient's cardiac enzyme levels.
- Anticipate giving a small bolus dose of regular insulin followed by a continuous insulin infusion.
- Anticipate giving the patient with HHNK syndrome less insulin than a patient with DKA. Even though the patient with HHNK syndrome has a higher blood glucose level, he's usually more sensitive to insulin.
- Monitor your patient's blood glucose levels hourly. A rapid drop in blood glucose can trigger cerebral edema, so expect to adjust the infusion rate to allow no more than an 80 to 100 mg/dl drop in the patient's blood glucose level each hour.
- When your patient's blood glucose level reaches 250 mg/dl, anticipate stopping the infusion and switching to subcutaneous insulin to prevent hypoglycemia. If hypoglycemia does occur during the infusion, stop the infusion and notify a physician.

Electrolyte replacement: Hyperglycemia-induced osmotic diuresis eventually leads to hyponatremia, hypokalemia, hypomagnesemia, and hypophosphatemia—imbalances that may not appear until fluid resuscitation has begun. Hypokalemia creates a special concern because it raises the risk of lethal arrhythmias. RAPID RESPONSE ► Include the following steps when providing electrolyte replacement for a diabetic patient with an MI:
- Administer electrolyte replacement therapy as prescribed. Replace sodium by infusing normal saline solution. Be aware that replacing magnesium may improve cardiac contractility. Start potassium replacement only after the patient's urine output has exceeded 30 ml per hour. You may administer phosphate in conjunction with the potassium as ordered. But don't give the potassium phosphate faster than 1.5 mEq/kg/24 hours. If you do, hypocalcemia can result as phosphate levels rise (phosphate and calcium are inversely proportional in the body).
- Monitor serum electrolyte levels hourly to assess the effectiveness of therapy.
- Continuously monitor heart rate and rhythm.
- Check for signs and symptoms of hypokalemia (tachycardia, tremors, spasms, cramping, drowsiness, nausea, vomiting, and flattened T waves on an ECG) and hyperkalemia (bradycardia, decreased cardiac output, weakness, lethargy, confusion, and peaked T waves), which indicate the patient is at increased risk for arrhythmias. Report such signs at once. Be prepared to administer an antiarrhythmic if necessary. ◄

Bicarbonate therapy: Acidosis can lead to arrhythmias and cardiac depression. Alkalosis can depress the central nervous system and shift the oxyhemoglobin curve to the left, decreasing the amount of oxygen released to the cells. Therefore, bicarbonate therapy is reserved for patients with an arterial pH of less than 7.

If your patient is receiving bicarbonate therapy, take these measures:
- Administer bicarbonate I.V. as prescribed until the patient's pH returns to 7 or the bicarbonate level is less than 10 mEq/dl.
- Monitor ABG values hourly.

- Every hour, monitor respiratory rate and depth, breath sounds, and breath odor.
- Monitor the patient for hypokalemia because bicarbonate shifts potassium into the cells.

Hypoglycemia

A diabetic patient may develop hypoglycemia after an MI if his dosage of insulin or oral hypoglycemic doesn't decrease to correspond with his decreased food intake and activity level. Plus, drugs such as beta blockers and salicylates can produce hypoglycemia, and beta blockers can mask its signs and symptoms.

The signs and symptoms of hypoglycemia are nonspecific and easy to mistakenly attribute to other conditions in a patient who's critically ill. Unless you begin treatment promptly, your patient could quickly fall into a coma. And if the hypoglycemia activates enough sympathetic response to cause tachycardia and hypertension, myocardial oxygen demand may increase, raising the risk of myocardial ischemia.

Confirming the complication

Confirm hypoglycemia by checking your patient's blood glucose level and correlating it with his signs and symptoms. Initially, he'll probably be apprehensive, unable to concentrate, or light-headed. Next, he may develop slurred speech, trembling, and diaphoresis. You'll have to watch carefully for these signs and symptoms and interpret them shrewdly to avoid confusing them with decreased cardiac output or hypoxia.

Nursing interventions

Your diabetic patient will need monitoring of his blood glucose level at least every 4 hours during the acute phase of his MI. He'll also need frequent assessment for signs and symptoms of hypoglycemia. Suspect hypoglycemia any time a patient receiving insulin begins to act in an uncharacteristic manner. Watch your patient closely if he's receiving a beta blocker because it can mask common signs and symptoms of hypoglycemia, including tachycardia, diaphoresis, anxiety, and trembling. Watch for other signs and symptoms, such as fatigue, shortness of breath, and palpitations.

If a hypoglycemic patient is conscious and can take food or fluid by mouth, give him 10 to 15 grams of an oral carbohydrate. For example, give 6 to 8 Lifesavers, 4 ounces of orange juice, 6 ounces of regular soda, or 6 to 8 ounces of skim or 2% milk. If the patient is unconscious or can't take food by mouth, give 50 ml of 50% dextrose I.V. The patient's LOC should improve within a few minutes. Check the blood glucose level in 10 to 20 minutes to determine if the hypoglycemia has been corrected. If the blood glucose level is still low, repeat the intervention. After the patient's blood glucose level stabilizes, give a snack of complex carbohydrate and protein (peanut butter crackers or half of a cheese sandwich, for instance) to restore glycogen and prevent recurring hypoglycemia. Also, continuously monitor the patient's ECG for ischemic changes throughout the hypoglycemic episode.

Acute arterial occlusion

The patient with an MI usually has underlying CAD and atherosclerosis and usually is in a hypercoagulable state, predisposing him to arterial occlusion. If he's also diabetic, the risk is even higher because diabetes increases the risk of atherosclerosis. Uncontrolled diabetes also increases the patient's hypercoagulable state because polyuria leads to dehydration if the patient's fluid intake is restricted, as may occur after an MI. Dehydration, in turn, can lead to stasis and subsequent thrombus formation.

All this makes a patient with diabetes and an MI more prone to pulmonary emboli from venous thrombi carried through the vascular system. Emboli that lodge in small pulmonary capillaries decrease arterial oxygenation and, therefore, myocardial oxygen supply. These life-threatening pulmonary emboli increase resistance to right ventricular ejection and decrease blood flow to the left side of the heart. This resistance decreases preload, cardiac output, and blood pressure. The sympathetic response causes tachycardia and increased myocardial workload, thereby worsening the myocardial ischemia.

Confirming the complication

A patient with peripheral arterial occlusion will have pain, paresthesia, paralysis, pallor, pulselessness, and poikilothermy in the affected limb. These signs and symptoms confirm the diagnosis.

Typical signs and symptoms of a pulmonary embolus include dyspnea, pleuritic chest pain, tachypnea, and cough. Other signs and symptoms include hemoptysis, syncope, nonpleuritic chest pain, and palpitations. The definitive test for a pulmonary embolus is an arteriogram; however, a recent MI contraindicates angiography. A ventilation-perfusion scan may suggest the probability of a pulmonary embolus, but it can't provide a definitive diagnosis. ABG values may indicate hypoxia, but they can't identify its cause.

Nursing interventions

If you suspect a pulmonary embolus, your nursing interventions will focus on maintaining ventilation, oxygenation, and circulation. If your patient requires surgery, you also need to provide postoperative care. To maintain ventilation and oxygenation, watch your patient closely for indications of hypoxia. Take his vital signs every 15 minutes until they're stable, auscultate his heart and lungs every 2 to 4 hours, and monitor ABG values. Help your patient breathe more easily by placing him in the semi-Fowler position and administering oxygen. Administer an analgesic, such as morphine, I.V. to ease his pain and anxiety as ordered.

To help maintain circulation, you'll need to administer fluids for hypotension. However, because your patient has had an MI, give them with caution and be prepared to perform CPR if necessary.

Expect to begin either anticoagulation therapy with heparin I.V. followed by oral warfarin or thrombolytic therapy. In either case, monitor your patient for bleeding as indicated and check his coagulation studies.

If you suspect an acute arterial occlusion, you'll need to focus on quickly alleviating the occlusion and preventing further injury. Although the occlusion must be removed to save the limb, the MI and diabetes increase your patient's risk during surgery. So expect the physician to order thrombolytic therapy first. Closely monitor the condition of the involved limb, making sure you don't apply too much pressure or jostle it.

If your patient needs thrombolytic therapy for a pulmonary embolus or arterial occlusion, take steps prevent complications. If your patient requires long-term thrombolytic therapy,

teach him about the precautions he'll need to take.

If your diabetic patient has had an embolectomy, arterial bypass, or another surgical procedure after an MI, take these measures:
- Assess the limb for color, temperature, sensation, movement, edema, capillary refill, and peripheral pulses hourly for 12 hours.
- Assess the incision site for redness, edema, and drainage.
- Remind the patient to avoid crossing his legs.
- Encourage the patient to move the limb.

Myocardial infarction and thyroid disease

The thyroid gland serves as the body's energy center by secreting hormones that act directly on cellular activity levels. Quite literally, an increasing level of thyroid hormone means increasing functional activity in all the body's cells. A decreasing level means decreasing functional activity in all the body's cells. Either problem has the potential to complicate the care of a patient with an MI.

Pathophysiology

Hyperthyroidism complicates your care of an MI patient for several reasons. The most obvious is that excessive thyroid hormone stimulates the cardiac system, which increases heart rate, stroke volume, and cardiac output. In addition, hyperthyroidism can increase your patient's metabolism greatly. By boosting myocardial oxygen consumption, hypermetabolism caused by hyperthyroidism may result in an extension of your patient's MI. Uncontrolled hyperthyroidism can lead to thyroid storm and heart failure (see *Cardiovascular effects of thyroid disorders*).

In contrast, hypothyroidism accelerates the development of atherosclerosis by increasing low-density lipoprotein cholesterol levels and decreasing high-density lipoprotein cholesterol levels. It also decreases stroke volume (from hypocontractility) and causes bradycardia, which may decrease cardiac output to as little as half the normal amount.

The patient may develop cardiomegaly as interstitial and intracellular edema occur. He may also develop hypertension from increased peripheral resistance brought on by the hypothyroidism.

The good news about hypothyroidism is that it may offer some protection from an MI by reducing oxygen demand more than it reduces oxygen supply. But even though hypothyroidism can protect the patient from an MI by lowering the heart's workload, excessive or inappropriate treatment for hypothyroidism can increase the danger of angina or even MI by increasing the patient's metabolic rate and the heart's demand for oxygen.

Severe hypothyroidism may stem from a physical or emotional stressor, such as severe illness or sedative use in a hypothyroid patient. Sedatives further depress a central nervous system already depressed from inadequate thyroid hormones. The patient also risks heart failure from ischemia in myocardial tissues already performing poorly because of lowered metabolism.

Cardiovascular effects of thyroid disorders

Thyroid disorder	Cardiovascular effects
Hyperthyroidism	• Increased cardiac output • Tachycardia at rest • Loud heart sounds • Supraventricular tachycardias
Hypothyroidism	• Reduced stroke volume and heart rate (causes decreased cardiac output) • Decreased blood flow to tissues during exercise • Decreased intensity of heart sounds • Electrocardiogram changes, including sinus bradycardia, depressed P waves, flattened or inverted T waves, low amplitude QRS complexes, and prolonged QT intervals • Cardiac tamponade (rare)

Adapting nursing care

The first priority in managing your patient with hyperthyroidism is to decrease his metabolic rate. Be prepared to administer antithyroid medications (such as propylthiouracil) to block the conversion of thyroxine to triiodothyronine. If the patient develops serious tachycardia, he may need propranolol. Don't give your patient aspirin because it increases the conversion of thyroxine to triiodothyronine.

Other priorities include decreasing your patient's blood pressure with an antihypertensive, temperature with acetaminophen, and agitation level with a sedative. These interventions decrease myocardial oxygen demand and reduce the risk of further ischemia. Watch your patient's ECG carefully for such changes as ST-segment elevation, T-wave inversion, and increased Q waves. These could indicate myocardial ischemia.

For your patient with hypothyroidism and an MI, focus on preventing life-threatening organ failure that could result from a decreased metabolic rate. Provide supportive care, and administer thyroid hormone carefully to avoid hyperthyroidism, extension of the MI, and heart failure. Your patient's slower metabolic rate may cause his body to metabolize cardiovascular drugs more slowly, prolonging their action. So monitor your patient closely, and expect his physician to order a lower dosage.

Complications

Common complications for patients with an MI and thyroid disease include arrhythmias, hypertension, and hypotension.

Arrhythmias
The patient with an MI and a thyroid disorder is at high risk for arrhythmias, which may decrease cardiac output or increase myocardial oxygen demand.

Hyperthyroidism places a great strain on the heart, causing tachyarrhythmias and heart failure. Supraventricular arrhythmias, especially

How to treat your patient's bradycardia

If your patient has bradycardia but doesn't have serious signs and symptoms, take these steps:
- Continue your assessment, determining if he has Type II second-degree atrioventricular (AV) heart block or third-degree AV heart block. If he doesn't, continue to observe him.
- If he has either type of AV heart block, prepare for the insertion of a transvenous pacemaker. After insertion, evaluate the patient's tolerance and the mechanical capture of the pacemaker. (On a cardiac monitor or 12-lead ECG, this would appear as a pacer spike followed by a QRS complex.)
- Give the patient an analgesic and a sedative, as needed.

If the patient has bradycardia accompanied by serious signs and symptoms, take these steps:
- Begin treatment immediately while assessing him to determine if he has Type II second-degree AV heart block or third-degree AV heart block.

- As ordered, administer 0.5 to 1 mg of atropine I.V. every 3 to 5 minutes for a total dose of up to 0.04 mg/kg.
- Depending on the patient's condition, give dopamine or epinephrine, as ordered. Dopamine can be given I.V. at 5 to 20 µg/kg/minute. If the patient's blood pressure is low, the rate can be increased. Administer an epinephrine infusion at 2 to 10 µg/minute.
- Give isoproterenol, if ordered. Although included in the advanced cardiac life support (ACLS) guidelines, isoproternol is rarely used for bradycardia. When it is, it's given in low doses and with extreme caution because seriously ill patients aren't usually able to tolerate its effects.
- If the patient's heart rate doesn't improve with atropine or he still has severe symptoms, a transcutaneous pacemaker may be applied.
- Monitor the patient continuously until his bradycardia resolves.

---

atrial fibrillation, are common. Left ventricular strain commonly shows up on the ECG as ST-segment depression and T-wave inversion. These arrhythmias typically don't respond to conventional treatment.

ECG changes seen most commonly in hypothyroidism include bradycardia, low voltage, a prolonged QT interval, and nonspecific T-wave changes. Atrial fibrillation with a slow ventricular response is common. Cardiac output is compromised by the decreased contractility and slow heart rate. The prolonged QT interval increases the risk that premature ventricular beats will fall on the vulnerable portion of the T wave and cause ventricular tachycardia.

Confirming the complication
Arrhythmias are confirmed by cardiac monitoring and 12-lead ECG analysis.

Nursing interventions
RAPID RESPONSE ▶ If your patient has had an MI, the bradycardia and tachycardia common to thyroid disorders require immediate intervention.

Perform the following interventions based on ACLS guidelines:
- Assess your patient's airway, breathing, and circulation.
- Ensure that your patient's airway is patent and secure.
- Begin oxygen therapy, as necessary.
- Insert and maintain an I.V. line.
- Begin continuous ECG monitoring, and attach a pulse oximeter and an automatic sphygmomanometer.
- Obtain vital signs.
- Review your patient's history, and assess his heart and breath sounds and peripheral pulses.
- Obtain a 12-lead ECG and a portable chest X-ray.
- Assess your patient for serious signs and symptoms, such as low blood pressure, shock, pulmonary congestion, heart failure, chest pain, shortness of breath, and decreased LOC. For further treatment guidelines, see *How to treat your patient's bradycardia* and *How to treat your patient's tachycardia.*

How to treat your patient's tachycardia

If your patient has atrial fibrillation or atrial flutter, he may not need treatment. But if either arrhythmia produces a rapid ventricular response with no other signs and symptoms, anticipate administering the following medications to slow his ventricular response:

- Calcium channel blockers or beta blockers.
- Digoxin, procainamide, or quinidine. Don't give propranolol I.V. less than 30 minutes after verapamil I.V. because profound bradycardia or asystole may occur.
- Anticoagulants to reduce the risk of arterial embolization if your patient converts to normal sinus rhythm.

If your patient has stable or borderline paroxysmal supraventricular tachycardia, take these steps:

- Begin with vagal maneuvers, such as carotid sinus massage, breath holding, and exertion of eyeball pressure, to redirect impulses back to the atrioventricular node. Other vagal maneuvers include immersing your patient's face in ice water; inserting a nasogastric tube; stimulating the gag reflex with tongue blades, fingers, or oral ipecac; and circumferential digital sweeping of the anus.
- If vagal maneuvers aren't successful, give your patient 6 mg of adenosine I.V. push over 1 to 3 seconds, followed by a 20-ml fluid flush. If that doesn't work after 1 to 2 minutes, give a 12-mg dose of adenosine I.V. push over 1 to 3 seconds. If necessary, repeat the 12-mg dose one more time after another 1 to 2 minutes has passed.
- If your patient's ventricular rate remains high, evaluate the width of the QRS complex on the electrocardiogram (ECG) as well as your patient's blood pressure. If the QRS complex is narrow and your patient's blood pressure is normal or elevated, give 2.5 to 5 mg of verapamil I.V. as prescribed. After 15 to 30 minutes, administer 5 to 10 mg of verapamil I.V. if needed.
- If the ventricular rate still remains high, other drugs—such as digoxin, beta blockers, and diltiazem—may be tried.
- If these measures don't work and the QRS complex is narrow but the patient's blood pressure is low or unstable, perform synchronized cardioversion. If the QRS complex is wide, regardless of the patient's blood pressure, administer 1 to 1.5 mg/kg of lidocaine I.V. push.

- If lidocaine isn't successful, administer 20 to 30 mg per minute of procainamide up to a maximum dose of 17 mg/kg.
- If procainamide isn't successful, perform synchronized cardioversion.

If your patient has stable or borderline ventricular tachycardia, take these steps:

- Begin with a 1-mg/kg to 1.5-mg/kg dose of lidocaine I.V. push. If necessary, give 0.5-mg/kg to 0.75-mg/kg doses of lidocaine I.V. push every 5 to 10 minutes up to a total dose of 3 mg/kg. If ventricular tachycardia ends, start a lidocaine drip of 2 to 4 mg per minute to prevent a recurrence.
- If your patient doesn't respond to lidocaine, administer a steady infusion of procainamide I.V. at a rate of 20 to 30 mg per minute up to a maximum dose of 17 mg/kg.
- If procainamide isn't effective, administer 5 to 10 mg/kg of bretylium I.V. over 8 to 10 minutes. If ventricular tachycardia ends, start a continuous bretylium infusion at a rate of 1 to 2 mg per minute for a maximum dose of 30 mg/kg over 24 hours.
- If bretylium isn't effective, perform synchronized cardioversion.

If your patient has unstable tachycardia, take these steps:

- Determine your patient's ventricular heart rate. If it's greater than 150 beats per minute, prepare him for immediate cardioversion. While that's happening, the physician may try a brief trial of medications. If the drugs work quickly, the patient won't need cardioversion. But cardioversion shouldn't be delayed just to give the drugs time to work.
- You usually won't need to perform immediate cardioversion for a patient with a ventricular heart rate below 150 beats per minute. Instead, perform the cardioversion in a controlled manner, as follows:
Insert an I.V. line and begin oxygen therapy.
Attach a pulse oximeter and an automatic blood pressure device to your patient.
Make sure that intubation and suction equipment is readily available.
If time permits, premedicate your patient with a combination of sedatives and analgesics, as ordered.
Begin cardioversion after these medications take effect.

- Remember that in a patient with an MI, propranolol may be used to treat tachycardia caused by hyperthyroidism. Although it's not usually given to MI patients, propranolol is the drug of choice for a patient with hyperthyroidism because it decreases heart rate and contractility. ◄

Hypertension

Hyperthyroidism can increase blood pressure enough to cause hypertension. In a patient who has had an MI, hypertension increases myocardial oxygen demand, which may extend the area of infarction and compromise cardiac output. In addition, the ischemic myocardium's decreased contractility may result in increased end-diastolic volume and pulmonary edema.

Confirming the complication

Two or more abnormally high blood pressure readings confirm hypertension. Occasionally, the patient may also complain of a headache, but hypertension generally produces no other symptoms.

Nursing interventions

If your patient has an MI and hyperthyroidism, your quick recognition of hypertension and immediate intervention could prevent hemodynamic compromise and a possible extension of his infarction.

RAPID RESPONSE ▶ Earlier in the chapter, you read about nursing interventions needed to prevent complications in a patient with an MI and hypertension. In addition to those steps, do the following for a patient with hyperthyroidism:

- Administer antithyroid drugs as prescribed. They'll control thyroid hormone levels, the underlying cause of your patient's hypertension.
- Monitor your patient's blood pressure. Watch his ECG for ST-segment changes that suggest myocardial ischemia.
- Provide a quiet environment and minimize activity to reduce your patient's emotional stress. Stress can cause a dangerous increase in blood pressure. ◄

Hypotension

Episodes of hypotension are common after an MI. Hypothyroidism raises that risk because it reduces cardiac output, stroke volume, heart rate, and pulse pressure, which can lower blood pressure.

Confirming the complication

Abnormally low blood pressure measurements confirm hypotension. The patient may also have such signs and symptoms as dizziness, light-headedness, pallor, a decreased LOC, and tachycardia.

Nursing interventions

RAPID RESPONSE ▶ Severe hypotension in a patient with an MI and hypothyroidism requires rapid intervention to prevent decreased tissue perfusion, extension of the infarction, and death. If your MI patient has hypothyroidism and develops severe hypotension, take these steps:

- Place your patient in a supine position. Elevate his legs to improve venous return.
- Administer small fluid boluses, about 200 to 500 ml, and monitor their effect on your patient's blood pressure and cardiac output. Because his heart has been weakened by the MI, he's also at increased risk for pulmonary edema. So assess him frequently for signs and symptoms of fluid overload: crackles, coughing, frothy sputum, and an S_3 heart sound.
- Administer volume expanders (such as albumin and hetastarch) as prescribed.
- Administer oxygen. Monitor your patient's oxygen saturation with pulse oximetry.
- Administer inotropic drugs as prescribed. Monitor your patient for signs of increased myocardial ischemia: angina, ST-segment changes, and T-wave changes.
- Monitor your patient's thyroid hormone levels and start thyroid hormone replacement therapy as prescribed. Although rapid replacement usually causes no problems for young adult patients, it may cause angina, cardiac arrhythmias, heart failure, and even sudden cardiac death in patients with underlying heart disease. Consequently, anticipate starting with small doses and increasing them gradually.
- If your patient doesn't respond to fluid boluses and inotropic drugs, a physician may order an intra-aortic balloon pump to improve coronary artery perfusion and decrease the

left ventricle's workload. If you're assisting with this procedure, monitor your patient's hemodynamic status closely. Maintain a quiet, calm atmosphere. Explain all procedures to your patient. To decrease his anxiety and reduce myocardial oxygen demands, administer anxiolytics as ordered. Complications of an intra-aortic balloon pump include immobility, infection, and bleeding. ◄

Suggested readings

Abboud CF, Giuliani ER. Endocrines and the heart. In: Giuliani ER, Gersh BJ, McGoon MD, Hayes DL, Schaff HV, eds. *Mayo Clinic practice of cardiology*. 3rd ed. St Louis, Mo: Mosby–Year Book; 1996.

Effat MA. Pathophysiology of ischemic heart disease: an overview. *AACN Clin Issues.* 1995; 6(3):369-374.

Gersh BJ, Chesbro JH, Clements IP, Berger PB. Acute myocardial infarction: management and complications. In: Giuliani ER, Gersh BJ, McGoon MD, Hayes DL, Schaff HV, eds. *Mayo Clinic practice of cardiology*. 3rd ed. St Louis, Mo: Mosby–Year Book; 1996.

Gersh BJ, Clements IP. Acute myocardial infarction: diagnosis and prognosis. In: Giuliani ER, Gersh BJ, McGoon MD, Hayes DL, Schaff HV, eds. *Mayo Clinic practice of cardiology*. 3rd ed. St Louis, Mo: Mosby–Year Book; 1996.

Grossman E, Messerli FH. Diabetic and hypertensive heart disease. *Ann Intern Med.* 1996; 125(4):304-310.

Huether SE, McCance KL. *Understanding pathophysiology*. St Louis, Mo: Mosby–Year Book; 1996.

Jick H, Derby LE, Gurewich V, Vasilakis C. The risk of myocardial infarction associated with antihypertensive drug treatment in persons with uncomplicated essential hypertension. *Pharmacotherapy.* 1996;16(3):321-326.

Keffer JH. Myocardial markers of injury: evolution and insights. *Am J Clin Pathol.* 1996;105(3):305-320.

Kinney M, Packa D, Andreoli K, Zipes D. *Comprehensive cardiac care*. 8th ed. St Louis, Mo: Mosby–Year Book; 1996.

Lauer JE, Heger JJ, Mirro MJ. Hemorrhagic complications of thrombolytic therapy. *Chest.* 1995;108(6):1520-1523.

Melchior T, Gadsboll N, Hildebrant P, Kober L, Torp-Pedersen C. Clinical characteristics, left and right ventricular ejection fraction, and long-term prognosis in patients with non-insulin-dependent diabetes surviving an acute myocardial infarction. *Diabet Med.* 1996; 13(5):450-456.

Phipps WJ, Sands J, Lehman MK, Cassmeyer VL. *Medical-surgical nursing: concepts and clinical practice*. 5th ed. St Louis, Mo: Mosby–Year Book; 1995.

Rakugi H, Yu H, Kamatini A, et al. Links between hypertension and myocardial infarction. *Am Heart J.* 1996;132(1)(pt 2): 213-221.

Schlant RC, Alexander W, eds. *Hurst's the heart: arteries and veins*. 8th ed. New York, NY: McGraw-Hill Book Co; 1994

Thelan LA, Davies JK, Urden LD, Lough ME. *Critical care nursing: diagnosis and management*. 2nd ed. St Louis, Mo: Mosby–Year Book; 1994.

Williams K, Morton PG. Diagnosis and treatment of acute myocardial infarction. *AACN Clin Issues.* 1995;6(3):375-386.

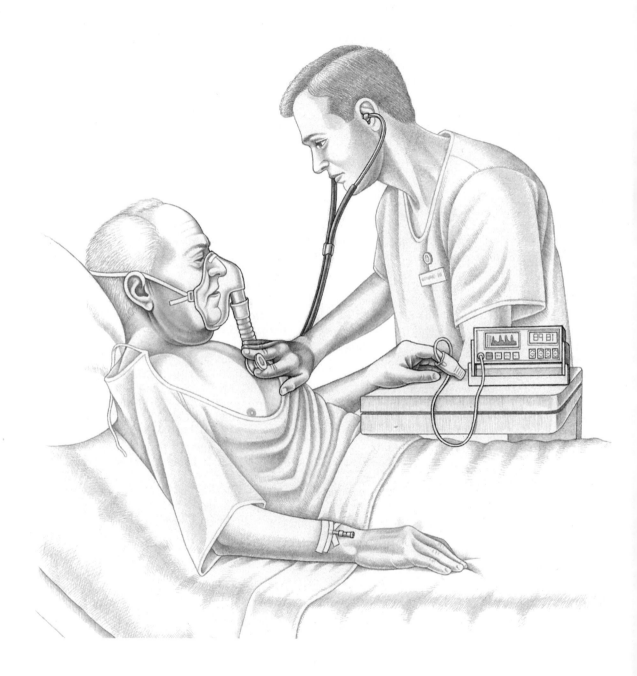

Heart Failure

4

In the United States, some 4 million people have heart failure, and about 200,000 die each year. The disease is particularly common among the elderly. In fact, it's the most common diagnosis among hospital patients over age 65—the very patients who are most likely to develop multisystem complications.

Other disorders common among patients with heart failure include myocardial infarction, pulmonary edema, and chronic obstructive pulmonary disease (COPD). In combination with heart failure, these disorders can give rise to such serious complications as reinfarction, cardiogenic shock, arrhythmias, cardiac arrest, deep vein thrombosis, atelectasis, respiratory failure, and renal failure.

Anatomy and physiology review

To understand what happens in heart failure, first briefly review the heart's structures and function. The key structures include the heart muscle, the heart valves, and the heart chambers. Together, these structures regulate the flow of blood throughout the heart and body.

Heart

Hollow and muscular, the heart lies in the mediastinum between the lungs. It lies slightly to the left of the midline and varies in shape and position according to a person's age and size. An average man's heart is roughly the size of a fist and weighs about 300 grams.

The heart is surrounded by the pericardium, which consists of the visceral and parietal layers separated by the pericardial space, a potential space lubricated by about 10 ml of serous fluid. The heart's muscular walls consist of three layers: the epicardium, or outermost layer contiguous with the pericardium; the myocardium, or middle, muscular layer; and the endocardium, or innermost layer contiguous with the valves and endothelial linings of the blood vessels.

The great vessels carry blood into and out of the heart chambers. The inferior and superior venae cavae return deoxygenated blood from the lower and upper portions of the body to the right atrium. The pulmonary artery arises from the right ventricle. Its right and left branches deliver deoxygenated blood to the right and left lungs, respectively. The pulmonary veins return oxygenated blood from the lungs to the left atrium. The aorta carries blood from the left ventricle to the rest of the body (see *Inside the heart*).

Heart valves

Consisting of dense connective tissue covered by the endothelial tissue of the endocardium, heart valves ensure that blood flows in only one direction through the heart. They open and close in response to pressure from cardiac contraction and relaxation.

The atrioventricular (AV) valves separate the atria and ventricles. The tricuspid valve separates the right atrium from the right ventricle. The bicuspid, or mitral, valve separates the left atrium from the left ventricle. Chordae tendineae, tendonlike chords on the AV valves, connect the valves to papillary muscles on the inner walls of the ventricles. Damage to the papillary muscle or chords can result in improper closure of the valves and backflow of blood into the atria during ventricular contraction.

The semilunar valves allow blood to flow from the arteries exiting the heart. They contain three moon-shaped cusps, which project into the blood vessel. As blood enters the vessels and the heart relaxes, these cusps tightly close, preventing a backflow of blood into the ventricles. The aortic semilunar valve lies between the left ventricle and the aorta. The pulmonary semilunar valve lies between the right ventricle and pulmonary artery (see *How the heart valves prevent backflow*, page 126).

Cardiac cycle

The cardiac cycle is a coordinated sequence of events that achieves one complete heartbeat. It consists of two phases: relaxation (diastole) and contraction (systole). During relaxation, blood fills the ventricles. During contraction, blood is pumped out of the ventricles and into the systemic circulation.

Deoxygenated blood enters the right atrium from the inferior and superior venae cavae, and oxygenated blood enters the left atrium from the pulmonary vein. The increased pressure opens the AV valves, allowing 70% of the blood to flow passively into the ventricles. Atrial contraction moves the remaining blood into the ventricles.

As blood fills the ventricles, ventricular pressures rise rapidly, closing the AV valves and preventing a backflow into the atria. This valve closure creates the first heart sound (S_1). When ventricular pressure becomes greater than aortic and pulmonary arterial pressures, the semilunar valves open. Blood is ejected from the ventricles into the aorta and pulmonary artery. As the ventricles relax, pressure begins to drop. When ventricular pressure

Inside the heart

The heart, a four-chambered muscle about the size of a fist, lies behind the sternum in the mediastinum, between the second and sixth ribs. Oxygen-depleted blood enters the heart's right side from the superior and inferior venae cavae. It then flows to the lungs by way of the pulmonary artery. Oxygen-rich blood enters the heart's left side from the pulmonary veins. The blood then flows into the systemic circulation by way of the aorta.

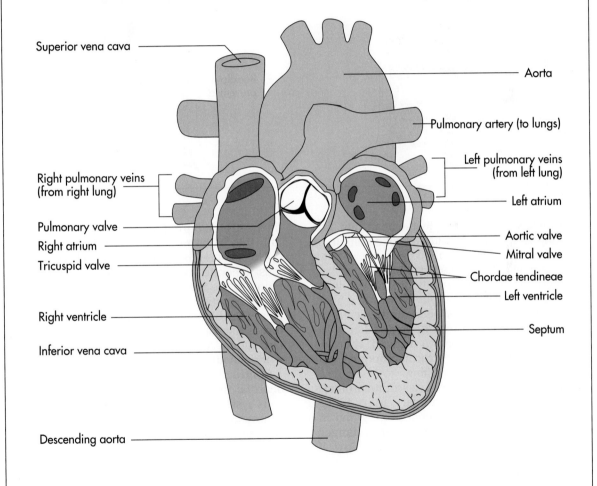

falls below the pressures in the aorta and pulmonary artery, the semilunar valves close, preventing a backflow of blood into the ventricles. This valve closure creates the second heart sound (S_2).

Cardiac output

Cardiac output is the volume of blood ejected from the left ventricle each minute—an amount that normally ranges from 4 to 7 liters. It's calculated by multiplying the stroke volume (the amount of blood ejected by the left

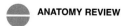

How the heart valves prevent backflow

Heart valves help ensure that blood flows in only one direction through the heart. Here's how: Rising pressure forces the cusps of the valve open, as shown in the illustration on the left. After blood passes through the valve, the cusps snap shut to prevent any backflow of blood, as shown in the illustration on the right.

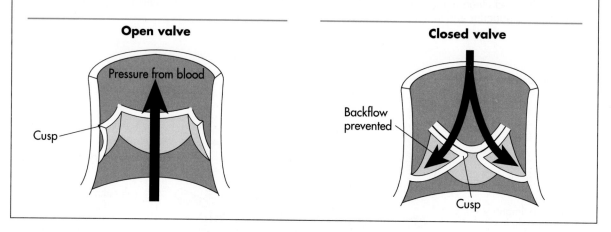

ventricle with each beat) by the heart rate. For example, in a patient with a stroke volume of 70 ml and a heart rate of 70 beats per minute, the cardiac output is 4,900 ml, or 4.9 liters.

Increases in the heart rate or stroke volume can increase cardiac output. However, a heart rate above 120 beats per minute or an increased heart rate in a damaged heart increases myocardial oxygen demand, shortens diastole (which reduces cardiac output), and reduces coronary artery filling.

Conversely, a decrease in heart rate prolongs diastole and increases coronary artery filling. It also enhances muscle contractility and increases stroke volume. However, a dangerously low heart rate (for instance, below 40 beats per minute) can reduce cardiac output because the ventricle can overfill and then can't force out the accumulated blood.

Factors affecting cardiac output

The three components of stroke volume ultimately affect cardiac output: preload, afterload, and contractility. Preload refers to the degree to which the left ventricular muscle stretches during diastole, specifically at the end of diastole. The more the ventricular muscle

fibers stretch during diastole, the more forcefully they'll contract during systole.

Afterload refers to the force the left ventricle must generate to open the aortic valve and eject blood to the rest of the body. Afterload is affected by total peripheral resistance, the diameter of the blood vessels, and blood viscosity—forces that resist blood flow in the peripheral circulation. As afterload increases, ventricular workload and oxygen demand also increase.

Contractility refers to the ability of the myocardial fibers to contract. Sympathetic nervous system stimulation increases the force of contraction, thus increasing stroke volume and cardiac output. Ischemia, hypoxia, and acidosis decrease contractility. A myocardial infarction (MI) decreases the amount of functional muscle tissue available for contraction, thus decreasing cardiac output. As cardiac output falls, the body attempts to compensate. Initially, increased sympathetic nervous system responses increase heart rate and stroke volume and cause arteriolar and venous vasoconstriction. The accelerated heart rate directly increases cardiac output by forcing more blood per minute from the left ventricle. The improved arteriolar tone leads to increased blood flow to the renal vessels and helps maintain blood pressure. The increased venous tone enhances venous return to the right side of the heart and improves cardiac output.

Pathophysiology

In heart failure, the heart can't pump enough blood to meet the body's metabolic needs. As cardiac output falls, perfusion to the organs decreases, resulting in tissue ischemia and, occasionally, infarction. As impaired contractility hinders the forward flow of blood, fluid retention and pulmonary congestion develop. Heart failure may develop slowly if compensatory mechanisms are activated, or rapidly if these mechanisms are overwhelmed.

Most commonly, heart failure results from ischemia caused by coronary artery disease (CAD). Ischemia causes heart failure by depriving the myocardium of sufficient oxygen to accomplish its work. Heart failure can also result if CAD leads to an MI, which decreases the amount of functioning muscle available to do the work. This, in turn, results in decreased stroke volume and cardiac output. The tissue surrounding the infarcted area may be ischemic, further impairing contraction.

Hypertension, the main cause of heart failure in African-Americans, is the second most common cause of heart failure overall. In many cases, it goes unrecognized or untreated. If untreated, hypertension increases afterload through vasoconstriction, increases myocardial workload, and causes muscle fiber hypertrophy. The hypertrophied muscle requires more oxygen, doesn't pump effectively, and eventually may fail. Sudden increases in blood pressure, as occur in malignant hypertension, may cause heart failure without left ventricular hypertrophy.

Mitral valve disease and septal defects can cause heart failure by interfering with the forward flow of blood. The heart fails when it's unable to compensate for the backup of blood.

Many patients with heart failure suffer from cardiomyopathy, which is classified as dilated, hypertrophic, or restrictive, depending on the nature of the myocardial dysfunction. In dilated cardiomyopathy, the ventricle enlarges, impairing systole. In hypertrophic cardiomyopathy, the thickened walls of the heart chamber, particularly the septum, obstruct aortic outflow and limit ventricular filling. In restrictive cardiomyopathy, the walls of the myocardium stiffen, compromising ventricular filling and weakening myocardial contractions.

Pulmonary diseases, such as COPD, also may lead to heart failure. In these diseases, hypoxemia leads to pulmonary vasoconstriction. This, in turn, causes the right ventricle to hypertrophy as it attempts to force blood through the pulmonary vasculature. Because of the congestion in the failing right ventricle, it can't collect all of the blood being returned to the heart. The result: organ congestion and peripheral edema.

Compensatory mechanisms

The body has several compensatory mechanisms that attempt to maintain cardiac output in the face of heart failure. These mechanisms increase stroke volume, cause vasoconstriction, increase fluid retention, redistribute blood flow, and produce ventricular dilation and hypertrophy. When the mechanisms can no longer overcome the effects of heart failure, decompensation occurs, and cardiac output again declines. Tachycardia, dyspnea, and organ dysfunction result.

Decreased cardiac output leads to decreased renal perfusion. Normally, the kidneys receive 20% to 25% of cardiac output. The juxtaglomerular cells of the kidneys react to decreased blood flow by secreting renin. The liver then produces angiotensin, which reacts with renin to form angiotensin I. Angiotensin-converting enzyme (ACE) then converts angiotensin I to angiotensin II. A potent vasoconstrictor, angiotensin II constricts the renal arterioles and stimulates the release of aldosterone from the adrenal cortex. Aldosterone causes sodium and water retention and potassium wasting. The increased fluid volume and increased preload further stretch the left ventricle, increasing cardiac output—at least temporarily.

However, when blood begins to stagnate in the heart, the walls of the atria and ventricles distend to accommodate the increased pressure and volume. Atrial distention triggers the release of atrial natriuretic factor. This substance increases sodium loss in urine, resulting in diuresis.

But at the same time, neurohormonal compensation for decreased cardiac output triggers the release of antidiuretic hormone (ADH) from the posterior pituitary gland. ADH stimulates the kidneys to retain fluid in the vascular space in an attempt to increase preload. The increased vascular volume eventually taxes the left ventricle and causes a further decrease in cardiac output.

Decreased cardiac output also activates the release of arginine vasopressin, another potent vasoconstrictor and inhibitor of water excretion. The release of prostaglandin E_2, a vasodilator, causes sodium retention.

In an effort to increase cardiac output, the body also stimulates the sympathetic nervous system to trigger the release of epinephrine and norepinephrine from the adrenal medulla. This leads to an increased heart rate and stroke volume, initially improving cardiac output. Venous constriction increases venous return, preload, and cardiac output. Arterial constriction decreases blood flow to the skin and peripheral tissues, allowing blood to be diverted to vital organs, such as the kidneys and brain.

The left ventricle dilates to accommodate more blood in an attempt to retain fluid and increase preload. Increased venous return and dilation of the left ventricle cause more forceful contractions. Eventually, as myocardial muscles are overstretched, the fluid retention and dilation overwhelm the heart muscle and decompensation occurs.

Another compensatory mechanism, ventricular hypertrophy occurs as the heart muscle works harder to eject blood. Initially, the larger ventricular muscle mass increases the force of contractions to propel the blood forward. Later, however, ischemia may develop as the enlarged myocardium's demand for oxygen increases and perfusion to the subendocardium is limited. A cycle of ischemia and increased diastolic dysfunction may result, leading to acute pulmonary edema.

Four ways of looking at heart failure

Heart failure can be classified according to the site of the failure, the effect on cardiac output, the effect on the direction of blood flow, and the acuity of the failure.

Site of failure

Each ventricle has its own role in maintaining circulation and is affected by its own stressors. Thus, one ventricle can fail while the other remains functional. Because the heart is part of a closed system, however, failure of one ventricle often progresses to failure of the other.

Left ventricular failure, commonly caused by CAD, hypertension, and other left ventricle disorders, results when the blood that isn't forwarded by the ventricle accumulates. As compensatory mechanisms are overwhelmed, the residual blood backs up across the mitral valve into the left atrium and pulmonary system, engorging the pulmonary vessels. This increases hydrostatic pressure within the vessels and causes fluid to shift into the alveoli. Pulmonary congestion and impaired gas exchange result. The impaired diffusion of oxygen leads to hypoxemia and such symptoms as dyspnea and anxiety. In the later stages of left ventricular failure, carbon dioxide can't exit, leading to respiratory acidosis.

Right ventricular failure results from pulmonary diseases, such as COPD and primary pulmonary hypertension. As the right ventricle fails, blood that's normally forwarded to the pulmonary artery and lungs backs up across the tricuspid valve into the right atrium. Because no valve controls the flow of blood from the venae cavae to the right atrium, back pressure continues to force blood into the venous circulation. Congestion of the liver's interstitial spaces develops, resulting in edema and weight gain. When the right ventricle fails to move enough blood to the left side of the heart, cardiac output from the left side decreases, even if the patient doesn't have left ventricular disease.

Cardiac output

When the body's metabolic demands are so great that normal or above-normal cardiac output can't meet them, the condition is called high-output heart failure. This occurs with sepsis, thyrotoxicosis, Paget's disease, and pregnancy. It may also develop when a large arteriovenous fistula is created for hemodialysis. When the left ventricle can't generate adequate stroke volume and cardiac output falls below normal, the condition is called low-output heart failure. This occurs with atherosclerosis, hypertension, MI, and valvular disorders.

Systolic failure refers to the inability of the left ventricle to contract adequately to eject enough blood into the arterial circulation. Diastolic failure results when the heart can't completely relax during diastole, causing insufficient filling. Because blood flows passively from the atria to the ventricles during diastole, the ventricle wall must relax fully to accommodate the incoming volume. In diastolic failure, the unyielding ventricles prevent complete filling and rely heavily on atrial contraction to receive blood. Therefore, any change in atrial contraction—from an atrial arrhythmia, for example—compromises ventricular filling and reduces cardiac output.

Direction of blood flow
Forward failure refers to the inability of the heart to pump blood to the body's organs to meet their metabolic needs. Reduced cardiac output results in decreased blood flow to vital organs and peripheral tissues. When this happens, mental confusion, muscle weakness, and sodium and water retention develop. Fluid retention increases circulating blood volume, further compromising the already failing heart.

Backward failure refers to the accumulation of blood in the ventricle, atria, and venous system that results from incomplete emptying or difficulty filling. Increased volume and pressure cause fluid to shift into the interstitial spaces, resulting in pulmonary congestion and peripheral edema. Because the heart is part of a closed system, forward failure eventually leads to backward failure—and vice versa.

Acute or chronic failure
Acute heart failure occurs suddenly and thus overwhelms the body's compensatory mechanisms. Usually it results from a myocardial injury, such as an acute MI. Chronic heart failure develops over months or years as the heart muscle is forced to work harder.

Assessment findings

Focus your initial assessment on the patient's ability to carry out activities of daily living. An older adult may attribute dyspnea and fatigue to aging rather than disease and simply limit his activities as these problems gradually develop.

New York Heart Association classification system

Classification systems, such as this one designed by the New York Heart Association, help you evaluate your patient's condition according to its effect on his ability to perform activities of daily living.

Class I
- No limitation on physical activity.
- Ordinary physical activity doesn't cause undue fatigue, palpitations, dyspnea, or angina.

Class II
- Slight limitation on physical activity.
- Comfortable at rest, but ordinary physical activity results in fatigue, palpitations, dyspnea, or angina.

Class III
- Marked limitation on physical activity.
- Comfortable at rest, but less than ordinary physical activity causes fatigue, palpitations, dyspnea, or angina.

Class IV
- Unable to carry on any physical activity without discomfort.
- Symptoms of cardiac insufficiency or angina may develop, even at rest.

Ask your patient about his typical daily activities and how they compare with those of several months ago. Use a classification system to document the degree of activity limitation (see *New York Heart Association classification system*).

Ask the patient about recent weight gain, nocturia, and the number of pillows he needs to sleep comfortably without shortness of breath (orthopnea). Also, ask about his typical diet. He may be especially thirsty because of aldosterone secretion.

The signs and symptoms of heart failure depend on which side of the heart is failing (see *Signs and symptoms of heart failure*, page 130).

Signs and symptoms of heart failure

Many signs and symptoms of heart failure result from rising capillary pressures. These pressure increases develop in the pulmonary circulation in left ventricular failure and in the peripheral circulation in right ventricular failure. Thus, the signs and symptoms of heart failure depend on which ventricle is failing.

Left ventricular failure	Right ventricular failure
• weakness	• weight gain
• fatigue	• peripheral or dependent
• confusion	edema
• shortness of breath	• abdominal distention
• orthopnea	• ascites
• paroxysmal nocturnal	• right upper-quadrant dis-
dyspnea	comfort
• cough	• anasarca
• crackles	• increased pulmonary
• tachycardia	artery pressure
• displaced point of maxi-	• hepatomegaly
mum impulse	• hepatojugular reflux
• alternating pulse	• jugular vein distention
• S_3 or S_4 heart sound	• indigestion
• increased pulmonary	• anorexia
artery wedge pressure	• nausea
• hypoxemia	• increased central ve-
• pleural effusion	nous pressure
• hemoptysis	• respiratory distress
• dependent edema	• nocturia
• tachypnea	• jaundice
• hypotension	
• oliguria	
• pallor or cyanosis	
• restlessness	
• anxiety	

Left ventricular failure

Fatigue typically results from reduced cardiac output; dyspnea results from pulmonary congestion. Dyspnea on exertion may progress to dyspnea at rest and to nocturnal dyspnea. Paroxysmal nocturnal dyspnea occurs several hours after the patient goes to bed, causing him to awaken with extreme shortness of breath that resolves when he sits up or walks. When the patient stands or sits, fluid pools in the legs and feet. When he lies down, the fluid is redistributed to the already congested pulmonary circulation, possibly causing orthopnea.

Other signs and symptoms of left ventricular failure include a dry, hacking cough and fine crackles, which you may hear first in the dependent lung fields. Chest pain may result from myocardial ischemia or ventricular hypertrophy. Tachycardia, arrhythmias, S_3 or S_4 heart sounds, confusion, pallor, and cyanosis also may develop. Cerebral hypoxia may result from the effect of decreased cardiac output on cerebral perfusion. The patient may be confused, weak, and dizzy. Hypoxemia from fluid-filled airways may cause restlessness, anxiety, or agitation. Premature ventricular contractions or ventricular tachycardia may indicate ischemia. Pink or frothy sputum may indicate pulmonary edema. Poor cardiac output may cause hypotension. You may also detect alternating pulse and a rapid respiratory rate. Inspection and palpation of the precordium may reveal an enlarged or left laterally displaced point of maximum impulse.

Right ventricular failure

Right ventricular failure is usually secondary to left ventricular failure and may produce peripheral edema, jugular vein distention, and weight gain. Bilateral pitting edema may occur in the feet, the ankles, and, if the patient is bedridden, the sacral area. As edema progresses, it moves up the legs and into the thighs, external genitalia, and lower portion of the trunk. Engorged tissues may cause the skin to crack from distention.

Weighing the patient is the most accurate way to assess fluid retention. A patient may gain 10 pounds or more before pitting edema develops. Abdominal distention, hepatomegaly, and mild jaundice may develop. With liver engorgement, the right upper abdominal quadrant becomes tender. As fluid accumulates in the abdomen, ascites develops. Eventually, the volume of fluid may displace the diaphragm, causing severe respiratory distress. The patient may report that his shoes feel tight, his abdominal girth is increasing, and his rings don't fit. Nausea and anorexia may result from liver and abdominal organ congestion. Usually, urine formation decreases during the day because blood pools away from the kidneys when the patient is upright. At night, when the patient is supine, nocturia may occur because urine formation increases as blood flow to the kidneys improves.

Diagnostic tests

A physician bases the diagnosis of heart failure on a patient's history and assessment findings. Diagnostic tests help to determine the underlying cause and the extent of the disease.

Chest X-ray
A chest X-ray helps determine the overall size and configuration of the heart. Typically in a patient with heart failure, it reveals cardiomegaly, pulmonary vascular prominence, alveolar or interstitial edema, or pleural effusions.

Multiple gated acquisition scanning
Multiple gated acquisition (MUGA) scanning helps detect abnormalities of wall motion and evaluate cardiac function, especially left ventricular function. In a patient with heart failure, a MUGA scan may reveal wall motion abnormalities and an ejection fraction (the percentage of blood emptied from the left ventricle during contraction) of less than 40%.

Electrocardiogram
An electrocardiogram (ECG) helps to identify problems with cardiac conduction, such as atrial fibrillation or tachycardia, which may result in impaired contractility. The ECG also shows left ventricular hypertrophy, left axis deviation, and patterns of infarction.

Hemodynamic measurements
Hemodynamic measurements provide information about blood volume, fluid balance, and the effectiveness of the heart's pumping action. In a patient with heart failure, hemodynamic measurements obtained by a pulmonary artery catheter may reveal a decreased cardiac output and index. In high-output failure, however, the cardiac output and index may be higher.

Along with congestion and increased circulating volume, heart failure also produces increased cardiac filling pressures, which may be detected by pulmonary artery pressure monitoring. Expect to find elevations in right atrial, right ventricular, pulmonary artery, and pulmonary capillary wedge pressures. Also, expect to find elevated systemic vascular resistance values, which reflect the rise in afterload and circulating blood volume.

Arterial blood gas analysis
Analysis of arterial blood gases (ABGs) may reveal a decreased partial pressure of arterial oxygen (PaO_2), indicating hypoxemia. Hyperventilation from hypoxemia may lead to respiratory alkalosis, indicated by an increase in pH levels. A drop in pH suggests that severe hypoxemia has lead to metabolic acidosis. A low bicarbonate level may also occur, reflecting metabolic alkalosis from diuretic use (hypochloremic alkalosis).

Serum electrolyte levels
Because of the fluid imbalance in heart failure, serum electrolyte levels commonly reflect dilutional hyponatremia and hypochloremia. Hypokalemia may result from potassium wasting caused by a diuretic. Or renal insufficiency may produce hyperkalemia. Hypomagnesemia may develop along with hyperkalemia, predisposing the patient to arrhythmias.

Albumin levels
As heart failure worsens, calorie and protein needs increase along with the body's increased metabolic needs. If albumin levels drop in response to malnutrition, decreased protein binding may allow increased amounts of therapeutic drugs to circulate in the blood, prolonging their action.

Renal and liver tests
Renal function studies evaluate the effects of decreased cardiac output on renal function. They may reveal increased blood urea nitrogen (BUN) and creatinine levels and decreased creatinine clearance. If blood flow to the kidneys

isn't restored, acute tubular necrosis may develop, leading to irreversible renal failure.

The results of liver function studies may reflect right ventricular failure. Serum lactate dehydrogenase, aspartate aminotransferase, alanine aminotransferase, and bilirubin levels may be elevated, and prothrombin time may be prolonged.

Medical interventions

The medical management of heart failure focuses on improving cardiac output, relieving dyspnea, and improving the patient's activity tolerance. Whenever possible, a physician corrects the underlying cause of heart failure.

Drug therapy
Typically, a physician prescribes a thiazide diuretic for mild heart failure and a loop diuretic, such as furosemide, for advanced heart failure. These drugs reduce vascular volume and cardiac workload.

Venous and arterial vasodilators may be given to decrease preload and afterload, respectively. Inotropic drugs increase the force of contractions and improve cardiac output.

A physician also may prescribe an anticoagulant if a patient is at risk for thromboembolism because of mural thrombi that form when blood stagnates in the left ventricle. An anticoagulant also may be administered prophylactically to a patient on bed rest. Higher doses of anticoagulants are used for patients with an acute MI, myocardial ischemia, or atrial fibrillation.

A physician may prescribe morphine to reduce preload and ease chest pain (see *Common drugs for heart failure*).

Diet
The cornerstone of treatment for patients with heart failure, a low-sodium diet enhances the effectiveness of diuretic therapy. Excessive sodium intake, on the other hand, triggers cardiac decompensation by increasing fluid retention. Many patients also benefit from restricting fluid intake to 1 to 2 liters per day.

For patients with cardiac cachexia caused by increased metabolic needs, a high-calorie diet may be recommended. These diets, typically high in protein and carbohydrates, provide increased energy for the activities of daily living and help to replace protein loss, which can worsen edema and affect drug levels in the blood. However, if the patient has renal insufficiency or failure, he'll need to restrict his protein intake.

Oxygen therapy
Oxygen may be prescribed to relieve hypoxemia and prevent myocardial ischemia. Usually, a patient receives 2 to 4 liters of oxygen per minute by nasal cannula to relieve dyspnea and myocardial ischemia. A patient with respiratory failure caused by pulmonary edema may require mechanical ventilation.

Activity
For a patient with heart failure, the goal is to balance exercise with rest periods. During acute exacerbations of heart failure, a patient may need bed rest or activity restrictions.

If the patient's condition permits, he can engage in an appropriate exercise program. Personnel in a cardiac rehabilitation program can work with the patient to develop an individualized exercise plan and monitor him for signs of distress.

Surgical and invasive procedures
If your patient's heart failure stems from ischemia, coronary artery bypass surgery may be used to restore blood flow and improve contractility and cardiac output. Or percutaneous transluminal angioplasty may be used to relieve obstructed coronary arteries and improve blood flow.

When the left ventricle fails to produce sufficient cardiac output, a physician may use an intra-aortic balloon pump. This procedure improves cardiac output in two ways. First, as the balloon inflates during diastole, blood flows into the coronary arteries, reducing ischemia.

Second, as the balloon deflates just before systole, aortic pressure drops, resulting in decreased afterload and ultimately increased forward blood flow. This temporary treatment is used until a patient's condition improves or he undergoes a procedure, such as heart transplantation.

Ventricular assist devices may also be used to support the heart until a patient recovers or undergoes surgery. These devices take over the pumping action of the left ventricle, the right ventricle, or both, restoring cardiac output and improving tissue perfusion. These devices may someday replace the need for heart transplantation (see *How ventricular assist devices work,* page 134). Transplantation is indicated for patients with end-stage cardiomyopathy or severe ischemic heart disease.

Nursing interventions

Nursing care for the patient with heart failure includes promoting oxygenation, maintaining fluid and electrolyte balance, administering drug therapy, and preventing complications. You'll also need to promote nutrition and elimination, provide a balance of activity and rest, and teach your patient about his condition and its management.

Oxygenation
Auscultate the patient's breath sounds for adventitious sounds, such as crackles, every 2 to 4 hours. Place the patient in the semi-Fowler or high Fowler position to relieve pulmonary congestion and shortness of breath.

Maintain the prescribed activity restrictions and promote a balance between exercise and rest. As your patient becomes more active, observe him for indications of worsening heart failure, such as increasing dyspnea. Also, watch for signs of hypoxemia, such as a dusky skin color and changes in mental status. Administer oxygen therapy, as ordered. Monitor oxygen saturation with pulse oximetry and check ABG values. Adjust oxygen therapy to maintain the oxygen saturation above 95% or the PaO_2 above 80 mm Hg.

Common drugs for heart failure

Diuretics
- thiazide diuretics (hydrochlorthiazide, metolazone)
- loop diuretics (furosemide, ethacrynic acid, bumetamide, torsemide)
- potassium-sparing diuretics (spironolactone, triamterene)

Inotropic drugs
- digoxin
- dopamine
- dobutamine
- amrinone
- milrinone

Drugs that reduce preload
- nitrates (nitroglycerin)
- morphine

Drugs that reduce afterload
- angiotensin-converting enzyme inhibitors (captopril, enalapril, lisinopril)
- hydralazine
- nitroprusside
- prazosin

Anticoagulants
- heparin
- warfarin

Fluid and electrolyte balance
Maintain precise intake and output records, and correlate your findings with your patient's daily weight. When you weigh your patient, use the same scale at the same time of day, preferably before breakfast, and make sure your patient wears similar clothing. Each kilogram of weight gained correlates to 1 liter of fluid retained. Maintain the prescribed fluid restrictions.

Decreased cardiac output causes fluid accumulation, particularly in the airways, thus reducing gas exchange. Anticipate administering a diuretic, such as furosemide I.V. at a rate of 20 to 40 mg over 1 to 2 minutes, to prevent hypotension and tinnitus. If refractory pulmonary congestion or edema develop, you may need to

How ventricular assist devices work

To improve a patient's cardiac output and organ perfusion, his surgeon may implant a ventricular assist device. The device, once called an artificial heart, will stay in place until the patient's heart recovers on its own or a donor heart becomes available for transplantation. These devices, which come in many different forms, are powered by air or electricity. This illustration traces the route of blood as it moves from the left ventricle through the pump of the ventricular assist device and into the aorta.

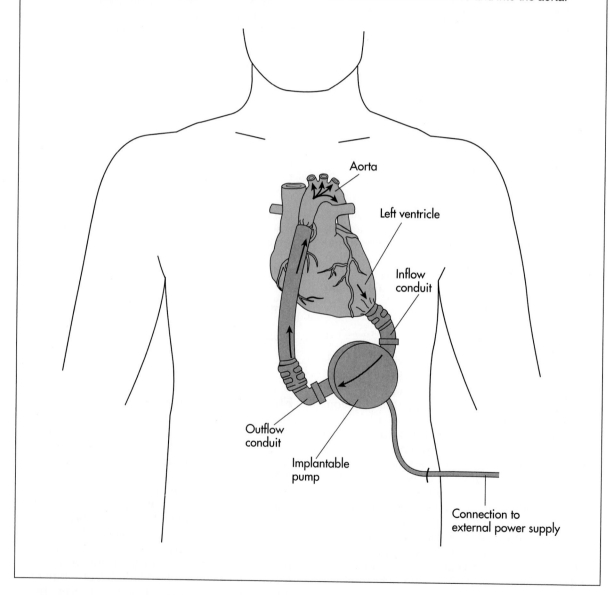

give a combination of diuretics. The physician may order oral metolazone to be given 30 to 60 minutes before a loop diuretic. For refractory oliguria, you may need to administer dopamine at 2 µg/kg/minute to improve renal and mesenteric artery flow and promote diuresis.

When giving diuretics I.V., you may need to insert an indwelling urinary catheter, so you can accurately monitor output hourly. The catheter also means that the patient will use less effort and less oxygen because he won't need to use the commode or make trips to the bathroom. Urine output should increase within 5 to 20 minutes of giving a diuretic I.V. Notify the physician if diuresis doesn't occur, if output is less than 30 ml per hour, or if crackles and dyspnea don't improve.

If your patient is receiving a thiazide or loop diuretic, monitor potassium levels frequently and be alert for hypokalemia. If you detect this electrolyte imbalance, the physician may order potassium replacement and switch to a potassium-sparing diuretic, such as spironolactone.

When administering a diuretic to correct fluid overload, watch for volume depletion that may lead to prerenal azotemia, renal failure, and hyperkalemia. Signs and symptoms of hyperkalemia include bradycardia and heart block, confusion, lethargy, anorexia, nausea, vomiting, visual disturbances, and peaked T waves on the ECG. Volume depletion also may cause hypovolemia and hypotension. Observe your patient for orthostatic hypotension and warn him to change positions slowly to prevent syncope.

Diuretics may also cause hypocalcemia. Watch for such signs and symptoms as irritability, seizures, muscle cramping, and respiratory stridor.

Additional drug therapy

Besides diuretics, drugs used to treat heart failure include nitrates, arterial vasodilators, ACE inhibitors, beta blockers, and inotropic and adrenergic drugs. When administering these drugs, monitor your patient closely to determine their effectiveness and any adverse effects. Auscultate his heart for S_3 and S_4 sounds, indications that heart failure is worsening despite drug therapy.

Nitrates

Nitrates cause vasodilation, thus reducing preload and, to a lesser extent, afterload. Topical, oral, or I.V. nitroglycerin or isosorbide may be prescribed. If the physician prescribes a topical nitrate, rotate the application sites and remove the old medication completely before applying new medication.

Monitor the patient's blood pressure and observe him for adverse reactions, such as headache, orthostatic hypotension, and dizziness. You may need to administer acetaminophen to relieve a nitrate-induced headache. Also, monitor the patient's heart rate and be alert for compensatory tachycardia as blood pressure decreases. To prevent nitrate tolerance, which reduces the medication's efficacy, the physician may prescribe a nitrate-free period of 8 to 12 hours, usually at night.

Arterial vasodilators

Arterial vasodilators such as hydralazine reduce afterload and thus decrease the workload of the left ventricle. Before administering a vasodilator, assess the patient's blood pressure. Although typically thought of as antihypertensives, vasodilators can be given to patients with systolic blood pressures as low as 80 mm Hg to decrease ventricular workload.

If other vasodilators fail, a physician may order I.V. nitroprusside. If he does, expect the patient to have an arterial line inserted for continuous blood pressure monitoring. Because nitroprusside is metabolized to thiocyanate, you'll also need to monitor your patient's serum levels and assess him for signs of thiocyanate toxicity, such as tinnitus and blurred vision.

Teach a patient who is receiving any vasodilator about orthostatic hypotension. Advise him to rise slowly from a sitting or lying position.

ACE inhibitors

ACE inhibitors decrease peripheral resistance, blood pressure, pulmonary artery wedge pressure, and pulmonary vascular resistance. Because these medications reduce the work of the left ventricle and improve blood flow, cardiac output improves.

Use ACE inhibitors cautiously in patients with renal failure and in those also receiving potassium-sparing diuretics because the risk of hyperkalemia increases. To prevent orthostatic hypotension, caution the patient to rise slowly from a sitting or lying position. To minimize the risk of hyperkalemia, tell him to avoid using salt substitutes that contain potassium as well as foods high in potassium, such as oranges. Expect to discontinue ACE inhibitor therapy if your patient develops a dry cough while taking the drug.

Beta blockers

To blunt the sympathetic release of catecholamines—which can dangerously increase heart rate and myocardial oxygen consumption and decrease diastolic filling in a patient with heart failure—the physician may order small doses of a beta blocker. Beta blockers also inhibit the renin-angiotensin-aldosterone system, the compensatory mechanism that increases sodium and water retention.

Never abruptly discontinue a beta blocker because rebound hypertension, angina, or myocardial decompensation may result. Beta blockers may be contraindicated in patients with COPD, bradycardia, or heart block and should be used cautiously in diabetic patients.

Inotropic drugs

Inotropic drugs, such as digoxin, are used to increase cardiac output. Digoxin increases the force of contraction and renal perfusion and reduces pulmonary and systemic congestion. Before administering digoxin, obtain baseline potassium, BUN, and creatinine levels. Expect to give an initial loading dose of 0.5 to 1.0 mg in two or three divided doses over 24 hours, followed by a daily dose of 0.125 to 0.25 mg.

Monitor your patient for indications of digoxin toxicity, including anorexia, nausea, vomiting, headache, malaise, visual disturbances, bradycardia, and arrhythmias. Be especially alert if your patient's renal function is diminished because digoxin is excreted through the kidneys. If he has renal insufficiency or renal failure, anticipate decreasing the dose or frequency to prevent toxic blood levels. If severe toxicity develops, administer digoxin immune Fab to neutralize the digoxin. If your patient will continue taking digoxin after discharge, teach him to prevent, recognize, and report digoxin toxicity. Warn him never to double a missed dose.

When a patient doesn't respond well to digoxin, a physician may order short-term use of amrinone and milrinone to relax vascular smooth muscle and improve cardiac output. Monitor the patient closely for adverse reactions, including thrombocytopenia and arrhythmias.

Adrenergic drugs

Low doses of dopamine, an adrenergic drug, may be administered to dilate renal and mesenteric blood vessels, promoting renal fluid loss. At intermediate and high dosages, dopamine improves myocardial contractility and increases arterial blood pressure, respectively. A physician may order dobutamine to improve cardiac output because it increases myocardial contractility with less tachycardia and peripheral resistance.

Expect to infuse dopamine or dobutamine through a central catheter to avoid extravasation. Be alert for adverse effects of these drugs, including arrhythmias, tachycardia, angina, and headache. Supervised by an infusion nurse, the patient may continue to receive intermittent infusions of dobutamine at home, using a central venous catheter or peripherally inserted central catheter.

Complications

As indicated, intervene to prevent or treat complications of heart failure, such as arrhythmias and thromboembolism. Be alert for the causes of arrhythmias, including myocardial ischemia, worsening heart failure, hypokalemia, and hypomagnesemia. To detect arrhythmias early, monitor the patient's cardiac rate and rhythm, check his vital signs frequently, and observe him for pulse deficits. Monitor the patient's ECG for arrhythmias, such as atrial fibrillation. Keep in mind that loss of atrial kick, which contributes as much as 30% to cardiac output, may exacerbate heart failure. Other ECG irregularities may indicate ventricular irritability from myocardial ischemia. Premature ventricular contractions may herald the onset of life-threatening arrhythmias.

To treat atrial fibrillation or atrial flutter, administer digoxin, as ordered. Digoxin controls the ventricular response by slowing conduction through the AV nodes. It also increases stroke volume and cardiac output, resulting in improved renal and systemic perfusion. Other treatments for atrial fibrillation and flutter include procainamide and cardioversion. Quinidine can be used for maintenance therapy after cardioversion.

Because blood tends to stagnate in the ventricles, blood clots can form. Eventually, clots can break off and travel through the circulation, possibly occluding blood flow to vital organs. To prevent this complication, a physician may prescribe an anticoagulant, such as heparin or warfarin.

Nutrition and elimination

Dyspnea, fatigue, and gastrointestinal (GI) circulatory congestion may prevent adequate nutrition. Offer your patient small, frequent meals, which may be better tolerated, require less energy to eat, and decrease oxygen consumption. Organize his activities and procedures to allow rest before and after meals. To decrease myocardial oxygen demand, administer bulk laxatives and stool softeners, as prescribed, and provide a bedside commode instead of a bedpan.

If your patient is taking a loop or thiazide diuretic, encourage him to consume high-potassium foods, such as bananas and orange juice.

Activity and rest

For a patient with heart failure, balancing activity and rest plays a crucial role in reducing the body's requirements for oxygen to levels that don't interfere with cardiac function. Until your patient's symptoms improve, he may need a program of rest or limited activity. As needed, help him perform self-care measures and activites of daily living. Allow for frequent rest periods.

If your patient has orthopnea, he may be more comfortable sitting up than lying down. If bed rest is needed, place him in the high Fowler position, using pillows for support. When he sits in a chair, keep his legs elevated to reduce venous pooling; if he has pulmonary edema, keep them dependent to decrease venous return. As his condition improves, increase his activities, as tolerated. A cardiac rehabilitation program may help increase his stamina and exercise tolerance.

Patient teaching

Effective patient teaching promotes independence and prevents readmission to the hospital. Teach your patient to recognize the signs and symptoms of heart failure. And tell him to notify his physician if he experiences a weight gain of 3 pounds or more in a week, progressive swelling of the feet and ankles, nausea, anorexia, palpitations, unusual shortness of breath or fatigue not relieved by rest, or a persistent cough. Review measures to modify such risk factors as smoking, sedentary lifestyle, and excessive alcohol consumption.

Teach your patient about his medication regimen, including the names of the prescribed drugs, their purposes, and their adverse effects. Help him develop an individualized dosage schedule. Try to identify any obstacles to compliance and develop strategies to overcome them. For example, when the patient begins to feel better, he may stop taking his medication because he doesn't think he needs it anymore. Reinforce the need to comply with drug therapy to prevent worsening heart failure and complications. Caution the patient to check with his physician before taking nonprescription drugs, even analgesics, laxatives, and cough remedies.

Teach your patient to check his pulse before, during, and after activity and before taking medications, such as digoxin. Advise him to have his blood pressure checked at regular intervals and to notify his physician if the readings remain elevated. If appropriate, teach him how to monitor his blood pressure at home.

Encourage your patient to balance rest and activity. Advise him to schedule at least two rest periods each day, during which he should sit quietly for 15 to 20 minutes with his legs elevated. Teach him to recognize the signs and symptoms of orthostatic hypotension and to minimize the risk by changing positions slowly and dangling his legs before getting out of bed.

Reinforce the physician's explanation of sodium restrictions. Tell the patient not to add salt to food while cooking or eating. Teach him how to read food labels to detect hidden sodium in foods, and advise him to avoid canned and processed foods. Warn him to check with his physician before using salt substitutes because they contain large amounts of potassium, which may be contraindicated in renal insufficiency and can increase the risk of

GOING HOME

Teaching a patient who has heart failure

Before your patient leaves the hospital, teach him to:

- Recognize the signs and symptoms of heart failure, such as nausea, unusual weight gain, and palpitations.
- Follow his medication regimen. Make sure he knows the names of his prescribed drugs, why he's taking them, when to take them, and what adverse effects they can cause.
- Check his pulse before and after activity and have his blood pressure checked regularly.
- Take at least two rest periods of 15 to 20 minutes every day.
- Restrict his sodium consumption. For example, advise him not to add salt while he's cooking and to use lemon juice and sodium-free herbs to enhance the flavor of foods.
- Restrict his fluid intake and keep a record of his fluid intake and output.
- Develop an exercise regimen that accommodates his heart condition. For example, advise him to avoid isometric exercises and exercise in extreme temperatures.

an electrolyte imbalance. Encourage him to use herbs and lemon juice to enhance flavor. And recommend cookbooks with healthy heart recipes, such as those published by the American Heart Association.

If your patient is receiving a vasodilator, tell him to avoid alcohol or to limit his consumption to one drink daily. Inform him that one drink is defined as 4 ounces of wine, 12 ounces of beer, or 1.5 ounces of hard liquor. Explain that alcohol is a myocardial depressant and may worsen heart failure.

Explain the importance of fluid restrictions to your patient. Translate the number of milliliters allowed per day into ounces, and show him how many cups of fluid he may have. Explain that gelatin, ice cream, and soups are considered fluids. If possible, have the patient record his own intake and output.

Help your patient develop a schedule that accommodates his exercise program—for example, walking 20 to 30 minutes at least four

times a week. Tell him to stop exercising and notify his physician if chest pain or severe shortness of breath develop and don't subside with rest. Caution him to avoid isometric exercise or any activity that requires him to hold his breath or perform Valsalva's maneuver. Also warn him not to exercise in extreme temperatures, which may cause blood pressure fluctuations. Advise him to exercise in an air-conditioned room when the weather is hot and humid.

Teach your patient about preventing exacerbations of heart failure (see *Teaching a patient who has heart failure*). Discuss precipitating causes, such as worsening ischemia, anemia, new arrhythmias, hypertension, progressing pulmonary disease, and nonsteroidal anti-inflammatory drugs. Inform him that two out of three readmissions for heart failure result because the patient didn't follow the regimen.

Help your patient learn to live with heart failure in a positive way. Emphasize the benefits of medications and treatments. Encourage him to express his thoughts and feelings about the medications, diet, and activity regimen. He may be afraid that heart failure means his heart will suddenly stop beating. Explain the cause of the failure and try to allay his anxiety. Discuss long-term treatment options with the patient and his family, including life-support measures, and encourage the patient to make his wishes known. By listening actively and offering emotional support, you can help your patient and his family make decisions about future treatment.

Heart failure and myocardial infarction

In a patient with heart failure, a myocardial infarction (MI) may result when compensatory mechanisms increase the cardiac workload. And the MI, in turn, worsens the heart failure because the heart is less able to meets its oxygen demands and pump blood to the body.

Pathophysiology

When coronary artery blood flow can't meet the oxygen demands of the myocardial cells, ischemia results. In a patient with heart failure, this problem stems from increased blood volume, decreased diastolic filling, increased heart rate, or increased thickness of the myocardium. Tachycardia or atrial fibrillation may worsen ischemia because they decrease diastolic filling time.

Ischemia hinders the heart's ability to pump. When myocardial perfusion is impaired, lactic acid accumulates, destroying the cells. Intracellular contents, including creatine kinase and potassium, are released into the systemic circulation. The release of potassium may predispose the patient to arrhythmias, further decreasing cardiac output.

Catecholamine release causes vasoconstriction, increasing afterload. Tachycardia develops, resulting in increased myocardial oxygen demand. When the coronary artery supplying the AV node is affected, bradycardia or heart block may develop. Hypotension and oliguria may result from decreased cardiac output.

Adapting nursing care

A patient with heart failure and an MI needs a cardiac monitor and a large-bore I.V. catheter. If he needs supplemental fluids, infuse 5% dextrose in water or lactated Ringer's solution, using microdrip tubing or an infusion pump. Unless the patient has hypovolemia or a right ventricular MI, infuse I.V. fluids at a keep-vein-open rate to prevent increasing vascular volume and heart failure. If your patient doesn't need supplemental fluids, you may use an intermittent infusion device to prevent further fluid excess.

Lowering oxygen demand

Other care measures focus on decreasing myocardial oxygen demand by decreasing pain and cardiac workload. Unrelieved pain produces further catecholamine release and may increase the size of the infarction, predisposing the patient to further heart failure. A physician may prescribe morphine because it relieves chest pain and decreases preload; it also has

the least effect on blood pressure of the narcotics. As ordered, administer morphine in 4 to 5 ml of normal saline I.V. over 4 to 5 minutes. Alternatively, administer 1 to 5 mg by I.V. push every 5 to 15 minutes until chest pain and shortness of breath diminish. Monitor the patient for bradycardia and heart block from enhanced vagal stimulation, which may further decrease cardiac output. Avoid intramuscular injections because they may alter creatine kinase levels, and the morphine may be poorly absorbed because of peripheral vasoconstriction. If your patient has a right ventricular MI, administer the prescribed nitrate and morphine cautiously because these drugs decrease preload and, thus, right ventricular volume. This lessens the amount of blood pumped to the left ventricle, further decreasing cardiac output.

Administer oxygen to relieve hypoxemia caused by pulmonary congestion and decreased coronary perfusion. Monitor oxygen saturation levels with pulse oximetry and check ABG results. Keep in mind that hypoxemia or myocardial ischemia may predispose the patient to an arrhythmia, further decreasing cardiac output. Be alert for signs and symptoms, such as increasing cough, exertional dyspnea, or feelings of impending doom, which may indicate that his condition is deteriorating.

As ordered, start an infusion of nitroglycerin to decrease myocardial oxygen demand and relieve chest pain. You may also need to administer a beta blocker, calcium channel blocker, anticoagulant, thrombolytic, and antiarrhythmic.

Checking for arrhythmias

Monitor serial enzyme results and ECG tracings to detect further myocardial damage. Also monitor the ECG for arrhythmias. Be especially alert for the following:
- six or more premature ventricular contractions (PVCs) per minute
- R on T phenomenon (QRS complex falls too close to the T wave)
- ventricular couplets (two PVCs in succession).

These arrhythmias may precipitate ventricular tachycardia and ventricular fibrillation, further reducing cardiac output.

RAPID RESPONSE ▶ If your patient develops ventricular tachycardia or ventricular fibrillation, you'll need to intervene immediately. Follow these advanced cardiac life support (ACLS) guidelines:

- To suppress PVCs, immediately administer lidocaine I.V. at 0.5 mg/kg every 2 to 5 minutes until the patient responds or he has received 3 mg/kg. If the patient responds, infuse lidocaine at a rate of 2 to 4 mg/minute.
- If the patient doesn't respond to lidocaine therapy, administer procainamide at 20 mg/minute until he responds or he has received 1 gram. Monitor him for hypotension and a widening QRS complex, which may indicate toxicity. If the patient responds, administer a continuous infusion of procainamide at 1 to 4 mg/minute using an infusion pump.
- Obtain serum digoxin and potassium levels and ABG results. Keep in mind that digoxin toxicity, hypokalemia, and hypoxia can cause PVCs.
- Administer supplemental oxygen, as ordered. Monitor the patient's oxygen saturation level. And continuously monitor his hemodynamic status for signs of worsening heart failure.
- After the patient's condition stabilizes, anticipate switching to an oral antiarrhythmic, such as procainamide, disopyramide, or quinidine. ◄

In some instances, an MI may precipitate heart block, which decreases cardiac output. If this occurs, anticipate that the physician will insert a pacemaker.

Monitoring the patient

Obtain the patient's vital signs every hour until his condition is stable, then every 4 hours thereafter. Listen for an S_3 heart sound, which may indicate early heart failure. Remember, an S_3 sound may precede pulmonary crackles by several hours. Auscultate the lungs for crackles every 2 hours until the patient's condition is stable, then every 4 hours thereafter. Notify the physician if the patient's temperature rises above 101° F (38.3° C) and request an antipyretic because fever increases the metabolic rate and oxygen demand and may decrease cardiac output.

Monitor the patient's intake and output, and insert an indwelling urinary catheter if necessary. Maintain bed rest or chair rest, as indicated. If heart failure worsens, anticipate that a pulmonary artery catheter will be inserted to assess preload and cardiac output. Maintain the pulmonary artery wedge pressure between 12 and 18 mm Hg (see *When your patient with heart failure and an MI needs pulmonary artery pressure monitoring*).

Expect a mild elevation of serum white blood cells (WBCs) after an MI. If it persists, assess the patient for other sources of infection. Also, keep in mind that the release of catecholamines may cause hyperglycemia.

Later care

During the acute phase, the patient should have a low-sodium diet and restrict fluids to 2 liters daily to limit vascular volume. Assess him for signs and symptoms of hypovolemia from diuretic use. Offer him small, soft meals to decrease the work of chewing and, thereby, oxygen demand. Suggest a stool softener to prevent vagal stimulation during defecation. Remember that such stimulation initially decreases venous return to the heart and causes bradycardia, followed by increased venous return, reflex tachycardia, and increased cardiac workload.

If the patient undergoes coronary artery bypass surgery, expect his cardiac performance to be depressed for 8 to 24 hours afterward. Observe him for arrhythmias, hypovolemia, increased heart rate, and hypoxia.

Be alert for a ventricular aneurysm, which may develop as a late complication of the MI. Paradoxic pulsations and persistent ST-segment elevation on the ECG suggest such an aneurysm, which can worsen heart failure. If thrombi form in the aneurysm, embolism may develop. Anticipate administering anticoagulant therapy to reduce the risk of embolism. If indicated, a surgeon may repair the aneurysm.

Complications

A patient with heart failure who sustains an MI risks developing complications, including reinfarction, cardiogenic shock, and renal failure.

ADAPTING YOUR CARE

When your patient with heart failure and an MI needs pulmonary artery pressure monitoring

Pulmonary artery pressure monitoring provides valuable information about your patient's blood volume and fluid status. It also helps determine the effectiveness of the heart's pumping ability. If your patient requires pulmonary artery pressure monitoring, prepare him for catheter insertion.

Catheter insertion
Begin by explaining the insertion procedure thoroughly to the patient and his family. By telling them what to expect and answering their questions, you can help allay their anxiety or fears. This, in turn, helps reduce the patient's stress and avoids increasing his myocardial oxygen demand, which could exacerbate his already fragile condition.

If your patient is experiencing dyspnea, position him with the head of the bed elevated. This improves his comfort and ventilation and allows him to concentrate on your explanation. Also, administer oxygen as needed.

Before, during, and after the procedure, check your patient's vital signs. Also, monitor his electrocardiogram (ECG) to detect changes in heart rate or rhythm. Look for ST-segment depression, which may indicate myocardial ischemia.

Normally, a patient will be placed in the Trendelenburg position if the catheter will be inserted into the subclavian or jugular vein. But in a patient who has heart failure, this position may cause increased dyspnea. If so, the physician will probably select a different insertion site.

During the insertion procedure, the patient will have to perform a vagal maneuver. Because such a maneuver can trigger bradycardia, closely watch the ECG. Also, when the catheter reaches the right ventricle, look for a ventricular arrhythmia. Usually, after the catheter reaches the pulmonary artery, this arrhythmia subsides. However, in a patient with heart failure and a myocardial infarction (MI), it may persist or worsen. Be ready to give lidocaine or perform cardioversion.

Monitoring the patient
After catheter insertion, monitor the patient closely for complications. Keep in mind that the catheter and the insertion site increase the risk of infection, which may increase myocardial oxygen demand.

Inspect the suture site frequently for redness and tenderness, and use strict aseptic technique during dressing changes.

Watch for signs of hemorrhage. If your patient is receiving a low-flow continuous heparin infusion to keep the catheter patent, his risk of hemorrhage is higher—especially if he's already taking an anticoagulant for his MI. Check the insertion site frequently for oozing and bleeding. Make sure all stopcocks are properly positioned and locked.

Throughout the patient's care, monitor his hemodynamic pressures. Be alert for pressure increases, which may indicate further cardiac decompensation. Continuously monitor oxygen saturation levels. Check the ECG for arrhythmias, especially ventricular arrhythmias. Reassure the patient and his family by providing frequent explanations and emotional support. Remind the patient about the reason for monitoring and the need to check his status often.

Reinfarction
A patient with heart failure and an MI risks developing a reinfarction, an extension of the infarcted area, because of the increased myocardial ischemia, decreased cardiac output, and increased workload of the heart.

An early reinfarction usually occurs 2 to 10 days after the original infarction. The amount of necrotic tissue increases, usually extending deeper into the affected muscle, further impairing the heart muscle's ability to contract. The risk of early reinfarction is especially great among women, patients with a subendocardial infarction, and patients with a large infarction resulting in cardiogenic shock. The risk is also high among those who have had an MI previously. A patient with an early reinfarction is at greater risk of arrhythmias, cardiogenic shock, and sudden death.

A late reinfarction occurs after the 10-day, immediate post-MI period. Typically, myocardial necrosis develops in regions adjacent to the original infarction. About 10% to 20% of people develop a late reinfarction. The risk is increased for patients who have surgery 3 to 6 months after MI.

Thrombolytic therapy, the standard treatment for an acute MI, increases the risk of early and late reinfarction. This therapy reestablishes coronary artery blood flow by dissolving the thrombus. But if if doesn't dissolve the thrombus completely, residual strands can reocclude the artery. Aspirin, heparin, warfarin, beta blockers, and ACE inhibitors reduce this risk of reocclusion.

Confirming the complication
Diagnosing a reinfarction may be difficult, depending on how much time has elapsed since the original infarction. Characteristic ECG changes and cardiac enzyme level elevations may still exist from the original infarction. Post-MI angina and ECG changes, such as PVCs, ventricular tachycardia, ventricular fibrillation, and accelerated idioventricular rhythm, suggest that reinfarction may be occurring.

Nursing interventions
Carefully monitor your post-MI patient for angina and ECG changes. Be alert for signs and symptoms of worsening heart failure and monitor laboratory studies. Closely monitor the patient's hemodynamic status for changes and provide supportive care, including oxygen therapy, dietary restrictions, and comfort measures.

After the patient's condition has stabilized, teach him about reinfarction, its contributing factors, and preventive measures he can take.

Cardiogenic shock
In cardiogenic shock, severe ischemia or infarction produces circulatory failure, severely compromising cardiac output. For a patient with heart failure and an MI, the risk of developing cardiogenic shock is especially great because he has both an infarction and decreased cardiac output. Usually, cardiogenic shock develops after a large anterior wall MI, when more than 40% of the left ventricle has been damaged, or when the papillary muscle ruptures.

In the early phases of cardiogenic shock, compensatory mechanisms may mask the initial decrease in cardiac output. As heart failure progresses, the heart can't eject its volume into the systemic circulation. Blood accumulates in the left ventricle and begins backing up into the pulmonary system, resulting in pulmonary edema. Eventually, blood backs up into the right ventricle and causes peripheral edema. Fluid in the alveoli interferes with gas exchange, leading to hypoxemia and hypercapnia. The sympathetic nervous system responds by constricting blood vessels to shunt blood to the heart and brain.

Cells turn to anaerobic metabolism, producing lactic acid, which contributes to lactic acidosis. Hyperkalemia results as the body attempts to buffer the acidosis by shunting hydrogen ions into the cells and releasing potassium to retain electroneutrality. The acidosis and hyperkalemia may precipitate arrhythmias, further reducing cardiac output. As hypoxemia progresses, myocardial ischemia further compromises pumping, creating a vicious circle.

Confirming the complication
A physician diagnoses cardiogenic shock based on the patient's signs and symptoms: profound hypotension, decreased level of consciousness (LOC), persistent sinus tachycardia, and oliguria or anuria. Metabolic and respiratory acidosis and hypoxemia help confirm the diagnosis. Hemodynamic findings show decreased cardiac output and cardiac index, elevated pulmonary artery and pulmonary artery wedge pressures, and increased right atrial pressures. Crackles, severe dyspnea, and cyanosis may develop.

Nursing interventions
Nursing care of a patient with heart failure and cardiogenic shock requires close monitoring to maintain a delicate balance among improving cardiac output, reducing cardiac workload and oxygen need, and preserving coronary perfusion.

Assess the patient's vital signs every 15 minutes until he's stable. Expect weak or thready peripheral pulses, prolonged capillary refill, and cool, pale, clammy skin. When auscultating the apical pulse, be alert for a pulse deficit, which may indicate an arrhythmia. An S_3 heart sound may indicate worsening heart failure. You may note a rapid respiratory rate and an increased work of breathing to increase oxygen supply. Watch carefully for signs of fatigue and worsening gas exchange, which may indicate the need for endotracheal intubation and mechanical ventilation.

Keep in mind that using a blood pressure cuff may give you inaccurate readings because of peripheral vasoconstriction. Thus, you may need to use Doppler ultrasound with a blood pressure cuff to determine systolic blood pressure. If circulation is severely impaired, you may need to measure blood pressure directly using an arterial line. Continuously monitor the patient's hemodynamic status, ECG waveforms, and oxygen saturation level for changes.

Expect to insert an indwelling urinary catheter. If urine output falls below 30 ml/hour, notify the physician. Monitor I.V. fluid intake and urine output hourly. Assess the patient for signs of excess fluid volume.

Assess cerebral perfusion by determining the patient's neurologic status. As shock continues, lethargy and confusion may be replaced by coma.

Unless the patient has hypotension, place him in the high Fowler position to allow the lungs to fully expand. If he has hypotension, place him in the semi-Fowler or supine position. Don't place a patient with heart failure and cardiogenic shock in the Trendelenburg or modified Trendelenburg position because it increases venous return and cardiac workload and inhibits lung expansion.

Auscultate the lungs for crackles and wheezes at least every 2 hours, as indicated. Administer oxygen by a Venturi mask for precise delivery. Observe the patient for accessory muscle use. Continuously monitor oxygen saturation levels and check ABG studies for hypoxemia and acidosis. Maintain the PaO_2 above 75 mm Hg.

If supplemental oxygen fails to correct hypoxemia and acidosis and your patient needs endotracheal intubation and mechanical ventilation, help decrease his anxiety by explaining all procedures. Because he can't speak when intubated, establish a means for him to communicate, such as using a picture board, paper and pencil, or magic slate.

Throughout the patient's care, monitor him for chest pain, ST-segment elevation, PVCs, and other arrhythmias. Administer nitroglycerin, as prescribed, to reduce preload and afterload and to increase collateral blood flow.

Monitor cardiac enzyme levels to detect a reinfarction. Support circulation with I.V. fluids, using minimal volume to avoid further increasing cardiac workload.

An intra-aortic balloon pump may be inserted to increase coronary artery perfusion and decrease afterload. As discussed earlier, a balloon-tipped catheter is inserted into the femoral artery until the tip reaches the aortic arch. The balloon is inflated during diastole and deflated just before systole.

When other therapies are unsuccessful, a ventricular assist device can be used to support the failing heart. A ventricular assist device temporarily decreases the workload of the ventricles and maintains perfusion, until the underlying defect is corrected.

Administer I.V. drug therapy, as prescribed. The physician may prescribe a diuretic, inotropic drug, and vasodilator in an effort to maintain systemic arterial pressure at 60 mm Hg or higher, preferably at about 90 mm Hg. If pressure falls below 60 mm Hg, perfusion will significantly decrease. As indicated, administer antiarrhythmics to control arrhythmias, which increase cardiac workload and decrease myocardial perfusion. You may also need to give the patient glucose-insulin-potassium solution and magnesium to improve left ventricular function and an H_2 blocker, such as famotidine, to prevent a stress ulcer caused by hypotension and decreased perfusion.

Reassure the patient and explain all procedures and treatments to decrease his anxiety, thereby decreasing oxygen demand.

Renal failure

When cardiac output decreases, renal perfusion and glomerular filtration decline, compromising kidney function. Severe episodes of reduced cardiac output and renal hypoperfusion may lead to mild azotemia or renal insufficiency and, eventually, acute tubular necrosis. Because the kidneys' ability to eliminate metabolic wastes is decreased, metabolic acidosis, hyperkalemia, hyperphosphatemia, and elevated BUN and creatinine levels may develop. Increased circulating blood volume overworks the left ventricle, further decreasing cardiac output. This, in turn, further decreases renal blood flow, worsening heart failure.

Recognizing acute renal failure

In a patient with heart failure and myocardial infarction, inadequate tissue perfusion may cause renal failure. Typically, the signs and symptoms result from the body's inability to excrete metabolic wastes, regulate electrolyte balance, and excrete fluid. Hematologic dysfunction also occurs because of the kidneys' role in producing erythropoietin. Expect your patient to have some or all of these signs and symptoms:
- increased serum blood urea nitrogen and creatinine levels
- worsening azotemia
- drowsiness
- confusion
- hyperkalemia
- metabolic acidosis
- hyperphosphatemia
- hypocalcemia
- oliguria or anuria
- crackles
- hypertension
- anemia
- leukopenia
- platelet dysfunction
- bleeding
- infection.

Conversely, renal failure may lead to heart failure and pulmonary edema when the failing kidney can't regulate sodium and water retention because of decreased glomerular filtration. This causes fluid volume excess and hypertension.

Confirming the complication
The diagnosis of renal failure is based on the patient's signs and symptoms and the results of laboratory tests. Typically, urinalysis reveals hematuria and proteinuria, and blood tests show increased BUN and creatinine levels, hyperkalemia, and metabolic acidosis (see *Recognizing acute renal failure*).

Nursing interventions
Maintain your patient's urine flow by administering furosemide or mannitol, as prescribed. Use caution when giving mannitol to your patient with heart failure because it increases vascular volume and cardiac workload.

If indicated, administer sodium polystyrene resin to treat hyperkalemia by exchanging sodium for potassium in the lumen of the bowel. Monitor your patient for arrhythmias and heart block until his potassium level stabilizes. To prevent hypokalemia, stop administering the exchange resin when the serum potassium level is between 4.5 and 5.0 mEq/liter. Also, if indicated, administer calcium acetate and aluminum hydroxide gel to control hyperphosphatemia and resulting hypocalcemia.

Because the kidneys excrete most drugs from the body, your patient's drug doses may need adjusting. Impaired renal function may prolong a drug's half-life, increasing the risk of toxicity. For example, many patients with heart failure take digoxin every day. But a patient with heart failure and renal failure may need to take digoxin every other day or even three times a week to prevent toxicity. Also, be aware that ACE inhibitors, commonly given to heart failure patients to reduce afterload, may worsen hyperkalemia and azotemia.

Examine the patient's stool and emesis for occult blood. Remember, renal failure patients are prone to stress ulcer formation, and severe stress ulcers may lead to hemorrhage, which further compromises the patient's cardiac status. As ordered, administer an H_2 blocker to prevent GI bleeding.

Evaluate the patient's mental status at least every 2 hours. Note any fatigue, lethargy, or confusion, which may indicate decreased cerebral perfusion caused by decreased cardiac output and hypoxia. In a patient with renal failure, fatigue, lethargy, or confusion may also result from increased BUN, acidosis, and hyperkalemia.

Maintain your patient's fluid balance. Remember to include both oral and I.V. fluids when calculating his fluid allowance.

Provide a diet that's liberal in calories, moderate in protein, low in sodium, and low in potassium. Encourage the patient to eat carbohydrates, which exert a protein-sparing effect. If he has severe azotemia, his protein intake may be limited to 0.7 to 1 gram/kg/day because protein accumulates in the blood as urea nitrogen. Warn your patient to avoid salt substitutes to minimize the risk of lethal hyperkalemia. If indicated, use special renal formulations for enteral or parenteral nutrition supplementation, such as amino acid infusions.

Observe the patient for signs and symptoms of increasing fluid overload, such as worsening dyspnea, weight gain, hypertension, tachycardia, and tachypnea. Listen for S_3 heart sounds, which may indicate worsening heart failure.

Also, assess the patient for Kussmaul's respirations, tachypnea, and hyperpnea, which may occur as compensation for metabolic acidosis. Assess your patient for increased work of breathing, pulmonary crackles, and mental status changes. Keep in mind that metabolic acidosis will worsen hyperkalemia as excess hydrogen ions are moved into the cell to buffer the acidosis.

Watch for signs of uremic pericarditis, including chest pain and tachycardia. Pericarditis decreases ventricular filling and further reduces cardiac output.

When fluid overload, acidosis, hyperkalemia, and pericarditis don't respond to conservative treatment measures, a physician may order dialysis. If so, prepare the patient and reinforce the physician's explanation of the procedure.

Because the damaged kidney can't produce erythropoietin—necessary for red blood cell (RBC) production—your patient may develop anemia early in renal failure, further decreasing his myocardial oxygen supply. As prescribed, administer subcutaneous recombinant erythropoietin to stimulate erythropoiesis. Monitor hemoglobin, iron, and folate levels and hematocrit. Also, keep in mind that synthetic erythropoietin may raise blood pressure, which may increase afterload and reduce cardiac output in a patient with heart failure.

Be prepared to intervene immediately if your patient develops pulmonary edema, an acute exacerbation of left ventricular dysfunction. As pulmonary lymphatic drainage is impeded, fluid is forced into the alveoli, causing acute respiratory failure. Auscultate the heart for S_3 heart sounds and crackles every 2 to 4 hours to allow for early intervention.

Because renal failure decreases immunologic responses, assess your patient for signs of infection, including fever, redness, and an elevated WBC count. Infection and sepsis increase myocardial oxygen demands and may worsen heart failure.

Heart failure and pulmonary edema

In pulmonary edema, excess fluid accumulates in the lungs. It's most commonly caused by left ventricular failure, which can result from an acute MI, hypertension, or mitral valve disease.

Pathophysiology

Pulmonary edema is a severe sign of cardiac decompensation. In a patient with heart failure, it occurs when the left ventricle can't eject all the blood that enters it. This increases left ventricular pressure, and blood is pushed back into the pulmonary circulation, distending the pulmonary vasculature and increasing pulmonary capillary hydrostatic pressure. As the process continues, fluid is forced first from the capillaries into the interstitial spaces and then from the interstitial spaces into the alveoli. After fluid enters the alveoli, it dilutes the surfactant, reducing surface tension and leading to alveolar collapse. As interstitial edema compresses some alveoli, intra-alveolar fluid impairs oxygen diffusion. Unoxygenated blood is then shunted through the lungs, causing hypoxemia (see *How heart failure leads to pulmonary edema*, pages 146 and 147).

The patient may develop pink, frothy, blood-tinged bronchiolar fluid. He also may experience extreme anxiety, tachycardia, tachypnea, and insomnia. And he may exhibit pallor and cyanosis with mottling of the arms and legs, possibly caused by an MI or worsening heart failure.

Later in pulmonary edema, hypercapnia results as carbon dioxide is unable to diffuse past the alveolar fluid. The interstitial fluid accumulation greatly increases the work of breathing, causing the lungs to stiffen and lose compliance. This increased work of breathing and inadequate gas exchange may lead to respiratory failure.

Pulmonary edema can also result when high-output heart failure that stems from infection

(Text continues on page 148.)

How heart failure leads to pulmonary edema

When heart failure affects the left side of the heart, blood backs up into the pulmonary vasculature, producing congestion and increased pressure. Because of this rise in pulmonary pressure, vascular fluid leaks into the interstitial spaces and alveoli, resulting in pulmonary edema.

1. Heart failure develops on the left side when the myocardium of the left ventricle is injured, as with a myocardial infarction, or when myocardial oxygen demand increases dramatically, as with ventricular tachycardia. Because the left ventricle isn't contracting forcefully or efficiently, blood begins to pool in it, and cardiac output is reduced.

2. Eventually, the left side of the heart fills with blood, and blood begins to back up into the pulmonary vein and the pulmonary vasculature (arterioles and venules). As blood volume in the pulmonary vasculature increases, so does the pressure. Plus, as cardiac output diminishes, the pulmonary vasculature compensates by vasoconstricting, further increasing the pressure. In response to volume and pressure, the vasculature distends, until it reaches its limit.

The lung has an extensive vasculature made up of many arterioles and venules, which are joined by capillaries. In this illustration, the lung's extensive vasculature is represented by three vessels.

3. The next step takes place in the capillaries, which join the arterioles and venules and surround the alveoli. The rising pressure in the vasculature causes pulmonary capillary hydrostatic pressure (the pressure that moves fluid out of the capillaries) to overcome plasma oncotic pressure (the pressure that holds fluid in the capillaries). This forces water and sodium into the interstitial spaces.

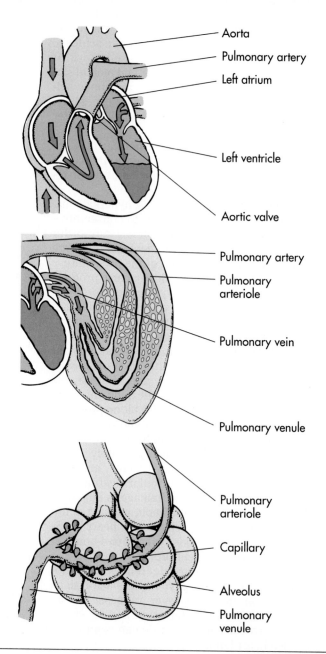

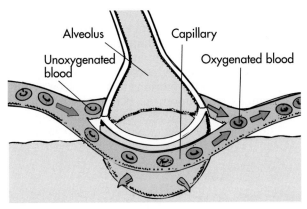

Alveolus Capillary

Unoxygenated blood Oxygenated blood

4. The transudation of water and sodium into the interstitial spaces results in interstitial edema and a rise in interstitial hydrostatic pressure. At this stage, normal gas exchange continues.

High interstitial hydrostatic pressure forces fluid from the interstitial spaces into the alveoli, causing alveolar edema.

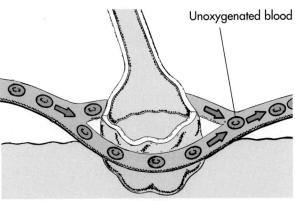

Unoxygenated blood

5. The fluid dilutes the surfactant, and eventually the alveoli collapse from the loss of surface tension. The fluid-filled, collapsed alveoli can't exchange oxygen and carbon dioxide; therefore, unoxygenated blood is shunted from the right side of the heart to the left side. The shunting produces hypoxia and hypercapnia.

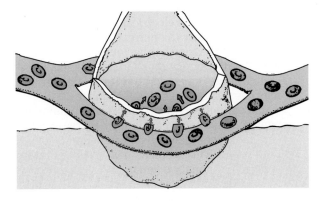

6. As pulmonary edema progresses, red blood cells leak from the pulmonary vessels into the alveoli, producing bloody or blood-tinged sputum.

leads to sepsis and septic shock. This hypermetabolic state results from catecholamine release in response to stress and may overwhelm a patient with coexisting cardiac or pulmonary problems.

Adapting nursing care

In patients at risk for pulmonary edema, be careful not to infuse I.V. fluids or blood products too rapidly. Always use an I.V. pump or microdrip tubing. Closely monitor the I.V. flow rate, especially if the patient is elderly. When transfusing blood to a patient with decreased cardiac output, you may need to administer a diuretic concurrently to promote fluid excretion.

RAPID RESPONSE ▶ Pulmonary edema is a medical emergency. The patient is literally drowning from fluid in the alveolar and pulmonary spaces. Without rapid intervention, severe tissue hypoxia will lead to organ failure and death.

- Place the patient in the high Fowler position to ease the work of breathing and enhance gas exchange. Encourage him to take slow, deep breaths.
- As indicated, administer high-flow oxygen through a nonrebreather mask. Continuously monitor the patient's oxygen saturation and ABG levels.
- Have emergency equipment available and be prepared to assist with endotracheal intubation and mechanical ventilation.
- Administer morphine I.V. to induce vasodilation, decrease venous return, and decrease the work of breathing.
- Monitor the patient's pulse and blood pressure every 15 minutes until they're stable. Watch for irregularities, such as increased heart rate and skipped beats, which can signal decompensation and decreased function.
- Prepare the patient to have a pulmonary artery catheter inserted for hemodynamic monitoring.
- Monitor the patient's ECG, noting any changes that may indicate worsening heart failure.
- Administer the prescribed diuretic, vasodilator, and inotropic drug. Monitor the patient's response to therapy. If pulmonary edema continues, respiratory failure and cardiogenic shock may result. ◄

After the crisis, teach your patient how to prevent exacerbations of heart failure that may lead to pulmonary edema. Reinforce all aspects of heart failure therapy, including medications, diet, and activity. Stress the importance of complying with a low-sodium diet and fluid restrictions, as appropriate. Make sure the patient's activity program allows for rest between activities, with at least two 15-minute rest periods each day. Teach him to sit upright in a chair or in the semi-Fowler or Fowler position to lower his diaphragm and increase oxygenation. To help ensure compliance with his diuretic therapy, encourage him to take the drug early in the morning to avoid sleep disturbances from nocturia. If diuresis interferes with his activities or work schedule, help him develop an acceptable schedule to promote compliance.

Complications

Common complications for a patient with heart failure and pulmonary edema include arrhythmias, respiratory failure, and cardiac arrest.

Arrhythmias
A disturbance or irregularity in the heart's conduction system, an arrhythmia may be benign or life-threatening. Generally, heart rates above 120 beats per minute impair diastolic filling, decreasing stroke volume and cardiac output. Extremely low heart rates prolong diastole, allowing extra filling time but, because residual blood remains in the ventricles, cardiac output decreases.

A disturbance in electrical activity may affect the heart's ability to contract in a synchronous manner, decreasing cardiac output. In a patient with heart failure and pulmonary edema, these arrhythmias consume additional oxygen and may cause more myocardial damage.

In a patient with heart failure and pulmonary edema, sinus tachycardia may increase myocardial oxygen demands by reducing diastolic filling time. This worsens heart failure and increases pulmonary edema.

With the exceptions of sinus bradycardia and sinus tachycardia, atrial arrhythmias occur when the conduction impulse originates in the atrial tissue outside the SA node, the heart's normal pacemaker. Common atrial arrhythmias include premature atrial contractions, supraventricular tachycardia, atrial fibrillation, and atrial flutter. Rapid by nature, these rhythms may be continuous or may start and stop abruptly. They worsen heart failure and, thus, pulmonary edema.

Ventricular arrhythmias—including PVCs, ventricular tachycardia, and ventricular fibrillation—originate in the ventricles. Usually caused by myocardial irritability or hypoxemia, these arrhythmias quickly affect cardiac output and impair tissue perfusion. A patient with heart failure and pulmonary edema is at increased risk for developing sudden cardiac arrest.

Atrioventricular heart block delays conduction through the AV node. Higher-grade blocks, such as Mobitz type II or third-degree block, may require pacemaker insertion. The very slow heart rates associated with higher-grade blocks can allow the ventricles to overdistend, decreasing cardiac output. This worsens existing heart failure and increases pulmonary edema.

Confirming the complication

The ECG waveform produces characteristic changes indicating the type of arrhythmia. Electrophysiologic studies may be performed to identify sites of ectopic conduction or evaluate the effectiveness of drug therapy.

Nursing interventions

Explain to the patient that the ECG will record the electrical activity of his heart. Obtain his vital signs every 2 to 4 hours. Also, monitor him for pulse deficits. Your patient with heart failure and pulmonary edema may report a sensation of skipped beats and his pulse force may vary. This results when premature beats cause the heart to eject a small amount of blood that's insufficient to perfuse distal areas; you may note a skipped beat when you palpate distal pulses.

Monitor the patient's hemodynamic status frequently during arrhythmias and when initiating I.V. antiarrhythmic therapy. Assess him for altered mental status, anxiety, tachypnea, hypotension, diaphoresis, oliguria, and decreased peripheral pulses. Monitor the ECG and record any findings. Administer digoxin and antiarrhythmic agents, as prescribed, watching carefully for possible interactions (see *Digoxin and antiarrhythmics: Dangerous interactions*, page 150).

Try to determine the underlying cause of the arrhythmia, such as hypoxia, an MI, a reinfarction, acidosis, or an electrolyte imbalance. Carefully evaluate your patient for electrolyte imbalances. Remember, potassium and magnesium may be deficient if your patient is taking a diuretic for heart failure and pulmonary edema. Anticipate routine electrolyte replacement therapy if your patient is receiving a loop or thiazide diuretic or if his potassium level is low (see *How electrolyte imbalances change ECG waveforms*, page 151).

When noting an arrhythmia for the first time, determine if the patient is hemodynamically stable and tolerating it. Take his vital signs, paying special attention to his blood pressure. If his vital signs are normal, continue monitoring the patient and notify his physician of any change in status. Keep the patient on bed rest until his condition is stable. Ensure his safety by elevating the side rails and observing him for dizziness and light-headedness.

If your patient develops atrial fibrillation or another supraventricular arrhythmia and drug therapy fails to convert it to a stable rhythm, prepare for cardioversion. If he develops a life-threatening arrhythmia, you'll need to intervene immediately. For more specific information, see *How to treat your patient's tachycardia*, page 119.

If your patient is apneic and without a pulse, he may be experiencing ventricular fibrillation or asystole. Immediately begin basic cardiac life support with cardiopulmonary resuscitation and follow your institution's protocol for cardiopulmonary arrest. If your patient is hemodynamically unstable, begin ACLS and implement standing emergency orders, as directed by your institution's policy.

DRUG ALERT

Digoxin and antiarrhythmics: Dangerous interactions

A patient taking digoxin for heart failure along with any of these antiarrhythmics may experience certain adverse effects from a drug interaction.

Antiarrhythmics	Adverse effects	Nursing actions
• Calcium channel blockers (diltiazem, verapamil) • Quinidine • Amiodarone • Esmolol • Flecainide	• Blood level of digoxin increases, heightening risk of digoxin toxicity.	• Administer digoxin immune Fab as ordered. • Monitor serum digoxin levels. • Monitor cardiac status. Evaluate electrocardiogram (ECG) for new arrhythmia. • Assess character and rate of apical pulse. • Monitor electrolyte levels and intake and output. • Instruct patient to report signs and symptoms of digoxin toxicity, such as loss of appetite, lower abdominal pain, diarrhea, weakness, drowsiness, headache, and blurred or yellow-green vision. • Instruct patient to eat a sodium-free, high-potassium diet to decrease risk of toxicity. • Teach patient how to take pulse. Tell him to notify physician if pulse rate is less than 60 or if pulse rhythm changes. • Anticipate switching to a different antiarrhythmic.
• Beta blockers	• Both drugs affect conduction through the atrioventricular node. Bradyarrhythmias, including third-degree heart block, may occur.	• Monitor heart rate. • Evaluate ECG. Assess PR interval every 4 hours. • Teach patient how to take pulse. Tell him to notify physician if pulse rate is less than 60 or if pulse rhythm changes. • Administer atropine for symptomatic bradycardia. • Be prepared to implement external pacing.

Patient teaching: Provide thorough patient teaching. Review with your patient all prescribed medications, including their purpose, action, and adverse effects. Teach him how to check his pulse before taking his medication and how to evaluate his response to treatment. Tell him to notify his physician if his pulse becomes irregular or falls below the designated parameters.

If an implantable cardioverter-defibrillator was inserted to treat recurrent ventricular tachycardia or fibrillation, discuss safety measures with the patient. Tell him to avoid magnetic fields, such as those found in magnetic resonance imaging machines or microwave ovens. Inform him that when the implantable cardioverter-defibrillator charges, he may feel a slight buzz or jolt, which may be uncomfortable but isn't harmful. Make sure he knows what to do when the device fires, including when to seek medical care.

Teach your patient to take his antiarrhythmic drug at regularly scheduled intervals—for instance, every 8 hours as opposed to three times a day with meals—to provide steady blood levels throughout the day. Warn him not to skip or double a dose. Discuss adverse effects of the drug, such as bradycardia and hypotension. Teach him safety measures to minimize the risk of injury from orthostatic hypotension. And emphasize the need for follow-up care, including monitoring of drug blood levels.

Respiratory failure
Acute respiratory failure results when the lungs can't provide sufficient oxygen and remove sufficient carbon dioxide when a person is at rest.

In a patient with heart failure and pulmonary edema, blood backing up into the pulmonary vasculature produces congestion and increased fluid volume, causing vascular fluid to leak into the interstitial spaces and alveoli. In acute respiratory failure, the fluid impairs gas diffusion across the alveolocapillary membrane, causing hypoxemia and hypercapnia. Hypoxemia leads to inadequate tissue perfusion and lactic acidosis; hypercapnia leads to respiratory acidosis. This results in chest pain and mental status changes, such as confusion and agitation. Hypercapnia also typically produces lethargy, confusion, and somnolence.

Confirming the complication
ABG measurements detect respiratory failure. Typically, respiratory failure occurs when the Pao_2 is less than 50 mm Hg and the partial pressure of arterial carbon dioxide ($Paco_2$) is greater than 50 mm Hg. The blood pH is less than 7.35, and the oxygen saturation is less than 90%.

Signs and symptoms of respiratory failure include severe dyspnea, orthopnea, anxiety, restlessness, tachycardia, arrhythmias, confusion, headache, and ashen skin. As respiratory failure progresses, a patient may become unresponsive.

Nursing interventions
If your patient with heart failure and pulmonary edema develops respiratory failure, establish a patent airway and administer oxygen to maintain his Pao_2 above 60 mm Hg. Be prepared to assist with endotracheal intubation and mechanical ventilation if the Pao_2 can't be maintained or if symptoms of hypercapnia appear. You also may need to administer morphine to decrease anxiety and preload, a diuretic to reduce fluid volume, and an adrenergic drug such as dopamine or dobutamine to improve contractility. Carefully monitor your patient's hemodynamic status and fluid and electrolyte balance for changes.

Your patient may be extremely anxious, which can increase oxygen consumption, thereby exacerbating impaired respiratory function. To help alleviate your patient's anxiety, explain all procedures and treatments and tell him what to expect, using a calm, quiet

How electrolyte imbalances change ECG waveforms

Electrolyte imbalance	ECG change
Hypokalemia	• depressed ST segment • flattened or inverted T waves • U waves present or superimposed on the T waves • peaked P wave
Hyperkalemia	• depressed ST segment • tall, tented T waves • prolonged PR interval
Hypocalcemia	• prolonged QT interval • prolonged ST segment
Hypercalcemia	• flattened or inverted T wave • slightly widened QRS complex • diminished voltage of P waves and QRS complex • prominent U wave • shortened QT interval • shortened ST segment
Hypermagnesemia	• widened QRS complex • prolonged PR interval • elevated T wave

tone of voice. Try to minimize disruptions and distractions so he can rest. Include the patient's family in all explanations and keep them informed of his progress.

If your patient needs mechanical ventilation, explain the reason for it. Inform him that it will help him breathe more effectively and will be used until his condition improves. Because he'll be unable to talk, establish a means of communication, such as using a pencil and paper. Closely monitor him for signs of improvement or deterioration. Look for nonverbal indicators of changes, such as grimacing, restlessness, and decreased responsiveness.

Cardiac arrest
Cardiac arrest can result from various arrhythmias, in particular ventricular fibrillation.

Ventricular fibrillation is a rapid, chaotic ventricular rhythm in which the ventricles quiver instead of contracting. Cardiac output disappears. Without immediate treatment, the person dies in 4 to 6 minutes.

Usually, ventricular fibrillation is triggered by severe myocardial ischemia or infarction. Half the time, it occurs without warning. Causes of ventricular fibrillation include PVCs, a deterioration of ventricular tachycardia, potassium imbalance, and metabolic acidosis. These conditions may develop in a patient with heart failure and pulmonary edema because of hypoxemia, adverse effects of medications, and renal insufficiency.

Confirming the complication
A patient with heart failure and pulmonary edema who suffers a cardiac arrest will be apneic, with no pulse or blood pressure. The ECG will show a grossly irregular pattern with no discernible rate or rhythm, or it will show a flat line.

Nursing interventions
RAPID RESPONSE ▶ A cardiac arrest requires immediate intervention.
- Establish that the patient is unresponsive and pulseless and call for help.
- Initiate ACLS, according to American Heart Association guidelines.
- Start cardiac monitoring.
- Intubate the patient and administer oxygen to support ventilation.
- Establish I.V. lines for fluid and drug administration; anticipate administering epinephrine, atropine, and lidocaine.
- Document the sequence of events and the patient's responses according to your institution's policy. ◀

After your patient has been resuscitated, provide emotional support to his family members and prepare them to see him. Describe any changes in his appearance. Inform them of the presence of any tubes or equipment. If the family wishes, contact a chaplain or clergy member to provide support.

After the patient's condition has stabilized, tell him what happened. Explain any lifestyle modifications, medications, treatments, or care measures that he requires.

Heart failure and chronic obstructive pulmonary disease

In chronic obstructive pulmonary disease (COPD), airflow into and out of the lung is obstructed. A progressive disorder, it's characterized by diffuse airway narrowing and resistance to airflow. The term COPD encompasses emphysema, chronic bronchitis, and asthma. About 15% to 25% of older adults have some degree of COPD. When it occurs with heart failure, your patient is at risk for developing atelectasis, deep vein thrombosis (DVT), and skin breakdown.

Pathophysiology

Chronic airway obstruction develops differently in the three disorders: emphysema, chronic bronchitis, and asthma.

Emphysema
Emphysema is characterized by the destruction of elastin in the lung parenchyma, which supports the distal airways and alveoli. As elastic recoil is lost, the lungs become hyperinflated. Increased lung compliance results in permanent overdistention of the lungs.

The loss of parenchymatous tissue also causes the terminal airways to collapse or narrow, particularly during expiration. Air becomes trapped in the distal airspaces, causing a further distention of the lungs. Ventilation diminishes as the overdistended lungs press against the diaphragm. As the patient works harder to force trapped air out of the lungs, intrapleural pressures increase, leading to more airway collapse.

In a patient with heart failure, dyspnea further increases the work of breathing and heightens the risk of airway collapse. The destruction of the alveolar and bronchiolar walls decreases the alveolocapillary membrane surface area, leading to impaired gas exchange.

Pulmonary congestion and vasoconstriction from heart failure further impede gas exchange. Hypoxemia, which causes generalized pulmonary artery constriction, and pressure from overdistended alveoli decrease the perfusion of the normal alveoli, impairing gas exchange even more. The patient hyperventilates to maintain oxygenation and expiration becomes prolonged. Eventually, the patient develops the barrel chest characteristic of emphysema because his lungs are hyperinflated.

Persistent hypoxemia resulting in pulmonary vasoconstriction may lead to right ventricular hypertrophy and cause or exacerbate right ventricular failure.

Chronic bronchitis

Chronic bronchitis results from respiratory irritants, which cause a hypersecretion of mucus from the goblet cells. The mucus impairs ciliary motion, which normally rids the respiratory tract of pathogens. Polymorphonuclear neutrophils migrate to the secretions, causing yellow sputum. Eventually, the inflamed bronchial walls are replaced by scar tissue, further obstructing the airway and predisposing the patient to repeated infections.

Infection and injury further increase mucus production. The bronchial walls become inflamed and thickened from edema and the accumulation of inflammatory cells. Eventually, all the airways become involved, and the bronchial smooth muscle becomes hypertrophied. The combination of hypertrophied smooth muscle and thick mucus obstructs the airway, especially during expiration, when the airways are already narrowed. This, in turn, leads to a ventilation-perfusion mismatch, hypoventilation, and hypoxemia. In a patient with heart failure, pulmonary shunting also occurs, thus increasing the ventilation-perfusion mismatch and worsening the patient's respiratory status.

Asthma

Asthma is characterized by reversible airway obstruction, inflamed airways, and an increased airway responsiveness to certain stimuli. During an asthma attack, airways sensitized by allergens react to a bronchospastic trigger, such as cold air or exercise, or an inflammatory trigger, such as dust or pollen. The result is bronchoconstriction. Histamine and related substances are released, resulting in contraction of smooth muscle in the bronchi, edema of the bronchial mucous membranes, changes in mucociliary function, and reduced clearance of respiratory tract secretions. In addition, expiratory airflow decreases, and gas becomes trapped in the airways, causing alveolar hyperinflation. The increased airway resistance leads to labored breathing.

Adapting nursing care

Nursing care for a patient with heart failure and COPD focuses on thorough assessment and intervention to decrease oxygen demands and improve cardiac and respiratory functioning.

Assessment

Obtain the patient's history, asking about exposure to irritants, including tobacco smoke. Ask the patient if he uses nonprescription breathing preparations. Look for signs and symptoms of hypoxemia, including anxiety, tachycardia, tachypnea, and cyanosis. Note somnolence, confusion, or lethargy, which may indicate hypercapnia caused by chronic bronchitis or an exacerbation of heart failure. Also, note any yellow sputum, which may indicate an infection. Ask the patient about any weight loss, possibly caused by increased work of breathing and anorexia. And assess him for weight gain, edema, and ascites, possibly indicating right ventricular failure.

Note whether the patient uses his accessory muscles to aid the work of breathing. Auscultate his lungs, noting any wheezing (rhonchi), which may indicate retained secretions.

Oxygen therapy

To relieve dyspnea and hypoxemia, place the patient in the semi-Fowler position and administer supplemental, low-flow oxygen, as needed. Remember, a patient with COPD may have chronic hypercapnia, so he may no longer respond to carbon dioxide as a stimulus to breathe. In such a patient, high levels of oxygen may suppress the hypoxic drive to breathe. Use oxygen saturation values to guide oxygen therapy. Maintain the saturation above 90% or the PaO_2 between 50 and 70 mm Hg and $PaCO_2$ in the patient's normal range.

Use ABG measurements to detect impending respiratory failure. A decrease in PaO_2 or an increase in $PaCO_2$ from the patient's baseline is significant. If oxygen therapy can't maintain his PaO_2 above 40 mm Hg and acidosis becomes severe, endotracheal intubation and mechanical ventilation may be needed.

Airway patency

If your patient has copious secretions, use a nebulizer to administer aerosolized treatments of saline and a bronchodilator. Be alert for tachycardia and palpitations, which increase oxygen demands. Monitor the patient's heart rate, ECG waveforms, and hemodynamic status closely for changes. If appropriate, increase his intake of fluids to about 2 liters daily to liquefy secretions and allow for easier expectoration. Assess him for signs and symptoms of increasing fluid overload. Monitor his intake and output, daily weight, and serum electrolyte, BUN, and creatinine levels. Perform nasotracheal suction, as needed.

To aid the drainage of secretions, perform percussion and postural drainage after the patient wakes up, before meals, and before he goes to bed. Always have suction equipment available. If your patient has dyspnea, place him in a position he can tolerate. A patient with heart failure, for example, may not tolerate the supine position. Continuously monitor his oxygen saturation for changes, especially with position changes and activity. Adapt your care according to his oxygen saturation levels. RAPID RESPONSE ▶ Provide frequent rest periods and help the patient perform activities of daily living, as needed, to decrease metabolic and myocardial oxygen demands. Teach him to use pursed-lip and diaphragmatic breathing to prevent air trapping and allow for complete expiration. During episodes of breathlessness and fatigue, place the patient in the high Fowler position with a pillow on the overbed table in front of him. Have him rest his arms and head on the pillow to relieve breathlessness. ◀

Nutrition

Fatigue, dyspnea, and the catabolic disease state make it difficult for a patient with heart failure and COPD to consume sufficient calories. Offer small, frequent meals to help your patient conserve energy. Encourage his family members and friends to visit during mealtimes. Provide a low-sodium diet with moderate amounts of carbohydrate and protein. Monitor his serum albumin levels to detect protein wasting. If he has severe hypercapnia, limit his carbohydrate intake because carbohydrate metabolism results in increased production of carbon dioxide. Administer liquid nutritional supplements such as Pulmocare, if indicated.

Provide mouth care to remove secretions and eliminate the metallic taste from inhalers. Have the patient perform coughing and deep-breathing exercises before meals to remove secretions, decrease dyspnea, and improve his appetite.

Drug therapy

Drug therapy includes bronchodilators, such as theophylline given systemically and albuterol given by inhalation to open the airways, a corticosteroid to reduce inflammation, and a diuretic to reduce edema.

When starting theophylline therapy, give a loading dose, as prescribed. Keep in mind that theophylline raises the heart rate and increases myocardial oxygen demand. Observe the patient carefully for tachycardia, which may decrease cardiac output and further exacerbate heart failure. Remember that a loop diuretic can interfere with theophylline absorption. If the patient is receiving a beta blocker along with theophylline, watch for theophylline toxicity. Monitor theophylline blood levels closely to maintain the therapeutic range of 10 to 20 mEq/ml.

Administer a corticosteroid, as ordered, to decrease airway inflammation. During an acute episode, you'll probably give the drug I.V. Otherwise, you'll probably use a metered-dose inhaler to minimize adverse systemic effects, such as fluid retention and blood pressure elevation, which may increase afterload. If the physician prescribes an inhaled bronchodilator and an inhaled corticosteroid, give the bronchodilator first to open the airways.

Teaching and supporting the patient

If your patient smokes, encourage him to stop. Also, advise him to avoid second-hand smoke. Refer him to a smoking cessation group, if appropriate. Keep in mind that a nicotine patch may be contraindicated for the patient with heart disease.

Tell the patient that exacerbations of COPD are usually caused by infection. Pneumonia can overwhelm a patient with alveolar secretions, leading to hypoxemia and myocardial ischemia. These effects are especially serious if a patient also has heart failure. Teach your patient to watch for signs of respiratory tract infection, including discolored, purulent sputum; fever; and increased dyspnea. Encourage him to receive a pneumococcal vaccine and yearly influenza vaccine to decrease the risk of infection. And explain that if an infection develops, his physician will prescribe a broad-spectrum antibiotic.

Allow your patient to make as many decisions about his care as possible. Discuss with him the possibility of endotracheal intubation and mechanical ventilation. Allow him and his family to express their feelings and concerns. Reassure him that when he feels breathless, he will receive help, and stay with him during times of breathlessness. Keep in mind that your patient may be clinically depressed, anxious, or frightened. He may experience feelings of hopelessness, loss of vitality, and powerlessness. To help alleviate these feelings, try to gain his trust and arrange for a mental-health consultation, if appropriate.

Provide thorough patient teaching. Before your patient leaves the hospital, obtain a referral for follow-up home care, if necessary. Arrange for home delivery of medical equipment, such as a home oxygen nebulizer, if necessary. Arrange for a home care nurse to assess the patient's cardiopulmonary status, educate him and his family about home care procedures, and provide reassurance (see *Teaching a heart failure patient who has COPD*, page 156).

Complications

A patient with heart failure and COPD is at risk for developing complications, including atelectasis, DVT, and skin breakdown.

Atelectasis

Atelectasis involves the collapse of alveoli. Both airway obstruction and ineffective ventilation contribute to its development. In patients with heart failure and COPD, atelectasis may result from compression by external pressure.

In airway obstruction, a mucous plug or retained secretions decrease ventilation to the alveoli. Air below the obstruction is absorbed into the pulmonary circulation through diffusion, and the alveoli collapse.

Ineffective ventilation may stem from respiratory muscle fatigue. In patients with heart failure and COPD, increased dyspnea adds to the problem, and hypoventilation causes atelectasis.

Compression atelectasis may result if a patient with heart failure and COPD develops pleural effusion. It's usually relieved by draining the fluid.

Confirming the complication

Because a patient with heart failure and COPD already has impaired gas exchange and hypoxemia, physical assessment alone may not confirm the diagnosis of atelectasis. However, observe the patient for increased dyspnea, restlessness, and tachycardia. With extensive atelectasis, a mediastinal shift toward the affected side may occur. You may hear crackles on auscultation. With a major collapse, you may hear decreased breath sounds—or you may not hear any breath sounds. An ABG analysis will reveal a decreased PaO_2. The extent of the hypoxemia will depend on the degree of shunting.

A chest X-ray helps confirm atelectasis. Findings can range from a subtle decrease in lung volume to an extensive volume loss and an elevation of the diaphragm.

Nursing interventions

Your primary nursing goal is to prevent atelectasis by incorporating prophylactic measures into the plan of care for your patient with heart failure and COPD. If your patient is confined to bed, perform frequent position changes and percussion and postural drainage. Encourage him to perform coughing, deep breathing, and incentive spirometry at regular intervals. When possible, increase your patient's activity, making sure to pace activities and provide adequate rest periods. Use humidification or administer

Teaching a heart failure patient who has COPD

For a heart failure patient who has chronic obstructive pulmonary disease (COPD), going home can be a relief—but it can also cause anxiety. Because of his breathing difficulties, he may be afraid that he'll stop breathing or die if he's left alone. To help relieve his anxiety, contact a visiting nurse's association. A home care nurse can provide appropriate care, assess his cardiopulmonary status, and help him adjust to living at home. In the meantime, prepare him for discharge by teaching him how to care for himself.

Activity and rest
Encourage your patient to use pursed-lip breathing when he performs activities or feels short of breath. Advise him to rest frequently and to pace his activities. Encourage exercise, such as walking, within his physical limits.

Teach your patient how to conserve his energy. Tell him to perform as many activities as possible while sitting on a stool or chair. Instruct him to climb stairs slowly. To help him decrease oxygen demand, teach him to exhale through pursed lips as he climbs each stair and to rest after exhaling. Tell him to resume climbing when he feels able.

Self-care measures
Review all aspects of your patient's medication regimen. Instruct him to inhale his bronchodilator before inhaling his corticosteroid. Tell him to wait 1 to 2 minutes between inhalations to allow the drugs to penetrate the lower airways more effectively. Emphasize the need for follow-up laboratory studies, especially if he's taking an oral bronchodilator, such as theophylline, or a diuretic.

Teach your patient how and when to monitor his pulse. Review with him the acceptable range for his pulse rate. And tell him to notify his physician if his pulse rate is out of that range or if his pulse rhythm changes.

Review the signs and symptoms of infection. Advise your patient to check his temperature daily. Tell him to notify his physician if he develops a fever higher than 100° F (37.7° C) or if the color or amount of his sputum changes.

Diet
Reinforce all aspects of your patient's prescribed diet. Teach him to eat low-sodium, high-potassium foods, to maintain any fluid restrictions, and to avoid salt substitutes. Encourage him to monitor his fluid output, noting any increase or decrease in the number of times he urinates. Advise him to weigh himself two or three times a week and to report any significant weight change.

When to get help
Teach your patient to recognize warning signs that may indicate an exacerbation of heart failure or COPD. Tell him to notify his physician immediately if he develops any of these signs and symptoms:
- weight gain of more than 3 pounds in 2 days
- leg or ankle swelling
- shortness of breath or cough not relieved by rest
- increased cough or shortness of breath
- irregular heartbeat
- change in mental status
- chest pain
- fever
- change in sputum color
- increased urination at night
- loss of appetite
- light-headedness or dizziness.

By teaching your patient with heart failure and COPD how to care for himself at home, you can help him leave the hospital with confidence. What's more, the knowledge you share empowers him to gain control over his condition and can help prevent serious complications.

mucolytics and bronchodilators, as prescribed, to help him expectorate secretions.

Untreated atelectasis places your patient at risk for infection, fibrosis, or decreased lung function, possibly leading to respiratory failure and worsening heart failure. Focus your care on improving ventilation and gas exchange. Auscultate heart and breath sounds at least every 2 hours and report a decrease in breath sounds, an increase in adventitious sounds, or S_3 or S_4 sounds. Continue to assess the patient for signs and symptoms of hypoxemia, such as restlessness, agitation, changes in LOC, and cyanosis. If a pulmonary artery catheter is in place, monitor the patient's hemodynamic status for changes indicating worsening heart failure.

Maintain a patent airway and encourage the patient to expectorate secretions, if possible. Use suction to remove accumulated secretions, as indicated. Also, encourage him to use incentive spirometry to expand the collapsed alveoli, thus improving gas exchange.

Administer medications to treat heart failure and COPD, as prescribed. Be alert for signs and symptoms of worsening heart failure, further respiratory or cardiac compromise, and respiratory failure. Continuously monitor pulse oximetry and obtain ABG measurements, as ordered, to evaluate oxygen saturation and PaO_2 levels.

Deep vein thrombosis

Typically, the thrombophlebitis associated with heart failure and COPD affects the deep veins. Venous stasis, vessel wall injury, and hypercoagulability of the blood can all cause DVT.

Bed rest heightens the patient's risk of developing DVT for several reasons. First, it decreases blood flow and causes venous pooling in the legs. Second, it eliminates the skeletal muscle pumping action that promotes venous return to the heart. Finally, it compresses the veins of the legs against the mattress, increasing venous pressure and damaging the intima of the vessel, causing platelets to adhere. Along with platelets, RBCs and fibrin may accumulate and attach to the vein wall, forming a thrombus. The proximal end of the thrombus floats freely in the lumen, ready to break apart and migrate into the circulation, causing an embolus. The decreased cardiac output associated with heart failure further increases the risk of DVT.

Confirming the complication

The patient's signs and symptoms depend on the level of the affected vein, the size of the thrombus, and the presence of collateral circulation. A patient may not even have signs and symptoms until he develops a pulmonary embolus. Or calf pain, edema, and increased calf circumference may develop. Other signs and symptoms include redness and warmth of the limb, tenderness along the vessel, dilated veins, and a low-grade fever. If the thrombus is at the level of the iliac and femoral veins, the patient may have pain and extensive swelling of the entire limb.

Venous duplex scanning shows the condition of the vein and confirms the diagnosis.

Nursing interventions

To prevent DVT, teach your patient what it is and how to reduce the risk factors. If DVT occurs, administer anticoagulant therapy, usually I.V. heparin followed by an oral drug, such as warfarin. Monitor your patient's coagulation studies to evaluate the effectiveness of therapy. Watch for signs of bleeding such as bruising, petechiae, hematuria, hematemesis, epistaxis, gingival bleeding, and blood in the stool.

During the acute stage, keep the patient on bed rest to prevent embolization and to avoid pressure fluctuations in the venous system that occur with walking and sitting. Keep in mind that bed rest can contribute to skin breakdown, especially in edematous areas. Inspect the skin carefully for signs of redness, irritation, and breakdown. Use protective devices, such as a bed cradle, heel protectors, and an air or water mattress.

Typically, you'd elevate a patient's legs above the level of his heart to promote venous return, thereby helping to relieve edema and pain and prevent venous stasis and new thrombi formation. In a patient with heart failure, however, elevating the legs may be contraindicated because the heart can't compensate for the increased venous return. Instead, you should use antiembolism stockings or sequential compression devices to facilitate venous return. Be sure to monitor the patient's circulation to the affected limb. Check pedal pulses, color, capillary refill, temperature, and sensation. Report any complaints of increased pain, numbness, or tingling. And measure the calf circumference at least once a day for changes. Report any increased circumference, edema, or circulatory changes.

After the threat of embolism has passed, help the patient walk and exercise in bed to decrease venous pressure and promote blood flow. As he increases his activity level, observe him closely for changes in oxygen saturation and ECG waveforms, which may indicate ischemia.

Apply warm, moist soaks to the affected limb, being careful not to burn the patient. Remember, his ability to feel heat may be decreased by impaired tissue perfusion.

If your patient will continue anticoagulant therapy at home, teach him how and when to take the medication. Also, make sure he knows the signs and symptoms to watch for. Encourage him to use a soft toothbrush and electric razor to minimize the risk of injury and bleeding. If he's taking warfarin, tell him to eat small but consistent amounts of foods high in vitamin K, which can interfere with the drug's intended action.

Skin breakdown

Skin breakdown is a deterioration of tissue integrity that impairs the exchange of oxygen and other nutrients. A patient with heart failure and COPD is at increased risk for developing skin breakdown, especially if he has activity restrictions and is on bed rest. Inactivity leads to venous pooling and stasis, which are made worse by the pitting edema caused by heart failure. Engorged tissues cause blood to pool, disrupting tissue perfusion and nutrient exchange. The skin may crack from the pressure, causing fluid to weep.

Minor trauma may cause tissue breakdown in a limb. Even the pressure of sheets and blankets can be great enough to initiate skin breakdown.

Confirming the complication

Typically, the affected area is swollen, pitted, pale, and cool to the touch. The skin appears taut and shiny, with visible cracks, weeping fluid, and, possibly, ulceration. Pulses may be diminished or absent.

Nursing interventions

Unfortunately, skin breakdown and ulceration may develop even with the best preventive care. Carefully assess the skin for signs and symptoms of infection, such as swelling, tenderness, and weeping fluid. Obtain a culture and begin antibiotic therapy, as necessary. Encourage the patient to drink fluids and maintain adequate nutrition to promote healing, keeping in mind the fluid and dietary restrictions needed for a patient with heart failure.

Keep the area clean and free from pressure, and use a bed cradle, heel pads, and an air or water mattress, as necessary. Place the patient in the Fowler position.

The patient should be on bed rest to decrease tissue oxygen demands. Monitor his oxygen saturation level. If the area of skin breakdown becomes infected, oxygen demands will increase and further compromise the patient's cardiac and respiratory status.

Change dressings as needed, using strict aseptic technique to prevent infection. Monitor the patient's response to treatments, such as wound care, which can increase oxygen demands, thus worsening his heart failure and COPD.

Maintain skin integrity in the unaffected limb, using lanolin creams to combat dryness and cracking. Reinforce skin care measures to minimize the extent of breakdown and to prevent problems in the unaffected limb.

Healing may be prolonged because circulation to the wound is impaired. Before your patient is discharged from the hospital, teach him how and when to change his dressings and care for the wound. Also, teach him to recognize signs and symptoms that may indicate infection or further wound deterioration, and tell him to notify his physician if they occur. A patient with severe dyspnea or activity intolerance may need to have a family member help him with dressing changes. Refer the patient to a home care nurse to help with wound care, if necessary.

Suggested readings

Beattie S, Pike C. Left ventricular diastolic dysfunction: a case report. *Crit Care Nurse.* 1996; 516(2):37-40.

Clark QK. *Pharmacologic basis of nursing practice.* 5th ed. St Louis, Mo: Mosby–Year Book, Inc; 1997.

Dennison RD. Making sense of hemodynamic monitoring. *Am J Nurs.* 1994;94(8):24-31.

Dressler DK. *Plans of care for specialty practice series: cardiovascular critical care nursing.* Albany, NY: Delmar Pubs; 1994.

Gleason M. Drug considerations in the elderly. *Crit Care Nurs Q.* 1996;19(2):7-12.

Ignativicious D. *Medical surgical nursing.* 2nd ed. Philadelphia, Pa: WB Saunders Co; 1996.

Juneau B. Special issues in critical care gerontology. *Crit Care Nurs Q.* 1996;19(2):71-75.

Lewis S, Collier I, Heitkemper M. *Medical-surgical nursing: assessment and management of clinical problems.* 4th ed. St Louis, Mo: Mosby–Year Book, Inc; 1996.

McKenry LM, Salerno E. *Mosby's pharmacology in nursing.* 19th ed. St Louis, Mo: Mosby–Year Book, Inc; 1995.

Moser DK. Maximizing therapy in the advanced heart failure patient. *J Cardiovasc Nurs.* 1996; 10(2):29-46.

O'Neal PV. How to spot early signs of cardiogenic shock. *Am J Nurs.* 1994;94(5):36-40.

Porth CM. *Pathophysiology: concepts of altered health states.* 5th ed. Philadelphia, Pa: Lippincott-Raven Pubs; 1998.

Ruppert SD, Kernicki JG, Dolan JT. *Dolan's critical care nursing: clinical management through nursing process.* Philadelphia, Pa: FA Davis Co; 1996.

Stark J. Dialysis choices: turning the tide in acute renal failure. *Nursing.* 1996;27(2):41-46.

Thompson CJ. Dysrhythmia formation in the older adult. *Crit Care Nurs Q.* 1996;19(2):23-33.

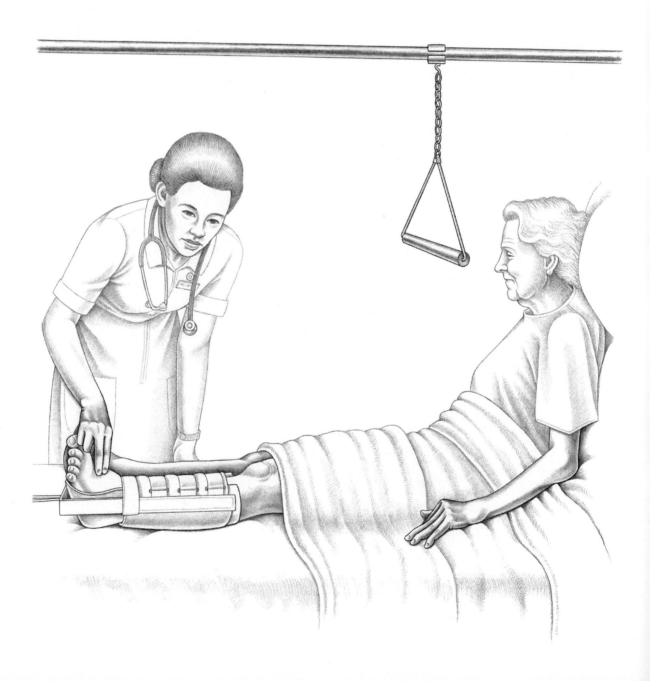

5

Rheumatoid Arthritis

A chronic, inflammatory disease, rheumatoid arthritis affects about 3% of the United States population. Primarily, it strikes postmenopausal women between ages 40 and 60, although it also affects some men and children. The most likely reasons for the high incidence of rheumatoid arthritis among women include the fluctuation of hormones, the use of birth control pills, the use of estrogen replacement therapy, and the effects of pregnancy.

When you think of rheumatoid arthritis, you may think of joint pain, stiffness, deformity, and limited mobility. But rheumatoid arthritis can affect more than just the musculoskeletal system. It may, for instance, produce arrhythmias or pleural effusion.

When a patient has rheumatoid arthritis and an associated disorder, such as atrial fibrillation or a hip fracture, you can face a complex nursing challenge. The combination of disorders can impose greater limits on your patient's mobility, restrict your treatment options, and produce further complications.

Anatomy and physiology review

Rheumatoid arthritis primarily affects the synovial joints, the most common joints in the body. Also called diarthroses, synovial joints provide skeletal flexibility and allow mobility of the hip, knee, ankle, shoulder, elbow, wrist, and finger. They consist of a fluid-filled joint cavity and a joint capsule that connects the joint's two bones. The joint capsule has two layers: the periosteum, an outer fibrous layer containing ligaments that anchor the bones of the joint and limit their movement, and the synovial membrane, an inner layer that lines the joint cavity and secretes synovial fluid.

Derived from blood plasma, synovial fluid is a viscous, yellow substance that protects the tendons from friction as they slide across the bone. (Fat pads in the joint capsule also cushion joint movement.) The synovial membrane can make the fluid more viscous by secreting hyaluronic acid. Synovial fluid absorbs the shock of movement and redistributes it to neighboring ligaments and tendons. It also provides nutrition to the articular surfaces and prevents bone formation in the capsule by keeping the blood vessels from invading the cartilage.

In certain joints, the synovial cavity extends beyond the joint, forming a fluid-filled pocket called a bursa. The outermost surfaces of the joint bones are covered with articular cartilage, which makes the surface tough and slippery (see *Inside the synovial joint*).

Pathophysiology

Although the cause of rheumatoid arthritis isn't known, we do know that it's an autoimmune disorder. An antibody called rheumatoid factor (RF) appears in the blood, synovial fluid, and synovial membrane of 70% to 90% of patients who have rheumatoid arthritis. In all likelihood, RF is an altered antibody produced by immunoglobulin G (IgG) in genetically predisposed people in response to an unknown trigger. RF responds to host tissues as though they were foreign, forming immune complexes with IgG and causing inflammation and eventual joint destruction.

No one knows exactly what triggers the production of RF. However, here are some possible explanations:

- Viruses may damage tissues, causing the release of antigens that don't normally circulate in the body. Also, viruses can damage T lymphocytes, altering the immune response.
- Hormones, such as estrogen, have immunomodulating properties and may trigger an immune response when their levels change.
- Genetic predisposition or errors also may influence the immune response. A genetic marker, human leukocyte antigen DW4, appears in many patients with rheumatoid arthritis.

Destruction of a joint

Whatever triggers the reaction, the formation of antigen-antibody complexes activates the complement system. This, in turn, triggers an inflammatory response in the synovial membrane. Polymorphonuclear leukocytes, monocytes, and lymphocytes migrate to the area to destroy the antigen-antibody complexes. During this process, the leukocytes, monocytes, and lymphocytes release lysosomal enzymes, which destroy the joint cartilage. This causes further inflammation, which attracts additional lymphocytes and plasma cells, creating a cycle of tissue damage and chronic inflammation.

Eventually, tissue destruction leads to hyperemia, swelling, and thickening of the synovial membrane. Then the synovial membrane penetrates the surrounding structures, including the cartilage, ligaments, tendons, and joint capsule, leading to the formation of a destructive, vascular, granulating tissue called pannus.

Pannus—a fibrous scar tissue composed of lymphocytes, macrophages, histiocytes, fibroblasts, and mast cells—forms in the joint capsule. This results in decreased joint mobility and, possibly, ankylosis, in which the joint becomes fixed in an abnormal position. Pannus erodes and destroys articular cartilage and subchondral bone and leads to the formation of bone cysts, fissures, spurs, and osteophytes. It also may result in the scarring and shortening of tendons and ligaments. The irreversible destruction of tissue and structural changes may ultimately lead to joint instability, stretching of the ligaments, and weakening of the tendons and muscles (see *Destructive effects of pannus*, page 164).

Effects on other body systems

Because rheumatoid arthritis is a systemic disease, other body systems also may be affected. Usually, problems develop in other systems if a patient has a high autoantibody titer to RF.

Subcutaneous nodules may develop in the lungs or meninges, possibly caused by local vasculitis. The nodules vary in size and consistency and are usually painless, unless they break or become infected.

Rheumatoid vasculitis (blood vessel inflammation in severe rheumatoid arthritis) can develop in any body system. This disorder can cause polyneuropathy, cutaneous ulceration, dermal necrosis, digital gangrene, and visceral infarctions. Commonly, vasculitis causes mild distal sensory neuropathy, small brown spots in the nail beds and digital pulp, and ischemic ulcers, especially in the legs. If vasculitis affects the coronary arteries, myocardial infarction may occur.

Inflammatory reactions may develop in the heart or lungs. In the heart, inflammation may lead to pericarditis or possibly myocarditis. In the lungs, inflammation may cause pleural effusions, interstitial fibrosis, pleuropulmonary nodules, pneumonitis, and arteritis.

A patient with rheumatoid arthritis also may develop osteoporosis, which can be aggravated by long-term corticosteroid therapy for rheumatoid arthritis. The combination of rheumatoid arthritis and osteoporosis causes a significant loss in bone mass and increases the risk of fractures.

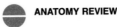 ANATOMY REVIEW

Inside the synovial joint

Each synovial joint contains a small space, a joint cavity between the articulating surfaces of the bones. This cavity is lined with synovial membrane, which secretes synovial fluid, a yellowish substance that cushions and nourishes the articular surfaces. In certain joints, the cavity extends beyond the joint itself, forming pockets of synovial fluid called bursae.

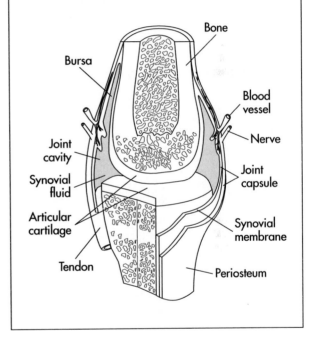

Assessment findings

Typically, a patient with rheumatoid arthritis experiences pain, stiffness, fatigue, and functional deficits. She also may experience systemic problems, such as fever, weakness, and changes in sleeping patterns. And rheumatoid arthritis can affect a patient's moods, causing mood swings, anger, frustration, depression, and changes in self-esteem (see *Recognizing rheumatoid arthritis*, page 165).

Joint swelling typically results from excess synovial fluid in the joint space and thickening of the synovial membrane. Persistent joint inflammation leads to deformities, such as radial

Destructive effects of pannus

As rheumatoid arthritis progresses, a fibrous scar tissue called pannus forms and eventually invades the bones. These illustrations show a normal joint and a joint being destroyed by pannus.

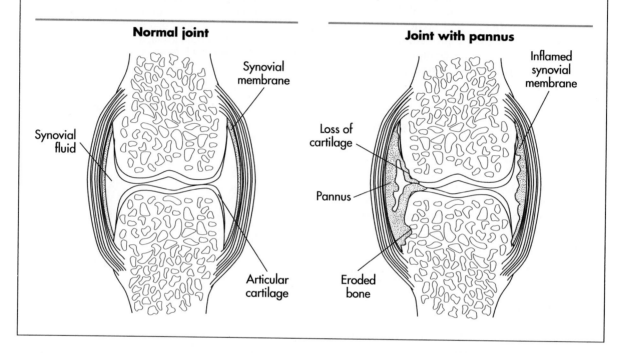

Normal joint

Synovial membrane

Synovial fluid

Articular cartilage

Joint with pannus

Inflamed synovial membrane

Loss of cartilage

Pannus

Eroded bone

deviation of the wrists, ulnar deviation of the fingers, palmar subluxation of the proximal phalanges (called the Z deformity), hyperextension of the proximal interphalangeal joints with compensatory flexion of the distal interphalangeal joints (swan-neck deformity), flexion deformity of the proximal interphalangeal joints (boutonnière deformity), and hyperextension of the first interphalangeal joints and flexion of the first metacarpophalangeal joints. Typical foot deformities include eversion of the hindfoot, plantar subluxation of the metatarsal heads, widening of the forefoot, hallux valgus, and lateral deviation and dorsal subluxation of the toes.

Expect to find a limited range of motion in the affected joints. Your patient may have a loss of thumb mobility and an inability to pinch because of a hyperextension of the first interphalangeal joints and flexion of the first metacarpophalangeal joints. You also may notice that your patient holds affected joints in the flexed position because doing so increases capsule volume and helps decrease distention and pain.

The area surrounding the joints may contain rheumatoid nodules. These firm, nontender nodules usually appear in the subcutaneous tissue and are composed of granulation tissue that surrounds a central core of fibrous debris. They tend to develop during exacerbations of the disease.

Some patients with rheumatoid arthritis develop arthritic changes in their temporomandibular joints, which lead to painful mastication. Because of this pain, your patient may not eat enough to maintain her body weight and so may appear underweight or even emaciated. What's more, poor calcium intake, corticosteroid use, and osteoporosis can lead to changes in posture, such as kyphosis.

Other signs of rheumatoid arthritis include a pericardial friction rub, an extra heart sound (such as S_3), and arrhythmias, such as atrial fibrillation. Your patient also may have adventitious breath sounds, such as crackles. Vasculitis may cause ischemia or necrosis in the arms and legs.

Diagnostic tests

A physician bases a diagnosis of rheumatoid arthritis on the results of a health history, physical examination, and diagnostic tests, including an RF titer, erythrocyte sedimentation rate (ESR), X-rays, and synovial fluid analysis. Although no one diagnostic test establishes the diagnosis of rheumatoid arthritis, a combination of several tests can help confirm it and determine its severity.

Rheumatoid factor titer
A blood test, the RF titer measures the antibodies directed at IgG. It's used to confirm the diagnosis of rheumatoid arthritis and to determine the patient's prognosis. Titers of 1:80 or higher usually indicate rheumatoid arthritis. The test detects such titers in 70% to 90% of patients who have rheumatoid arthritis and in about 5% of patients who don't have it. Typically, patients with higher RF titers have more severe musculoskeletal symptoms and a higher risk of developing symptoms in other body systems.

Erythrocyte sedimentation rate
The ESR measures the time needed for erythrocytes in a whole blood sample to settle to the bottom of a test tube. An increased ESR isn't diagnostic for any one disease, but it may indicate an ongoing disease process. In a patient with rheumatoid arthritis, the ESR usually is increased because inflammation and necrosis alter blood proteins, causing red blood cell (RBC) aggregation, and, thus, heavier RBCs. Usually, the higher the ESR, the greater the inflammation. However, higher rates normally appear in patients over age 50. Also, rates may be falsely elevated by stress from various sources, including excessive exercise, anxiety, pain, or dehydration.

Recognizing rheumatoid arthritis

The signs and symptoms of rheumatoid arthritis can appear similar to those of other diseases, such as osteoarthritis. However, if you note all or most of the following findings, your patient probably has rheumatoid arthritis:
- joint stiffness in the morning
- soft-tissue swelling and fluid in three joints, at least one of them in the hand
- symptoms in the same joint on both sides of the body
- rheumatoid nodules
- elevated serum rheumatoid factor
- rheumatoid changes on X-ray.

X-rays
X-rays help confirm rheumatoid arthritis by revealing evidence of soft-tissue swelling and joint destruction. The joint spaces may be narrowed, and articular surfaces may appear eroded. Bone cysts and subchondral bone erosion also may appear. As the disease progresses, X-rays may show subluxation and misalignment of the joints.

Synovial fluid analysis
Synovial fluid analysis detects inflammation in the joint space. If the joint is inflamed, the synovial fluid will appear turbid and will have an increased protein content and a decreased viscosity and glucose concentration. The white blood cell (WBC) count may range from 5 to 50,000 cells per microliter.

Medical interventions

For most patients, treatment consists of drugs that relieve pain, decrease inflammation, slow the disease progression, and ultimately preserve joint function. Some patients, however, need surgery to have their joints fused, reinforced, or replaced to improve their mobility and quality of life.

Common nonsteroidal anti-inflammatory drugs

Several nonsteroidal anti-inflammatory drugs (NSAIDs) are used to treat rheumatoid arthritis, including:
- aspirin
- diclofenac
- diflunisal
- etodolac
- fenoprofen
- ibuprofen
- indomethacin
- ketoprofen
- nabumetone
- naproxen
- oxaprozin
- piroxicam
- sulindac
- tolmetin.

Drug therapy

The primary drugs used to treat rheumatoid arthritis include nonsteroidal anti-inflammatory drugs (NSAIDs), immunosuppressants, corticosteroids, and gold preparations.

Nonsteroidal anti-inflammatory drugs

These drugs are widely used to treat the joint pain and inflammation caused by rheumatoid arthritis. They work by blocking the activity of the enzyme cyclooxygenase, thus inhibiting prostaglandin synthesis and decreasing inflammation (see *Common nonsteroidal anti-inflammatory drugs*).

The most common adverse effects of NSAIDs are gastrointestinal (GI) irritation, GI bleeding, and renal insufficiency. A patient may be able to control GI irritation by taking the prescribed NSAID with food, a full glass of water, or an antacid. A physician also may prescribe an H_2 blocker, such as cimetidine, or a proton-pump inhibitor, such as omeprezole, to help protect the GI mucosa. If the patient develops severe GI irritation, another NSAID, such as ibuprofen, may be prescribed. If the patient develops renal insufficiency, her physician will reduce the dose or replace the drug.

In elderly patients, age-related changes—such as diminished serum albumin levels, hepatic blood flow, and liver enzyme production—may decrease the body's ability to clear an NSAID. This, in turn, can lead to adverse effects.

Immunosuppressants

Immunosuppressants may be used for long-term therapy or for intermittent therapy to reduce symptoms during rheumatoid arthritis flare-ups. Such drugs as methotrexate, azathioprine, and cyclosporine suppress the proliferation of T and B lymphocytes, which destroy antibody-antigen complexes and joint tissue.

When methotrexate is used, the physician is likely to prescribe an NSAID, too. That's because methotrexate takes 4 to 6 weeks to produce therapeutic effects, and the NSAID offers some relief in the interim. Treatment with methotrexate usually begins with a dose of 7.5 mg per week. The dose increases at 1-month to 2-month intervals until the drug achieves maximum efficacy.

Some patients can't tolerate the high doses needed for therapy. Others can't take methotrexate because of its adverse effects, including liver, pulmonary, and renal toxicity. If renal insufficiency develops, the kidneys will no longer be able to clear the drug effectively, and the methotrexate blood level may climb dangerously high. The risk of toxicity increases when methotrexate is used with an NSAID.

Azathioprine and cyclosporine also cause adverse effects, including hyperglycemia, leukopenia, and renal insufficiency. Plus, their immunosuppressive effects increase the patient's risk of developing infections.

Corticosteroids

Corticosteroids used to be the treatment of choice for patients with rheumatoid arthritis. In low doses, they produce anti-inflammatory effects; in higher doses, they exert an immunosuppressive effect on T-helper cells. However, because corticosteroids also produce significant adverse effects—especially hyperglycemia and osteoporosis—they've been replaced by NSAIDs and immunosuppressants as a first-line treatment.

Prednisone in doses of up to 7.5 mg per day may be given to treat acute exacerbations of rheumatoid arthritis symptoms. The dose may be increased if the patient has severe vasculitis or other major systemic complications.

In addition to hyperglycemia and osteoporosis, the adverse effects of corticosteroids include an increased risk of bleeding from platelet dysfunction and GI irritation, an increased risk of infection from bone-marrow suppression and agranulocytosis, and fluid retention. Also, sudden discontinuation of a corticosteroid can be life threatening. Because long-term therapy with these drugs can cause adrenal suppression, they must be discontinued gradually to prevent adrenal insufficiency and crisis.

Gold preparations

Gold preparations appear to reduce acute and chronic inflammation. Usually, they also reduce the ESR. Although gold preparations produce some positive results, they also cause several adverse effects, including dermatitis, stomatitis, alopecia, and diarrhea, which limit the time a patient can safely and comfortably take them. Also, they may not produce a therapeutic response for up to 6 months.

Gold preparations also may trigger a nitrate reaction—a vasomotor response characterized by dizziness, sweating, weakness, nausea, flushing, and tachycardia—10 to 20 minutes after an intramuscular injection. The reaction can be diminished by having the patient lie flat during the injection or by injecting an oil-based gold preparation. Gold also can be given orally. Although a patient may better tolerate an oral dose, it's not as effective as the intramuscular preparation.

Surgery

Surgery may be indicated when pain, swelling, and stiffness lead to functional impairment that interferes with the patient's normal activities. If the patient's condition permits, joint replacement surgery may be performed.

Surgery may be contraindicated because the systemic effects of rheumatoid arthritis place the patient at risk for complications, such as infection, bleeding, and skin breakdown. The immunologic effects of rheumatoid arthritis increase the risk, as do the drugs used to treat the disease, including NSAIDs, methotrexate, and corticosteroids.

Nursing interventions

Nursing care focuses on assessing your patient's condition, keeping her comfortable, coordinating activity and rest periods, maintaining range of motion, and teaching her about her disorder. Because rheumatoid arthritis is chronic, your patient must understand the need to comply with long-term treatment. For best results, try to integrate her treatment plan with her lifestyle.

Assessment

Ask your patient about her symptoms and how they affect her lifestyle. Try to determine the nature of her pain, stiffness, fatigue, and functional deficits.

When assessing pain, ask your patient to describe the type, location, duration, severity, and onset. Find out if the pain is constant or intermittent, and if it builds gradually or strikes suddenly. Ask how long it lasts and if it occurs with movement or upon awakening. Find out which joints are affected and whether the patient has associated symptoms, such as stiffness or swelling. Also, ask about precipitating factors. Try to determine what makes the pain better or worse. Ask your patient how pain or stiffness affects her ability to perform normal activities of daily living.

Assess your patient's level of fatigue by asking her to describe its character and extent. If she complains that she feels tired all the time, try to pinpoint the severity of the fatigue and her ability to cope. Keep in mind that fatigue may be a symptom of depression.

If possible, schedule a physical examination after your patient has received her prescribed arthritis drug to avoid causing pain during joint movement. Carefully inspect each joint, keeping in mind that rheumatoid arthritis affects several joints simultaneously, usually in a symmetrical pattern. The most severely affected joints are the smaller ones of the hands, wrists, ankles, and feet, including the proximal interphalangeal and the metacarpophalangeal joints. In some patients, the upper cervical spine also may be affected.

Because movement aggravates joint pain, swelling, and tenderness, you may not be able to check your patient's range of motion accurately. Ask her to show you which joints she can move and to what extent. Her ability to flex and extend her joints may vary with the time of the day, disease severity, and drug administration. After inspecting the joints, inspect and gently palpate the surrounding tissue for rheumatoid nodules.

Also perform a head-to-toe assessment to check for signs of rheumatoid arthritis in other body systems. Start by noting general characteristics, such as your patient's body weight and posture. Listen to her heart rate and rhythm to detect arrythmias, such as atrial fibrillation. Also, listen for a pericardial friction rub, which may result from pericarditis, and for an S_3 or another extra heart sound, which may indicate myocarditis-induced heart failure.

When auscultating the lungs, note adventitious breath sounds, such as crackles. In rare cases when rheumatoid arthritis affects the cervical spine, subluxation of the vertebrae leads to diaphragmatic paralysis, which may result in respiratory failure.

To check for visceral organ infarctions, carefully palpate the abdomen for pain and tenderness. Auscultate bowel sounds and check the stool for occult blood.

Carefully examine the arms and legs for signs of ischemia or necrosis, which may result from vasculitis. Feel the skin of the arms and legs for coolness. Note any pallor or prolonged capillary refill time in the nail beds.

Rest and activity

Physicial rest decreases the stress on the joints and helps relieve inflammation and pain. Emotional rest helps relax muscles, which increases comfort. It also may prevent exacerbation of the disease.

The amount of rest your patient needs depends on the severity of her inflammation. With severe inflammation, she may need complete bed rest; with mild inflammation, intermittent rest periods and activity limitations may be sufficient. Assess your patient closely and implement rest measures as prescribed.

To promote rest, support the joints, and prevent contractures, use splints on all affected joints during flare-ups. When placing a splint,

make sure the affected hand, arm, or leg is positioned comfortably, with the joint and limb in the correct anatomic position and alignment. Periodically remove the splints and gently exercise the joints.

If your patient is on bed rest, monitor her closely for complications of immobility, such as atelectasis, deep vein thrombosis (DVT), constipation, and urine retention. Gradually increase her activity as tolerated, balancing activity with rest periods to protect the joints. Anticipate the use of an assistive device, such as a cane, walker, crutches, or braces.

Remember to provide emotional rest. Encourage the use of relaxation techniques, and minimize distractions. Also, provide for diversionary activities, such as listening to soft music, reading, conversing with visitors, and working on crafts (which also helps maintain finger mobility and function).

Comfort measures

When caring for a patient with rheumatoid arthritis, providing comfort and controlling pain are primary goals. Pain interferes with mobility, which can lead to further deformity and loss of function.

Monitor your patient's pain regularly, noting the location, type, and severity. Administer the prescribed antiarthritic drugs and monitor your patient for signs of their effectiveness. If inflammation is severe, anticipate the need for increased analgesia. Although not routinely used, narcotic analgesics may be administered to a patient who has undergone surgery or who has severe pain caused by an acute exacerbation. Be alert for adverse reactions, especially if your patient is immobile and receiving a narcotic analgesic.

As appropriate, use heat and cold therapy to help relax muscles and promote analgesia. Most commonly, you'll administer moist heat because it's usually the most effective. If your patient has stiffness in her hands, the physician may order a paraffin bath. Before applying heat or cold therapy, check the temperature to prevent injury. Use the therapy only for the prescribed time. Be sure to monitor your patient's response to therapy and notify the physician of any complaints.

Other nonpharmacologic pain-relief measures include relaxation techniques, guided imagery, and transcutaneous electrical nerve stimulation (TENS). Use the method or methods that work best for your patient. Commonly, these measures are most effective if they're used after a patient has taken her antiarthritic drug.

Therapeutic exercise

Therapeutic exercise helps maintain joint and muscle strength, endurance, and mobility—all of which are as important as receiving adequate rest. Work with a physical or occupational therapist to plan a program of progressive exercise and activity for your patient. Explain that it encourages purposeful movements and promotes self-care activities.

Before exercise, apply moist heat using hydrotherapy or a paraffin bath to reduce pain and stiffness. Initially, help your patient perform passive range-of-motion and isometric exercises. As her activity tolerance increases, help her perform active range-of-motion and progressive resistance exercises. Continually assess her tolerance of the exercise routine. Monitor her vital signs and be alert for signs of pain. Encourage your patient to continue her exercise program at home.

Patient teaching

Your teaching can help a patient cope with rheumatoid arthritis, maintain optimal function, and prevent complications.

As you teach, emphasize that although rheumatoid arthritis can't be cured, the symptoms can be managed, so that your patient can enjoy a better quality of life. Remember, she may be afraid that she'll become disabled because of immobility and pain. Address this concern by providing realistic information about her condition and prognosis and stressing the need to comply with her treatment regimen. Because rheumatoid arthritis affects not only your patient but also her family, include family members in your teaching. Try to enlist their aid in promoting compliance.

Carefully review your patient's drug schedule with her. Make sure she knows each drug's name, dosage, and adverse effects. Tell her to check with her physician before taking any nonprescription drug to avoid an overdose. For example, if she takes aspirin, explain that it contains salicylates, which also are found in certain antacids and other nonprescription drugs.

Advise your patient to take her drug with food to minimize GI irritation. Teach her to recognize the signs and symptoms of GI bleeding, such as dark, tarry stools and weakness. If GI irritation occurs, advise her not to stop taking her drug abruptly—especially if it's a corticosteroid. Instead, instruct her to notify her physician, who'll tell her how to taper the dosage gradually.

If your patient is taking an immunosuppressant, such as methotrexate or azathioprine, inform her that she'll need frequent blood tests to evaluate her kidney and liver function and to assess her bone-marrow function. Warn her that she'll be more susceptible to infection, and make sure she knows the signs and symptoms of infection, such as fever.

Reinforce all instructions about activity, rest, comfort measures, and exercise. Tell the patient to modify her exercise or activity if it produces pain that persists for more than 1 hour. If appropriate, refer her to a home care agency for a home physical therapy evaluation.

Teach your patient to protect her joints by:
- conserving energy whenever possible
- using smooth, continuous motions and avoiding sudden, jarring motions
- using large muscles for movement to avoid placing stress on the joints
- alternating easy and strenuous tasks
- allowing for rest between tasks
- decreasing exercise during acute bouts of inflammation
- using assistive devices, such as a cane or a raised toilet seat.

Finally, discuss the impact of lifestyle changes on the disease. Emphasize the need to reduce emotional stress, which can exacerbate an acute arthritic attack. Discourage smoking and unhealthy dietary habits. If your patient is obese, explain how added weight can place further stress on the joints and hamper her mobility. If she's malnourished, stress the importance of consuming sufficient calories and nutrients to increase her sense of well-being and provide enough energy to perform daily activities. Help your patient and her family incorporate lifestyle changes into her routine to promote optimal functioning and a positive self-image.

Rheumatoid arthritis and atrial fibrillation

Because rheumatoid arthritis is a systemic disorder, the associated inflammation can affect many body tissues and organs. When the heart becomes inflamed, the patient may develop cardiac complications, such as pericarditis, pericardial effusion, and valve deformities—all of which can precipitate atrial fibrillation. The risk is especially great among older women and patients with a history of rheumatic fever.

Pathophysiology

Pericarditis (inflammation of the pericardial sac) develops in 30% to 50% of all patients with rheumatoid arthritis, particularly in men who have subcutaneous nodules. In some cases, pericarditis leads to pericardial effusion (a collection of fluid in the pericardial sac). Pericarditis or pericardial effusion can cause disorganized electrical activity in the atria, which leads to atrial fibrillation.

In some patients, rheumatoid arthritis leads to inflammation and granuloma formation of the mitral and aortic valves, which can cause valvular deformity and regurgitation. A patient with a history of rheumatic fever during childhood may already have valve damage, especially mitral valve damage. If mitral valve damage causes mitral valve regurgitation, atrial enlargement may occur. This enlargement and stretching of atrial myocardial tissue fibers leads to ectopic atrial impulses, and, in turn, atrial fibrillation.

Sometimes, a patient with rheumatoid arthritis may develop vasculitis, which can lead to vessel occlusion. If the coronary arteries become occluded, the patient may suffer a myocardial infarction, which can precipitate atrial fibrillation.

A common cardiac arrhythmia, atrial fibrillation occurs when several irritable sites in the atria produce impulses that supercede the heart's normal pacemaker, the sinoatrial (SA) node. These abnormal impulses, which can fire at rates faster than 350 beats per minute, cause the electrical activity of the atria to become disorganized. The atria can't recover from one atrial contraction to the next. Thus, instead of contracting, the atria simply quiver. Without atrial contraction, the ventricles don't receive sufficient blood, and cardiac output diminishes.

The number of atrial impulses that actually reach the ventricles determines how many times the ventricles contract per minute. But because the atrioventricular (AV) node acts as a gatekeeper, it only allows a fraction of the atrial impulses to reach the ventricles. For instance, if the atrial rate is 400 beats per minute, the AV node may allow only 70 impulses to reach the ventricles. If, however, the AV node fails to block the ectopic atrial impulses, the ventricular rate will quicken. If it climbs to 150 beats or more per minute, cardiac output diminishes further.

Without atrial contractions, blood pools in the atria. In a patient with chronic atrial fibrillation, mural thrombi can form, putting her at high risk for cerebral embolism. However, anticoagulant drugs, such as warfarin, can significantly reduce the risk of this complication.

Atrial fibrillation is confirmed with an electrocardiogram (ECG) tracing of the patient's heart rhythm (see *Recognizing atrial fibrillation*).

Adapting nursing care

Start by performing a thorough assessment. A patient with atrial fibrillation may be asymptomatic, or may complain of palpitations, such as a fluttering or pounding feeling in the chest or a sensation of skipped heart beats. Because cardiac output is decreased, the pre-existing fatigue from rheumatoid arthritis may become more severe.

Upon physical examination, you'll usually feel an irregular pulse rate. Because your patient's cardiac output may vary with each beat, you also may feel a variable pulse force—some beats will feel strong and others will be barely palpable. Upon auscultation, you'll hear an irregular

Recognizing atrial fibrillation

In atrial fibrillation, several sites of atrial irritability trigger a rapid succession of abnormal impulses. These impulses take over the sinoatrial (SA) node's role as the heart's pacemaker. Fortunately, the atrioventricular (AV) node usually can block enough of the atrial impulses to maintain a normal ventricular rate.

The illustration below shows how atrial fibrillation affects electrical conduction in the heart. The normal atrial conduction pathway is shown in black; the abnormal atrial conduction pathways are shown in color.

The waveform shows the electrocardiogram (ECG) characteristics of atrial fibrillation: irregular QRS complexes, a wavy baseline, and indiscernible P waves. Typically, the atrial rate is 350 to 500 beats per minute, but because of indiscernible P waves, it's impossible to measure on an ECG.

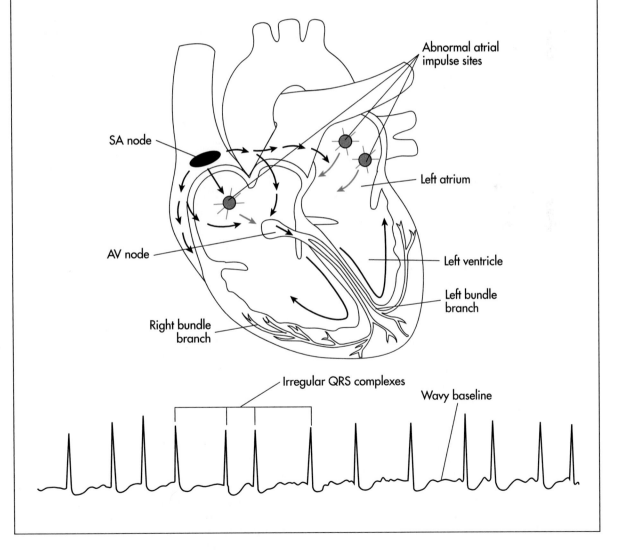

DRUG ALERT

Antiarthritic and antiarrhythmic drugs: Dangerous interactions

Antiarthritic drugs	Antiarrhythmic drugs	Adverse effects	Nursing actions
• Methotrexate	• Digoxin	• Decreased serum levels of digoxin and decreased therapeutic effectiveness	• Monitor serum levels of digoxin. • Monitor ECG for changes that indicate a return to atrial fibrillation, increased ventricular rate, or new arrhythmia. • Anticipate need to increase digoxin dosage.
• Indomethacin	• Digoxin	• Increased serum levels of digoxin with a risk of digitalis toxicity	• Monitor serum levels of digoxin. • Monitor patient for signs and symptoms of digitalis toxicity, including halo vision, nausea, vomiting, diarrhea, and slow pulse rate. • Anticipate need to decrease digoxin dosage.
• Nonsteroidal anti-inflammatory drugs, methotrexate	• Warfarin	• Increased anticoagulant effect with increased risk of bleeding	• Encourage patient to take antiarthritic drug with food. • Assess patient for signs and symptoms of bleeding, including oozing from injection and insertion sites and bruising. • Monitor vital signs. • Monitor hemoglobin levels, hematocrit, and coagulation studies. • Check urine and stool for occult blood. • Anticipate giving H_2 blocker or mucosal protectant to minimize risk of gastric irritation and bleeding. • Protect patient from injury. • Have vitamin K (antidote for warfarin) available.

rhythm, and if the patient has valve disease, you'll probably hear a murmur.

After your patient is diagnosed with atrial fibrillation, expect her to undergo transesophageal echocardiography to help pinpoint the cause of the arrhythmia. Prepare her by explaining that an ultrasound transducer will be placed in her esophagus next to her heart to allow a physician to view her heart and its structures. If indicated, inform her that the physician may order serum thyroid function tests to ensure that thyroid problems aren't causing the arrhythmia.

Maintaining hemodynamic stability
Because atrial fibrillation adversely affects a patient's cardiac output, interventions are aimed at controlling the ventricular rate and restoring the sinus rhythm. For chronic atrial fibrillation, treatment may include anticoagulant therapy. If your patient needs such therapy, her physician may discontinue her antiarthritic drug or reduce the dosage because of the increased risk of bleeding.

Ventricular rate control
If the patient has a rapid ventricular rate and is experiencing hypotension or other symptoms, expect to administer I.V. drugs to slow the conduction of impulses through the AV node. A

physician may prescribe a calcium channel blocker, such as diltiazem or verapamil, which directly impairs AV node conduction; a beta blocker, such as metoprolol, which reduces sympathetic control of AV node conduction; or digoxin, which increases vagal inhibition of AV node conduction.

If your patient has mild signs and symptoms, expect to administer one or more of these drugs orally. Typically, digoxin is the drug of choice for long-term rate control. Calcium channel blockers and beta blockers may be used with digoxin to achieve optimal ventricular rate control.

Monitor your patient's blood pressure for hypotension, particularly if she's receiving a beta blocker or calcium channel blocker. Also, monitor her pulse rate for bradycardia, particularly if she's taking digoxin. Be aware that some antiarthritic drugs can interfere with the action of antiarrhythmic drugs (see *Antiarthritic and antiarrhythmic drugs: Dangerous interactions*).

In a patient with chronic or intermittent atrial fibrillation, drug therapy may not effectively reduce ventricular rates or relieve symptoms. In this case, a physician may order implantation of a permanent pacemaker, a device that provides an electrical stimulus to the heart. The stimulus may fire at a constant rate or may be programmed to fire on demand, at a rate based on physical activities, such as walking and climbing stairs. After the patient undergoes pacemaker insertion, monitor the incision site for signs of bleeding or infection, such as redness and purulent drainage. Your patient also may need anticoagulant therapy because the atria are still in fibrillation and the risk of mural thrombi remains.

Sinus rhythm restoration

In some patients, a physician uses drugs instead of electrical cardioversion to convert the arrhythmia to the normal sinus rhythm. Commonly used drugs include quinidine, procainamide, disopyramide, sotalol, and amiodarone. Often, they convert the arrhythmia within 24 hours. Then they can be used to maintain the rhythm, although they may produce adverse effects. For example, quinidine, the most commonly used drug, may cause nausea, vomiting, and diarrhea. Procainamide may cause a lupuslike syndrome and thrombocytopenia. Disopyramide typically produces anticholinergic effects, particularly in men. And sotalol may cause a prolonged QT interval.

If drug therapy doesn't convert the arrhythmia or if your patient becomes hemodynamically unstable, a physician may perform electrical cardioversion. This procedure aims to completely disrupt the aberrant electrical foci in the atria with an external electrical charge, so that the SA node can resume the heart's pacemaker function.

If your patient is scheduled to receive electrical cardioversion and if time permits, have her fast for 6 hours before the procedure to reduce the risk of aspiration. Administer the prescribed sedative before the procedure and take measures to protect her from injury during the procedure. Be sure you have cardiopulmonary resuscitation equipment on hand (see *When your patient with rheumatoid arthritis and atrial fibrillation needs electrical cardioversion*, page 174).

Anticoagulant therapy

If your patient remains in atrial fibrillation despite electrical cardioversion, the physician probably will prescribe an anticoagulant to prevent thromboembolism, particularly to the brain. Warfarin, the most commonly used oral anticoagulant, interferes with vitamin K–dependent clotting factors, including prothrombin (factor II) and factors VII, IX, and X. Thus, it effectively prevents thrombus formation and the subsequent embolism that can occur from atrial blood pooling.

If your patient is receiving warfarin, evaluate the results of her baseline coagulation studies, such as her prothrombin time (PT), and monitor subsequent results to detect abnormal changes. Typically, the warfarin dosage is based on the PT results. Assess your patient for signs of bleeding, such as increased bruising; blood in the stool, urine, or sputum; hypotension; increased pulse rate; and neurologic changes.

If your patient is taking a gold preparation for rheumatoid arthritis, be aware that it can destroy platelets, which can lead to blood clotting abnormalities and hemorrhage. The risk increases if your patient also is taking warfarin. Be sure to monitor this patient's platelet count.

ADAPTING YOUR CARE

When your patient with rheumatoid arthritis and atrial fibrillation needs electrical cardioversion

Electrical cardioversion involves delivering an electric charge to convert an arrhythmia, such as atrial fibrillation, to normal sinus rhythm. A patient with rheumatoid arthritis and atrial fibrillation may need cardioversion if her ventricular rate is high and she develops complications, such as hypotension.

Before cardioversion

- If time and the patient's condition permit, explain the procedure thoroughly to her and her family. She may be frightened by the thought of electricity being used to shock her heart or by the television or movie image of a defibrillator being used to bring someone back to life. Emphasize that, although the procedure is similar, much lower energy levels are used.
- Make sure that a signed consent form has been obtained and is included in the patient's medical record.
- Confirm that digoxin has been withheld for at least 48 hours to avoid predisposing the patient to ventricular arrhythmias.
- Obtain baseline serum electrolyte levels, including a potassium level. A low serum potassium level increases the patient's risk of developing lethal arrhythmias, such as ventricular tachycardia. Expect to administer potassium replacement before cardioversion.
- Make sure the patient has had nothing by mouth for several hours before the procedure.
- Perform cardiac monitoring to evaluate the patient's heart rate and rhythm. Keep in mind that the QRS complex must be high enough to be sensed by the defibrillator for successful cardioversion. The electrical burst of energy is timed to coincide with the peak of the R wave.

- Start an I.V. infusion to administer the prescribed antiarrhythmic drug. To reduce fear and help relax the patient, administer the prescribed sedative, but only if her blood pressure is stable.
- Be sure to keep the patient's airway open, which may require tilting her neck slightly. Keep in mind that if the patient has cervical spine changes from her rheumatoid arthritis, this positioning may induce pain or severe injury. With such a patient, try opening the airway by lifting the chin without tilting the head.
- If necessary, administer supplemental oxygen and monitor oxygen saturation levels with pulse oximetry to decrease the risk of hypoxemia and further arrhythmias.
- Properly position the patient and use pillows for support to reduce straining deformed or immobile joints and to prevent stiffening.
- Make sure you have emergency equipment on hand.

During and after cardioversion

- Closely assess the heart rhythm and pulse. If the normal rhythm is restored, continue to monitor the patient and provide supplemental oxygen as needed.
- Be especially alert for ventricular fibrillation or tachycardia. If either occurs and the patient has no pulse, prepare for defibrillation.
- As soon as possible after the procedure, resume the patient's drug therapy.
- If she experiences any discomfort from the procedure or from the required immobility and positioning, assist her with repositioning and performing passive or active exercise, as tolerated.

Usually, platelets return to normal levels several weeks after a gold preparation is discontinued.

Aspirin may be used to prevent clotting because of its antiplatelet and analgesic effects. Because high doses of aspirin can predispose a patient to salicylate toxicity, monitor her for complaints of tinnitus and hearing loss.

Patient monitoring

If appropriate, institute continuous cardiac monitoring. Evaluate the ECG waveform for changes, such as an increased ventricular rate; widening of the QRS complex; or other arrhythmias, such as premature ventricular contractions, which may indicate a deterioration of the patient's condition. Notify the physician of any changes. Also, monitor the effectiveness of drug therapy by evaluating the ECG tracing.

The patient's heart rate should be sufficient to sustain effective blood pressure, usually a systolic pressure above 100 mm Hg.

During continuous ECG monitoring, be sure the monitor cable doesn't interfere with your patient's ability to move in her bed or chair. If she's being monitored by telemetry, attach the transmitter so that it doesn't cause pulling or tugging that may further limit her movement or exacerbate joint stiffness and pain. When she's in bed, position the transmitter so that she won't roll onto it during sleep.

Monitor the patient's vital signs at least every 4 hours. Be alert for signs of insufficient cardiac output, such as hypotension, chest pain, increased heart rate, and tachypnea. Also, check for decreased level of consciousness (LOC) and urine output. Auscultate lung sounds every 4 hours and be especially alert for crackles, which may indicate heart failure. Notify the physician of any abnormal findings.

If you're using an automatic blood pressure monitoring device, try to minimize discomfort caused by physical limitations. Remove the cuff regularly to allow the patient to move her arm freely. If she's receiving an anticoagulant, check her arm for bruising caused by cuff inflation. If bruising occurs, avoid using the automatic blood pressure cuff and check her PT results for an abnormally high level.

Promoting comfort

If the physician discontinues your patient's antiarthritic drug or reduces the dosage to avoid bleeding complications, your patient may experience increased inflammation, pain, and joint and muscle stiffness. Talk with the physician about other analgesics and alternative treatments, such as massage. Encourage your patient to change position often to reduce the complications of immobility. Also, perform passive range-of-motion exercises, as needed.

To combat fatigue, encourage your patient to rest frequently between activities and to perform the most taxing activities at the time of day when she feels best.

Patient teaching

Teach your patient how to check her pulse, and tell her to notify her physician of any abnormal changes. Review with her the antiarrhythmic drug she's taking, making sure she knows its purpose, dosage, adverse effects, and drug interactions. If she's taking an anticoagulant, review safety measures to decrease the risk of bleeding. For example, using a soft toothbrush or electric razor can minimize the risk of bleeding. Teach her to recognize the signs and symptoms of bleeding. Advise her to notify her physician of increased bruising or black, tarry stools. Encourage her to have laboratory studies performed, as directed, so that the physician can evaluate her response to treatment.

Complications

A patient with rheumatoid arthritis who also has atrial fibrillation risks developing certain complications, including GI bleeding and shock.

Gastrointestinal bleeding

Antiarthritic drugs, such as NSAIDs, immunosuppressants, corticosteroids, and gold preparations, increase the patient's risk of GI bleeding from GI mucosal damage or drug-induced coagulopathies. The risk is even greater if the patient develops atrial fibrillation and needs anticoagulant therapy.

The NSAIDs inhibit prostaglandin E, which normally protects the GI mucosa from being digested by gastric secretions. This lack of protection can result in GI ulceration and bleeding. Most NSAIDs also interfere with platelet function and therefore tend to prolong bleeding time. About 50% of patients who take NSAIDs develop gastritis. Of these, fewer than 25% develop symptoms of bleeding, such as black, tarry stools and decreased hemoglobin levels.

Immunosuppressants, such as methotrexate, can decrease the inflammation associated with rheumatoid arthritis. Unfortunately, the most common adverse effect of methotrexate is GI mucosal irritation.

Corticosteroids inhibit prostaglandin synthesis, increase gastric acid and pepsin secretion, reduce gastric mucosal blood flow, and weaken the protective mucous membane, thereby increasing the patient's risk of GI ulceration. Also, these drugs can mask the signs of ulcer formation and delay healing.

Although gold preparations can cause other adverse GI effects, such as diarrhea, they usually do not produce GI bleeding.

Because of its anticoagulant effect, warfarin places a patient at an increased risk for bleeding, especially GI bleeding. The risk increases when warfarin is administered with other anti-inflammatory drugs.

Confirming the complication

A physician bases the diagnosis on the patient's signs and symptoms and the results of certain diagnostic tests. The signs and symptoms depend on the source and rate of bleeding. If the patient is taking antiarthritic drugs, bleeding usually stems from an ulcer in the stomach or proximal duodenum. Most patients who experience upper GI tract ulcers complain of epigastric distress that's usually relieved by eating or taking an antacid. The patient may vomit blood; pass black, tarry stools or bright red blood through the rectum; or experience dizziness, faintness, and pallor.

If the patient loses a significant amount of blood, shock may result. Signs and symptoms of shock include decreased blood pressure; increased heart rate; pale, cool, clammy skin; slight confusion and disorientation; dizziness; fatigue; and, occasionally, chest pain.

Laboratory analysis of a patient's stool sample may detect occult blood, which indicates GI bleeding. The patient may undergo gastroscopy, gastroduodenoscopy, or esophagogastroduodenoscopy to help a physician locate the source of upper GI tract bleeding, or a patient may undergo sigmoidoscopy to help a physician locate the source of lower GI tract bleeding. An upper GI tract X-ray may reveal gastric mucosal abnormalities and the source of bleeding.

If a patient is bleeding, serum hemoglobin levels, hematocrit, and the RBC count may be decreased. The serum blood urea nitrogen (BUN) level may be elevated because excess blood in the GI tract is catabolized in the liver to urea, which is then deposited in the blood and transported to the kidneys for excretion.

Nursing interventions

Monitor the patient's vital signs and assess her for signs of GI bleeding, such as black or tarry stools, increased pulse rate, and postural hypotension. If she loses a significant amount of blood, her cardiac output, which is already decreased by atrial fibrillation, will decrease even more. If she's taking a beta blocker for atrial fibrillation, it may mask the signs of bleeding, such as an increased heart rate.

Monitor the results of blood tests, including hemoglobin, hematocrit, BUN, and PT. Prepare the patient for endoscopy or sigmoidoscopy, as indicated. Make sure she takes nothing by mouth for 8 to 12 hours before the endoscopy. Administer the prescribed sedative to relax her, an analgesic to relieve her discomfort, and atropine to reduce GI secretions and help prevent aspiration. After the procedure, make sure the patient takes nothing by mouth for 2 to 4 hours to allow her gag reflex to return.

RAPID RESPONSE ▶ If your patient experiences acute GI bleeding, do the following:

• Expect to discontinue her anticoagulant and to discontinue or reduce the dosage of her antiarthritic drugs.
• Prepare to administer an H_2 blocker, a mucosal protectant, or an antacid, as prescribed.
• Keep the patient from taking anything by mouth until the bleeding stops.
• Consult with her physician about using alternatives to antiarthritic drugs for pain relief, such as I.V. narcotic analgesics.
• Monitor the patient's ECG for changes in her heart rate and rhythm. Be especially alert for premature ventricular contractions, which can arise from myocardial ischemia caused by decreased cardiac output.
• Monitor the patient carefully for increased bleeding. Check her stools for occult blood, and, if a nasogastric tube is in place, check the drainage for blood or a coffee-ground appearance.
• Perform gastric lavage, as needed, to help stop the bleeding and keep her stomach clear of blood. Monitor her vital signs, especially her blood pressure and pulse. Carefully measure the patient's intake and output, including nasogastric drainage. ◀

After the patient's bleeding is under control and she's resumed taking her antiarthritic drug, try to prevent repeat episodes of GI irritation. If possible, have her take her antiarthritic drug with food or meals. Also, give an antacid 1 to 2 hours after giving other oral drugs to prevent the antacid from interfering with their absorption. And administer a mucosal protectant, if indicated.

To help promote comfort, especially if your patient is on bed rest during the bleeding episode, position her properly and provide adequate support to her arms and legs. Change her position frequently. Try splinting her arms and legs, especially if they're deformed, to maintain functional ability and provide support and rest for the joints. Obtain an occupational or physical therapy consultation to help the patient learn to use assistive devices. Try alternative pain-control methods, such as diversionary activities (including reading, watching television, and visiting), guided imagery, biofeedback, self-hypnosis, and other relaxation techniques.

After the patient's pain is under control, begin gentle range-of-motion exercises to help maintain mobility and function. Apply heat, ice, or a combination to help reduce pain and stiffness.

Help your patient establish a schedule that maximizes the absorption of all prescribed drugs. If she's taking aspirin, tell her about the various formulations. For example, explain that buffered aspirin is no different from plain aspirin in its effect on the GI mucosa. Point out that enteric-coated preparations are less irritating to the mucosa, although their absorption rate is slower. If the patient resumes warfarin therapy, emphasize the need to return for follow-up laboratory tests, as directed. Also, advise her of dietary restrictions when taking warfarin. For example, she should eat a small but consistent amount of foods that are high in vitamin K, such as leafy green vegetables, to avoid interfering with the action of warfarin and to keep the PT consistent.

Shock

Anything that alters blood volume, blood pressure, or the heart's ability to function can disrupt tissue perfusion. When the body tissues and cells aren't adequately perfused with oxygenated blood, the result is hypoxia—and eventually shock. If shock goes untreated or the body can't compensate, shock progresses to organ failure and death.

Hypovolemic shock, the most common form, occurs when the fluid volume in the vascular compartment decreases. This may happen if a patient experiences prolonged bleeding or rapid loss of a large amount of blood, as in acute GI bleeding. Thus, patients with rheumatoid arthritis and atrial fibrillation are particularly at risk for hypovolemic shock.

Hypovolemic shock develops when intravascular blood volume decreases by 15% to 25%. Initially, the body tries to compensate by releasing catecholamines, thereby increasing systemic vascular resistance and heart rate— and improving cardiac output and tissue perfusion. Interstitial fluid also moves to the vascular compartment to increase volume. The liver and spleen release stored RBCs and plasma, adding to the blood volume. The renin-angiotensin-aldosterone system is initiated, resulting in sodium and water retention. Antidiuretic hormone also increases water retention. If the blood loss continues or becomes massive, these compensatory mechanisms fail, and tissue perfusion decreases further. The result is impaired cellular nutrition and metabolism (see *How the body tries to prevent hypovolemic shock*, page 178).

Confirming the complication

In the early stages of shock, your patient may experience few signs and symptoms. She may be restless, apprehensive, or slightly confused. Her pulse and respiratory rates may be increased, but her blood pressure may be normal or slightly low. Urine output may be slightly decreased, and the patient may complain of thirst.

As shock progresses, respirations become shallow, and crackles or other adventitious breath sounds may indicate pulmonary congestion. Blood pressure decreases, and the pulse may become weak and thready. The patient appears pale, with cool, clammy skin. Cerebral hypoxemia causes increased lethargy that may progress to coma. Oliguria or anuria may develop as kidney perfusion decreases. Arterial blood gas (ABG) analysis reveals respiratory and metabolic acidosis.

Nursing interventions

Hypovolemic shock is an emergency that requires prompt intervention.

RAPID RESPONSE ▶ If your patient develops hypovolemic shock, you'll need to act quickly:

PATHOPHYSIOLOGY

How the body tries to prevent hypovolemic shock

When a patient with rheumatoid arthritis and atrial fibrillation receives antiarthritic and anticoagulant drugs, gastrointestinal bleeding—and ultimately, hypovolemic shock—may result. When cardiac output drops, the body attempts to compensate, as shown in the flowchart below.

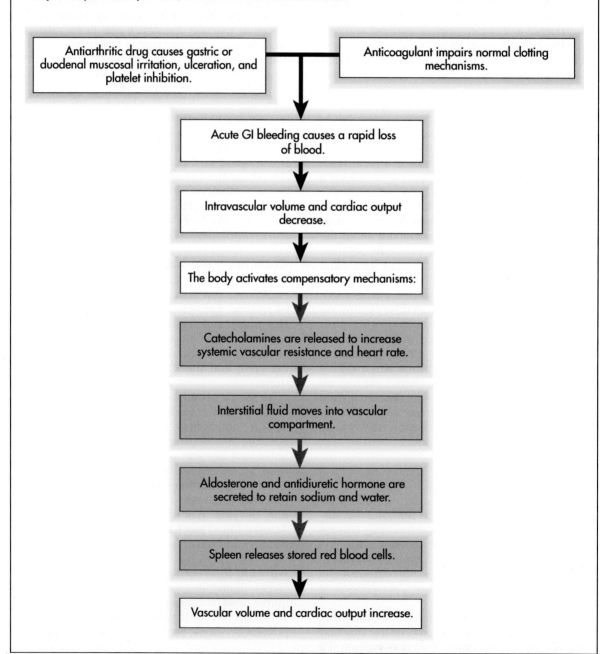

- Insert at least two large bore I.V. catheters for rapid fluid volume replacement and drug administration.
- Begin continuous cardiac monitoring to evaluate your patient for worsening atrial fibrillation and for lethal arrhythmias, such as ventricular tachycardia.
- Anticipate the insertion of a pulmonary artery catheter to monitor her hemodynamic status and an arterial line to monitor arterial blood pressure and obtain samples for ABG analysis.
- Replace lost volume by administering fluids, such as blood, blood products, albumin, and crystalloids (lactated Ringer's solution or normal saline solution), as prescribed.
- Continuously monitor vital signs, ECG waveforms, and hemodynamic measurements.
- Administer supplemental oxygen and monitor oxygen saturation levels, using pulse oximetry and ABG analysis results, as indicated. Anticipate the need for endotracheal intubation and mechanical ventilation if oxygen saturation decreases or cardiac arrest occurs.
- If indicated, insert an indwelling urinary catheter and monitor urine output at least hourly. Obtain creatinine, BUN, and electrolyte levels, as ordered, to evaluate renal function.
- Prepare to administer inotropic drugs, such as dopamine, to maintain blood pressure and promote renal perfusion. ◄

After your patient's condition stabilizes, take measures to prevent a recurrence. Expect the physician to reduce the antiarthritic or oral anticoagulant drug dosage or to replace one of these drugs. Prepare the patient for the possibility of taking another drug, such as an H_2 blocker, to decrease the risk of bleeding. Reinforce all instructions about adverse effects and the need for follow-up care, especially laboratory studies.

Rheumatoid arthritis and hip fracture

Certain common antiarthritic drugs increase the patient's risk of developing osteoporosis, a condition characterized by loss of bone density or mass. Such losses, particularly from the axial skeleton, can be rapid and profound during the first year of treatment for rheumatoid arthritis. They make a patient who has rheumatoid arthritis more vulnerable to bone fracture, particularly of the hip.

The risk of a bone fracture doubles among patients who take more than 7.5 mg of a corticosteroid daily because corticosteroids decrease osteoblastic (bone-building) activity. Immunosuppressants, such as methotrexate, also increase the risk of a bone fracture. Even when administered in low doses for a short time, methotrexate causes osteopathy and increases the risk of fracture.

Pathophysiology

When the rate of bone resorption exceeds the rate of bone formation, a patient loses cancellous and compact bone tissue. This weakens the meshwork of intercommunicating spaces that are filled with bone marrow. As a result, the bone becomes more fragile and prone to fracture (see *Effects of osteoporosis*, page 180).

Most commonly, osteoporosis in patients with rheumatoid arthritis results from corticosteroid or immunosuppressant drug use. Immobility, which disrupts osteoblastic and osteoclastic activity, can contribute to osteoporosis. Immobility also depletes bone mass by eliminating skeletal stress from muscle contraction and weight bearing. Also, poor nutrition can reduce the level of calcium, which is necessary for bone growth.

Adapting nursing care

Nursing care focuses on prevention—that is, slowing the rate of calcium and bone loss. This includes monitoring your patient's serum calcium levels frequently and encouraging her to eat a well-balanced diet that's high in calcium (up to 1,500 mg/day) and vitamin D, which increases calcium absorption. Also, encourage regular, moderate, weight-bearing exercise because it stimulates bone formation. Using appropriate assistive devices, such as a cane or walker, decreases the risk of falls.

Effects of osteoporosis

Most bones contain cancellous and compact tissue, and a patient with osteoporosis loses bone mass from both. The illustration on the left shows a cross-section of normal bone, including the locations of cancellous and compact bone tissue.

The close-up view on the left shows normal trabeculae, the meshwork of bone matrix that makes up cancellous bone. The illustration and close-up view on the right show how the trabeculae and compact bone diminish in osteoporosis.

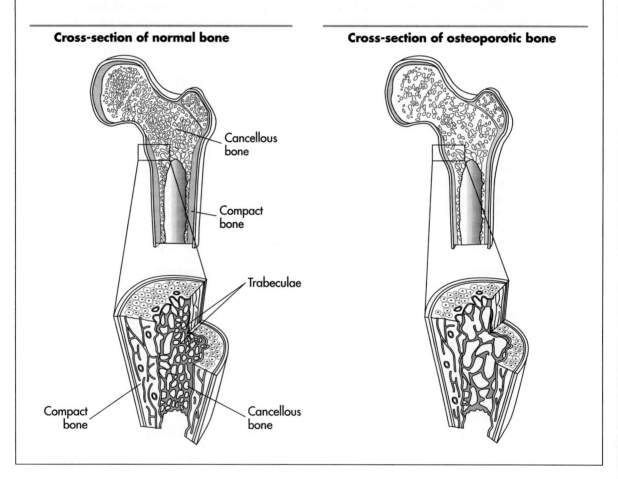

Cross-section of normal bone

Cancellous bone

Compact bone

Trabeculae

Compact bone

Cancellous bone

Cross-section of osteoporotic bone

Treatment for hip fracture depends on the type of fracture and the presence of other injuries or conditions. Obtain a health history, which may include a report of a sudden fall, and perform a thorough physical examination. The affected limb may have ecchymosis and tissue trauma and appear shortened and externally rotated. Anticipate the need for an X-ray to confirm the hip fracture. Then prepare the patient for surgery, as appropriate.

Hip surgery

If your patient has been taking an oral corticosteroid, she may receive I.V. corticosteroid therapy before, during, and after surgery. This decreases the risk of a steroid crisis or secondary adrenocortical insufficiency from abrupt withdrawal of the oral drug.

Before surgery, the patient may be placed in traction to provide comfort, immobilize the joint, help decrease the risk of further soft-tissue damage, realign the fractured bone, and reduce muscle spasms in the limb. During this time, be sure to monitor your patient's vital signs, skin integrity, fluid balance, mental status, nutritional status, and coping skills.

Surgical options include hip pinning or nailing, hemiarthroplasty, and complete joint replacement. The choice of procedure depends on the type and area of the fracture and the patient's condition and bone stock. The choice of procedure also determines how soon she'll be mobile after surgery. For example, a joint replacement may allow the patient to bear weight while ambulating sooner than the use of hip pins, which may require the use of crutches to prevent weight bearing.

After surgery, perform routine postoperative care, being especially alert for signs of infection, which may be masked by corticosteroid use. Remember, corticosteroids alter the immune response and may decrease your patient's resistance to local infection. Monitor her temperature closely and check the incision sites carefully for redness and drainage.

Corticosteroids also may increase the risk of peptic ulcer disease and its associated complications: perforation and hemorrhage. Similarly, long-term use of NSAIDs and the stress of surgery can increase the patient's risk of GI bleeding and stress ulcers. Therefore, monitor your patient's vital signs carefully and check her stool for occult blood.

Corticosteroids can increase your patient's risk of skin breakdown because they make the skin thin and fragile and may increase sweating, which can impair wound healing. Inspect the wound regularly and note any changes in color or shape. Change your patient's position at least every 2 hours or encourage her to use the overbed trapeze to shift her weight. Help her walk as soon as possible, and enlist the aid of a physical therapist to plan an exercise program that can minimize the effects of immobility on the joints.

Because of the sodium-retaining properties of corticosteroids, your patient may retain fluid, causing a fluid imbalance. Monitor her fluid intake and output at least every 4 hours after surgery. Also, monitor her serum electrolyte levels and weigh her daily. Auscultate the lungs to detect crackles, which may indicate fluid accumulation. Encourage your patient to cough, deep-breathe, and use incentive spirometry to prevent pulmonary complications related to immobility.

Before discharge, reinforce all aspects of the patient's drug regimen. Also, review specific instructions about her recovery from surgery (see *Recovering from hip surgery at home*, page 182).

Complications

A patient with rheumatoid arthritis and a hip fracture is at increased risk for developing complications, such as DVT, pulmonary embolism, fat embolism, atelectasis, chronic venous insufficiency, and skin breakdown.

Deep vein thrombosis

DVT develops when platelets come in contact with a damaged vessel wall and adhere to it. As more platelets adhere to the vessel wall, they become more permeable and then rupture, releasing clotting factors for fibrin formation. The fibrin strands trap RBCs, WBCs, and more platelets, forming a thrombus. Eventually, the enlarging thrombus decreases blood flow through the vessel. As a result, the patient is at risk for venous insufficiency and embolism.

Several factors—including clotting mechanism disorders, venous insufficiency, and immobilization—increase the risk of DVT. For a patient with rheumatoid arthritis, the risk is even greater, especially if she's immobilized with a hip fracture.

Confirming the complication

Signs and symptoms of DVT include pain and swelling in the affected limb, deep muscle tenderness, and warmth and redness in the area of the thrombus. The patient may have a slightly elevated temperature and a positive Homans' sign (calf pain elicited by dorsiflexing the foot).

Recovering from hip surgery at home

A patient with rheumatoid arthritis who undergoes hip surgery needs to take special care to ensure adequate healing and proper joint alignment. Before your patient is discharged, provide thorough teaching.

- Teach her to position her body properly when sitting, standing, and walking. Caution her to avoid crossing her legs because doing so increases the risk of venous stasis. Advise her to sit in a chair with a straight back and a raised seat to prevent flexing her hip beyond 90 degrees. Suggest that she use a raised toilet seat.
- Instruct her not to stay in one position for a prolonged period. Tell her to get up and walk around or to change her position to improve circulation and relieve stiffness.
- Explain that joints affected by rheumatoid arthritis should be splinted or positioned for support and comfort.
- Teach her how to modify her home to avoid safety hazards. For example, advise her to keep hallways adequately lit, avoid using throw rugs, have safety bars installed in the tub or shower, and use nonskid floor mats.
- Review activity precautions. Teach her to perform appropriate exercise. Advise her to take the prescribed analgesic before exercising. Also,

remind her to pace her activities and to rest frequently to minimize fatigue.
- Warn her to avoid sudden jarring movements to prevent straining swollen, painful joints and dislocating the hip.
- Teach her how to use assistive devices—such as long-handled shoe horns or reachers, zipper pulls, and Velcro closures—to ease stress on arthritic joints and encourage independence.
- Teach her to care for her incision to prevent infection and promote healing. Tell her to notify her physician if she detects signs of infection, such as redness, swelling, or drainage.
- Review her drug regimen. Tell her to take her antiarthritic drug with food to decrease stomach irritation. Advise her to take her anticoagulant at the same time each day.
- Teach her to assess herself daily for signs of bleeding, such as bruising, rectal bleeding, and black, tarry stools. Tell her to notify her physician immediately if she notes these signs. Discuss bleeding precautions, such as avoiding injury and using a soft toothbrush and an electric razor.
- Stress the importance of keeping follow-up appointments with her physician. Also, explain the need for frequent blood tests to determine if anticoagulant therapy is effective.

Venous duplex scanning, which allows visualization of the vein, confirms the diagnosis of DVT. Doppler ultrasonography may be used to evaluate blood flow and blood vessel patency. However, it isn't as accurate in confirming DVT because the results are affected by the ultrasound technician's skill. Also, Doppler ultrasonography can't identify the extent of an occlusion and can't evaluate the deep veins of the thigh and pelvis.

Plethysmography may be used to evaluate volume changes in the legs during venous filling and emptying. However, it's associated with false-negative results because it requires the patient to lie perfectly still and hold deep inhalations to cause venous pooling in the deep veins.

Nursing interventions
The key to nursing care is to prevent DVT by promoting venous return to the heart and preventing blood from stagnating in the leg veins. While your patient is in bed, apply antiembolism stockings or use sequential compression devices to improve venous flow. Perform range-of-motion exercises with the unaffected leg every 2 hours.

As soon as possible after hip surgery, encourage the patient to walk to improve venous return from the legs. Monitor her vital signs, LOC, and respiratory status closely. Also, perform neurovascular checks on both legs, assessing them for pain, pallor, pulselessness, paresthesia, and paralysis. Immediately report signs or symptoms of DVT to the physician.

Treating DVT usually includes administering anticoagulants, such as heparin and warfarin.

COMFORT MEASURES

Relieving the pain of rheumatoid arthritis, hip fracture, and deep vein thrombosis

Rheumatoid arthritis, hip fracture, and deep vein thrombosis (DVT) each produce pain. When a patient has all three disorders, the pain can become unbearable. To make matters worse, your patient may need to stop taking her antiarthritic drug while she receives anticoagulant therapy for her hip fracture and DVT. This helps decrease the risk of bleeding but heightens the pain of rheumatoid arthritis. To help relieve your patient's pain, try these interventions:

• Perform thorough and frequent pain assessments. In particular, pay attention to the type of pain, its location, severity, intensity, and duration. Try to determine its source. For example, is it joint, incision, or calf pain? Keep in mind, however, that your patient may experience pain from all three conditions simultaneously and be unable to distinguish the source.

• Give the prescribed analgesic at the first sign of pain. Emphasize to your patient the importance of reporting pain when she first feels it. If she understands that the analgesic will be more effective if given early in the pain cycle, she'll be more likely to request it.

• Closely monitor your patient's reaction to pain-relief measures. Use ones that are most effective.

• Discuss alternate pain-relief treatments with the physician. For example, your patient may obtain relief from epidural analgesia administered by continuous infusion or by intermittent direct injection. Or she may respond to the use of transcutaneous electrical nerve stimulation (TENS). Sometimes, a patient needs a narcotic analgesic to relieve intense pain.

• Try nonpharmacologic measures with your patient, including guided imagery, relaxation, and distraction. You can use more than one nonpharmacologic method as part of the patient's treatment plan. For example, distraction may work better in the morning when the patient is well rested; guided imagery may be more helpful later in the day.

• Look for sources of irritation that can start the pain cycle. For example, your patient may begin to experience pain when she lies in one position for too long. Or she may become uncomfortable if the moist compress used to treat DVT leaks, making the bed linens wet. Take corrective action immediately to make your patient more comfortable. Then monitor her comfort level frequently.

• If your patient doesn't tolerate a particular position well or if she achieves better pain control with a specific type of therapy, share this information with other members of the health care team to increase your patient's comfort.

• Be your patient's advocate. Discuss her pain-relief needs with the physician as often as necessary. Ask your patient and her family how she managed her pain at home, and try to implement these measures in the hospital.

In a patient with rheumatoid arthritis, give these drugs with extreme caution because antiarthritic drugs can adversely affect blood clotting and platelet formation, and anticoagulants increase the risk of bleeding. During treatment, monitor the patient's vital signs and assess her for signs of bleeding. Obtain the results of baseline coagulation studies and compare them with subsequent results.

To minimize the risk of injury, take safety precautions, such as having the patient use a bed cradle and heel protectors to prevent pressure ulcers. Determine which pain relief measures are most effective for your patient (see

Relieving the pain of rheumatoid arthritis, hip fracture, and deep vein thrombosis).

Before your patient's discharge, review all aspects of her care, including her drug and exercise regimens. Teach her to recognize and report the signs and symptoms of complications.

Pulmonary embolism

Pulmonary embolism occurs when a thrombus dislodges—as a result of muscle action, limb injury, or a change in blood flow—and travels in the bloodstream until it reaches the lungs, causing a partial or complete obstruction. Pulmonary emboli originate in the veins (most commonly in the deep veins of the legs) and in the right side of the heart. A patient with rheumatoid arthritis and a hip fracture is at increased risk for developing pulmonary embolism because of clotting mechanism disorders, venous insufficiency, and immobilization.

Confirming the complication

Changes in pulmonary status depend on the extent of pulmonary artery obstruction and on the patient's previous cardiopulmonary condition. Signs and symptoms include unexplained shortness of breath, a dry or productive cough with bloody sputum, pleuritic or anginal chest pain, cyanosis, hypoxemia, tachycardia, tachypnea, pleural friction rub, fever, and diaphoresis. The patient may experience confusion, loss of consciousness, increased anxiety, apprehension, or a sense of impending doom. A ventilation-perfusion scan helps confirm the diagnosis.

Nursing interventions

Focus your care on reducing your patient's risk of developing a pulmonary embolism. Assess her thoroughly whenever she reports new symptoms. Also, place her in a position that maximizes breathing while preventing acute hip flexion. For example, try elevating the head of the bed 30 degrees.

RAPID RESPONSE ▶ When pulmonary embolism develops, you'll need to act quickly. A patient can die rapidly from right ventricular failure, shock, dyspnea, hyperventilation, arterial or pulmonary hypertension, or pulmonary infarction.

- Assess the patient's airway, breathing, and circulation. Establish your patient's airway, auscultate her breath sounds, and assess her oxygen saturation level with pulse oximetry and ABG analysis.
- Notify the physician, and administer supplemental oxygen, as appropriate.
- If your patient's oxygen saturation level falls or if severe respiratory distress develops, prepare for endotracheal intubation and mechanical ventilation.
- Anticipate the need for the insertion of a central venous line and the administration of I.V. heparin.
- Be alert for signs and symptoms of embolism in other parts of the body. ◄

Throughout your nursing care, provide support to your patient and her family. Explain what's happening to help alleviate fear and anxiety.

After your patient's condition stabilizes, the physician will order a ventilation-perfusion scan to confirm the pulmonary embolism. Because the chance of recurrence is high, expect to give your patient prophylactic anticoagulant therapy.

Fat embolism

Fat embolism is the presence of fat globules in the bloodstream. In this condition, embolic fat is deposited in the capillaries of the lungs, causing an acute pulmonary disorder similar to acute respiratory distress syndrome (ARDS).

The exact cause of fat embolism isn't known. One theory suggests that after a long bone (such as the head of the femur) has been fractured, fat globules are released from the bone marrow and enter the venous circulation. These fat globules (along with free fatty acids and neutral fats) are released, leading to platelet aggregation and fat embolism (see *Understanding fat embolism*).

For a patient with rheumatoid arthritis who needs a total hip replacement, the risk of fat embolism is increased. That's because during the surgery, the intermedullary canal must be reamed to allow for placement of the prosthesis. This surgical reaming allows fat to enter the venous circulation.

Confirming the complication

Typically, on the patient's buccal mucosa, hard palate, conjunctivae, and chest, you'll see petechiae that don't blanch with pressure. Other signs and symptoms include neurologic changes and subtle behavior changes, such as confusion, restlessness, apprehension, agitation, irritability, and a decreased LOC. Your patient also may have chest pain, tachycardia, dyspnea, tachypnea, crackles or wheezes on auscultation, an unexplained fever, and hypoxemia. Hemoglobin levels and platelet counts will be decreased, and lipuria will be present.

If fat embolism progresses to ARDS, a chest X-ray will show consolidation, and a ventilation-perfusion scan may be performed to rule out

PATHOPHYSIOLOGY

Understanding fat embolism

After a long bone is fractured, fat globules are released from yellow bone marrow into the blood. These illustrations show how such a bone fracture can lead to respiratory failure.

---

1. Following a hip fracture, fat globules are released into the bloodstream.

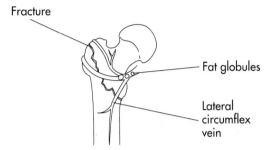

---

2. Fat globules enter the venous circulation, as shown, then travel to the inferior vena cava and pass through the right side of the heart.

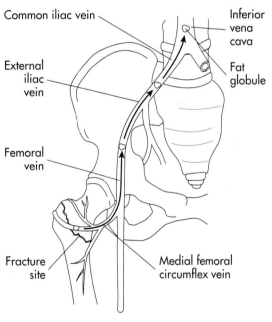

---

3. From the right side of the heart, the fat globules enter the lungs via the pulmonary artery. In the lungs, they obstruct the capillaries and arterioles. As a compensatory mechanism, lipase is secreted to break the fat globules into fatty acids. However, the fatty acids damage the alveolocapillary membrane, as shown in this close-up of an alveolus and a capillary. This damage leads to impaired gas exchange, which, if severe, can result in life-threatening respiratory failure.

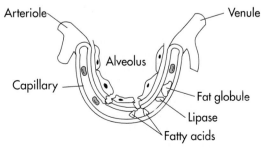

Comparing fat embolism and pulmonary embolism

The assessment findings for fat embolism and pulmonary embolism can be quite similar. Use the table below to help distinguish between the two types of embolism.

Assessment finding	Fat embolism	Pulmonary embolism
Onset	• 1 to 4 days after fracture	• 4 to 10 days after injury or development of deep vein thrombosis; can be much later
Typical signs and symptoms	• Petechiae on buccal mucosa, hard palate, conjunctivae, and chest • Confusion • Restlessness • Agitation • Apprehension • Irritability • Decreased level of consciousness • Chest pain • Dyspnea • Fever • Hypoxemia • Tachycardia • Tachypnea • Crackles or wheezes • Decreased hemoglobin level and platelet count • Lipuria	• Anxiety • Apprehension • Sense of impending doom • Confusion • Loss of consciousness • Sudden severe anginal or pleuritic chest pain • Tachycardia • Tachypnea • Shortness of breath • Cough • Hemoptysis • Cyanosis • Hypoxemia • Fever • Diaphoresis • Pleural friction rub
Contributing factors	• Fluid loss • Shock • Delayed immobilization of fracture • Multiple fractures	• Venous stasis or deep vein thrombosis • Immobility • Obesity • Traumatic injury or major surgery • Heart disease • Previous pulmonary thrombosis

pulmonary embolism (see *Comparing fat embolism and pulmonary embolism*).

Nursing interventions

When a patient with rheumatoid arthritis fractures her hip, immobilize the joint immediately and help prepare her for surgery. To reduce the risk of fat embolism, handle the affected leg gently, especially when turning and positioning the patient.

If you suspect that your patient is developing a fat embolism, notify her physician immediately. Administer fluids to maintain adequate circulation and perfusion. Monitor the patient's fluid intake and output at least every hour,

weigh her every day, and monitor her hemodynamic status.

Administer supplemental oxygen and anticipate the need for mechanical ventilation with positive end-expiratory pressure (PEEP) if ARDS develops. If your patient needs mechanical ventilation, administer a sedative and a neuromuscular blocker, as prescribed, to ease discomfort, decrease anxiety, and reduce oxygen demands. Provide emotional support and frequent explanations to your patient and her family to help relieve anxiety.

Treatment also includes administering a corticosteroid to reduce inflammation that develops with vascular occlusion. Corticosteroids are thought to reduce pulmonary edema and stabilize the pulmonary membrane. If your patient already takes a corticosteroid for rheumatoid arthritis, her physician will adjust the dosage to minimize sodium retention, potassium loss, muscle wasting, delayed healing, increased susceptibility to infection, and an increased risk of bleeding. Closely monitor your patient for signs and symptoms of these complications.

Atelectasis

Atelectasis, the collapse of lung tissue, may result from external pressure exerted by a tumor, air, or fluid in the pleural space. Or it may result when alveoli are obstructed or hypoventilated. When atelectasis develops, debris can become trapped in the collapsed airways, stimulating an inflammatory reaction that can lead to pneumonia.

A patient with rheumatoid arthritis and a hip fracture is at increased risk for developing atelectasis for several reasons. First, rib cage deformities and rheumatoid nodules can interfere with chest expansion. Second, during hip surgery, the patient is positioned in a way that decreases the expansion of dependent lung fields, leading to decreased ventilation, decreased alveolar gas exchange, and decreased aeration. Third, after surgery, immobility leads to pooling of pulmonary secretions, which can obstruct the airway and impair ventilation.

Confirming the complication

The signs and symptoms of atelectasis depend on how fast the collapse develops, how much of the lung is affected, and whether there's an infection. A patient with mild atelectasis may have no symptoms. One with severe atelectasis and lung collapse may report dyspnea and pain on the affected side. You may detect decreased chest expansion and decreased or absent breath sounds on the affected side. Also, the patient may have cyanosis, fever, tachycardia, and decreased blood pressure. She even may be in shock.

ABG analysis may reveal hypoxemia. A chest X-ray can help confirm the diagnosis of atelectasis. Findings depend on the extent and cause of the collapse. They can range from a subtle decrease in lung volume with opacification to complete opacification of a lung segment, lobe, or entire lung.

Nursing interventions

To prevent atelectasis, help your patient with rheumatoid arthritis and a hip fracture avoid immobility. If she's on bed rest, turn and reposition her frequently, keeping in mind the need for proper body alignment and positioning after hip surgery. Also, encourage her to cough, deep-breathe, and use an incentive spirometer. Chest physiotherapy, humidified oxygen therapy, and treatment with a bronchodilator and mucolytic may help mobilize secretions.

If your patient develops atelectasis, focus your care on improving ventilation and gas exchange and on removing the cause of atelectasis. If the suspected cause is a mechanical obstruction that can't be removed by coughing or vigorous chest physiotherapy, the physician may use bronchoscopy.

Auscultate the patient's heart and breath sounds at least every 2 hours and report any decrease in breath sounds or increase in adventitious sounds. Also, note S_3 or S_4 heart sounds, which may indicate heart failure. Continue assessing your patient for signs and symptoms of hypoxemia and monitor her oxygen saturation levels using pulse oximetry or ABG analysis.

Keep in mind that your patient's risk of infection is increased if she's receiving long-term corticosteroid therapy. If she develops an infection, administer the prescribed antibiotic.

Chronic venous insufficiency

Chronic venous insufficiency results from DVT. As the vein walls thicken from DVT, the valves of the vein thicken and constrict. As a result, the valves lose their ability to prevent blood from flowing backward.

The immobility associated with rheumatoid arthritis and hip surgery promotes venous stasis, which leads to DVT—and ultimately to chronic venous insufficiency.

Confirming the complication

Chronic venous insufficiency causes a dull ache in the affected leg that's worsened by prolonged standing and relieved by elevating the leg. Other characteristics include superficial varicose veins, swollen and reddened legs, dermatitis and skin ulceration (usually near the malleoli), and cellulitis.

Doppler ultrasonography and plethysmography may reveal vessel obstruction or valve incompetence.

Nursing interventions

For patients with insufficiency of the superficial veins, treatment may include surgical ligation and stripping of the veins. For most patients, however, chronic venous insufficiency is not curable. Therefore, treatment focuses on improving venous flow and preventing complications, such as skin breakdown. Early mobilization, ambulation, and an exercise program help prevent complications.

Assess your patient's legs for color changes, and check her peripheral pulses. Help her perform range-of-motion exercises with the unaffected leg to improve venous return. When she's sitting in a chair, make sure that her legs don't dangle and that she keeps her hips even with her knees.

Inspect the skin frequently, especially at pressure areas, such as the heels and sacrum. Keep the skin clean and dry. Evaluate the skin closely for any signs of redness and perform skin care to prevent breakdown.

Teach the patient to avoid standing in one place for a long time and to elevate her legs when seated. Instruct her to use antiembolism stockings and sequential compression devices to help promote venous return, especially after hip surgery. Also, explain which areas are prone to breakdown and how to prevent it by using proper footwear.

Skin breakdown

A patient with rheumatoid arthritis and a hip fracture is at risk for developing skin breakdown because of the immobility associated with both disorders. Also, the long-term use of a corticosteroid can impair the skin's function as a primary defense. Corticosteroid use also may delay wound healing and predispose your patient to infection.

Confirming the complication

A patient's signs and symptoms depend on the stage of the breakdown. Initially, the affected area may become reddened, but the skin is warm, firm, and intact. Eventually, breaks appear in the skin, and the area becomes discolored. If the breakdown penetrates the subcutaneous layer, the area is painful and visibly swollen.

Continued breakdown results in an opening that, if infected, will ooze green or yellow foul-smelling fluid. If the muscle is affected, eschar may appear at the edges. If the sore extends to the bone, the area may appear necrotic. You may note foul drainage and tunneling.

Nursing interventions

The key to nursing care is prevention. Turn the patient frequently, encourage her to walk as soon as possible, and provide meticulous skin care. Be sure to maintain the skin integrity of unaffected areas. To minimize dryness, apply moisturizing cream.

If skin breakdown does develop, keep the area clean, dry, and free from pressure to prevent further breakdown. Keep in mind that healing may be delayed if your patient is receiving a corticosteroid to treat rheumatoid arthritis.

Monitor the patient for signs and symptoms of infection. Obtain a wound culture, if necessary, and anticipate antibiotic therapy.

Also, anticipate the need for wound care, using strict aseptic technique and standard precautions. Prepare your patient for possible mechanical or surgical debridement, as appropriate. Encourage fluid intake and adequate nutrition to promote healing. Also, check the wound for signs of bleeding because antiarthritic drugs may interfere with clotting and increase the risk of bleeding.

Suggested readings

Ceccio CM. Autoimmune and inflammatory disorders. In: Maher AB, Pellino TA, Salmond SW, eds. *Orthopaedic nursing.* Philadelphia, Pa: WB Saunders Co; 1994.

Cooper C, Coupland C, Mitchell M. Rheumatoid arthritis, corticosteroid therapy and hip fracture. *Ann Rheum Dis.* 1995;54(1):49-52.

Corrao S, Salli L, Arnone S, et al. Cardiac involvement in rheumatoid arthritis: evidence of silent heart disease. *Eur Heart J.* 1995;16(2):253-256.

Diker E, Aydogdu S, Ozdemir M, et al. Prevalence and predictors of atrial fibrillation in rheumatic valvular heart disease. *Am J Cardiol.* 1996;77(1):96-98.

Fiore LD. Anticoagulation: risks and benefits in atrial fibrillation. *Geriatrics.* 1996;51(6):22-24, 27-28, 31.

Gabriel SE. Update on the epidemiology of the rheumatic diseases. *Curr Opin Rheumatol.* 1996;8(2):96-100.

Henderson NK, Sambrook PN. Relationship between osteoporosis and arthritis and effect of corticosteroids and other drugs on bone, *Curr Opin Rheumatol.* 1996;8(4):365-369.

Hirschowitz BI. Nonsteroidal antiinflammatory drugs and the gastrointestinal tract, *Gastroenterologist.* 1994;2(3):207-233.

Kirwan JR, Lim KK. Low dose corticosteroids in early rheumatoid arthritis: can these drugs slow disease progression? *Drugs Aging.* 1996;8(3):157-161.

Klippel JH, Dieppe PA. *Rheumatology.* 2nd ed. St Louis, Mo: Mosby–Year Book, Inc; 1997.

Kremer JM. The changing face of therapy for rheumatoid arthritis. *Rheum Dis Clin North Am.* 1995;21(3):845-852.

Lyssy KJ, Escalante A. Perioperative management of rheumatoid arthritis: areas of concern for primary care physicians. *Postgrad Med.* 1996;99(2):191-194.

Michel BA, Bloch DA, Wolfe F, Fries JF. Fractures in rheumatoid arthritis: an evaluation of associated risk factors. *J Rheumatol.* 1993;20(10):1666-1669.

Moncur C, Williams HJ. Rheumatoid arthritis: status of drug therapies. *Phys Ther.* 1995;75(6):511-525.

Morley J, Marinchak R, Rials SJ, Kowey P. Atrial fibrillation, anticoagulation and stroke, *Am J Cardiol.* 1996;77(3):38A-44A.

Orsinelli DA. Current recommendations for the anticoagulation of patients with atrial fibrillation. *Prog Cardiovasc Dis.* 1996;39(1):1-20.

Rankin JA. Pathophysiology of the rheumatic joint. *Orthop Nurs.* 1995;14(4):39-46.

Rudd JH, Maxwell S, Kendall M. The causes and management of atrial fibrillation. *J Clin Pharm Ther.* 21(1):37-43, 1996.

Star VL, Hochberg MC. Osteoporosis in patients with rheumatic diseases. *Rheum Dis Clin North Am.* 1994;20(3):561-576.

Turpie AG, Connolly SJ. Antithrombic therapy in atrial fibrillation. *Can Fam Physician.* 1996; 42:1341-1345.

Weisman MH. Corticosteroids in the treatment of rheumatologic diseases. *Cur Opin Rheumatol.* 1995;7(3):183-190.

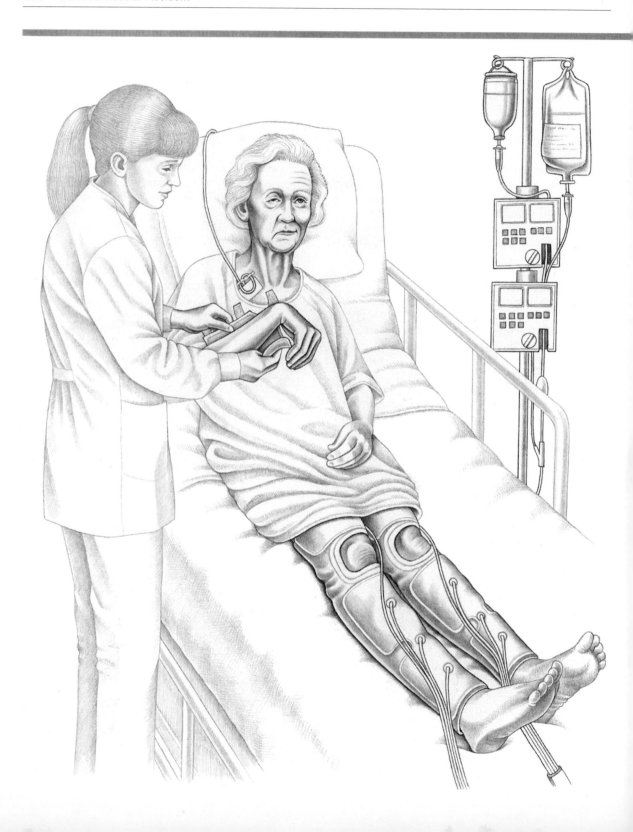

6

Cerebrovascular Accident

Few medical conditions evoke the level of fear produced by the prospect of a cerebrovascular accident (CVA). Commonly known as a stroke, CVA is the third leading cause of death in the United States, outranked only by heart disease and cancer.

Cerebrovascular accidents are also the nation's leading cause of disability. Of the nearly 550,000 Americans who have a CVA each year, about 150,000 die. Most of those who survive must learn to live with some level of impairment. Some patients face profound disability from a permanent reduction of their mental or physical function.

The good news is that fewer people experience CVAs than just a few years ago. And those who do have a greater chance of a full recovery. Still, several common disorders—hypertension, diabetes, pneumonia, atherosclerosis, and osteoarthritis, for example—can raise the risk of a CVA and complicate its outcome. Specifically, they can increase the likelihood of hemorrhage, occlusion, neurologic deficit, and nutritional and mobility problems.

Anatomy and physiology review

The brain, the seat of the central nervous system (CNS), sits at the top of the spinal cord and is surrounded and protected by the skull. Formed of roughly 100 billion neurons and related structures, the brain coordinates and regulates CNS function through the spinal cord and countless nerves that traverse the body.

The brain itself is composed of three main parts: the cerebrum, cerebellum, and brain stem (see *Two views of the brain*). The cerebrum is the largest and uppermost portion. It's divided into hemispheres by a deep longitudinal fissure. The cerebrum's outer layer—less than a quarter inch thick—is called the cerebral cortex.

The cerebrum is divided into four paired lobes: frontal, parietal, temporal, and occipital. Although all the lobes perform some similar functions, they each dominate different functional areas.

The frontal lobes are responsible for conceptualizing, forming abstract thoughts, making judgments, starting and stopping motor activity, forming and writing words, and ensuring higher-level autonomic functions.

The parietal lobes coordinate the perception and interpretation of sensory information, including the ability to recognize body parts and tell left from right.

The temporal lobes form the primary auditory receptive area. The left temporal lobe contains Wernicke's area, which allows for the understanding of spoken and written language. The temporal lobes also interpret visual and somatic input. And they store memories that require more than one sense.

The occipital lobes receive and interpret visual images.

The cerebellum contains several types of neurons and complex interconnections. From its position in the posterior fossa, it coordinates fine movements and muscular activities, allows for the estimation of distances and speeds, and maintains balance and equilibrium.

The brain stem lies between the cerebellum and the spinal cord and includes the midbrain, pons, and medulla oblongata. It controls alertness and the autonomic functions of such organs as the heart, blood vessels, lungs, stomach, and intestines.

Cerebral blood flow

Continued function in all areas of the brain depends on a steady supply of oxygen and nutrients. Naturally, that supply comes by way of a network of arteries—one that carries about 800 ml of blood to the brain every minute.

Oxygenated blood reaches the brain by two distinct routes: the anterior route by way of the carotid arteries and the posterior route by way of the vertebral arteries. The two routes join in an arterial structure called the circle of Willis (see *A look at blood supply to the brain*, page 194).

The carotid arteries provide the bulk of the brain's blood supply. After entering the skull, each internal carotid artery divides into the anterior and middle cerebral artieries. The anterior cerebral arteries supply the basal ganglia, corpus callosum, medial surfaces of the cerebral hemispheres, and superior surfaces of the frontal and patietal lobes. The middle cerebral arteries primarily supply the cortical surfaces of the frontal, parietal, and temporal lobes.

The vertebral arteries originate at the subclavian artery and travel upward in the foramina of the cervical vertebrae. They enter the skull through the foramen magnum and join at the level of the medulla and pons to form the basilar artery. The basilar artery then branches into the anterior and posterior inferior cerebellar arteries, which supply the brain stem and cerebellum. At the level of the midbrain, the basilar artery branches again to form the posterior cerebral arteries, which supply the diencephalon and the temporal and occipital lobes.

The anterior, middle, and posterior cerebral arteries join to form the circle of Willis around

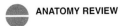 **ANATOMY REVIEW**

Two views of the brain

These two illustrations show the major areas and structures of the brain.

Surface view

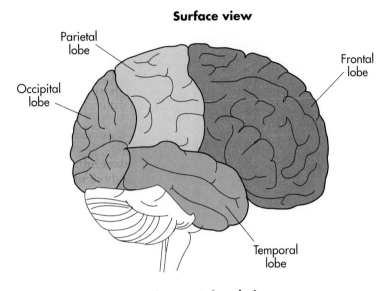

Cross-sectional view

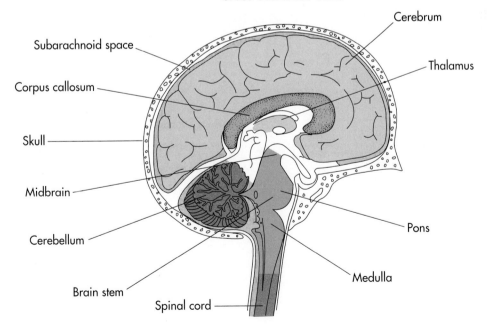

ANATOMY REVIEW

A look at blood supply to the brain

A complex series of arteries brings a steady supply of oxygenated blood to the brain, as shown in these illustrations.

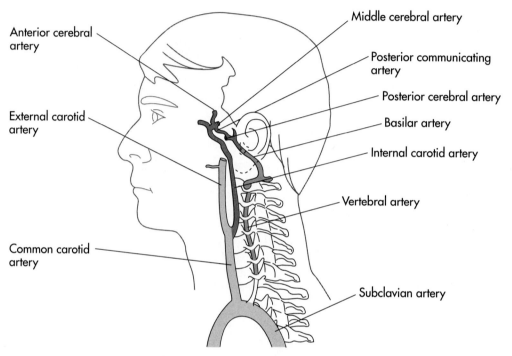

Middle cerebral artery

Anterior cerebral artery

Posterior communicating artery

Posterior cerebral artery

External carotid artery

Basilar artery

Internal carotid artery

Vertebral artery

Common carotid artery

Subclavian artery

Base of the brain

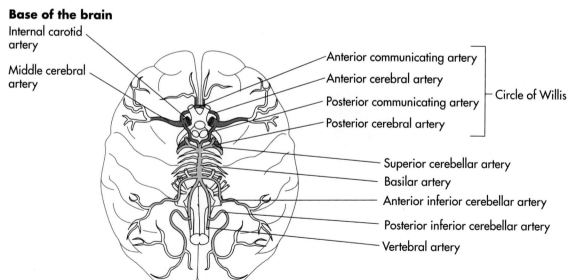

Internal carotid artery

Middle cerebral artery

Anterior communicating artery

Anterior cerebral artery

Posterior communicating artery

Posterior cerebral artery

Circle of Willis

Superior cerebellar artery

Basilar artery

Anterior inferior cerebellar artery

Posterior inferior cerebellar artery

Vertebral artery

the optic chiasm, which stabilizes blood flow throughout the brain by establishing communication between the anterior and posterior circulation routes.

Blood drains from the cerebrum by superficial and deep cerebral veins that empty into venous holding areas between the inner and outer dural layers. From there, venous blood returns to the superior vena cava through the internal jugular veins at the base of the skull.

Cerebrospinal fluid flow

The brain also relies on the cushioning effect of a clear, colorless liquid called cerebrospinal fluid (CSF). The choroid plexus of the brain's ventricles produces about 600 ml of CSF every day; 125 to 150 ml circulate around the brain and spinal cord at any given time. That volume of fluid creates about 12 mm Hg of pressure inside the skull.

Once produced, CSF flows from the lateral ventricles through the foramen of Monro into the third ventricle, then through the cerebral aqueduct to the fourth ventricle. It then passes through either the foramen of Luschka or the foramen of Magendie and into the subarachnoid space. The subarachnoid space has one-way, pressure-sensitive valves (arachnoid villi) that open to allow CSF to move out of the skull and into the venous drainage system of the dura (see *Following the flow of cerebrospinal fluid*, page 196).

Regulating the cerebral environment

To function properly, the brain must maintain and regulate pressure inside the skull. It also must maintain the flow of oxygen and nutrients to its tissues. The brain does both by balancing changes in blood flow and CSF volume.

Cerebral blood vessels constrict and dilate to maintain pressure and nutrients in response to carbon dioxide concentration, oxygen concentration, and hydrogen ion concentration. When the carbon dioxide concentration rises, carbon dioxide combines with body fluids to form carbonic acid and, eventually, hydrogen ions. A rising hydrogen ion concentration triggers vasodilation in the cerebral vessels, which increases cerebral blood flow and brings the hydrogen

ion concentration back down. A drop in oxygen concentration also triggers vasodilation, increasing cerebral perfusion and delivering more oxygen to the brain.

Usually, autoregulatory mechanisms control cerebral blood flow. When these mechanisms fail, however, the sympathetic nervous system takes over. During strenuous exercise, for example, as blood pressure rises, sympathetic stimulation causes large and medium-sized cerebral arteries to constrict. This constriction prevents high blood pressure from reaching the small vessels and injuring them.

Like changes in blood flow, fluctuations in CSF volume also help maintain intracranial pressure (ICP) at optimal levels. A rise in ICP of only 5 mm Hg is enough to force the arachnoid villi to open and drain a portion of the CSF into the venous system, thus maintaining normal ICP.

The blood-brain barrier provides another mechanism for regulating and maintaining a stable environment in the brain. This barrier results from tight junctions between endothelial cells in the cerebral vessels and supporting neuroglia cells, especially the astrocytes. A relatively impermeable membrane, the blood-brain barrier protects the brain from most toxins, but it allows the passage of substances needed for metabolism, based on their size, solubility, and chemical charge. The barrier also helps regulate volume in the skull by restricting the flow of water from blood.

Pathophysiology

When an area of brain tissue is denied its usual supply of oxygen and glucose, the cells immediately stop functioning. They do so because, unlike other body tissues, the brain can't store glucose or glycogen, and it can't engage in anaerobic metabolism. Within minutes, the person begins to show neurologic deficits that may include motor weakness, speech impairment, visual disturbances, altered gait, sensory loss, and dizziness.

If cerebral blood flow resumes promptly, these neurologic deficits may resolve in minutes or hours. If they resolve within 24 hours,

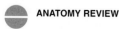 **ANATOMY REVIEW**

Following the flow of cerebrospinal fluid

The choroid plexus of the lateral ventricles produces cerebrospinal fluid, which flows to the subarachnoid space and then into the blood by way of the superior sagittal sinus.

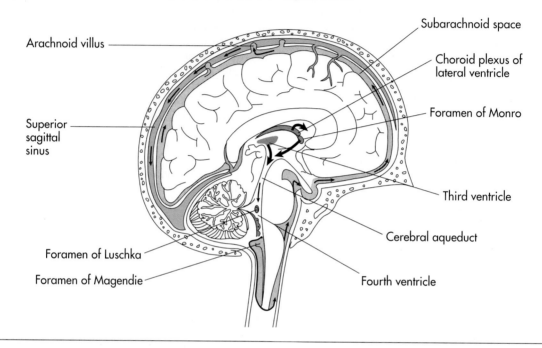

the patient had what's called a transient ischemic attack (TIA). If the restricted blood flow lasts long enough to kill some of the patient's brain cells, however, some level of neurologic deficit becomes permanent. In this case, the patient has experienced a CVA.

Even though a TIA resolves completely, it's a warning sign of an impending CVA. In fact, the risk of a CVA after a TIA ranges from 24% to 29% over the following 5 years. However, only about half of CVA patients experience a warning TIA.

Most CVAs involve the brain's anterior circulation route and typically result from one of two problems: ischemia or hemorrhage involving the cerebral circulation. Ischemia causes about 75% of all CVAs. About 15% stem from intracerebral or subarachnoid hemorrhage. The remaining 10% result from various other causes, including artery dissection, fibromuscular dysplasia, systemic lupus erythematosus, giant cell arteritis, polyarteritis, granulomatous angiitis, acquired immunodeficiency syndrome, polycythemia, sickle-cell disease, and hyperviscosity syndrome.

Ischemic CVA

An ischemic CVA results from an occlusion caused either by a thrombus or an embolus. It also may result from decreased perfusion. In all cases, reduced or blocked blood flow causes brain tissue to become ischemic distal to the blockage.

Thrombotic CVA

In many cases, a thrombotic CVA results from atherosclerosis. Early in atherosclerosis, the intimal walls of arteries become lined with lipids and, eventually, fatty streaks develop between layers of smooth-muscle cells. Over time, the fatty streaks become raised fibrous plaques or erosions into the arterial lining. The roughened vessel walls may cause platelets and fibrin to begin collecting. The same may happen if the artery's endothelial lining becomes injured by hypertension, smoking, genetic factors, immune reactions, or toxic substances in the blood. If the resulting thrombus becomes large enough, it may block blood flow to distal branches of the artery.

A CVA results from this blocked blood flow when the thrombus forms in extracranial or intracranial vessels, decreasing flow to the cerebral cortex. In cerebral circulation, fibrous plaques tend to develop in large vessels. Usually, they develop in:

- the bifurcation of the carotid arteries
- the distal intracranial portion of the vertebral arteries
- the proximal basilar artery.

The carotid artery is the most commonly affected extracranial vessel. The middle cerebral artery is the most commonly affected intracranial vessel.

Lacunar CVA: A specific type of thrombotic CVA, a lacunar CVA usually is caused by vascular changes resulting from hypertension. It's called a lacunar CVA because it creates small cavities deep within the white matter of the brain. Affected structures may include the internal capsule, basal ganglia, thalamus, and pons.

The underlying pathologic changes result from a condition called lipohyalinosis, in which a hyaline-lipid material coats the small penetrating arteries and arterioles, thickening—and weakening—their walls. Damage to these walls can cause subintimal dissections and microaneurysms that encourage thrombus formation. If a thrombus occludes the arteriole, microinfarction and small cavitations may result.

Not all lacunar CVAs cause signs and symptoms. In fact, many are discovered incidentally on a computed tomography (CT) or magnetic resonance imaging (MRI) scan. Some patients with dementia have, in fact, suffered a lacunar CVA. When a lacunar CVA creates neurologic deficits, it affects the arms, face, and legs equally. Other types of CVAs cause varying levels of deficit in the arms and legs.

Embolic CVA

An embolic CVA occurs when an embolus from the heart or extracranial arteries floats into the cerebral bloodstream and lodges in the middle cerebral artery or one of its branches. Typically, this type of CVA arises during activity and isn't preceded by a warning sign.

Most emboli originate in the heart, most commonly from atrial fibrillation. Other cardiac problems that tend to cause emboli include valve lesions, atrial septal defect, a patent foramen ovale, hypokinetic heart disease (such as cardiomyopathy), atrial myoma, infective endocarditis, arrhythmia, and previous myocardial infarction (MI) or cardiac surgery.

Decreased perfusion

Decreased perfusion that causes a CVA may result from cardiopulmonary bypass surgery, heart failure, hypotension, blood loss, or hypovolemia. Brain tissue supplied by more than one artery is most vulnerable to a CVA caused by decreased perfusion. For example, distal regions supplied by the anterior and middle cerebral arteries receive the least amount of blood during low perfusion and, consequently, become ischemic first. This ischemic area is known as the watershed or border zone.

Hemorrhagic CVA

As its name implies, a hemorrhagic CVA results from intracranial bleeding from an artery or vein. Bleeding may involve the parenchymatous tissue (intracerebral hemorrhage) or the spaces surrounding the brain (subdural, subarachnoid, or ventricular hemorrhage). A hemorrhagic CVA usually results from hypertension, a ruptured saccular aneurysm, an arteriovenous malformation, trauma, a hemorrhagic disorder (such as leukemia), or a septic embolism.

When bleeding begins, the brain's regulatory mechanisms try to maintain equilibrium. The stress response and the release of catecholamines trigger an increase in blood pressure in an attempt to maintain cerebral perfusion pressure. As ICP rises, CSF exits the system.

With minor bleeding, these compensatory mechanisms may be enough to keep the patient alive and minimize neurologic deficits.

With heavy bleeding, however, increased pressure in the skull halts cerebral perfusion rapidly, and the patient loses consciousness. The patient may regain consciousness as increased blood pressure restores cerebral perfusion, but a large number of brain cells may become ischemic, swell, and die.

Risk factors for a CVA

The risk factors for a CVA fall into three categories: uncontrollable factors, treatable factors, and lifestyle factors.

Uncontrollable factors

People can't alter their age, ethnic background, sex, or family history. Yet all these factors raise a person's risk of a CVA. For example, 66% of CVAs affect people over age 65. And after age 55, the risk of a CVA doubles with each passing decade. Those with a family history of a CVA or a TIA face an even higher risk.

African-Americans have a 60% higher risk of CVAs than whites and Hispanics of the same age. In African-Americans, CVAs usually result from disease in the small cerebral vessels. In whites, CVAs usually result from disease in the large carotid arteries.

Men of all races have a 30% higher risk of a CVA than women and a higher likelihood of death as a result.

Treatable factors

Hypertension is the single most important risk factor for a CVA, and the level of risk is related to the severity of the hypertension. Cardiac conditions—including arrhythmias, coronary artery disease (CAD), acute MI, dilated cardiomyopathy, and valvular disease—also increase the risk of a CVA.

Nonvalvular atrial fibrillation, the most common arrhythmia in people over age 60, is the most common cause of an embolic CVA; in fact, it increases a person's risk sixfold. Left ventricular hypertrophy increases the risk of ischemic CVA threefold. Patients who've had an MI, especially those who've had an acute anterior-wall MI, face the highest risk of a CVA 1 to 3 weeks after the infarction.

Diabetes not only increases the risk of such vascular diseases as hypertension and CAD—which, in turn, increase the risk of CVA—but is also an independent risk factor.

Families with hyperlipidemia have an increased risk of CVA, probably because elevated blood lipid, cholesterol, and triglyceride levels lead to atherosclerosis. Treating hyperlipidemia helps decrease the risk of vascular disease and may help reduce the risk of a CVA.

Lifestyle factors

A number of lifestyle factors can affect the risk of having a CVA. For example, cigarette smoking increases the risk of ischemic and hemorrhagic CVAs by 40% in men and 60% in women. The risk is strongly related to the number of cigarettes smoked. People who smoke more than 40 cigarettes a day have twice the risk of nonsmokers. Within 5 years after a person quits smoking, the risk from smoking is eliminated.

Alcohol also increases the risk of a CVA if it's consumed heavily every day or in periodic binges. Heavy consumption means more than 3 ounces of hard liquor, more than 8 ounces of wine, or more than 24 ounces of beer a day.

Obesity may contribute to the risk of a CVA because excess body weight commonly is associated with hypertension. Women over age 35 who use an oral contraceptive face an increased risk of a CVA, especially if they also smoke or have hypertension.

Physical activity may help reduce the risk of a CVA by lowering blood pressure, raising high-density lipoprotein levels, lowering low-density lipoprotein levels, and improving glucose tolerance.

Assessment findings

The signs and symptoms of a CVA vary with the location and extent of the occlusion. The more anterior the occlusion, the more likely it will produce motor or speech problems. The more posterior, the more likely it will produce sensory and visual-field impairments. The most common signs and symptoms of a CVA are those produced by an occlusion of the middle cerebral artery (see *Linking signs and symptoms to CVA location*). Specific signs and symptoms also may be related to the cerebral hemisphere that sustained the damage.

Linking signs and symptoms to CVA location

Affected artery	Signs and symptoms
Anterior route	
Internal carotid artery	• Paralysis and sensory deficits of the arm, leg, and face on contralateral side • Aphasia (if dominant hemisphere affected) • Hemianopia and episodes of blurred vision or temporary blindness on ipsilateral side • Carotid bruit
Anterior cerebral artery	• Hemiparesis or hemiplegia of foot and leg on contralateral side • Sensory loss over toes, foot, and leg • Mental status impairment, including confusion, amnesia, perseveration, apathy, and flat affect • Abulia (inability to make decisions or perform voluntary acts)
Middle cerebral artery	• Hemiparesis or hemiplegia of arm and face on contralateral side • Sensory loss of arm and face on contralateral side • Hemianopia of contralateral side • With damage in left hemisphere, aphasia and difficulty reading, writing, and calculating • With damage in right hemisphere, neglect of left visual field, inability to feel stimuli on left side, and spatial disorientation

Affected artery	Signs and symptoms
Posterior route	
Vertebral and basilar arteries	• Hemiplegia and hemiparesis or quadriplegia and quadriparesis • Numbness and weakness of face on ipsilateral side • Dysarthria and dysphagia • Vertigo, nausea, and dizziness • Ataxic gait and clumsiness • Diplopia, homonymous hemianopia, nystagmus, conjugate paralysis, and ophthalmoplegia • With occluded basilar artery, akinetic mutism, locked-in syndrome
Posterior cerebral artery	• Homonymous hemianopia, cortical blindness, lack of depth perception, loss of peripheral vision, visual hallucinations • Memory deficits • Perseveration and dyslexia • With thalamic or subthalamic involvement, diffuse sensory loss, mild hemiparesis, and intentional tremor • With brain stem involvement, pupillary dysfunction, nystagmus, and loss of conjugate gaze
Cerebellar artery	• Nystagmus • Unsteady gait, vertigo, and ataxia • Loss of balance on the affected side • Horner's syndrome on ipsilateral side • Nausea and vomiting • Loss of pain and temperature sensation on one or both sides

In general, if you detect one or more of the following problems, your patient may have had a CVA:
• sudden hemiparesis or monoparesis
• acute dysphasia or dysarthria
• sudden loss of vision in one or both eyes
• sudden onset of double vision
• ataxia
• clumsiness or lack of motor coordination
• sensory loss
• facial weakness
• altered consciousness or severe headache.

Most patients with an ischemic CVA don't lose consciousness. If your patient did lose consciousness, she probably had a CVA-related seizure, a hemorrhagic CVA with increased ICP, or a CVA involving the brain stem.

Diagnostic tests

After a CVA, the patient should have a series of laboratory tests to help determine the etiology of the CVA, the extent of injury, and treatment options. Tests include a complete blood count (CBC) with differential, a platelet count, prothrombin time (PT), activated partial thromboplastin time (APTT), and a serum osmolality test. Also, electrolyte, creatinine, blood urea nitrogen (BUN), blood glucose, and triglyceride levels should be measured. And the patient should have a urinalysis.

The patient also will undergo diagnostic procedures, such as a CT scan, an arteriography, a carotid duplex scan, an echocardiogram, a chest X-ray, and a lumbar puncture.

CT scan
As soon as the patient is hemodynamically stable, she'll probably have a CT scan to rule out a hemorrhage. Usually, an ischemic CVA and edema won't show up on a CT scan until 12 to 24 hours after the start of symptoms, unless the patient has a large infarction. On the other hand, an intracerebral hemorrhage larger than 1 cm shows up on the scan right away. A CT scan diagnoses more than 95% of subarachnoid hemorrhages from an aneurysm because the blood is clearly visible in the subarachnoid space.

Arteriography
If there's evidence of blood in the subarachnoid space or if a patient with a nonhemorrhagic CVA that's less than 6 hours old exhibits neurologic symptoms, the patient will probably undergo arteriography. This test can help a physician decide on an appropriate treatment for an aneurysm. It may also help in diagnosing stenosis or an acute thrombotic occlusion in the head and neck. Plus, it can help determine if the patient is a candidate for thrombolytic therapy. Used later, arteriography helps evaluate whether the patient can benefit from surgery to repair carotid artery stenosis.

Carotid duplex scanning
This noninvasive test, which can be used to view the internal carotid arteries, identifies stenosis that exceeds 60%. If the test detects such stenosis, the patient probably will undergo arteriography before having a carotid endarterectomy.

Echocardiogram
A CVA patient may have a transesophageal echocardiogram to detect atrial thrombi, an atrial septal defect, or a patent foramen ovale. Patients with a history of cardiac problems, a recent MI, or atrial fibrillation are at high risk for atrial thrombi. Before performing a transesophageal echocardiogram, a physician makes sure the patient is a candidate for long-term anticoagulation therapy or surgery to repair any cardiac lesions.

Transthoracic echocardiography can detect ventricular thrombi and may help evaluate ventricular function in a CVA patient.

Chest X-ray
A physician may order a chest X-ray to check the size of the patient's heart and to rule out pneumonia, the second most common cause of death in CVA patients.

Lumbar puncture
If the CT scan results are normal, but the patient's signs and symptoms suggest a subarachnoid hemorrhage, a physician may perform a lumbar puncture. If the CSF contains blood, the patient probably has a hemorrhage.

Medical interventions

Medical management of a CVA can include drug therapy, management of ICP, and surgery.

Drug therapy
Thrombolytic drugs are the treatment of choice for an acute CVA. Patients who've had a CVA and patients at risk for a CVA also may benefit from an anticoagulant to prevent an arterial occlusion or antiplatelet therapy to prevent thrombus formation.

Thrombolytic drugs
For the first few hours after a CVA begins, thrombolytic drugs can help minimize cerebral damage by opening vessels blocked by blood clots, thus restoring the blood supply. Doing so minimizes the size of the infarcted area and,

consequently, minimizes the patient's neurologic deficits.

Thrombolytic drugs include streptokinase, urokinase, recombinant tissue plasminogen activator (TPA), and anisoylated plasminogen streptokinase activator complex. They all activate the conversion of plasminogen to plasmin, which, in turn, lyses the clot.

Streptokinase: Streptokinase, the oldest of the thrombolytic drugs, depletes fibrinogen throughout the circulatory system, not only at the clot. Because it's a bacterial product, streptokinase may cause an allergic response that includes a fever, rash, and hypotension. To counteract this response, a patient may need treatment with diphenhydramine and a corticosteroid. A patient also may produce antibodies to streptokinase that would prevent its use in the future.

Urokinase: Like streptokinase, urokinase affects the entire circulatory system. The drug works by converting both fibrin-bound and circulating plasminogen into plasmin.

Urokinase, which can be given up to 6 hours after CVA symptoms begin, produces lysis for 24 hours. Urokinase doesn't produce an allergic response, and no antibodies are formed, so it can be used repeatedly.

Tissue plasminogen activator: TPA converts plasminogen into plasmin on the surface of a clot. Except when given in doses larger than 100 mg, it doesn't affect circulating plasminogen.

This drug must be given within 3 hours of the first signs of a CVA. Before it's given, however, a patient must be evaluated because any of the following may rule out the use of TPA:
- hemorrhage visible on a CT scan or suggested by the patient's signs and symptoms
- PT greater than 15 seconds, platelet count less than 100,000 mm, or fibrinogen less than 100 mg/dl
- gastrointestinal (GI) or genitourinary bleeding in the past 21 days
- trauma, surgery, or cardiopulmonary resuscitation in the past 14 days
- arterial puncture at a noncompressible site in the past 7 days
- lumbar puncture in the past 7 days

- diastolic blood pressure more than 130 mm Hg.

Anisoylated plasminogen streptokinase activator complex: This drug also converts plasminogen to plasmin. Derived from streptokinase, it also carries a risk of an allergic response. The risk is lower than that for streptokinase.

Anticoagulant and antiplatelet drugs

If more than a few hours have passed since CVA symptoms began, an anticoagulant or antiplatelet drug may be needed after thrombolytic therapy to maintain the patency of the vessel. These drugs also may help prevent another TIA or CVA. However, anticoagulant treatment remains controversial both because the drug may not halt a CVA's progression and because it could convert an ischemic CVA to a hemorrhagic CVA.

Despite the controversy, anticoagulants are the first choice for treating an embolic CVA. And heparin is the first line anticoagulant treatment because of its immediate action. Usually, a patient receives an initial bolus to achieve therapeutic blood levels quickly and then she's given a continuous infusion. As soon as the APTT reaches the desired therapeutic level, the patient receives warfarin—the drug of choice for preventing cardiogenic emboli. The patient's international normalized ratio should be maintained at 2.5 to 3.0. Warfarin also may be effective for patients who continue to experience cerebral ischemia while they're taking an antiplatelet drug.

Aspirin, an antiplatelet drug, is the drug of choice for treating noncardiogenic TIAs. Aspirin decreases platelet aggregation by inhibiting cyclooxygenase. Adverse GI effects can be reduced by using enteric-coated aspirin or by giving aspirin after the patient eats.

For patients who can't tolerate aspirin or who continue to have cerebral ischemia while taking it, a physician may prescribe the antiplatelet drug ticlopidine. It inhibits platelet aggregation by blocking the action of adenosine diphosphate. Ticlopidine's adverse effects include bone marrow suppression, diarrhea, and rash. Neutropenia commonly occurs during the first 3 months but reverses when therapy stops. The patient will need a CBC with differential every 2 weeks for 3 months to check for neutropenia.

Intracranial pressure management

The goals in managing patients with cerebral edema include reducing ICP, maintaining cerebral perfusion, and preventing brain herniation. Immediate treatment includes using hyperventilation to decrease the partial pressure of arterial carbon dioxide ($Paco_2$) by 5 to 10 mm Hg, which lowers ICP by 25% to 30%. The patient also may receive an osmotic diuretic, such as mannitol. If she has hydrocephalus, she may need an intraventricular catheter to drain CSF.

Surgical and invasive procedures

If the patient has a large cerebellar infarction that's compressing her brain stem, treatment may involve removing the infarcted brain tissue to help decompress the remaining live tissue.

If the patient has a subarachnoid hemorrhage caused by an aneurysm, she may undergo surgery to cut off the aneurysm from circulation. This is done by fastening a clip across the neck of the aneurysm. As an alternative, the patient may undergo a procedure that uses a coated platinum coil to fill and obliterate the aneurysm. In this procedure, a neuroradiologist places a small catheter in the aneurysm and then threads a coated platinum strand through the catheter and into the aneurysm. He may use several coils of varying lengths and diameter to fully occlude the aneurysm. The risks of the procedure include aneurysm rupture, malocclusion of the aneurysm, coil compression over time, and emboli. Postprocedure management may include giving heparin I.V. to prevent emboli formation.

If the patient's signs and symptoms stem from stenosis in the carotid or vertebrobasilar arteries, she may benefit from percutaneous transluminal angioplasty or the placement of a stent in the occluded vessel. Percutaneous transluminal angioplasty may be especially useful for treating stenosis of the posterior circulation because these vessels are difficult to reach surgically.

For a conscious patient who has experienced an acute minor stroke, stenosis in the carotid arteries can also be treated with carotid endarterectomy. However, this procedure can't be performed if the arteries are totally occluded.

Nursing interventions

Obtain vital signs and perform a neurologic assessment every hour for the first 8 hours. To perform this assessment, you can use the Glasgow Coma scale (see *Using the Glasgow Coma scale*). If your patient's level of consciousness (LOC), respiratory pattern, pupillary response, or other neurologic signs change, notify her physician immediately.

Your patient faces the highest risk of increased ICP during the first week after a CVA. Cerebral edema is more common after an occlusion of a major intracranial artery or a large multilobar infarction. Monitor the patient for seizures; if not controlled, they may be life-threatening. Treat seizures with phenytoin or phenobarbital, as prescribed.

Monitor your patient's cardiac function carefully for the first 48 hours after a CVA. Many CVA patients have underlying cardiac problems, which may raise their risk of an MI during the acute stages of a CVA.

Maintain your patient's airway, and use a pulse oximeter to check her oxygen saturation. If it dips below 90%, give her oxygen at 2 to 4 liters per minute to maintain a saturation level of at least 90%. If it drops below 90%, expect to obtain arterial blood gas (ABG) levels and a chest X-ray.

Auscultate your patient's breath sounds frequently and evaluate her for signs and symptoms of aspiration and respiratory compromise, such as dyspnea, cyanosis, and tachypnea. Make sure her gag reflex is intact and evaluate her for signs of dysphagia.

Because fever is common after a CVA, either from infection or from neurogenic causes, monitor your patient's temperature. When associated with cerebral edema, even a small temperature increase can worsen the tissue damage. Treat your patient's fever with an antipyretic, such as acetaminophen, as prescribed. If she has a persistent fever above 101° F (38.3° C), use hypothermia blankets. Because CVA can interfere with bladder function, evaluate your patient for signs and symptoms of urinary tract infection, such as urinary frequency and foul-smelling urine, and intervene appropriately.

Controlling blood pressure

During the acute stage of an ischemic CVA, check your patient's blood pressure frequently. In many patients, blood pressure will increase during the first 48 hours because the brain tries to enhance blood flow to damaged tissues by boosting cerebral perfusion. If your patient's systolic pressure exceeds 220 mm Hg or her diastolic pressure exceeds 120 mm Hg for three readings taken 15 minutes apart, a physician will probably prescribe an antihypertensive. But remember, reducing blood pressure too much or too fast could decrease blood flow to tissues surrounding the infarction and worsen your patient's neurologic deficits.

Ideally, you'll want to maintain a systolic pressure of 160 to 170 mm Hg for normotensive patients and 180 to 185 mm Hg for hypertensive patients. Try to keep diastolic pressure at 95 to 100 mm Hg for normotensive patients and 105 to 110 mm Hg for hypertensive patients. The physician probably won't use vasodilators because they increase ICP along with cerebral perfusion pressure. Instead, the drug of choice is labetalol, which doesn't increase ICP.

The patient who has a hemorrhagic CVA—particularly in the subarachnoid area—needs her blood pressure carefully controlled before surgery. Try to maintain blood pressure within 20 mm Hg of her baseline pressure. However, if she's comatose, she'll need her blood pressure maintained at a higher level to ensure adequate cerebral perfusion but low enough to prevent rebleeding. After surgery, let her blood pressure seek its own level, and take steps to prevent vasospasm.

For most patients, blood pressure returns to normal within 48 hours after a CVA. If it doesn't, notify a physician and evaluate your patient for factors that could contribute to hypertension, such as a full bladder or pain. Before getting your patient out of bed, check her blood pressure when she's lying down and sitting up. And check her standing pressure the first time she gets out of bed.

Managing fluids and nutrition

Hydration and nutrition are crucial elements of your patient's care. Most CVA patients receive nothing by mouth for the first 12 to 24 hours. Infuse the prescribed I.V. solution to maintain

Using the Glasgow Coma scale

Use this scale to help assess your patient's level of consciousness. Assign a score to each of the three responses, then add the three scores to find your patient's total score. A patient who scores 15 points is fully alert and oriented; one who scores 3 points is deeply comatose. A patient who scores 8 points is generally considered comatose and may require endotracheal intubation.

Eye opening response	Patient opens eyes spontaneously.	4
	Patient opens eyes to verbal command.	3
	Patient opens eyes to pain.	2
	No response.	1
Verbal response	Patient is oriented and converses.	5
	Patient is disoriented and converses.	4
	Patient uses inappropriate words.	3
	Patient makes incomprehensible sounds.	2
	No response.	1
Motor response	Patient obeys verbal commands.	6
	Patient localizes pain.	5
	Patient withdraws from pain.	4
	Patient exhibits abnormal flexion.	3
	Patient exhibits abnormal extension.	2
	No response.	1

hydration, but do so cautiously because overhydration can worsen edema.

Because many CVA patients have an increased risk for life-threatening aspiration, monitor your patient carefully for dysphagia. This complication is more common in those with a brain stem infarction, large hemispheric lesions, or decreased consciousness. Dysphagia also is common in patients who've had more

How to prevent aspiration

Many patients have an increased risk of aspiration after a cerebrovascular accident. If the patient can swallow, take these steps to help reduce that risk:

- Monitor your patient closely during the first few meals. Keep suctioning equipment nearby in case you need it quickly.
- Perform mouth care before meals to enhance sensations and salivation, which can improve swallowing.
- Place your patient in the high Fowler position or have her sit in a chair for meals.
- Tell your patient or her caregiver to place foods on the unaffected side of the patient's mouth.
- Offer small portions and provide plenty of time for the patient to chew and swallow.
- Teach the patient to touch her chin to her chest to minimize the chance of aspiration when she swallows.

- Urge your patient not to use drinking straws. Never let her drink thin fluid from a straw while she's lying flat in bed.
- If your patient has a visual-field deficit, tell her to scan left and right, so she can see everything on her plate.
- Keep your patient in an upright position for 30 minutes after each meal.
- Assess your patient's respiratory status after she eats.
- To find out if your patient is pocketing food between her cheek and gum, perform mouth care after meals. Retained food fragments can lead to aspiration later.
- Make sure your patient's family knows all the steps needed to reduce the risk of aspiration.

than one CVA. Watch for coughing, choking on saliva or food, garbled speech, weak facial muscles, a delayed or absent swallow reflex, drooling, and gurgling.

Keep in mind that some patients at risk for aspiration show none of these signs. Because you may see signs of trouble only when your patient actually tries to swallow something, give her ice chips and watch her swallow them.

If your patient can swallow well enough to eat, start feeding her by mouth as soon as possible. Consider giving her thickened liquids to help prevent aspiration (see *How to prevent aspiration*). Special adaptive devices—such as thick-handled utensils, plate guards, and suction-based dishes—can promote independence.

If difficulty swallowing places your patient at risk for aspiration, the physician may order a feeding tube. Or if she needs long-term feeding, she may have a percutaneous endoscopic gastrostomy tube inserted.

If your patient needs enteral nutrition, provide frequent oral care to maintain hygiene and protect the oral mucosa from breakdown and discomfort. To help ease your patient's anxiety about having a feeding tube, encourage her and her family to participate in the feeding routine.

If your patient needs oral medications, take into account her ability to swallow when determining how to give the medications. For instance, you may need to crush them or use a liquid form. If necessary, have a speech therapist evaluate the patient's ability to swallow. A videofluoroscopy swallowing examination can verify whether the patient is a "silent aspirator." If she is, the speech therapist can teach her ways to swallow to help prevent aspiration. You can also have a dietitian evaluate the patient's nutritional needs. To ensure that your patient is getting adequate nutrition, monitor her caloric intake and weigh her two or three times a week.

Controlling glucose levels

Monitor your patient's blood glucose levels during the acute stages of an ischemic CVA. If she develops hypoglycemia, expect to administer an I.V. bolus of 50% dextrose. Hyperglycemia, especially in diabetic patients, may worsen the infarction. If necessary, use insulin to maintain your patient's glucose levels between 140 and 180 mg/dl.

Ensuring elimination

Constipation is a common problem among CVA patients, so auscultate for bowel sounds and watch for abdominal distention. Assess your patient's elimination pattern. And every 2 days check for fecal impaction if her elimination pattern changes.

To prevent constipation, work high-fiber foods (or high-fiber formula), bulk-forming laxatives, and stool softeners into your patient's diet. You can start giving stool softeners as prescribed as soon as you've confirmed your patient's ability to swallow. If these measures don't stop constipation, try giving your patient a tablespoon of magnesium hydroxide at bedtime as prescribed.

If your patient develops urinary incontinence during the acute stage of the CVA, she may require an indwelling urinary catheter. To avoid infection, remove the catheter as soon as your patient is stable. Based on the results of a bladder scan, you may need to perform intermittent catheterization to retrain her bladder. Watch carefully for signs of a urinary tract infection.

Preserving mobility

Your patient with a CVA faces several complications of immobility, including contractures, atrophy, deep vein thrombosis (DVT), pneumonia, and pressure ulcers.

Proper positioning can help prevent contractures, atrophy, nerve pressure palsies, and other orthopedic complications. Watch carefully for signs of deformity on the affected side, including:

- shoulder adduction
- subluxation of the affected shoulder
- flexion contractures of the hand, wrist, and elbow
- external rotation of the hip
- plantar flexion of the foot.

Shoulder subluxation can lead to a painful shoulder-hand syndrome that occurs when the humoral head slides down in the shoulder and compresses the brachial nerve. To help prevent this syndrome, support the patient's shoulder with pillows and armrests. Also, don't pull on her affected arm during transfers and passive range-of-motion exercises or force the joint past the point where she complains of pain.

To help decrease the risk of DVT, pneumonia, and pressure ulcers, help your patient become mobile as soon as possible. In addition to passive range-of-motion exercises, urge her to perform active range-of-motion exercises, when appropriate. If she can't walk, she'll probably benefit from sequential pneumatic compression devices or antiembolism stockings on her legs during the acute stage. Unless contraindicated, give subcutaneous heparin or low-molecular-weight heparin during rehabilitation, as prescribed.

Providing skin care

Several factors increase your CVA patient's risk of skin breakdown, including a loss of sensation, impaired circulation, and immobility. Related complications, such as incontinence, can cause skin breakdown as well.

To prevent skin problems, examine your patient's pressure points regularly. Reposition her at least every 2 hours and keep her skin clean and dry. If necessary, use an air or water mattress to prevent pressure ulcers. Be careful to avoid excessive friction, shear, or pressure when moving your patient.

Assessing mental health

Monitor your patient for signs and symptoms of depression, including:

- a consistently depressed appearance (for instance, not changing clothes daily or attending to personal grooming, flat affect, gazing downward or closing eyes)
- lack of interest in friends, family, or usual activities
- loss of energy or appetite
- sleep disturbances or agitation
- inability to concentrate
- expressed feelings of worthlessness or suicidal thoughts.

If your patient has several of these warning signs or symptoms and there's no drug-related cause, consider setting up a mental health consultation. Treatment depends on the cause of the depression and may involve psychotherapy, antidepressant medications, or both.

How a CVA can affect vision

A cerebrovascular accident (CVA) can cause one of several types of visual impairment, depending on where the cerebral damage occurs. This illustration shows the kinds of visual impairment that can develop when a CVA affects the right optic nerve, the optic chiasm, the right optic tract, the right temporal lobe, the right parietal lobe, and the right occipital lobe. The shading in the visual fields represents loss of vision.

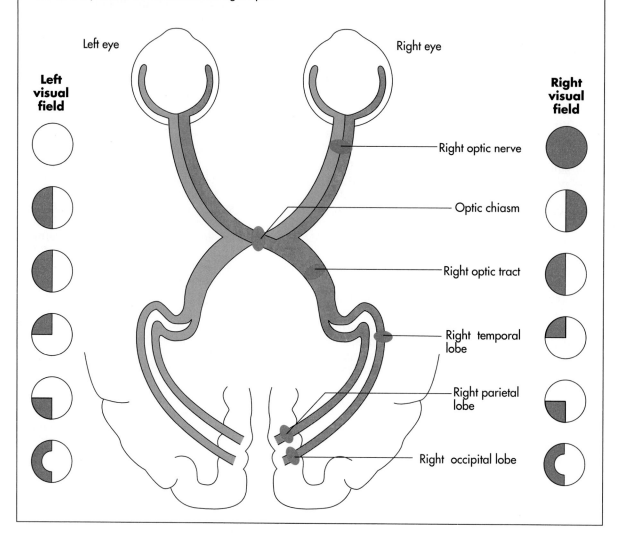

Although less common than depression, other psychological problems may develop in CVA patients. These problems include emotional lability, mania, delusions, hallucinations, obsessive-compulsive disorder, and personality changes. Depending on the cause, the patient may be treated with medications, psychotherapy, or both.

Promoting sensory function

A CVA can affect your patient's sensory function and awareness. Many patients develop homonymous hemianopia. Others develop conjugate paralysis, visual-field defects, or diplopia. Naturally, such visual defects complicate your patient's rehabilitation (see *How a CVA can affect vision*).

A patient with a right-hemisphere CVA may develop a condition called unilateral neglect. She'll ignore sensory stimuli on the left half of her body. She may deny problems created by the CVA, or she may not recognize her own body parts on that side. When asked to describe a picture, she may ignore the left half. When you approach this patient, you may find her head turned to the right; if you're on her left side, she may ignore you.

A patient with unilateral neglect faces many problems. She may not perform hygiene on the left side of her body. She risks falling because she won't see obstacles on her left. And she won't recognize her motor deficits because she doesn't recognize her affected side. Obviously, this patient requires special attention and considerable rehabilitation.

Your CVA patient also may have trouble communicating—either speaking or understanding speech. Work with such a patient to devise a set of verbal or nonverbal cues to help her communicate. Make sure her family or caregiver knows the cues. Sometimes, patients who can't speak can use a pen and paper to communicate their needs. Talking boards or magnetic alphabet letters offer other options. Set up a communication system that works for your patient.

Encourage your patient to be as independent as possible. Show her how to use assistive devices to aid in self-care and activities of daily living. For example, specialized splints can help support her joints. Long-handled mirrors and brushes can increase her ability to ensure good hygiene and grooming. If your patient has trouble with fine-motor activity, such as fastening buttons, suggest that she use Velcro closures instead. If weakness or hemiplegia makes it difficult for your patient to open medicine containers, try to obtain containers that she can open by herself.

Patient teaching

A CVA patient may be discharged to one of several locations, depending on her needs, abilities, and rehabilitation prognosis. Some patients are discharged to a long-term care facility, some to another type of health care facility (such as a rehabilitation center), and some to their homes.

Whether your patient goes home or to a health care facility, you'll need to educate her and her family thoroughly about her condition and needs. As much as possible, adapt your approach to meet their educational and cultural background, the patient's mental status, and the distracting emotions that are a part of this disorder. Make referrals to local support groups and social service organizations as needed (see *Teaching topics for CVA patients*, page 208).

Cerebrovascular accident and atherosclerosis

About 80% of the time, an ischemic CVA results from atherosclerosis and thrombus formation. Even the aneurysms associated with hemorrhagic CVA commonly result from atherosclerotic changes.

Pathophysiology

As described earlier in the chapter, atherosclerosis contributes to the development of a CVA by causing irritation of the arterial lining, thrombus formation, and occlusion of the vessel.

Adapting nursing care

Because atherosclerosis raises your patient's risk of hypertension, which can complicate CVA treatment, you'll need to monitor the patient's blood pressure closely.

While your patient is bedridden, concentrate on preventing thrombophlebitis, pulmonary embolism, and arterial occlusion. Encourage

GOING HOME

Teaching topics for CVA patients

Before your patient with a cerebrovascular accident (CVA) is discharged, cover these teaching topics with her and her family.

Topic area	Specific topics
Basic CVA education for patient and family	• Description of a CVA • Cause of a CVA • Effects of a CVA on the patient • Effects of a CVA on the family
Routine care in hospital, rehabilitation setting, or home	• Nutrition and hydration • Bowel and bladder care • Sleep and rest • Medications and need for compliance • Position and movement in bed • Blood-clot prevention • Skin-breakdown prevention • Safety measures to prevent falls • Exercise during and after rehabilitation • Techniques for performing specific tasks, such as transfers and personal hygiene • Specific skill training • Social functioning
Possible complications	• Swallowing problems • Complications of indwelling urinary catheter and feeding tube use • Respiratory complications • Speech or language deficits • Depression and other psychological disturbances
CVA prevention	• Blood-pressure monitoring • Lifestyle modifications • Medical or surgical methods for preventing another CVA
Postdischarge concerns	• Caregiver concerns • Family functioning • Support groups and respite care • Sexual function • Recreational and vocational pursuits • Automobile operation • Vocational counseling

early mobility, active and passive range-of-motion exercises, frequent repositioning, and adherence to the rehabilitation plan. If your patient receives an anticoagulant, monitor her for signs and symptoms of bleeding. Take precautions to keep her safe from injury.

After your patient's condition is stable, help her make lifestyle modifications to reduce her risk of CAD. Start by discussing diet changes. Encourage your patient to adopt a diet in which saturated fats make up less than 10% of her daily caloric intake. Urge her to consume fewer than 300 mg of cholesterol daily. Check her serum lipid levels and monitor them over time, if possible.

Also, stress the benefits of exercise and weight control. Help your patient develop an exercise program tailored to her abilities as part of her rehabilitation plan. Explain that these changes in diet and activity can help her lose weight and lower her lipid levels. If your patient smokes, urge her to stop. If changes in diet and exercise don't reduce her lipid levels, a physician may prescribe an antilipemic drug.

Complications

Common complications for patients with a CVA and atherosclerosis include thrombophlebitis, pulmonary embolism, and acute arterial occlusion.

Thrombophlebitis

In general, thrombophlebitis develops when at least two elements of Virchow's triad exist. The triad includes:
• stasis
• vascular damage
• hypercoagulability.

Patients with CVA and atherosclerosis face an increased risk of thrombophlebitis because their decreased mobility can lead to stasis and hypercoagulability and because of the vessel damage caused by atherosclerosis. Vessel damage is even more likely if the patient fell or injured herself during the CVA or if a venous access site or injected medication irritates a vein.

Thrombophlebitis that arises in a superficial vein probably will correct itself. DVT, however, can become life-threatening if a piece of a thrombus dislodges and pulmonary embolism results.

Confirming the complication
Thrombophlebitis may or may not cause signs and symptoms. If it does, the patient may

complain of an aching or burning pain in the affected limb. If she has DVT, she may complain of calf or groin tenderness. You may see redness and swelling at the site, and it may feel warm and cordlike. The patient also may experience malaise and a fever.

If you suspect thrombophlebitis despite the absence of signs and symptoms, venography, Doppler studies, or impedance phlebography can be used to confirm the diagnosis.

Nursing interventions

For superficial thrombophlebitis, provide supportive treatment: keep the patient on bed rest, elevate the affected limb, apply warm compresses to the site, and give nonsteroidal anti-inflammatory drugs, as prescribed. Be especially careful when applying warm compresses because a patient with a CVA and atherosclerosis may not be able to tell if the compress is too hot. Encourage mobility early on, use a sequential pneumatic compression device or antiembolism stockings, and ensure frequent position changes and range-of-motion exercises.

For DVT, treatment should focus on preventing pulmonary emboli. Treatment usually involves giving an anticoagulant such as heparin for the existing clot and drugs such as aspirin to prevent additional clots. Obtain baseline coagulation study results and monitor them throughout treatment. Other treatment measures include those used to treat superficial thrombophlebitis.

Before discharge, review all aspects of your patient's care, including risk-factor modification, medications, the rehabilitation plan, and the need for follow-up treatment. If your patient is receiving long-term anticoagulant therapy, remind her about the need for follow-up laboratory studies and safety measures. Urge her to wear a medical identification bracelet that indicates that she takes an anticoagulant.

Pulmonary embolism

Because a patient with atherosclerosis and a CVA has an increased risk of DVT, she also has an increased risk of pulmonary embolism. A piece of the thrombus may break free and float into the pulmonary circulation, partially or completely blocking a branch of the pulmonary artery. In most patients, the thrombus originates in a deep leg vein.

Confirming the complication

Signs and symptoms of pulmonary embolism include dyspnea, anxiety, pleuritic chest pain, cough, and hemoptysis. Physical findings include tachypnea, crackles, tachycardia, an S_3 or S_4 heart sound, diaphoresis, and fever. Hyperventilation from hypoxia and pain may lead to respiratory alkalosis, which is confirmed by low $Paco_2$ and high pH values on ABG studies. If treatment is delayed, blood continues to be shunted without being oxygenated, leading to respiratory acidosis.

Pulmonary embolism can be diagnosed with a ventilation-perfusion lung scan. If the scan is inconclusive, the patient will undergo pulmonary angiography. Electrocardiogram findings include T-wave and ST-segment changes as well as left-axis and right-axis deviations.

Nursing interventions

Establish and maintain your patient's airway, and administer supplemental oxygen as necessary. Monitor her oxygen saturation levels using pulse oximetry. Check ABG study results regularly.

Administer heparin, as prescribed. When the patient's APTT reaches 2 to 2.5 times normal, the physician may prescribe warfarin. Assess the patient continually for signs and symptoms of bleeding.

If your patient develops respiratory distress, anticipate intubation to prevent respiratory arrest. Expect to administer furosemide to control pulmonary edema. Prepare for mechanical ventilation with positive end-expiratory pressure (PEEP). And give morphine, as prescribed, to relax your patient. Provide support to the patient's family and keep them informed.

Acute arterial occlusion

Arterial occlusion can be caused by a thrombus but more commonly results from an embolus that arises in the heart or a free-floating piece of plaque from a distal artery. Patients with a CVA and atherosclerosis have an increased risk of acute arterial occlusion because of the underlying vascular changes that damage vessel walls.

Confirming the complication

A patient with an acute arterial occlusion typically has severe pain below the occlusion, and her limb is pale and cool. The limb also may be pulseless or mottled. The severity of the signs and symptoms depends on the clot's origin and size and on the extent of the disease process.

Nursing interventions

The best way to detect a problem quickly is to monitor your patient's arms and legs routinely. Evaluate them for changes in temperature, color, capillary refill, and pulses. Also, investigate any complaints of pain or sensory changes. Remember that your patient with a CVA and atherosclerosis may have sensory impairment and may not notice that a limb has changed color or become cool.

If a clot has formed, give heparin as prescribed. Expect to give a bolus of up to 10,000 units followed by a continuous low-dose infusion. Monitor your patient's APTT regularly.

If necessary, your patient may undergo a thrombectomy or embolectomy. Monitor her closely after surgery to detect complications, such as muscle spasm and swelling. Instead of surgery, your patient may receive local intra-arterial thrombolytic therapy with urokinase. If so, monitor her closely for signs of bleeding.

Cerebrovascular accident and hypertension

Hypertension contributes to both ischemic and hemorrhagic CVA by altering vessels directly and by accelerating the development of atherosclerosis.

Pathophysiology

In hypertension, arteries undergo hypertrophy and hyperplasia to compensate for higher blood pressure. In larger vessels, these changes maintain arterial flexibility and protect the microcirculation and blood-brain barrier from increased pressure. When smaller arteries can no longer compensate for the increased blood pressure, however, changes occur in the vessel walls. Plasma components begin to leak into the walls, marking the first step in the development of degenerative vascular and perivascular lesions. Leaking vessels lead to a dysfunctional blood-brain barrier and increased cerebral edema. Vascular lesions lead to the development of lacunar infarcts and lacunar hemorrhages.

Also, a patient with chronic hypertension has a higher-than-normal mean arterial pressure—which, in turn, leads to increased cerebral perfusion pressure. The increased pressure is necessary to maintain cerebral perfusion in the hypertensive patient, but it increases her risk for CVA.

Of course, hypertension also contributes to the development of atherosclerosis. Atherosclerotic changes begin in the carotid and vertebral arteries, and then they develop around the circle of Willis. Over time, small cerebral arteries are affected. Atherosclerosis in large vessels can lead to severe stenosis or occlusion. In small vessels, it can lead to a lacunar CVA.

Hypertension also is a precursor to heart failure. Thus, the hypertensive patient has a higher risk of a CVA from left ventricular hypertrophy and reduced cardiac output.

Adapting nursing care

If your CVA patient also has hypertension, be sure to monitor her blood pressure closely. If her blood pressure drops too much or too fast, her cerebral perfusion could decrease, causing an infarction and worsening the effects of the CVA.

An arterial line may be inserted so you can monitor your patient's blood pressure directly. Usually, a CVA causes a greater rise in blood pressure in a hypertensive patient than it does in a normotensive patient. A patient with hypertension can tolerate a systolic blood pressure above 160 mm Hg. However, if the systolic pressure falls below 120 mm Hg, the patient may show neurologic signs related to decreased cerebral perfusion.

Because of the increased blood pressure, a patient with a CVA and hypertension risks increased ICP (see *When your patient with a CVA and hypertension needs ICP monitoring*, page 212). Watch carefully for signs and symptoms, including a decreased level of consciousness, headache, visual disturbances, changes in blood pressure or heart rate, and changes in respiratory pattern. Late signs and symptoms of increased ICP include pupillary abnormalities, persistent changes in vital signs, more serious changes in respiratory pattern, and abnormal ABG levels. If these signs and symptoms appear, take steps to reduce ICP as appropriate:

- Administer an osmotic diuretic as prescribed to decrease cerebral edema and vascular fluid volume and improve cerebral perfusion pressure.
- Raise the head of your patient's bed to 30 degrees or, if your patient's blood pressure is stable, place her in the reverse Trendelenburg position.
- To prevent cerebral vasodilation produced by hypercapnia, maintain a $Paco_2$ of 30 to 35 mm Hg.
- Administer 100% oxygen before suctioning. To prevent hypoxia, limit your suctioning time to 15 seconds.
- Provide adequate pain control. Narcotics and sedatives may mask signs and symptoms of neurologic deterioration, so they probably won't be prescribed.
- Organize your patient's activities to avoid tiring or overstimulating her.
- Maintain your patient's normal body temperature.
- Monitor intake and output. Check urine output hourly. Assess your patient's renal function studies and her serum electrolyte, BUN, and creatinine levels for changes.

After your patient's condition stabilizes, focus on preventing complications from the CVA. Maintain the patient's nutritional status, help her compensate for perceptual difficulties, promote activity, encourage communication, and provide emotional support and patient education. Continue to monitor your patient's blood pressure frequently. Adjust her drug doses as prescribed and plan for appropriate exercise.

Before discharge, review all aspects of your patient's care and make sure she or her caregiver understands your instructions. Emphasize lifestyle changes your patient should make to reduce or manage her hypertension and help her implement your suggestions, as needed.

Complications

Common complications for patients with a CVA and hypertension include intracerebral hemorrhage and increased neurologic deficits.

Intracerebral hemorrhage

An intracerebral hemorrhage results primarily from hypertension. It typically occurs in the basal ganglia, thalamus, pons, cerebellum, or deep hemispheric white matter of the brain. Usually, it occurs because long-term hypertensive changes weaken the walls of small vessels and cause them to rupture.

As hypertensive changes progress, the vessel lumens narrow, microaneurysms form in small cerebral arteries and arterioles, and necrosis may develop from atherosclerotic changes. If blood leaks from the weakened vessels into the surrounding brain tissue, it displaces and compresses that tissue, resulting in ischemia, edema, and increased ICP. Blood may seep or rupture into the cerebral ventricles as well.

The amount of damage caused by an intracerebral hemorrhage depends on the amount of blood. If a small hemorrhage is untreated, the blood will resorb on its own. After macrophages help clear away the blood, a cavity surrounded by neuroglia cells remains.

Confirming the complication
Patients with an intracerebral hemorrhage usually experience a sudden headache, vomiting, and seizures. About 75% have a decreased LOC; 25% become comatose. Other signs and symptoms are similar to those for an ischemic CVA. A CT scan confirms the hemorrhage.

Nursing interventions
Assess your patient's airway, LOC, blood pressure, and neurologic status. Remember, bleeding can continue for several hours, so assess her neurologic status every 30 to 60 minutes to check for deterioration. If she scores less than 8 on the Glasgow Coma scale, expect her to undergo endotracheal intubation.

ADAPTING YOUR CARE

When your patient with a CVA and hypertension needs ICP monitoring

A patient with a cerebrovascular accident (CVA) and hypertension needs careful assessment of her cerebral perfusion pressure. If it falls too low, more of her brain could become ischemic. Therefore, her physician may decide to insert a sensor to monitor intracranial pressure (ICP).

By adapting your care to the needs of this patient and her family, you can help maximize her functional outcome and minimize the anxiety that usually accompanies ICP monitoring.

Before ICP monitoring
Explain to your patient and her family that because of her CVA and high blood pressure, she requires a special device to monitor the pressure inside her skull. Explain that a sensor will be placed in her brain through a small hole in her skull.

Understandably, the prospect of this procedure may frighten your patient and her family. But because your patient's fear can increase her blood pressure and oxygen demands, you should try to keep her as relaxed as possible. And keep her family calm, too. Explain to family members that their calmness and support can make a difference in the patient's recovery.

Explain the procedure carefully and in as much detail as the patient and family want. Let them ask questions. Make sure they know that ICP monitoring will allow the health care team to spot problems early and provide prompt treatment.

During ICP monitoring
After the physician inserts the sensor, determine your patient's cerebral perfusion pressure by subtracting her ICP reading from her mean arterial blood pressure. Remember that hypertensive patients need a higher-than-normal cerebral perfusion pressure to maintain cerebral function.

Even though your patient has a monitoring device in place, don't let that stop you from assessing her carefully and regularly for other signs that might point to a complication. Also, check her ICP frequently and note whether it's going up or down over time. To ensure accurate ICP readings, make sure the transducer is at the level of the foramen of Monro (at the outer canthus of the eye or the top of the ear).

Your patient faces a significant risk of infection during ICP monitoring. And infection will increase her oxygen demands and raise her risk of continued ischemia and further neurologic deficits. To help prevent infection, use aseptic technique when caring for the insertion site and make sure that all connections are tightly closed.

Patients with an intracerebral hemorrhage are at risk for increased ICP. Those with severe hypertension and intracerebral hemorrhage will require continuous blood pressure monitoring. Anticipate the insertion of an arterial line to monitor blood pressure and an ICP catheter to monitor cerebral perfusion pressure during antihypertensive treatment.

To control the bleeding, you need to control your patient's blood pressure. Start by finding out if the patient was hypertensive before the CVA. If so, find out her baseline blood pressure. Use this baseline as your guide.

If your patient was hypertensive before the CVA, a physician probably will want to continue the established antihypertensive regimen and add a short-acting, easily titrated drug to control the increased blood pressure in the early stages of the CVA. Labetalol, a combined alpha and beta blocker, is the antihypertensive of choice because it can be given I.V. and doesn't adversely affect ICP or local cerebral blood flow. After giving this drug, especially after the first dose, monitor your patient's blood pressure closely. Keep in mind that you shouldn't give a vasodilator or calcium channel blocker because cerebral vasodilation could increase ICP.

Increased neurologic deficits
Because uncontrolled hypertension forces a larger volume of blood into the cerebral vasculature and continues to weaken blood vessels, the risk of rupture and bleeding increases. This in turn can lead to a severe CVA, an extension of an existing CVA, and subsequent CVAs. The

result is increased neurologic deficits for the patient.

Confirming the complication

Such indications as a change in LOC or thought processes, visual deterioration, increasing weakness or paralysis on either side, or difficulty in speaking point to a new or worsening neurologic deficit. A CT scan that shows renewed bleeding or reinfarction helps confirm the diagnosis.

Nursing interventions

After a CVA, help your patient prevent increased neurologic deficits by encouraging her to follow her antihypertensive drug regimen and urging her to make lifestyle changes designed to reduce hypertension.

If this strategy fails and renewed bleeding leads to further neurologic deterioration, she'll need prompt, aggressive treatment to minimize the effects. Once her condition is stable, help her begin the recovery process. Start by supporting her affected arms and legs with pillows, and change their position frequently. Also, make sure her head remains in alignment with her body.

As soon as possible, begin an aggressive rehabilitation program to maximize your patient's functional ability. Arrange for physical, speech, and occupational therapy. Show your patient how to use assistive devices, as needed. Help her communicate in a manner that promotes independence and minimizes frustration. Include the patient and family in the plan of care. Be sure to allow additional teaching time, so your patient can participate as much as possible.

If your patient develops new visual deficits, encourage her to move her head from side to side and to scan the room frequently. Make sure that necessary items—such as the telephone, call bell, and food on her meal tray—are placed within her field of vision and reach.

If your patient develops new alterations in thought processes, reorient her. Use clocks and calendars as needed. Take steps to minimize noise, confusion, and distraction. Maintain her safety and be sure to keep the side rails up when she's unattended.

Recognize that new or worsening neurologic deficits may be frustrating—possibly devastating—to your patient's family. Provide supportive care. Allow your patient and her family to express their feelings. If indicated, consult with a mental health professional, such as a psychiatric clinical nurse specialist, to provide support and guidance.

Cerebrovascular accident and diabetes mellitus

Patients with Type I or Type II diabetes face a higher risk of cerebral thrombosis than patients who don't have diabetes. Plus, diabetic patients tend to have more severe CVAs and a higher risk of death from CVAs.

Pathophysiology

Diabetes raises the risk of a CVA—especially a lacunar CVA—because it produces widespread changes in the patient's vasculature. Microvascular changes include thickening of the basement membrane throughout the body, including the kidneys, eyes, and brain. Macrovascular changes include atherosclerotic variations in large blood vessels. These atherosclerotic variations occur at an earlier age and advance more rapidly in diabetic patients than they do in nondiabetic patients.

Other factors also increase the risk of a CVA for a diabetic patient. For example, serum lipid levels may be high, especially triglyceride levels. Plus, many Type II diabetic patients are obese. Diabetic patients also have hematologic changes that tend to produce hypercoagulation, a condition that increases the risk of an ischemic CVA. These changes include increased plasmin fibrinogen levels, increased hematocrit, and increased platelet aggregation and adhesion.

In addition to raising the risk of a CVA, diabetes also may complicate its outcome. When a

CVA occurs, it induces a stress response, which increases endogenous glucose production and may lead to hyperglycemia. As a result, a diabetic patient may become dehydrated and develop electrolyte imbalances that could lead to severe diabetic ketoacidosis. Type I diabetic patients may develop hyperglycemic hyperosmolar nonketotic (HHNK) syndrome, which causes severe dehydration and electrolyte imbalances stemming from osmotic diuresis. In both cases, dehydration can lead to hypotension, which decreases cerebral perfusion pressure and may widen the area of infarction.

Adapting nursing care

If you have a patient with a CVA and diabetes, check her blood glucose levels regularly. If she develops an unexplained focal neurologic sign or a change in her LOC, check her blood glucose immediately.

Responding to hyperglycemia

If your patient develops hyperglycemia, you'll need to respond rapidly with an I.V. infusion of regular insulin. If you have only one I.V. access line, piggyback the insulin into the main I.V. line. That way, you can change the primary I.V. fluid without affecting the insulin dose. If the patient has diabetic ketoacidosis, administer small doses of insulin hourly by infusion, as prescribed. If the patient has HHNK syndrome, expect to start with a loading dose of insulin.

Monitor blood glucose levels hourly. The goal is to reduce the glucose level by 80 to 100 mg/dl per hour until you reach the desired level.

During insulin treatment, watch for signs and symptoms of hypoglycemia: irritability, headache, confusion, restlessness, tremors, diaphoresis, pallor, and stupor. If they develop, check your patient's blood glucose level right away. Decrease the infusion rate as needed. If the glucose level drops below 50 mg/dl, administer 50 ml of 50% dextrose I.V., as prescribed. Recheck the patient's glucose level in 20 minutes.

Remember that a patient who uses an oral hypoglycemic drug to control her glucose levels may need insulin during periods of acute illness.

Responding to hypoglycemia

After a CVA, a diabetic patient can become hypoglycemic if her food intake declines and her oral hypoglycemic drug or insulin dose stays the same. In a critically ill patient, hypoglycemia produces nonspecific signs and symptoms. Your patient may become lethargic and confused or exhibit abnormal behavior that mimics other conditions, such as a CVA or alcohol intoxication. Hypoglycemia also may cause seizures.

RAPID RESPONSE ▶ If you suspect hypoglycemia, check your patient's blood glucose levels. If test results show that she's hypoglycemic, take the following actions:

- If a hypoglycemic patient is conscious and can take fluids by mouth, give her 10 to 15 grams of carbohydrate, such as 6 to 8 Lifesavers, 4 ounces of orange juice, 6 ounces of regular soda, or 6 to 8 ounces of skim or low-fat milk.
- If the patient is unconscious or can't take fluids by mouth, give her 50 ml of 50% dextrose I.V., as prescribed. She should improve within in a few minutes.
- Recheck your patient's blood glucose levels in 20 minutes. If they're still low, repeat the intervention. ◀

After your patient's glucose levels stabilize, give her a snack that contains carbohydrate and protein to rebuild her glycogen stores and prevent recurring hypoglycemia.

Remember, hypoglycemia activates a sympathetic response that causes tachycardia and hypertension, both of which increase oxygen demand and can increase the risk of extending the infarction. If hypoglycemia goes untreated, your patient can slip into a coma within hours.

Reducing the risks

If your diabetic patient needs a cerebral angiography, she faces an increased risk of nephropathy from the dye used in the procedure. Therefore, the physician should use the smallest possible amount of dye. Also, you should give the patient fluids I.V. before and after the test as prescribed to enhance renal excretion of the dye. Monitor your patient's renal function studies closely, including serum BUN and creatinine levels, for abnormal changes.

As the patient gradually increases her activity, she'll have her medication or insulin dosage adjusted to prevent hypoglycemia and hyperglycemia. Monitor her blood glucose levels frequently as she begins her rehabilitation program. Your patient may need frequent small snacks throughout rehabilitation to reduce the chance of hypoglycemia.

Patient teaching

When caring for a diabetic patient after a CVA, observe her abilities and assess the effect of any neurologic deficits caused by the CVA. Help her relearn her diabetic regimen, if necessary, by presenting information one step at a time. Don't skip steps or assume that the patient remembers them. Don't move on to the next step until you're sure she has learned the previous one. Set realistic learning goals.

If necessary, teach your patient how to use memory aids. Involve the patient's family in your teaching, but encourage them to let the patient remain as independent as possible in caring for herself and performing activities of daily living.

Complications

Common complications for patients with a CVA and diabetes mellitus include venous stasis ulcers, thrombophlebitis, and malnutrition.

Venous stasis ulcers

Diabetes and CVA increase the risk of venous stasis ulcers in a couple of ways. First of all, diabetes commonly causes chronic venous insufficiency, which can lead to venous stasis. In chronic venous insufficiency, prolonged venous hypertension causes leg veins to stretch. Over time, venous valves fail to close properly, resulting in retrograde venous blood flow and stasis. Fluid eventually infiltrates the surrounding tissues and, over time, causes edema, cellulitis, and venous stasis ulcers. The hemiplegia and weakness caused by a CVA make the patient especially prone to venous stasis—and thus to venous stasis ulcers—because the skeletal muscles may not contract strongly enough to force venous blood out of the lower legs. The immobility and bed rest imposed by an acute CVA also hinder venous circulation.

The second way diabetes and CVA increase the risk for venous stasis ulcers stems from the sensory deficits these disorders can cause. They may make it difficult for a patient to detect the signs of skin breakdown, including bruises, scrapes, pressure points, and ulcerations on the legs and feet. Retinopathy and neuropathy, both complications of diabetes, reduce the patient's ability to see and feel these signs. When the patient also has a CVA, sensory perception may be reduced even more.

Confirming the complication

Look carefully for wounds or ulcerations on the patient's feet or lower legs. Venous stasis ulcers usually have irregular borders and appear over the medial malleolus. Venous insuffiency also typically causes edema and hyperpigmentation of the feet and ankles (stasis dermatitis). You may or may not be able to palpate pulses in the patient's lower legs.

Nursing interventions

To promote venous return and prevent venous stasis ulcers from forming, take the following steps:

- Encourage the patient to move, exercise, and walk as early as possible after the CVA.
- Use sequential pneumatic compression devices or antiembolism stockings.
- Elevate your patient's feet above heart level. Don't let her legs dangle when she sits in a chair.
- Warn your patient to avoid sitting in a chair for more than an hour without shifting her weight frequently.
- Use a bed cradle to lift linens off her feet and lower legs.
- When your patient gets out of bed, make sure she wears well-fitting shoes or slippers with nonskid soles.
- Evaluate the skin on her legs regularly for reddened areas and provide skin care during her hospitalization.

If your patient does develop venous stasis ulcers, she's at increased risk for delayed healing and infection. Keep the area clean, dry, and free from pressure to prevent it from worsening. Monitor her for signs and symptoms of infection.

Guidelines for chemically debriding a wound

If your patient develops a venous stasis ulcer, you may need to chemically debride the wound with a combination of topical drugs such as fibrinolysin and desoxyribonuclease (Elase). This combination drug can be applied as an ointment or a solution. To enhance its effectiveness and avoid complications, follow these guidelines:

- Before applying the drug, check your patient's history for hypersensitivity to the drug or to bovine or mercury products.
- Before each application, clean the wound with sterile water or normal saline solution.
- If you're using the ointment form, apply a thin layer to the entire area. To work effectively, the ointment must be in constant contact with the wound.
- If you're using the solution form, prepare it immediately before application. To make the solution, mix one vial of the drug in dry powder form with 10 to 50 ml of normal saline solution, as prescribed.
- Apply the solution directly to the affected area as a liquid or a spray or on a wet dressing. Never inject it into the tissue because fibrinolysin may be antigenic.
- If you're using the solution with wet-to-dry dressings, saturate strips of gauze with the solution and apply them to the wound. Allow the gauze to dry for about 8 hours. Remove the dried dressing, clean the wound, and repeat the procedure.
- With each application, observe your patient for signs of hypersensitivity. If your patient's skin becomes irritated or inflamed, notify her physician.

To promote healing, encourage fluid intake, adequate nutrition, and blood glucose control. You may need to obtain a culture from the ulcer so that a physician can prescribe an antibiotic. Appropriate wound dressings include oxygen-permeable hydrocolloid dressings and oxygen-impermeable hydrocolloid dressings. For an ambulatory patient, you may use an Unna's boot made from gauze saturated with zinc oxide.

The ulcer may also need debridement. Four basic methods exist. Surgical debridement involves cutting away the necrotic tissue. Mechanical debridement uses wet-to-dry dressings. Chemical debridement uses topical biologic enzymes to break down necrotic tissue (see *Guidelines for chemically debriding a wound*). In the autolytic method, moisture-retaining dressings allow the enzymes that naturally occur in wound fluid to digest dead tissue.

Always use strict aseptic technique and follow standard precautions when treating an ulcer. Monitor your patient's blood glucose levels frequently because the stress response causes catecholamine release, which can result in hyperglycemia and worsen the CVA.

Before discharge, teach your patient and her family how to assess vulnerable skin areas and prevent problems at home. If your patient has an ulceration, teach her and her family how to care for the wound. Be sure to teach your patient foot care, especially if she'll be fitted with special shoes or braces to promote rehabilitation after a CVA. Show your patient and her family how to inspect the patient's feet. Urge them to inspect both feet every day and to take special care when inspecting the weaker leg. Also, show them how to maintain skin integrity on the unaffected leg. Suggest using creams to minimize dryness, but not so much that they macerate the skin.

Thrombophlebitis

Diabetes raises the risk of thrombophlebitis, especially DVT, by causing endothelial injury and increasing platelet aggregation, platelet adhesion, and venous stasis. Both a CVA and diabetes impair physical mobility and venous circulation, further raising the risk of thrombophlebitis and, consequently, pulmonary embolism.

Confirming the complication

Signs and symptoms of thrombophlebitis vary with the level of the occlusion, the size of the thrombus, and the amount of collateral circulation. The patient may have calf pain, localized edema and warmth, increased calf circumference, a low-grade fever, and tachycardia. You also may detect tenderness along the course of the vessel. Homans' sign may be present.

If a physical examination doesn't confirm thrombophlebitis, a physician may order venography, Doppler ultrasonography, or impedance phlebography.

Nursing interventions

If your patient has diabetes and a CVA, take steps to prevent thrombophlebitis from developing. Encourage your patient to move around as soon as possible after the CVA. And use sequential pneumatic compression devices or antiembolism stockings to improve circulation. Give subcutaneous heparin, as prescribed. If the patient is also taking aspirin to minimize platelet aggregation, watch for possible drug interactions, such as a significantly increased risk of bleeding.

Assess your patient's legs at least once every 8 hours and compare her calf circumference bilaterally. Check pedal pulses, color, temperature, capillary refill, and sensation in both legs. If your patient has neuropathy, she may have paresthesia and some numbness. Remove the antiembolism stockings or sequential compression devices to check for pressure areas.

If your patient develops thrombophlebitis, expect a physician to reduce the dosage of her anticoagulant. Instead of subcutaneous administration, your patient may require intermittent I.V. injections or infusions. Monitor her coagulation studies carefully and watch for signs of bleeding.

During the acute phase of thrombophlebitis, your patient will be on bed rest to help reduce the risk of pulmonary emboli. However, bed rest also raises the risk of venous stasis, pressure ulcers, and hypoglycemia. Monitor her blood glucose levels closely and modify her insulin dosage as needed.

To help prevent venous stasis and the formation of new thrombi, raise your patient's legs above the level of her heart, so gravity can aid blood flow and relieve edema and pain. Also, apply warm, moist soaks to the affected leg. Take special precautions to avoid burns, however, because your patient may have neuropathy from the diabetes, sensory deficits from the CVA, or both.

If your patient will be discharged while taking anticoagulant therapy, teach her about the medication. Be sure to discuss the proper dosage, adverse effects, and safety measures to reduce the risk of bleeding. If your patient is taking warfarin, warn her to eat small but consistent amounts of foods high in vitamin K, which can interfere with the drug's intended action.

Anticoagulant therapy also raises the risk of hematoma. Encourage your insulin-dependent diabetic patient to rotate injection sites carefully to reduce this risk. Also, warn this patient to avoid injecting insulin into a bruised area because these areas absorb insulin poorly. Reinforce all aspects of your patient's blood glucose management and any adaptations needed to compensate for her neurologic deficits.

Malnutrition

The effects of a CVA and diabetes can combine to increase your patient's risk for malnutrition. Many CVA patients have some level of dysphagia. And most have weakness or paralysis that can result in fatigue, frustration, and difficulty in preparing meals. Visual deficits caused by both a CVA and diabetes can reduce the patient's ability to see or recognize the foods in front of her. Plus, many patients with both disorders become depressed by the incurable nature of their illnesses and the seemingly endless effort required to manage them. The depression results in a suppressed appetite.

Confirming the complication

A malnourished patient typically shows a significant weight loss. She may appear thin and pale, with reduced muscle mass. She'll probably complain of weakness, lethargy, cold intolerance, ankle edema, and dry skin.

Laboratory tests can be used together with physical findings to confirm malnutrition. A low hemoglobin level may indicate anemia secondary to catabolism and low serum albumin levels associated with malnutrition. Serum albumin and transferrin levels can help assess visceral protein stores and determine the amount of protein depletion. A low serum cholesterol level, usually one below 160 mg/dl, also indicates malnutrition.

Nursing interventions

If your patient has a CVA and diabetes, take steps to prevent malnutrition before it develops. Check your patient's weight at least twice weekly. Ask a dietitian to evaluate your patient's nutritional needs, then work with the dietitian, your patient, and her family to establish a sound dietary plan.

If your patient can swallow but has motor deficits from the CVA, ask an occupational therapist for adaptive devices that the patient can use to simplify eating and cooking. Suggest that the family allow extra time for meals. If necessary, your patient may benefit from smaller, more frequent meals and snacks.

If your patient has dysphagia, she'll probably need enteral feedings. If she has severe protein wasting, she'll probably need total parenteral nutrition. Closely monitor her blood glucose levels if she's receiving enteral or parenteral nutrition; many enteral formulas are high in calories, and parenteral solutions are high in glucose. Depending on the results of the blood glucose tests, your patient's insulin dosage may need adjustment. Monitor your patient closely to prevent hypoglycemia as physical activity increases during rehabilitation.

Before discharge, review all aspects of your patient's care with the patient and her family. Make referrals for home follow-up care, so the patient's diet and the effects of the CVA on her nutritional status can be evaluated.

Cerebrovascular accident and pneumonia

A CVA can readily lead to pneumonia, from either the increased risk of aspiration or the prolonged immobility associated with a CVA. When the effects of a CVA and pneumonia are combined, the risk for such further complications as atelectasis and respiratory acidosis increases.

Pathophysiology

In a CVA patient, pneumonia typically develops when oropharyngeal secretions are aspirated into the lungs, either because of decreased consciousness or dysphagia. When aspirated secretions carry bacteria into the lungs, an inflammatory response occurs. Fibrin deposits then form on the pleural surfaces, which causes phagocytosis in the alveoli. In a healthy person, macrophages remove debris from the lung tissues and resolve the infection. In a CVA patient, however, the pneumonia may continue and further complicate the delivery of oxygen to an already ischemic brain (see *How pneumonia can develop after a CVA*).

The CVA may also leave the patient immobile for some time, preventing her from breathing deeply. This makes her airway clearance ineffective and allows the buildup of secretions, which can lead to pneumonia.

Adapting nursing care

The best way to handle pneumonia in a patient with a CVA is to prevent it. Start by assessing your CVA patient for a decreased LOC and dysphagia, both of which raise the risk of aspiration. If your patient has already aspirated secretions, a physician will order a chest X-ray, ABG studies, and possibly bronchoscopy to remove debris from the lung and prevent further damage. Give your patient nothing by mouth and expect a physician to insert a temporary or permanent feeding tube or an endotracheal tube.

Help your patient clear any aspirated secretions by encouraging deep breathing and coughing exercises, incentive spirometry, early mobility, and frequent position changes. Watch closely for signs and symptoms of developing pneumonia, including a fever, chills, cough, malaise, and an elevated white blood cell (WBC) count. Keep in mind, however, that your patient's WBC count may already be elevated because of neurologic injuries and inflammation caused by the CVA.

Obtain a sputum culture specimen and give the prescribed antibiotic. The duration of antibiotic therapy depends on the bacteria, the possibility of aspiration as a cause of the infection, and the patient's response to treatment. Start treatment as early as possible to limit further injury to the brain from ischemia.

PATHOPHYSIOLOGY

How pneumonia can develop after a CVA

After a cerebrovascular accident (CVA), many patients have difficulty swallowing. If impaired swallowing sends food or fluid down the trachea instead of the esophagus, the patient could develop pneumonia. Here's how:

1. Normally, cranial nerves and the medulla coordinate the movements of the tongue, soft palate, and epiglottis so that foods and fluids move into the esophagus. If the swallowing reflex is impaired, however, food, fluids, or secretions can slip into the trachea instead.

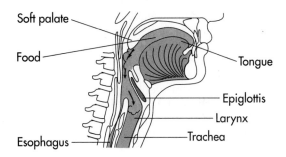

2. Aspirated material travels through the trachea and into the bronchi and bronchioles, triggering an inflammatory response. Mucus gathers in the affected airways, cilia cease to function properly, and the patient may experience bronchospasm. If the CVA has weakened the patient's chest muscles or impaired her cough reflex, mucus continues to accumulate, further occluding the airways.

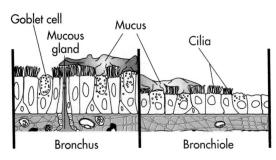

3. The inflammatory response attracts neutrophils to the area, inflammatory mediators are released, and exudate, red blood cells, and bacteria accumulate. These reactions begin to take place in the alveoli as well.

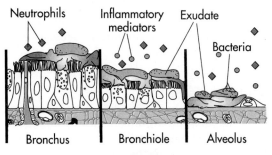

4. In the alveolus, lung tissue begins to transform into a solid mass, and fibrin is deposited. Macrophages attempt to ingest neutrophils, fibrin, and bacteria. In the patient weakened by a CVA, however, phagocytosis can't resolve the infection. Eventually, the alveolocapillary membrane becomes damaged, and the lungs become stiff and noncompliant from disrupted surfactant production. Gas exchange becomes impaired.

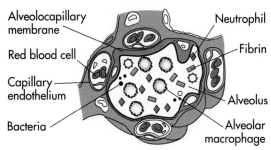

Also, give a bronchodilator to enhance the patient's ability to cough and breath deeply. Aerosol treatments may be prescribed to open your patient's airways and help her expectorate secretions. If your patient can't clear secretions on her own, you may need to use suction. Perform postural drainage and percussion every 4 hours to help loosen secretions and aid expectoration. Keep your patient well hydrated to make secretions as liquid as possible.

Give the prescribed antipyretic, which will not only reduce the patient's fever but also improve oxygen delivery and use in the brain. Monitor your patient's oxygen saturation levels frequently. Administer supplemental low-flow oxygen and monitor her ABG studies as indicated.

Give your patient an analgesic to relieve muscle aches associated with the CVA. Monitor her neurologic and respiratory status closely.

Aspiration caused by a CVA may resolve on its own by the time the patient is discharged. Even so, teach your patient and her family about her condition, including the risks of aspiration and her need for ongoing care. Make a referral for follow-up home care if appropriate (see *Teaching a CVA patient who has pneumonia*).

Complications

Common complications for patients with a CVA and pneumonia include atelectasis and respiratory acidosis.

Atelectasis

A patient who's had a CVA has a risk of atelectasis because immobility leads to impaired ventilation. If the patient also has pneumonia, muscle weakness further impairs ventilation. Also, the increased secretions caused by pneumonia can obstruct airways.

If an airway becomes obstructed by gastric secretions, a mucous plug, or consolidation, air becomes trapped beyond the obstruction. The air then diffuses into the bloodstream, allowing the distal airway to collapse. Any debris trapped in that airway can trigger an inflammatory response and worsen the pneumonia.

Confirming the complication

A patient with atelectasis may have tachypnea, tachycardia, dyspnea, cyanosis, hypoxemia, decreased chest expansion, decreased or absent breath sounds, and intercostal retractions. She also may have a fever and other signs of infection.

A chest X-ray can confirm atelectasis. A physician may use bronchoscopy to obtain a specimen, remove debris or mucous plugs, and assess the inflammation.

Nursing interventions

To prevent atelectasis in your patient with a CVA and pneumonia, encourage early mobility, deep breathing and coughing, and incentive spirometry.

Depending on the amount of airway collapse, treatment for atelectasis may mirror these preventive measures. Monitor your patient's respiratory status closely. Assess her oxygen saturation levels and ABG studies. Anticipate the need for supplemental oxygen and be alert for the signs and symptoms of hypoxemia.

You may need to use aerosol therapy, nasotracheal suctioning, and postural drainage and percussion. In severe atelectasis, your patient may need endotracheal intubation with mechanical ventilation, possibly with high tidal volumes or PEEP.

Respiratory acidosis

Respiratory acidosis is an increase in arterial carbon dioxide caused by decreased ventilation. A CVA and pneumonia raise the risk of respiratory acidosis because they produce muscle weakness and immobility that interfere with ventilation. Also, aspiration caused by a CVA can further decrease ventilation. And infection associated with pneumonia can impair gas exchange and obstruct the airways.

Because respiratory acidosis dilates blood vessels, it can worsen a CVA by increasing cerebral congestion and decreasing cerebral oxygenation.

Confirming the complication

A patient with respiratory acidosis has a blood pH under 7.35 and a $Paco_2$ over 50 mm Hg.

Teaching a CVA patient who has pneumonia

If your patient has had a cerebrovascular accident (CVA) and is recovering from pneumonia, you'll need to teach her and her caregiver how to keep her recovery on track and prevent further complications at home.

Instruct the caregiver to monitor the patient's temperature daily and to call the physician if it's higher than 99.5° F (37.5° C). Also, the caregiver should check the color, consistency, amount, and odor of respiratory secretions. Greenish yellow, thick, copious, or malodorous secretions may indicate a recurrence of pneumonia or another respiratory infection.

If the patient is immobile, explain the importance of changing her position at least every 2 hours around the clock to prevent stasis of respiratory secretions, which may lead to a recurrence of pneumonia. During meals, the patient should sit upright with her head forward and neck slightly flexed. Tell her to remain upright for at least 30 minutes after eating or receiving an enteral tube feeding. If she has difficulty swallowing, instruct her to try soft foods or thick liquids to reduce the risk of aspiration.

Advise the patient not to see visitors who may be contagious, and emphasize that visitors should not smoke. Instruct the caregiver to change the water in the respiratory reservoirs every 8 to 24 hours to prevent bacteria from migrating to the respiratory tract. After every meal, the patient or caregiver should perform mouth care.

If a physician has prescribed an oral antibiotic, emphasize the importance of taking all the prescribed medication. If the patient has a feeding tube, ask the pharmacist if the antibiotic can be broken or crushed and mixed with food.

If the patient isn't allergic to eggs or the preservative thimerosal, she should receive a flu vaccination before the flu season. Also, advise her to obtain a pneumococcal vaccination.

Referrals

If your patient will need further assistance after discharge—for instance, if she'll need instruction on taking her medications or using equipment or if she'll be receiving medications I.V. at home—obtain a referral for home care.

If the patient needs medical equipment at home (such as supplemental oxygen equipment, feeding tubes, or a commode), social services can help with the arrangements. A social worker also can assess the patient's situation to determine if she'll need financial aid or help with her home care.

To help the patient maintain her mobility, you may need to set up a consultation with a physical therapist. The therapist will assess the patient and either arrange for home visits or outpatient rehabilitation.

She'll have shallow, rapid breathing that progresses to slow, deep breathing. She may complain of a headache, blurred vision, and nausea, and you may note irritability, vomiting, and muscle twitching. As the carbon dioxide level increases, the lethargic patient may slide into a coma.

Nursing interventions

For the patient with a CVA and pneumonia who develops respiratory acidosis, focus on improving ventilation. If your patient has a normal neurologic status, assess her respiratory drive. Give supplemental oxygen, as needed, and monitor her ABG studies to see how she responds. Also, monitor her oxygen saturation continuously using pulse oximetry.

If your patient has a depressed neurologic status, she may need endotracheal intubation to maintain a patent airway, allow suctioning, and increase tidal volumes to open small collapsed airways. Also, by providing moist air, intubation may make it easier to remove mucus and debris. A physician may order bronchoscopy as well to remove debris and mucous plugs.

Encourage your patient to do deep-breathing and coughing exercises and to use the incentive spirometer. Watch for aspiration, especially when she's eating. Warn your patient and her family against overusing analgesics for pain and anxiety because they can lead to respiratory acidosis and may mask the signs of neurologic deterioration.

Cerebrovascular accident and osteoarthritis

Osteoarthritis, an inflammatory condition, places a patient at risk for immobility and its associated complications. If that same patient has a CVA, the likelihood of complications from immobility increases.

Pathophysiology

In osteoarthritis, peripheral and axial joints progressively lose articular cartilage, possibly from overuse or traumatic injury. Over time, the cartilage develops fissures and pitting, and it becomes thin and begins to erode. Joint spaces narrow and bone spurs form. Inflammatory exudate or blood may enter the joint. Eventually, the cartilage begins to swell from increased synovial fluid or fragments of osteophytes in the synovial cavity.

A patient with osteoarthritis commonly complains of pain that increases with weight bearing and improves with rest. Her joints will be stiff, especially in the morning and after a period of rest. You'll hear cracking when the joints move, and you'll usually find decreased range of motion and muscle atrophy from disuse.

Naturally, most patients respond to osteoarthritis by moving the painful joints as little as possible. For the CVA patient however, immobility can lead to more complications.

Adapting nursing care

Treatment goals for your patient with a CVA and osteoarthritis include reducing inflammation and pain, preserving function, and preventing deformity.

In most cases, you'll give nonsteroidal anti-inflammatory drugs (NSAIDs) to combat the inflammation and pain, usually ibuprofen or ketoprofen. Corticosteroid injections can provide rapid, dramatic relief of pain and inflammation, but adverse effects limit their use.

To protect your patient's joints and promote joint function, encourage rest, exercise, and lifestyle changes. Obtain a physical therapy consultation and work with the therapist to develop a rehabilitation program that's specific to your patient's needs.

You'll also need to apply heat or cold therapy as prescribed. Be especially careful when applying heat or cold to a CVA patient because her senses may be impaired. Be sure to check your patient for areas of redness or skin breakdown because of the potential for decreased sensation.

Perform active and passive range-of-motion exercises on your patient at least twice daily to maintain her muscle tone. And encourage your patient to participate in as much self-care as she can tolerate without experiencing additional pain. This will increase her strength, decrease her pain, and make her more independent.

If your patient experiences back discomfort from her immobility and osteoarthritis, make sure her mattress is firm, so it provides optimal lumbosacral support. For neck stiffness or pain, ask the physician if the patient can wear a cervical collar. And if the patient uses crutches, a walker, braces, or other assistive devices, make sure they're adjusted for the proper fit.

Finally, before discharge, make sure your patient and her family understand the need for mobility and the risks of the drug regimen. Urge them to use nondrug measures to relieve pain whenever possible. Outline important safety precautions to prevent bleeding and avert injury from assistive devices and heat therapy. Also, review the signs and symptoms of bleeding and tell your patient to report them to her physician.

Complications

Common complications for patients with CVA and osteoarthritis include hemorrhage, pressure ulcers, and contractures.

Hemorrhage

If your patient takes an NSAID for arthritis and receives a thrombolytic, anticoagulant, or antiplatelet drug for a CVA, she faces a considerable

DRUG ALERT

Drugs for CVA and osteoarthritis: Dangerous interactions

Drugs for cerebrovascular accident (CVA)	Drugs for osteoarthritis	Adverse effects	Nursing actions
• Thrombolytics • Anticoagulants (heparin, warfarin)	• Nonsteroidal anti-inflammatory drugs (NSAIDs)	• Increased anticoagulant effect and increased risk of bleeding	• Check vital signs to detect indications of bleeding, such as tachycardia and hypotension. • Monitor laboratory studies, including complete blood count and coagulation profile. • Check for signs and symptoms of bleeding: petechiae, bruising, oozing from injection or I.V. sites, and occult blood in urine or stool. • Anticipate reducing thrombolytic or anticoagulant dosage.
• Antiplatelet drugs (aspirin)	• Corticosteroids	• Decreased plasma salicylate concentration • Increased risk of gastrointestinal (GI) ulceration	• Assess effectiveness of antiplatelet drug. • Check for signs and symptoms of GI bleeding. • Anticipate use of H_2 blocker or mucosal protectant to minimize risk of ulceration. • Administer aspirin with food to minimize GI irritation.
	• Fenoprofen, flurbiprofen, indomethacin, meclofenamate, naproxen, sulindac	• Decreased serum level of NSAID • Increased risk for adverse GI effects	• Evaluate effectiveness of pain relief. • Use nondrug measures for pain. • Monitor patient for increased GI upset and irritation. • Check for signs and symptoms of GI bleeding. • Administer both drugs with food to decrease GI irritation. • Anticipate switching to another NSAID, antiplatelet drug, or both.
	• Ketoprofen, tolmetin	• Increased serum levels of NSAID • Increased risk of aspirin toxicity	• Monitor patient for tinnitus, visual changes, and nephrotoxicity. • Monitor patient's urine output. • Anticipate switching to another NSAID.

risk of bleeding (see *Drugs for CVA and osteoarthritis: Dangerous interactions*).

The acute stress of a CVA also makes the patient prone to stress ulcers, which can further raise the risk of a hemorrhage. If a hemorrhage does develop, volume depletion may worsen the neurologic deficits of a CVA.

Confirming the complication
If your CVA patient with osteoarthritis develops severe bleeding from the prescibed therapy, the signs and symptoms will depend on the site of the bleeding. For instance, lower GI bleeding may cause bright red blood or tarry stool; upper GI bleeding may cause the patient to vomit bright red blood or material that resembles coffee grounds. If your patient develops cerebral hemorrhage, you may note a decrease in her LOC as well as other signs of increasing ICP. And, of course, if the patient is hemorrhaging from a wound or puncture, you'll see overt signs of profuse bleeding. Regardless of the bleeding site, the patient will develop hypotension, tachycardia, dyspnea, and, eventually, decreased urine output.

Hemorrhage also can be confirmed with certain diagnostic tests. For example, a physician may perform endoscopy to directly view the source of GI bleeding. To confirm cerebral bleeding, a physician may order CT or MRI scanning.

Other tests, such as serum hemoglobin, hematocrit, and red blood cell count, may help confirm the complication.

Nursing interventions

When caring for a patient with a CVA and osteoarthritis, monitor her closely for signs and symptoms of bleeding. Check all of her puncture sites and dressings for oozing, and look for epistaxis, bruising, and petechiae. Test your patient's urine and stool for occult blood. Assess her vital signs and hemodynamic measurements for changes. And monitor her CBC, hemoglobin, and hematocrit.

RAPID RESPONSE ▶ If your patient begins to hemorrhage, intervene quickly to prevent shock.

- Insert a large-bore I.V. catheter for rapid volume replacement with lactated Ringer's or normal saline solution.
- Prepare to administer blood and blood products as ordered.
- Give supplemental oxygen as necessary. Monitor your patient's oxygen saturation continuously. Obtain ABG study results as indicated to identify hypoxemia and acidosis. If your patient's condition worsens, anticipate endotracheal intubation and mechanical ventilation.
- Begin cardiac monitoring to detect arrhythmias.
- Monitor your patient's vital signs and hemodynamic measurements frequently. Check her urine output hourly.
- Anticipate direct arterial blood pressure monitoring.
- Administer an H_2 blocker, such as cimetidine, as prescribed.
- If your patient's systolic blood pressure drops below 120 mm Hg or her cerebral perfusion pressure drops below 60 mm Hg, prepare to give dopamine or norepinephrine to increase mean arterial pressure, which will in turn maintain cerebral perfusion pressure. ◀

After your patient's condition stabilizes, evaluate her to determine what caused the bleeding. Anticipate adjusting her drug dosages. Many NSAIDs can be taken with food to decrease gastric irritation. And a physician may prescribe an H_2 blocker or a mucosal protectant to help decrease the risk of ulcer formation and GI bleeding.

Pressure ulcers

A patient usually remains on bed rest during the acute phase of a CVA. Even after the acute phase, neurologic and motor deficits may keep her immobile and place her at risk for pressure ulcers. If the patient also has osteoarthritis, self-imposed immobility increases the risk of pressure ulcers.

Pressure ulcers result from high pressure applied for a short time or low pressure applied for a long time. In both cases, the pressure impairs circulation and deprives tissues of oxygen and nutrients. Untreated ulcers can lead to deep ulceration and infection.

Most pressure ulcers develop over bony prominences, where friction and shear combine with pressure to break down skin and underlying tissues. Common sites include the sacrum, coccyx, ischial tuberosities, and greater trochanters. Other common sites include the skin over the vertebrae, scapulae, elbows, knees, and heels in bedridden and relatively immobile patients.

Confirming the complication

A developing pressure ulcer will begin with a change in skin color, temperature, and sensation. But remember, a CVA patient may not be able to feel the growing pressure.

Nursing interventions

To prevent pressure ulcers in a patient with a CVA and osteoarthritis, assess her skin frequently. Also, turn and reposition your patient every 1 to 2 hours, unless contraindicated. When turning your patient, lift her rather than slide her. Sliding increases friction and shear forces. Ask for help and use a turning sheet, if necessary.

Post a turning schedule at your patient's bedside, and emphasize the importance of regular position changes to the patient and her family. They can help prevent pressure ulcers by learning how to turn the patient properly.

If your patient can't be turned every 1 to 2 hours, use a pressure-reducing device such as

Stages of a pressure ulcer

If your patient develops a pressure ulcer, you'll base your treatment on the stage of development. Use the following illustrations and descriptions to identify the four stages.

Stage I

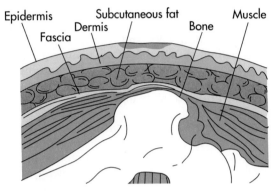

- Epidermis is intact.
- Area of redness over pressure area doesn't blanch.
- Redness remains 30 minutes after pressure relief.
- Sore is usually reversible if pressure is relieved.
- Treatment includes cleaning with plain water and applying transparent films or hydrocolloid dressings over reddened areas.

Stage II

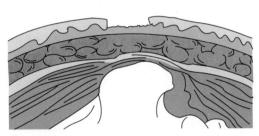

- Partial-thickness skin loss.
- Wound looks like a superficial abrasion, blister, or shallow crater.
- Skin loss may affect epidermis and dermis, but doesn't extend through dermis.
- Wound base is moist and pink, without necrotic tissue.
- Wound is painful.
- Treatment includes cleaning with normal saline solution and applying dressings that help retain moisture.

Stage III

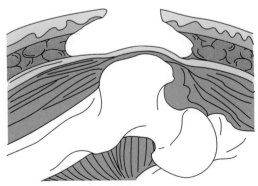

- Full-thickness skin loss with damaged or lost subcutaneous tissue.
- Wound may extend down to but not through underlying fascia.
- Wound looks like a deep crater.
- Usually the wound isn't painful.
- Treatment includes cleaning with normal saline solution and applying dressings that help retain moisture.

Stage IV

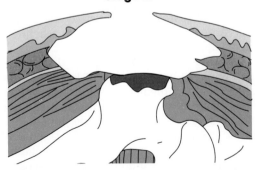

- Full-thickness skin loss with major tissue destruction.
- Damage to muscle, bone, or supporting structures.
- Wound looks like a deep crater with sinus tracts.
- Usually the wound isn't painful.
- If wound isn't necrotic, treatment includes irrigating with normal saline solution, loosely packing with gauze or absorptive dressing, and covering with another dressing.
- If wound is necrotic, treatment includes irrigating with normal saline solution and debridement.

an air or water mattress. To reduce excessive pressure and promote the evaporation of excess moisture, use a low-air-loss device. To relieve pressure and promote circulation, use passive range-of-motion exercises.

Use pillows to position your patient and increase her comfort. Smooth wrinkles in the sheets that could increase pressure and cause discomfort. Avoid placing the patient directly on her trochanter. Instead, position her on her side, at an angle of about 30 degrees.

To promote blood flow to compressed tissues, tell your patient to shift her weight every 30 minutes when sitting in a chair. If she has trouble understanding you because of her neurologic deficits, help her. Provide pressure-relieving cushions, as appropriate. Don't use a rubber or plastic doughnut, however, because they increase sweating and the risk of skin breakdown.

Provide a diet that includes adequate calories, protein, and vitamins. Consult a dietitian as needed.

If your patient is incontinent, keep her skin as clean and dry as possible. Use a protective moisture barrier to prevent skin maceration.

If a pressure ulcer develops, continue measures to relieve pressure, maintain circulation, and manage the underlying disorders. You'll also need to clean and debride the ulcer and apply dressings. The effectiveness and duration of such treatment depend on the stage of the ulcer (see *Stages of a pressure ulcer*, page 225). An enterostomal therapist can help devise an appropriate wound care plan.

Clean the ulcer to help remove dead tissue and debris, as ordered. Expect to use normal saline solution; commercial solutions may contain chemicals that can harm sensitive skin, and hydrogen peroxide and povidone-iodine solutions are toxic to living cells. Document the size and appearance of the ulcer, including the color, odor, and amount of any drainage. If the wound needs irrigation, use just enough force to clean the wound; too much force could traumatize the tissue or force surface bacteria into the wound. Hydrotherapy may also be ordered for wound cleaning. The ulcer also may need debridement.

Apply the prescribed dressing, changing it as needed. Keep in mind that moist dressings promote healing better than dry dressings. Monitor the patient for signs of infection, and watch for excessive draining, which may necessitate a switch to an absorptive dressing. Throughout your care, follow standard precautions.

Before discharge, educate the patient and her family about wound care and prevention.

Contractures

In combination, CVA and osteoarthritis place your patient at high risk of not using her joints and ligaments. The longer such immobility continues, the more ligaments fibrose. Eventually, the affected joints may fuse.

Confirming the complication

A patient who is beginning to develop contractures will have a limited range of motion in the affected joint. The joint will seem somewhat deformed.

Nursing interventions

You can help avoid contractures or reduce their severity by supporting and positioning the patient's joints and using range-of-motion exercises. Immediately after a CVA and throughout the recovery period, position your patient's joints properly. Use pillows as supports and make sure to align her joints carefully in their normal functional position. Doing so may reduce the need for resting splints.

During passive or active range-of-motion exercises, include the digit joints and the large joints. If necessary, give your patient an analgesic before these exercises. As soon as possible, involve your patient in activities of daily living. And help her learn to manage her osteoarthritis together with the effects of her CVA.

Teach your patient and her family about the importance of pain management and continued movement and exercise. Home visits from a physical or occupational therapist can help maximize your patient's joint function, mobility, and independence while minimizing the risks of immobility.

Suggested readings

Adams HP Jr, Brott TG, Crowell RM, et al. Guidelines for the management of patients with acute ischemic stroke: a statement for healthcare professionals from a special writing group of the Stroke Council, American Heart Association. *Stroke.* 1994;25(9):1901-1914.

Barnett HJ, Eliasziw M, Meldrum HE. Drugs and surgery in the prevention of ischemic stroke. *N Engl J Med.* 1995;332(4):238-248.

Bell DS. Stroke in the diabetic patient. *Diabetes Care.* 1994;17(3):213-219.

Bronner LL, Kanter DS, Manson JE. Primary preventing stroke. *N Engl J Med.* 1995;333(21):1392-1400.

Department of Health and Human Services. Agency for Health Care Policy and Research. *Post-stroke rehabilitation, clinical practice guideline no. 16* (AHCPR Publication No. 95-0062). Rockville, Md: Department of Health and Human Services; 1995.

Fisher M, Jonas S, Sacco RL. Prophylactic neuroprotection for cerebral ischemia. *Stroke.* 1994;25(5):1075-1080.

Hacke W, Stingele R, Steiner T, Schuchardt V, Schwab S. Critical care of acute ischemic stroke. *Intensive Care Med.* 1995;21(10):856-862.

Hernandez CA, Grinspun DR. The challenges of teaching clients with cerebrovascular accidents to manage their diabetes. *Diabetes Educ.* 1994;20(4):311-316.

Huether SE, McCance KL. *Understanding pathophysiology.* St Louis, Mo: Mosby–Year Book, Inc; 1996.

Lewis S, Collier I, Heitkemper M. *Medical-surgical nursing: assessment and management of clinical problems.* 4th ed. St Louis, Mo: Mosby–Year Book, Inc; 1996.

Macabasco AC, Hickman JL. Thrombolytic therapy for brain attack. *J Neurosci Nurs.* 1995;27(3):138-149.

Maklebust J, Sieggreen MY. Attacking on all fronts: how to conquer pressure ulcers. *Nursing.* 1996:26(12):34-39.

McKenry LM, Salerno E. *Pharmacology in nursing.* 19th ed. St Louis, Mo: Mosby–Year Book, Inc; 1995.

Polaski AL, Tatro SE. *Luckmann's core principles and practice of medical-surgical nursing.* Philadelphia, Pa: WB Saunders Co; 1996.

Shephard TJ, Fox SW. Assessment and management of hypertension in the acute ischemic stroke patient. *J Neurosci Nurs.* 1996;28(1):5-12.

Sherman DG, Dyken ML Jr, Gent M, Harrison JG, Hart RG, Mohr JP. Antithrombotic therapy for cerebrovascular disorders: an update. *Chest.* 1995;108(4Supp):444S-456S.

Thompson DW, Furlan AJ. Clinical epidemiology of stroke. *Neurol Clin.* 1996;14(2):309-315.

Weber CE. Stroke: brain attack, time to react. *ACCN Clin Issues.* 1995;6(4):562-575.

Whitney F. Drug therapy for acute stroke. *J Neurosci Nurs.* 1994;26(2):111-117.

Wojner AW. Optimizing ischemic stroke outcomes: an interdisciplinary approach to poststroke rehabilitation in acute care. *Crit Care Nurs Q.* 1996;19(2):47-61.

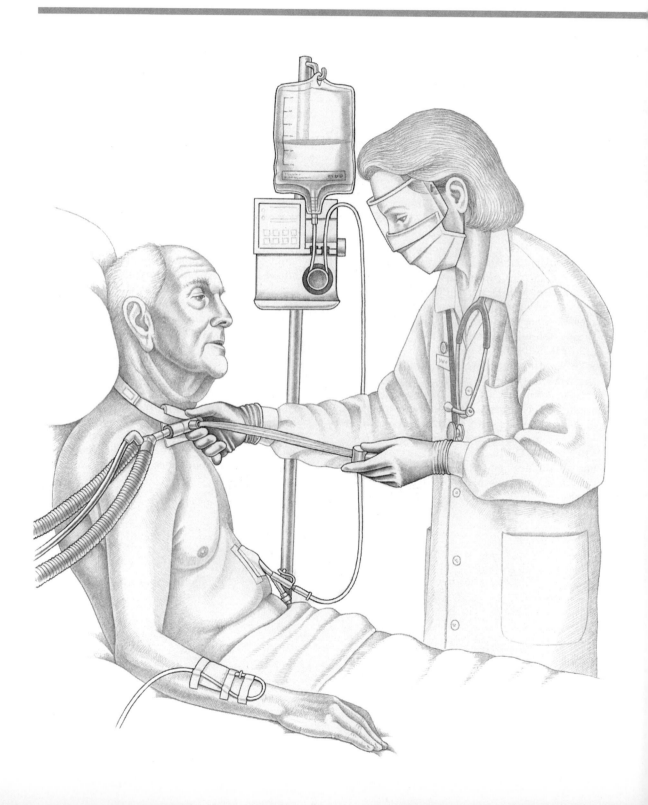

7

Emphysema

Several chronic diseases can limit air-flow into or out of the respiratory system. Grouped under the term *chronic obstructive pulmonary disease* (COPD), these diseases include emphysema, chronic bronchitis, and asthma. Together, they affect 15% to 25% of Americans. And they represent the fifth leading cause of death in the United States, after heart disease, cancer, cerebrovascular accident, and fatal accidents.

Commonly, emphysema occurs in combination with other disorders—such as bronchitis, asthma, pneumonia, hypertension, and cirrhosis—which can make both the diagnosis and treatment complex. Plus, patients with emphysema risk a number of life-threatening complications, such as hypoxemia, respiratory acidosis, pneumothorax, pleural effusion, respiratory failure, cardiac arrhythmias, cardiomyopathy, and heart failure.

Anatomy and physiology review

The complex structures of the respiratory system work together to accomplish one goal: the exchange of oxygen and carbon dioxide. Also, the respiratory system maintains the body's acid-base balance, regulates internal water levels, manages body temperature, and contributes to the ability to speak and smell.

Upper respiratory tract

Made up of the nose, mouth, pharynx, and larynx, the upper respiratory tract directs air into the respiratory system and begins the process of warming, cleansing, and humidifying it (see *Inside the respiratory system*).

Air usually is inhaled through the nose, which is lined by stiff hairs in the front and a mucous membrane in the back. The nose blocks most large and many small foreign particles from passing into more vulnerable areas of the respiratory system. Turbinates, covered with a mucous membrane richly supplied by warm blood from the carotid arteries, project into a cavity called the vestibule just behind the nose. The turbinates begin the process of warming and humidifying the inspired air.

Once inspired air moves through the nose, it passes through the three areas of the pharynx: first the nasopharynx, then the oropharynx, then the laryngopharynx. In the nasopharynx, inspired air passes the pharyngeal tonsils (adenoids) and the openings of the eustachian tubes. In the oropharynx, it passes the palatine tonsils and the uvula. At the back of the oropharynx lies the epiglottis, a small flap of cartilage at the base of the tongue that covers the larynx during swallowing. The laryngopharynx extends from the tip of the epiglottis to the larynx.

The larynx, which extends from the laryngopharynx to the trachea, is protected by nine rings of cartilage (three paired and three single) and houses the vocal cords. Once past the larynx, inspired air enters the lower respiratory tract.

Lower respiratory tract

By the time inspired air reaches the trachea, it's been warmed and humidified. In fact, no matter what the environmental temperature is, air reaches the lungs at about 97° F (36.1° C). And only the tiniest debris remain.

Trachea

In front of the esophagus and held open by 6 to 10 C-shaped rings of cartilage, the trachea is a flexible, muscular tube. It contains many mucus-producing goblet cells and is lined with fine cilia. The trachea extends from the larynx to about the level of the fourth or fifth thoracic vertebra, where it divides into two mainstem bronchi at a point called the carina or angle of Louis.

Bronchi and bronchioles

The mainstem bronchi are somewhat smaller in diameter than the trachea. They, too, are surrounded by C-shaped rings of cartilage. The right bronchus is shorter, wider, and more vertical than the left, making it easier for foreign objects to be aspirated into it. The mainstem bronchi extend from the mediastinum to the lungs. They enter each lung through a structure called the hilum.

Once inside the lungs, the bronchi divide and subdivide; in fact, they look like inverted trees. The mainstem bronchi first divide into five lobar bronchi. Then they divide again and again into segmental and subsegmental bronchi. As they continue branching toward the lung bases, the bronchi become progressively smaller. The smallest bronchi are called bronchioles.

Like the trachea and bronchi, most bronchioles contain embedded pieces of cartilage that hold the airways open. After the bronchioles divide into the terminal bronchioles, however, they lose that protective cartilage. Here, they're made up only of smooth muscle. Because they lack cartilage, the terminal bronchioles can expand, constrict, and even collapse.

Terminal bronchioles branch into lobules (also called the acini), which contain the respiratory bronchioles, alveolar ducts, and alveolar sacs.

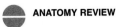

Inside the respiratory system

The respiratory system consists of airways extending from the mouth and nose to the tiny alveoli in the lungs, as shown in the main illustration below. The inset gives a close-up view of a terminal bronchiole and acini, also called the gas-exchange airways.

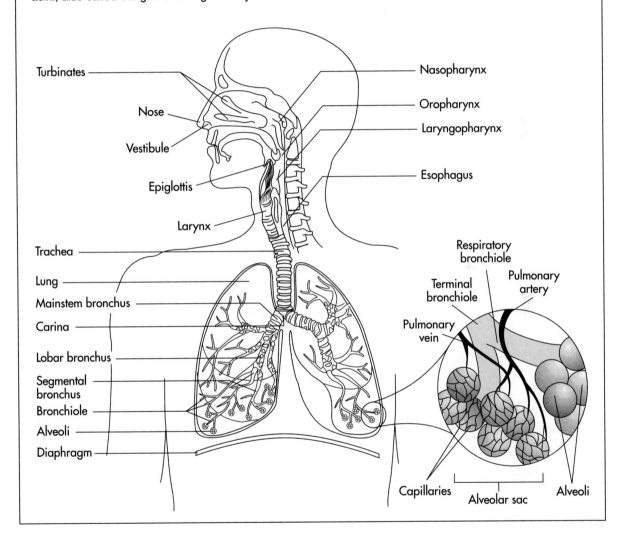

Alveoli

Branching from the respiratory bronchioles are the alveolar ducts. From these ducts arise alveolar sacs that contain clusters of alveoli. Imagine the alveoli as roughly 300 million tiny bubbles, each about 0.3 mm in diameter. If you flattened all these alveoli and spread them in a single layer, they'd be about the size of a tennis court. Along this large surface, gas exchange occurs. If this surface is diminished, gas exchange will be impaired.

Each alveolus contains two cell types. Type I cells provide structure. Type II cells produce a compound called surfactant that lowers surface tension inside the alveolus, which makes it easier to keep the alveoli inflated.

The alveolar sacs are surrounded by beds of pulmonary capillaries. Across a membrane that varies from 0.4 μm to 2 μm thick, gas exchange takes place between air in the alveoli and blood in the capillaries.

Lungs

The lungs are surrounded and protected by 12 pairs of ribs that make up the thoracic cavity. Additional protection is afforded by the sternum and clavicles to the front and the vertebral column and scapulae to the back. Inside the thoracic cavity, the lungs are separated from each other by the mediastinum, which contains the trachea and esophagus, the heart and its great vessels, the thymus gland, and the vagus and phrenic nerves. The lung bases rest on the diaphragm.

The lungs themselves are two cone-shaped masses of spongy, elastic tissue. The right lung has three lobes; the left lung has two. Both are covered by the visceral pleura, a thin serous membrane. The inside of the thoracic cavity also is lined by a thin serous membrane, this one called the parietal pleura. In the potential space between these two membranes is a small amount of fluid, typically less than 30 ml, that allows the membranes to move smoothly across each other during respiration.

Respiratory circulation

Two separate circulatory systems—the bronchial system and the pulmonary system—interact with the lungs and the alveoli. Bronchial arteries, which don't participate in gas exchange, arise from the thoracic aorta and bring oxygenated blood to nourish the lung tissues.

The pulmonary system arises from the pulmonary arteries and brings oxygen-depleted blood from the systemic circulation to the alveoli for reoxygenation. These arteries rapidly decrease in size until they become the pulmonary capillary beds. Here, oxygen and carbon dioxide trade places across the alveolocapillary membrane, and freshly oxygenated blood returns to the left atrium and ventricle through the pulmonary veins. From there, it enters the systemic circulation.

Normally, the pressure needed to pump blood through the pulmonary circulation is much lower than that needed to pump blood through the body. In fact, the typical pulmonary blood pressure is only about 25/8 mm Hg; the typical systemic blood pressure is 120/80 mm Hg. Thus, the thin-walled right ventricle can easily move blood through the pulmonary circulation.

Respiratory mucosa

Lining almost all of the respiratory system is a layer of mucosa that's crucial for removing foreign debris from inspired air before it reaches the alveoli. Goblet cells that line the respiratory tract secrete about 100 to 125 ml of mucus each day—enough to form a continuous sheet over the respiratory structures.

As air enters the respiratory system, even the most minute airborne particles stick to the mucous lining. Then, millions of tiny, continuously beating cilia work to move the mucus, and the foreign particles, upward toward the pharynx. Once in the pharynx, the mucus can be expectorated or swallowed. This system effectively cleans inspired air of pollens, dust, insects, bacteria, and other potentially harmful contaminants before they reach the alveoli.

Understanding respiration

Respiration, the exchange of gases between body cells and the atmosphere, involves three processes:
• ventilation—the movement of air into and out of the lungs
• diffusion, or gas exchange—the transfer of oxygen and carbon dioxide across the alveolocapillary membrane
• gas transport—the movement of oxygen from the lungs to cells and the movement of carbon dioxide from cells to lungs.

Ventilation takes place when the diaphragm and external intercostal muscles contract in response to signals from the brain and various chemical and mechanical receptors. Diaphragmatic contraction enlarges the thoracic cavity from top to bottom. Contraction of the external intercostal muscles enlarges it from front to back and from side to side. As a result, negative pressure in the thoracic cavity draws atmospheric air into the lungs. Expiration takes place when the diaphragm and external intercostal muscles relax, and elastic recoil causes the lungs to spring back to their former position. For a more complete explanation of ventilation, see Chapter 8.

Diffusion, or gas exchange, relies on the pressure gradient of oxygen and carbon dioxide in the alveoli and the pulmonary capillaries. When oxygen pressure is higher in alveoli than in the capillaries, oxygen moves across the alveolocapillary membrane into the capillaries. Likewise, when carbon dioxide pressure is higher in the capillaries than in the alveoli, carbon dioxide moves across the alveolocapillary membrane into the alveoli. Several factors can alter diffusion, including changes in atmospheric pressure and changes in the amount of surface area available for gas exchange.

Gas transport depends largely on heart function and hemoglobin. Anything that affects cardiac output also can affect the amount of oxygen available to the tissues. Although 1% to 2% of oxygen is dissolved in plasma, most of the oxygen in the blood clings to hemoglobin molecules. Thus, anything that affects the availability of hemoglobin can also affect the amount of oxygen delivered to tissues.

Carbon dioxide travels through the blood as a carbaminohemoglobin. It can also be dissolved in plasma. Carbon dioxide is more soluble than oxygen and can diffuse from the tissues into the blood quickly. The amount of carbon dioxide that enters the blood depends on the amount of oxygen that leaves the blood and enters the tissues.

Pathophysiology

Emphysema affects the smallest respiratory structures: the bronchioles and the alveoli. In general, it's characterized by a narrowing of the bronchioles, destruction of the alveolar walls, and enlargement of the air spaces.

Types of emphysema

Two major types of emphysema exist: centrilobular and panlobular (see *Comparing types of emphysema*, page 234).

In centrilobular (also called centriacinar) emphysema, the more common type, the respiratory bronchioles become inflamed and enlarged, but the alveolar ducts and sacs are spared. This type of emphysema usually starts in the upper lung lobes and moves downward. Typically, it affects men who smoke.

Panlobular (also called panacinar) emphysema involves the respiratory bronchioles, alveolar ducts, and alveolar sacs. Over time, the disease destroys the whole lobule, creating a progressive loss of lung tissue and a decreasing alveolocapillary surface. Panlobular emphysema occurs randomly throughout the lung but usually affects the front of the lower lobes. It's most common in elderly people and in those with an inherited deficiency of the plasma protein alpha$_1$-antitrypsin.

Development of emphysema

Four processes contribute to the development of emphysema:
- loss of elasticity
- airway collapse
- hyperinflation
- bullae formation.

Successful expiration depends on the ability of the lungs to recoil when the diaphragm and external intercostal muscles relax. In emphysema, that elastic recoil is reduced when proteolytic enzymes break down elastin and collagen fibers in the small airways. Air can move into the lungs normally, but the lack of elastic recoil prevents air from exiting normally. Instead, air becomes trapped in the alveoli and the patient must begin to use the accessory muscles in an attempt to forcefully drive air from the lungs. That forceful exhalation results in increased intrathoracic pressures, which cause small unsupported bronchioles to collapse and air to become trapped in the alveoli. Some alveoli are destroyed in the process; others become enlarged. Eventually, trapped air causes the lungs to become hyperinflated and press down against the diaphragm, flattening it and reducing its ability to function.

Comparing types of emphysema

Centrilobular emphysema primarily affects the respiratory bronchioles. Panlobular emphysema affects the respiratory bronchioles and the alveoli. The illustrations below show a normal acinus, one affected by centrilobular emphysema, and one affected by panlobular emphysema.

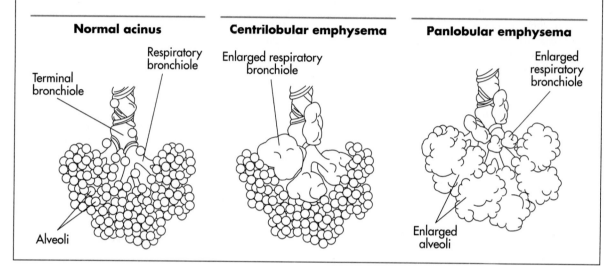

Normal acinus — Terminal bronchiole, Respiratory bronchiole, Alveoli

Centrilobular emphysema — Enlarged respiratory bronchiole

Panlobular emphysema — Enlarged respiratory bronchiole, Enlarged alveoli

As the alveolar walls continue to deteriorate, alveolar ducts and sacs may coalesce into bullae. Not only do bullae raise the risk of pneumothorax, they also reduce the amount of alveolocapillary membrane available for gas exchange and increase dead-space ventilation (the movement of air that never participates in gas exchange).

The reduced gas exchange and the increased dead-space ventilation mean that the patient must attempt to compensate—by breathing deeper and faster—to maintain oxygenation. Breathing deeper (increasing tidal volume) usually doesn't help because the patient's lungs already are hyperinflated. Breathing faster usually does help because it increases gas exchange in the functioning alveoli. However, the increased effort required by the respiratory muscles raises the patient's energy requirements and oxygen use, further increasing the work of breathing.

Role of alpha$_1$-antitrypsin

The inflammation, overinflation, and destruction of lung tissue results in large part from the body's reaction to inhaled toxic substances, especially cigarette smoke, over a long period of time. In response to this inflammation, the body releases proteolytic enzymes, specifically elastase.

In normal lungs, a plasma protein called alpha$_1$-antitrypsin protects tissues from the damaging effects of elastase. When inflammation develops or when elastase increases in the lung tissue, alpha$_1$-antitrypsin increases to counteract its effects. If alpha$_1$-antitrypsin is diminished, however, elastase may overwhelm the lungs and damage lung tissue.

Why is smoking so central to the development of emphysema?
- Cigarette smoke paralyzes the cilia that line the respiratory tract, reducing their ability to remove toxins.
- Cigarette smoke increases the number of polymorphonuclear neutrophils and macrophages, which release proteolytic enzymes in lung tissue.

- Cigarette smoke decreases the level of alpha$_1$-antitrypsin stored in the body.

In about 2% of patients, emphysema results from a congenital deficiency of alpha$_1$-antitrypsin. These patients usually develop emphysema by the time they reach age 45, even if they never smoked.

Assessment findings

Usually, emphysema progresses slowly over several decades, and a patient first seeks medical care because he has become short of breath.

If your patient is in the early stages of emphysema, he may have no symptoms at all or only a slight shortness of breath on exertion. Over time, however, more signs and symptoms will appear. Besides shortness of breath on exertion or at rest, you may note the following:
- pursed-lip breathing with minimal exertion or even at rest
- a tendency to lean forward when sitting and place the elbows on the knees
- severe weight loss from poor eating habits, usually because a full stomach makes breathing more difficult
- chronic cough with little sputum production
- severely decreased or absent breath sounds
- slightly pink skin color
- finger clubbing
- barrel chest (see *Recognizing barrel chest,* page 236).

In the late stages of emphysema, you may note dependent edema.

Diagnostic tests

A diagnosis of emphysema is based on a thorough history and physical examination and on certain diagnostic tests, including a chest X-ray, an electrocardiogram (ECG), arterial blood gas (ABG) studies, and pulmonary function tests.

Chest X-ray

If your patient has emphysema, a chest X-ray will show hyperlucent, overinflated lungs with a flattened or scalloped diaphragm and a decreased costal angle. The X-ray will also show increased intercostal spaces and an increased anterior-posterior diameter.

Electrocardiogram

Early in the disease, your patient's ECG will remain unchanged. As the disease progresses, however, you'll notice peaked P waves, especially during flare-ups. If your patient has right ventricular heart failure, you may see right-axis deviation and R waves over the right precordial leads.

ABG studies

A patient's ABG measurements may indicate an increased partial pressure of arterial carbon dioxide (Paco$_2$), a decreased partial pressure of arterial oxygen (Pao$_2$), and respiratory acidosis. However, some patients with emphysema have normal ABG measurements because they compensate by breathing more rapidly and deeply. In fact, some patients may overcompensate, creating a slight respiratory alkalosis from hyperventilation. The Paco$_2$ level usually is normal or slightly decreased, also from the hyperventilation.

Pulmonary function tests

Some simple pulmonary function tests can also help confirm the diagnosis of emphysema and determine the extent of the disease, especially if your patient has no symptoms. These tests include measurements of forced vital capacity (FVC), forced expiratory volume in 1 second (FEV$_1$), total lung capacity (TLC), and residual volume (RV). Essentially, pulmonary function tests for emphysema patients reveal an increased resistance to expiratory airflow: decreased FVC and FEV$_1$ and increased TLC and RV.

Additional tests

If the patient's physician suspects a respiratory tract infection, she may order a sputum culture. The physician may also order serum electrolyte and blood glucose levels. A complete blood count may be performed to determine if your patient has polycythemia, a common condition in hypoxemic patients. To assess the

Recognizing barrel chest

Emphysema causes hyperinflated lungs and requires the patient to use his accessory muscles to breathe. Over time, using these muscles changes the shape of the patient's chest. First, the costal angle changes. Then, the anterior-posterior chest diameter becomes larger than the transverse diameter, giving the patient's chest a characteristic barrel shape.

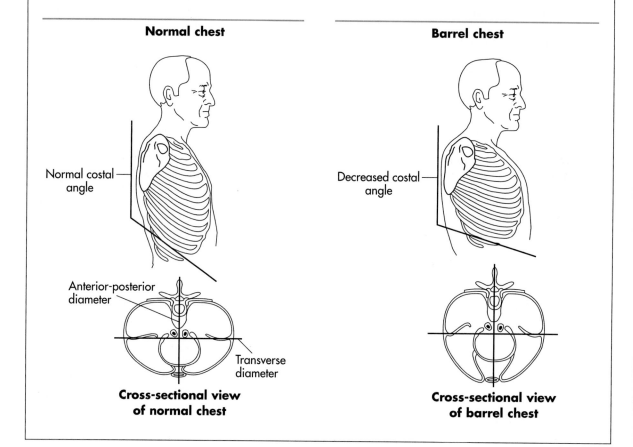

Normal chest

Normal costal angle

Anterior-posterior diameter

Transverse diameter

Cross-sectional view of normal chest

Barrel chest

Decreased costal angle

Cross-sectional view of barrel chest

patient's nutritional status, a physician may order measurements of serum albumin, magnesium, and phosphorus levels.

Medical interventions

Emphysema treatment may include drug therapy, oxygen therapy, pulmonary rehabilitation, diet therapy, and surgery.

Drug therapy

No drug therapy can halt the progression of emphysema. However, several drugs can help reduce the symptoms and improve the patient's activity tolerance. These drugs include bronchodilators to relieve bronchospasm, corticosteroids to reduce airway inflammation, and antibiotics to treat recurrent pulmonary infections.

Bronchodilators usually are inhaled, using an inhaler or a nebulizer. If the patient can't or won't use the inhaled drug properly, oral theophylline may be prescribed. Theophylline improves the function of the respiratory muscles, stimulates the central respiratory center, and reduces inflammation (see *Adverse effects of common bronchodilators*).

Corticosteroids decrease airway inflammation and improve airflow and gas exchange during flare-ups of emphysema. They may also be prescribed for a patient who doesn't respond to bronchodilator therapy. A corticosteroid may be inhaled or taken orally.

The air trapping and excess mucus production caused by emphysema places the patient at risk for pulmonary infections. Usually a physician will order a sputum specimen for culture, sensitivity, and Gram's stain. Antibiotics used to treat pulmonary infections include ampicillin, tetracycline, and cephalosporins.

Oxygen therapy

If the patient can't maintain a PaO_2 of 55 mm Hg or more at rest or if he can't accomplish his daily activities without becoming short of breath, he'll need supplemental oxygen. Usually oxygen is delivered at 1 to 2 liters per minute by nasal cannula. Oxygen can be given continuously, while sleeping, or during exercise.

Pulmonary rehabilitation

Pulmonary rehabilitation helps the emphysema patient build endurance and activity tolerance and helps prevent complications of the disease. Training should be gentle and gradual, incorporating endurance, flexibility, and some aerobic training. Training can include breathing exercises, leg-raising exercises, and conditioning activities such as walking and riding a stationary bicycle. The patient probably will benefit from portable oxygen during the training sessions.

Diet therapy

Because patients with emphysema risk weight loss and muscle wasting, they need to maintain an adequate nutritional intake. Usually, these patients need a high-protein, high-calorie diet,

Adverse effects of common bronchodilators	
Drug	**Adverse effects**
Albuterol	• bad taste in the mouth and nausea • nervousness, tremors, and headache • pallor, flushing, and sweating • cardiac arrhythmias, including tachycardia
Bitolterol	• bad taste in the mouth and nausea • apprehension, nervousness, tremors, and insomnia • cough • cardiac arrhythmias
Metaproterenol	• bad taste in the mouth, nausea, vomiting, and heartburn • restlessness, apprehension, and nervousness • sweating, pallor, and flushing • cardiac arrhythmias
Pirbuterol	• nausea • nervousness, tremors, insomnia, headache, and dizziness • tachycardia
Terbutaline	• nausea • anxiety, nervousness, tremors, headache, and dizziness • pulmonary edema • palpitations and arrhythmias including tachycardia
Theophylline	• loss of appetite, nausea, vomiting, and diarrhea • headache, insomnia, irritability, and restlessness • tachypnea and respiratory arrest • life-threatening ventricular arrhythmias
Ipratropium	• dry mouth • headache • eye pain • urine retention • urticaria • palpitations and tachycardia

possibly with vitamin supplements. For some patients, a physician also may order a liquid dietary supplement.

Surgery

A surgical procedure called lung-volume reduction may help increase a patient's activity tolerance and, consequently, his quality of life.

During the procedure, a surgeon removes diseased sections of the patient's lung to reduce overall lung volume. Doing so reduces air trapping, making the lungs work more efficiently. Also, this surgery allows the chest wall and diaphragm to take a more normal position. And functioning tissue has more room to expand as the patient breathes.

Good candidates for lung-volume reduction surgery include patients who:
- have emphysema that severely restricts their activities
- have a fully distended thorax and a fully flattened diaphragm
- haven't smoked for at least 6 months
- have failed to respond to other therapies
- don't have contraindications, such as asthma, bronchiectasis, pulmonary fibrosis, or pulmonary hypertension.

Nursing interventions

While your emphysema patient is hospitalized, assess him at least every 4 hours. Be sure to auscultate his lungs and listen for changes in his breath sounds. If you hear wheezes or crackles, he may have secretions or fluid in his airways. Also, observe your patient for increased or decreased use of his accessory muscles, paradoxical respirations, and changes in his level of consciousness (LOC). A decreasing mental status may be an early indication of hypoxemia or hypercapnia.

Monitor your patient's vital signs frequently. Keep in mind that bronchodilators tend to cause tachycardia, which increases oxygen demand. Begin cardiac monitoring, as ordered, to check for new or worsening arrhythmias. Also, assess your patient for signs and symptoms of right ventricular heart failure, such as dependent edema and jugular vein distention. If your patient's temperature rises, check for signs of respiratory infection, such as a productive cough, increased sputum production, or a change in the color or viscosity of sputum. An infection increases oxygen demand and also places your patient at risk for further respiratory compromise.

As you care for your patient, keep in mind that he must deal with emotional challenges as well as physical ones. Besides having a disorder that requires attentive care, he also has a disorder that causes great anxiety. And anxiety can worsen his symptoms.

Oxygenation

To ease breathing and relieve dyspnea, place your patient in the semi-Fowler or high Fowler position. If he still has trouble breathing, place pillows across his overbed table and have him lean forward with his arms resting on the pillows.

Administer the prescribed drug therapy to improve your patient's oxygenation. Observe him carefully to ensure its effectiveness and detect any adverse effects.

Use pulse oximetry, ABG measurements, or both to monitor your patient's oxygen levels. Keep his oxygen saturation level above 90% by giving supplemental oxygen. Keep in mind, however, that a patient with long-standing emphysema may be chronically hypercapnic, and his respiratory drive may be stimulated only by low levels of oxygen. If you give him oxygen at a flow rate that's too high, you'll actually decrease his drive to breathe. Therefore, monitor his oxygen saturation levels closely as you change oxygen flow rates. If supplemental oxygen won't keep your patient's oxygen saturation above 90% and he's in respiratory distress, anticipate endotracheal intubation and mechanical ventilation.

If your patient has copious secretions, perform chest physiotherapy. Remember, though, that he may not be able to tolerate the full range of positions. Give a bronchodilator as prescribed to open his airways and promote expectoration.

Finally, show your patient that slowing his breathing rate will help decrease the work of breathing and control his dyspnea. To encourage deep breathing and strengthen respiratory muscles, have him perform incentive spirometry every 2 hours. Urge him to use his diaphragm and abdominal muscles for breathing because they use less oxygen and distribute a greater volume of air. To reduce air trapping, encourage him to inhale through his nose and exhale slowly through pursed lips.

Adequate nutrition
Patients with severe dyspnea commonly feel that they don't have enough breath to eat. Plus, a full stomach presses upward against the diaphragm, making breathing more difficult. And some bronchodilators can leave an unpleasant metallic taste in the mouth. Consequently, you'll need to make sure your patient consumes enough calories and fluids.

Work with the dietitian, the patient, and his family to create a customized nutritional plan. Encourage small, frequent meals and snacks. Don't give your patient too much food and don't hurry him through his meals. Use liquid supplements as prescribed.

Encourage your patient to drink 2 to 3 liters of fluid daily, especially if he has copious secretions. But watch for fluid overload, especially if your patient takes an oral corticosteroid, which causes sodium and water retention. Monitor your patient's intake, output, weight, and serum electrolyte levels every day.

Rest and activity
Emphysema causes severe fatigue, so give your patient plenty of time to perform activities and an opportunity to rest afterward. Also, space his activities throughout the day. During activities, monitor your patient's oxygen saturation levels and encourage him to use pursed-lip breathing. Progress to more strenuous activities only if your patient can tolerate them.

To alleviate the anxiety that accompanies shortness of breath, teach your patient relaxation techniques. Help your patient and his family develop a plan that maximizes his independence and minimizes dyspnea and functional limitations. For example, encourage him to sit rather than stand at the bathroom sink when he shaves and brushes his teeth. Gradual progressive activity coupled with energy conservation can help improve your patient's self-esteem as well as his ability to function.

Patient teaching
Teach your patient how to take medications properly, use supplemental oxygen, maximize his breathing while minimizing complications, maintain an adequate diet, and avoid toxins and infections.

Medications
Most emphysema patients take a bronchodilator using a metered-dose inhaler. But many patients have difficulty using the inhaler correctly, so spend time teaching your patient how to use it. If necessary, have him use a spacer so he receives the full dose (see *Teaching your patient to use a metered-dose inhaler*, page 240).

Instead of a metered-dose inhaler, your patient may need an aerosol nebulizer. If so, teach him and his family how to use it. Make sure they know how to dilute the medication and clean the equipment properly. Warn them that the mouthpiece, solution chamber, and tubing are excellent reservoirs for bacterial growth. If they're not cleaned properly, the patient risks infection.

Supplemental oxygen
If your patient is going home with supplemental oxygen, explain that oxygen will do the most good if it's used as directed by his physician. Reinforce the safety precautions that need to be taken when using oxygen. And instruct your patient to notify his local fire department and power company that oxygen is being used in his home. Make sure your patient is familiar with the method of oxygen delivery he's using, the oxygen flow rate, and what he should do if a problem arises. To make sure he's using the equipment correctly, arrange for a nurse to visit your patient at home.

Breathing efficiency
During your patient's hospitalization, a physical therapist or an occupational therapist will teach him pursed-lip breathing, diaphragmatic breathing, and energy conservation techniques for walking and activities of daily living. Reinforce these instructions before your patient goes home.

Also, show him positions that can ease exhalation, such as leaning forward over a table with his arms supported on pillows, sitting forward with his elbows on his knees, and leaning

Teaching your patient to use a metered-dose inhaler

To help your emphysema patient use his metered-dose inhaler correctly, instruct him to take these steps.

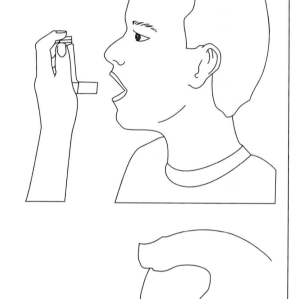

- Shake the inhaler.
- Remove the cap from the inhaler.
- Tilt your head back a little and breathe out.
- Hold the inhaler upright about an inch in front of your mouth. Open your mouth.
- Press down on the inhaler to release the medication.
- As the medication is released into the air in front of you, breathe in through your mouth for 3 to 5 seconds.
- Hold your breath for 10 seconds, so the medication can spread through your lungs.
- If your doctor prescribed more than one inhalation, wait at least a full minute before taking the next one.

Using a spacer
- If you have trouble using your inhaler, attach a spacer to it.
- Close your lips around the mouthpiece of the spacer.
- Discharge the medication into the spacer. Then inhale.

Ongoing care
- Rinse your inhaler every day and clean it with mild soap once a week. Use a second inhaler while the first one is drying.
- To check how much medication you have left, remove the canister from the inhaler. Then place it in water and match its position to the illustration shown here.

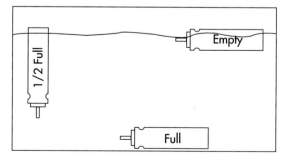

against a wall with his shoulders sagging forward and arms relaxed.

If your patient has copious secretions, show his family how to perform chest physiotherapy, including postural drainage and percussion. Tell them to perform these procedures in the morning, before meals, and at night.

Although pulmonary rehabilitation probably doesn't improve lung function, it can help build your patient's tolerance for activity, bolster his feelings of independence, and reduce his chances of future hospitalizations. So that he doesn't lose the conditioning he's gained in the hospital, encourage your patient to take part in outpatient pulmonary rehabilitation.

Diet guidelines
To help your patient maintain an adequate diet at home, teach him these tips:
- Eat 30 to 60 minutes after taking medications.
- Eat smaller, more frequent meals to prevent a full stomach that can press against the diaphragm.
- Eat high-protein snacks between meals.
- Drink a high-calorie dietary supplement.
- Space food and fluid intake throughout the day.

If your patient needs continuous oxygen, help him devise a system to keep it flowing during meals. For example, if he normally wears a mask to receive oxygen, suggest that he switch to a nasal cannula while he eats.

If your patient has late-stage emphysema and is beginning to retain carbon dioxide, advise him to avoid high-carbohydrate foods. Explain that eating such foods may further increase his carbon dioxide blood levels because carbohydrate metabolism produces carbon dioxide.

Toxins and infections
If your patient smokes, urge him to stop. And encourage him to avoid secondhand smoke. If family members smoke, urge them to quit or at least to smoke well away from your patient. Refer your patient and his family to community resources that can help them stop smoking.

Remind your patient to be alert to air pollutants. Suggest that he listen to weather reports and stay indoors when the air quality is poor. And encourage him to avoid extreme changes in temperature. Recommend that he clean the air in his home by using a high-efficiency, particulate air filter. Also, advise him to avoid crowds and people who have upper respiratory tract infections.

Emphysema and pneumonia

Pneumonia, an acute inflammation and consolidation of lung tissue, can result from a wide variety of organisms and conditions. The most common cause is bacterial infection. But pneumonia also can result from viruses, mycoplasms, and protozoans. And it can stem from therapies that affect lung tissue (such as radiation), inhalation of noxious fumes, and gastric aspiration.

A patient with emphysema is more susceptible to pneumonia and more apt to suffer from its effects than most people. He's more susceptible because of his retained secretions, ineffective breathing, and altered lung defense mechanisms. If he's taking a corticosteroid to treat his emphysema, his risk of pneumonia increases even more.

Pathophysiology

The emphysema patient's reduced defenses allow an invading pathogen to spread quickly through lung tissues to the distal airways. The lungs then react to the pathogen, releasing a large number of cells and increasing inflammatory exudate. White blood cells release enzymes and mediators in an attempt to kill the pathogen, further increasing the inflammatory reaction. Endotoxins produced by the pathogen damage bronchial mucous and alveolar membranes, leading to edema, further inflammation, and the accumulation of exudate and debris in the terminal bronchioles and alveoli. These reactions may occur in diffuse patches throughout both lungs or as local consolidation. Either way, the effects of the invasion and the body's reaction to it further reduce the emphysema patient's lung volume, ventilation, and blood flow.

PATHOPHYSIOLOGY

How emphysema and pneumonia reduce gas exchange

Emphysema reduces gas exchange by destroying the alveolocapillary membrane; pneumonia reduces gas exchange by covering the alveolocapillary membrane in exudate. The three illustrations below show the progression from healthy alveoli and capillaries to those affected by both emphysema and pneumonia.

1. This illustration shows normal alveoli and capillaries. Oxygen and carbon dioxide move easily across the undisturbed alveolocapillary membrane.

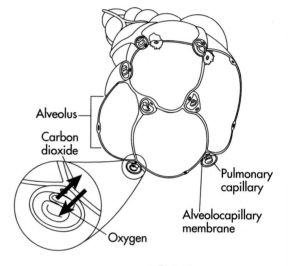

Alveolus
Carbon dioxide
Oxygen
Pulmonary capillary
Alveolocapillary membrane

2. Emphysema weakens and destroys alveolar walls, creating enlarged air spaces distal to the terminal bronchioles. What's more, as alveolar walls are destroyed, the adjacent pulmonary capillaries also are destroyed. Thus, the alveolocapillary membrane is markedly decreased, and less gas exchange can take place.

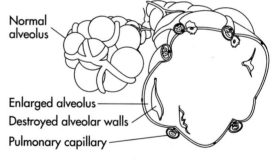

Normal alveolus
Enlarged alveolus
Destroyed alveolar walls
Pulmonary capillary

3. In pneumonia, the inflammatory reaction to the pathogen causes the alveoli to fill with exudate—including serum, red blood cells, and other debris. Also, leukocytes migrate to the affected area to destroy bacteria, and macrophages move in to help remove cellular and bacterial debris. Sometimes they're successful. But sometimes the alveoli remain filled with the exudate, further reducing the size of the functioning alveolocapillary membrane.

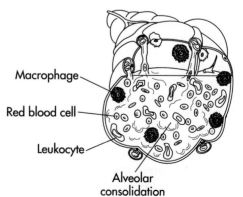

Macrophage
Red blood cell
Leukocyte
Alveolar consolidation

Developing pneumonia on top of emphysema increases the patient's work of breathing by further reducing the alveolocapillary surface area available for gas exchange. Here's how: When the inflammatory process increases capillary permeability, interstitial and alveolar fluids increase. The affected alveoli fill with an exudate of bacteria, fibrin-containing fluid, red blood cells, and polymorphonuclear leukocytes. These interstitial and alveolar fluids make the lungs harder to inflate, increasing the work of breathing (see *How emphysema and pneumonia reduce gas exchange*).

Adapting nursing care

Nursing care for a patient with emphysema and pneumonia should focus on reducing the risk of hypoxemia by maintaining his airway and improving gas exchange. Start by assessing your patient's respiratory status frequently. Check his respiratory rate, depth, and character. Use pulse oximetry or ABG measurements to monitor his oxygen saturation. Give a low concentration of supplemental oxygen, as ordered, to avoid depressing his respiratory drive. To control the flow of oxygen more precisely, use a Venturi mask as needed (see *Using a Venturi mask*).

Auscultate your patient's lungs for changes that warn of increasing secretions or deteriorating respiratory status, such as increased crackles, wheezing, or decreased or absent breath sounds. Help your patient breathe easier by elevating the head of his bed so that he's upright. Encourage him to use pursed-lip and diaphragmatic breathing.

If your patient produces more than 30 ml of sputum daily, his physician may order incentive spirometry and chest physiotherapy—or increase their frequency. A physician also may order the use of a flutter device (see *Teaching your patient to use a flutter device*, page 244).

Make sure your patient gets adequate rest and nutrition. Avoid activities, treatments, and procedures for at least 1 hour before and after meals. Encourage coughing and deep breathing before he eats to remove secretions, decrease dyspnea, and improve his appetite. And provide frequent mouth care to remove secretions and improve taste sensation.

Using a Venturi mask

Using a Venturi mask allows you to give your patient precise oxygen concentrations at high flow rates. It's especially good for delivering low, constant concentrations to a patient with emphysema. The mask is lightweight, and you can add an adaptor to humidify the inspired air. Keep in mind, however, that the large mask may be uncomfortable for your patient and may make communication difficult. Also, he'll have to remove it to eat.

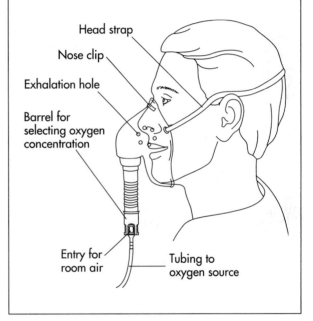

Head strap

Nose clip

Exhalation hole

Barrel for selecting oxygen concentration

Entry for room air

Tubing to oxygen source

Administering medications

If your patient was using a metered-dose inhaler to take a bronchodilator before he developed pneumonia, he may benefit from a switch to an aerosolized nebulizer. If so, clean the nebulizer parts carefully to prevent bacterial growth.

Besides his bronchodilator therapy, your patient also may benefit from a mucolytic drug, such as acetylcysteine, to help loosen secretions. Of course, hydration also helps loosen secretions. So, unless contraindicated, be sure your patient gets 2 to 3 liters of fluids daily. Monitor his daily intake, output, and weight. And watch for signs of fluid overload.

ADAPTING YOUR CARE

Teaching your patient to use a flutter device

Your patient with emphysema and pneumonia may have trouble keeping his airway clear because of his copious, sometimes tenacious, secretions. Plus, the stress of pneumonia added to the muscle fatigue of emphysema may make it tough for him to cough effectively. To help your patient loosen and remove secretions, teach him to use a flutter device.

Preparing to use the flutter device
- Show your patient the flutter device and explain how it works. Tell him the device goes in his mouth. Point out that, as he exhales, the steel ball inside the device moves, causing vibrations. These vibrations extend to his lungs, loosening the secretions clinging to his airways.
- Tell the patient that repeated use of the device will help his lungs move secretions upward, so he can more easily cough them out.
- Place the patient in a comfortable position that maximizes chest expansion. If possible, use the high Fowler position. Urge him to keep his back straight and tilt his head back a little to maximize chest expansion and help keep his airway open.
- If your patient has severe dyspnea, pad his overbed table with pillows and have him lean forward with his elbows on the pillows. Again, have him tilt his head back a little bit.
- For practice, ask your patient to inhale deeply, hold his breath for 2 to 3 seconds, then exhale forcefully but steadily. Explain that this is what he should do when the device is in his mouth.
- While your patient practices this breathing pattern, place your hand on the muscles of his upper abdomen to see how much he's using his

diaphragm. Encourage him to use his large abdominal muscles to breathe.
- Make sure you have suction equipment nearby in case the patient loosens secretions but can't cough them up.

Using the flutter device
- When you think your patient is ready to use the device, ask him to inhale deeply and hold his breath for 2 to 3 seconds. Then place the device in his mouth.
- To enhance the vibratory sensation during exhalation, tell your patient to hold the device parallel to the floor or tilted upward no more than 30 degrees.
- When the device is in place, tell your patient to exhale forcefully, at a steady, consistent speed. Encourage him to exhale as much air as possible to clear the lower airways.
- Make sure he doesn't puff out his cheeks when exhaling because doing so reduces the device's effectiveness. If he puffs out his cheeks, place your hands over them so he can feel what he's doing.
- Check to make sure the device is working properly by placing one hand on the patient's chest and the other on his back. You should be able to feel the vibrations as he exhales.
- Assess your patient carefully while he uses the flutter device. Watch for increasing dyspnea, changes in mental status, and increasing pallor.
- If your patient receives supplemental oxygen, make sure he keeps receiving it when he uses the flutter device. Monitor his oxygen saturation frequently.

A physician may prescribe an antibiotic for your patient before the pneumonia-causing pathogen has been identified. To check if the appropriate drug is being given, the physican will order a sputum culture and Gram's stain. If your patient takes theophylline for his emphysema, watch for interactions with the antibiotic. Antibiotics that contain erythromycin can increase the effects of theophylline and raise the risk of toxicity. Monitor your patient's serum theophylline levels regularly. If they exceed 20 µg/ml, he may experience nausea,

vomiting, diarrhea, headache, insomnia, and irritability. If they exceed 30 µg/ml, he may develop severe hypertension and life-threatening arrhythmias.

Patient teaching
Before your patient with emphysema and pneumonia leaves the hospital, reinforce all aspects of his care. Specifically, be sure to cover his medication therapy, breathing exercises, energy conservation measures, the signs

and symptoms of infection, infection prevention measures, nutrition, activity limitations, and oxygen use.

If your patient will continue taking an antibiotic at home, make sure he knows the drug's name, dosage, and adverse effects. Reinforce the need to finish the entire prescription and comply with follow-up care. Obtain a referral for home care as appropriate, so a nurse can evaluate your patient's respiratory status and provide continuing education and support.

Complications

Common complications for patients with emphysema and pneumonia include hypoxemia, respiratory acidosis, pneumothorax, pleural effusion, and respiratory failure.

Hypoxemia
In a patient already compromised by the reduced gas exchange of emphysema, the development of pneumonia raises the risk of hypoxemia.

Emphysema causes the enlargement of terminal bronchioles, the fragmentation of alveoli, and the destruction of alveolar septa. These three factors cause the destruction of lung elastin, which leads to the loss of elastic recoil. The terminal airways collapse or narrow, leading to air trapping and lung distention. Thus, ventilation is impaired, and the patient has to work harder to force the trapped air out of his lungs.

Additional destruction occurs to the alveolar and bronchiolar walls, which decreases the surface area of the alveolocapillary membrane and impairs oxygen and carbon dioxide exchange. In response, the pulmonary arteries constrict. This, coupled with the increased pressure from over-distended alveoli, leads to a further decrease in perfusion and gas exchange.

Pneumonia further impairs gas exchange in the patient with emphysema. The inflammatory process of pneumonia leads to edema, inflammation, and the accumulation of exudate and debris in the terminal bronchioles and alveoli. These changes further decrease lung volume, blood flow, and the surface area of the aveolocapillary membrane. As a result, oxygen and carbon dioxide exchange is even more impaired, exacerbating the patient's hypoxemia.

Confirming the complication
A pulse oximetry reading below 86% oxygen saturation confirms hypoxemia. If you're not using pulse oximetry, the first sign may be a change in your patient's mental status. He may become confused or combative, for instance, and you'll find that his heart rate and blood pressure have increased. Later, he may become lethargic. At this stage, his heart rate and blood pressure will be reduced, and he may develop respiratory failure. His PaO_2 will fall below his baseline levels.

Nursing interventions
In a patient who develops hypoxemia, your main goal is to promote oxygenation. Give supplemental oxygen by nasal cannula at 2 to 4 liters per minute or by Venturi mask at no more than 40% oxygen. If your patient's $PaCO_2$ is chronically elevated, too much oxygen can depress his respiratory drive. Usually, a physician will try to avoid endotracheal intubation and mechanical ventilation because it may be difficult to wean your patient from the ventilator after the hypoxemia resolves. Expect to use ABG measurements and pulse oximetry frequently to monitor your patient's condition.

Other nursing interventions include:
- bronchodilator, mucolytic, and antibiotic drug therapy
- coughing, deep breathing, incentive spirometry, and breathing exercises
- positioning for maximum chest expansion
- hydration
- energy conservation and rest.

Respiratory acidosis
Respiratory acidosis develops in conditions in which hypoventilation leads to inadequate carbon dioxide excretion. Emphysema and pneumonia are two such conditions. Emphysema commonly leads to a weakening of respiratory muscles; pneumonia only worsens the problem by increasing secretions and raising the risk of airway obstruction.

Emphysema by itself tends to cause chronic respiratory acidosis, and pneumonia by itself tends to cause acute respiratory acidosis. Together, they may cause or exacerbate either condition.

Confirming the complication

A change in your patient's mental status may be the first sign of respiratory acidosis. He may become confused, combative, even unresponsive. If he's in the late stages of emphysema and losing his ability to compensate for a chronically elevated carbon dioxide level, however, he may not show these signs.

Your patient's ABG measurements provide the definitive diagnosis. He'll have a pH under 7.35, a $Paco_2$ over 45 mm Hg, and a bicarbonate level that's normal or only slightly elevated. His Pao_2 may be normal or decreased. In late-stage emphysema, your patient's $Paco_2$ may top 60 mm Hg. And his bicarbonate level will be elevated, a sign of renal compensation.

Nursing interventions

To prevent respiratory acidosis, focus on improving your patient's ventilation and gas exchange, which will increase carbon dioxide excretion. Reposition your patient frequently, perform chest physiotherapy, and encourage him to cough, breathe deeply, and use an incentive spirometer. Use supplemental low-flow oxygen, and give the prescribed bronchodilator, mucolytic, and antibiotic drugs.

Monitor your patient closely for signs and symptoms of respiratory acidosis. Use pulse oximetry to check his oxygen saturation levels frequently. And evaluate his ABG measurements. Because a rapid rise in $Paco_2$ levels can alter your patient's vital signs, check his pulse, respiratory rate, and blood pressure frequently. Also, note any changes in mental status, such as confusion or lethargy. Your patient may complain of weakness, a dull headache, and increased shortness of breath—symptoms of chronic respiratory acidosis caused by his emphysema.

If your patient develops these signs and symptoms of respiratory acidosis, notify his physician immediately. If your patient's respiratory status is compromised, anticipate endotracheal intubation and mechanical ventilation. Besides maintaining a patent airway,

endotracheal intubation allows easier suctioning of secretions that may be a major cause of the patient's hypoventilation. Mechanical ventilation increases your patient's tidal volume, opens collapsed small airways, and, by providing moist air, may help to loosen secretions.

If your patient doesn't need intubation or mechanical ventilation, continue to assess his respirations carefully. Give low-flow supplemental oxygen and obtain serial ABGs, as ordered. And continue to monitor his oxygen saturation levels by pulse oximetry.

Pneumothorax

A pneumothorax occurs when air gets into the pleural space and separates the visceral and parietal pleural layers. By changing the force of negative pressure in the pleural space, a partial pneumothorax raises the danger of a collapsed lung.

A patient with emphysema faces an increased risk of pneumothorax because air-filled bullae form in the lung. If these bullae rupture, as they tend to do with emphysema, air may escape into the pleural space and cause a tension pneumothorax. Depending on the amount of lung tissue involved, a patient may develop a ventilation-perfusion mismatch and, as a result, acute hypoxemia. A patient with pneumonia may also develop a ventilation-perfusion mismatch and hypoxemia as fluid and exudate fill the alveoli, causing alveolar consolidation.

If a patient has both emphysema and pneumonia and he develops pneumothorax, he's at risk for hypoxemia that could quickly become life threatening.

Confirming the complication

If a patient with emphysema and pneumonia develops a small pneumothorax, he may not even realize it. Generally, however, he'll have sudden, severe shortness of breath and pleuritic chest pain that's referred to his shoulder, arm, face, back, or abdomen. When you examine him, you'll find that chest wall movement on the affected side is decreased or absent. And his trachea will be shifted toward the unaffected side.

A patient with a large pneumothorax may have subcutaneous emphysema. On the affected

GOING HOME

Teaching a patient who has had a pneumothorax

If your patient is being discharged after treatment for a pneumothorax, teach him to avoid complications at home and to reduce his risk of another pneumothorax. Start by finding out who'll be taking care of him at home. Then involve this primary caregiver in all your patient teaching.

Review all your patient's medications. Write down what they're for, when and how the patient should take them, and how much he should take. Tell your patient and his caregiver how to detect drug interactions and emphasize that even over-the-counter drugs can cause reactions. Urge your patient to check with his physician before taking any over-the-counter drugs.

If your patient will be using supplemental oxygen at home, tell him to think of it as one of his drugs and include it in your discussion of his drugs. Review key safety measures for home oxygen use. Explain to your patient and his caregiver that the oxygen concentrator runs on electrical current. Make sure they have a backup oxygen source—such as a portable oxygen tank—in case the electricity goes off. Show your patient how to use a portable tank for outdoor activities.

Teach your patient and his caregiver how to reduce the risk of infection at the chest tube insertion site. Demonstrate how to clean and dress the site, then have the caregiver repeat the demonstration. Review the signs and symptoms of infection, including increased sputum, a change in the color of sputum, increasing dyspnea, and fever. If your patient develops redness, swelling, discharge, or drainage at the site, he should notify his physician. Urge the caregiver to take the patient's temperature at least twice daily and to call the physician if it goes above 99° F (37.2° C).

As necessary, review the importance of coughing, deep breathing, pursed-lip breathing, and the use of an incentive spirometer.

To make sure your patient has all the supplies and equipment he needs at home, refer him to a home health provider. A home health nurse will make sure the patient has an appropriate follow-up schedule for physician visits and laboratory tests. This nurse will also schedule periodic visits to the patient's home.

---

side, breath sounds will be decreased or absent, and you'll hear hyperresonance on percussion. A chest X-ray confirms the diagnosis.

Nursing interventions
A small pneumothorax may need no intervention. Simply assess your patient's condition frequently and make sure he maintains a clear airway. Monitor his oxygen saturation levels and ABG measurments. And check his breath sounds at least once a day.

If your patient has a large pneumothorax or if his signs and symptoms worsen, prepare to assist with the insertion of a chest tube. This patient will probably need oxygen therapy, but keep the flow rate low.

Remember that a patient with emphysema and pneumonia risks a recurrence of pneumothorax because a new infection or a worsening of the emphysema can lead to a ruptured bulla (see *Teaching a patient who has had a pneumothorax*).

Pleural effusion
Normally, only a small amount of fluid exists in the pleural space. When excessive fluid accumulates, the patient has a pleural effusion. Emphysema patients who also have pneumonia run an increased risk of pleural effusion because of the pleural inflammation caused by the invading pathogen.

Confirming the complication
A small amount of excess fluid in the pleural space may cause no specific signs and symptoms. An amount large enough to compress the lung will increase your patient's shortness of breath. You'll find chest expansion reduced on the affected side, and tactile fremitus may be decreased or absent over the affected area. Percussion reveals dullness or flatness over the effusion. On auscultation, breath sounds may be decreased, and you may note bronchial breath sounds, egophony, and whispered pectoriloquy.

Easing the anxiety of chest-tube insertion

Having a chest tube inserted can cause anxiety in any patient. To help your patient through the procedure while minimizing his risk of complications, take the following steps.

Before chest-tube insertion
- Clearly explain the procedure to your patient.
- To reduce the risk of hypoxemia, begin oxygen therapy.
- Because your patient's anxiety may worsen his respiratory status, his physician may prescribe a mild antianxiety drug that won't depress respirations—for example, alprazolam, clorazepate, or hydroxyzine.
- Gather all the necessary equipment, including a thoracotomy tray. Prepare the closed-chest drainage system, so it can be connected immediately after the chest-tube insertion.
- Monitor your patient's vital signs and oxygen saturation levels.

During chest-tube insertion
- Offer emotional support and encouragement to your patient during the procedure. Repeat your earlier explanation of the procedure as it's happening.
- As soon as the tube has been inserted, connect it to the closed-chest drainage system.

- Cover the insertion site with an occlusive bandage.
- Monitor your patient's vital signs and oxygen saturation levels closely for changes.

After chest-tube insertion
- Prepare your patient for a chest X-ray. Make sure he understands that this routine procedure is used to confirm the proper placement of the chest tube.
- Tell your patient that you'll be checking his drainage system frequently to make sure the connections are tight and that the system is working properly.
- Monitor your patient's vital signs closely. Note any changes in his respiratory rate or breath sounds because they could indicate hypoxemia. Use pulse oximetry or arterial blood gas measurements to check his oxygen saturation levels.
- Immediately report to the physician any subcutaneous emphysema, respiratory distress, or cyanosis.
- Keep the dressing over the insertion site dry and intact.
- Ask your patient if the insertion site is painful. If it is, give him an analgesic, as prescribed.

A chest X-ray confirms the effusion. A physician also may perform a thoracentesis to evaluate the fluid, identify the underlying cause, and determine if a chest tube is necessary.

Nursing interventions

If your patient begins to complain of increasing shortness of breath, notify his physician immediately. It may be a sign that an effusion is growing. Monitor your patient's respiratory function closely and check his oxygen saturation levels by pulse oximetry. Also, monitor his ABG measurements.

If a pleural effusion is large or your patient experiences considerable respiratory distress, anticipate thoracentesis or chest-tube insertion to drain the excess fluid (see *Easing the anxiety of chest-tube insertion*). If your patient is

scheduled for thoracentesis, give him an analgesic, as prescribed, to alleviate the pain of the procedure. If a chest tube is inserted, monitor and record the amount of drainage regularly. Provide supplemental low-flow oxygen therapy, as needed. Because pneumonia usually is the underlying cause of the pleural effusion, continue to administer antibiotic therapy, as prescribed.

Respiratory failure

As discussed, emphysema impairs gas exchange by reducing the amount of effective alveolocapillary membrane. Pneumonia worsens this impairment by filling alveoli with fluids and exudate. If these disorders severely limit gas exchange, the patient may develop respiratory failure.

Confirming the complication

A physician uses ABG measurements to confirm respiratory failure. Usually, a patient is considered to be in respiratory failure when his PaO_2 drops below 50 mm Hg and his $PaCO_2$ exceeds 45 mm Hg. However, a patient with emphysema may have chronically elevated $PaCO_2$ levels. So look for significant increases in his baseline level. Other signs and symptoms depend on the extent of tissue hypoxia. As hypoxia increases, mental status changes such as restlessness, anxiety, and confusion may worsen. Early in respiratory failure, your patient's blood pressure may be elevated; later, it will drop. The patient also may have tachycardia and other arrhythmias. He may complain of shortness of breath and appear diaphoretic. His skin may be pale, bluish, or flushed. And he may use his accessory muscles to breathe.

Nursing interventions

Respiratory failure requires immediate action. You must maintain your patient's airway and ventilation to prevent cardiac and respiratory arrest.

RAPID RESPONSE ▶ If your patient is in respiratory failure, take these steps:

- Place him in an upright position to maximize chest expansion and maintain a patent airway.
- Immediately obtain ABG measurements to verify pulse oximetry values. Continuously monitor your patient's oxygen saturation levels using pulse oximetry.
- Make sure suction equipment and emergency equipment are readily available.
- Begin cardiac monitoring and evaluate the ECG for changes in heart rate and rhythm and for ischemic changes.
- Monitor your patient's vital signs for evidence of impending cardiac arrest, including hypotension, decreasing heart and respiratory rates, and decreasing respiratory effort.
- Anticipate the insertion of a pulmonary artery catheter to evaluate your patient's hemodynamic status directly.
- Administer supplemental oxygen if it's not already in use. If it is, increase the flow rate or switch to a Venturi mask, as indicated.

- If supplemental oxygen therapy can't maintain adequate PaO_2 levels, provide respiratory assistance with a manual resuscitation bag and oxygen and prepare for endotracheal intubation and mechanical ventilation.
- Repeat ABG measurements, as ordered.
- As prescribed, give an antibiotic for the pneumonia and a bronchodilator and other drugs to open your patient's bronchioles and promote gas exchange. Evaluate your patient's response to all drugs. ◄

Emphysema and hypertension

Hypertension commonly develops with emphysema, particularly in people who smoke. Nicotine, a potent vasoconstrictor, further impairs gas exchange when it's combined with emphysema. Also, the vasoconstriction of nicotine increases vascular resistance, which may impair pulmonary perfusion and increase the heart's workload. The combination of emphysema and hypertension is especially dangerous because it affects both the respiratory and cardiovascular systems.

Pathophysiology

The impaired gas exchange caused by emphysema leads to hypoxemia and increases the patient's work of breathing. Hypertension complicates the patient's condition by increasing the heart's workload and raising the heart's need for oxygen, possibly beyond the amount that the diseased lungs can provide.

The increased peripheral resistance of hypertension may cause left ventricular failure that leads to pulmonary edema, further compromising gas exchange. If pulmonary vasoconstriction develops, it'll raise the workload on the right side of the heart. Over time, as the left ventricle hypertrophies, the risk of myocardial infarction increases.

Adapting nursing care

As you would with any emphysema patient, take action to promote gas exchange and increase the efficiency of breathing. Maintain an oxygen saturation level of 90% or more by giving supplemental oxygen. Use pulse oximetry to monitor the oxygen saturation levels. Place the patient in an upright position to maximize lung expansion. Encourage him to cough, breathe deeply, and use the incentive spirometer. Perform chest physiotherapy, as ordered, and assess his respiratory status regularly to detect developing problems. Give prescribed medications, such as a bronchodilator and mucolytic.

Monitor your patient's blood pressure closely and give prescribed antihypertensive drugs to keep it within the target range. Be alert for interactions between antihypertensive drugs and the bronchodilators and corticosteroids used to treat emphysema (see *Drugs for emphysema and hypertension: Dangerous interactions*).

Because your patient with emphysema and hypertension is at increased risk for cardiac ischemia, obtain a baseline ECG. If you note ischemic changes on later ECGs, be prepared to start continuous cardiac monitoring. Assess your patient's heart rate and heart sounds regularly. Note the presence of S_3 or S_4 heart sounds because they may be a sign of heart failure.

Sometimes, a treatment for one disorder can negatively affect the other disorder or the patient's overall condition. Nutrition is a case in point. Typically, patients with hypertension must limit their sodium intake. But the resulting bland-tasting food may reduce the patient's desire to eat, further impairing a nutritional status already impaired by the effects of emphysema. To help correct this problem, suggest ways to add flavor to foods without adding sodium. Work with a dietitian, the patient, and his family to develop a meal plan that meets the patient's nutritional needs and the requirements of his therapy.

Activity is another example. For the hypertensive patient, exercise provides an effective way to reduce blood pressure. But exercise can exacerbate emphysema. To help deal with this problem, work with a physical therapist and an occupational therapist to develop an exercise program that can lower your patient's

blood pressure without causing overexertion. Encourage your patient to use supplemental oxygen and assistive devices during any activity. And monitor your patient's oxygen saturation levels for changes that suggest developing hypoxemia.

Smoking cessation may cause a similar problem. Of course, you'll want to encourage your patient to quit smoking. But if he uses a nicotine patch as an aid to quitting, it could adversely affect his blood pressure by causing peripheral vasoconstriction. If he decides to use a smoking cessation aid that contains nicotine, tell him to have his blood pressure monitored closely.

Clearly, education is an extremely important aspect of nursing care for your patient with emphysema and hypertension. Reinforce all aspects of his treatment program, including information on the drugs he needs to take. Specifically, review adverse effects and drug interactions. Also, review energy-conservation measures, diet restrictions, lifestyle modifications, and the planned exercise program. Stress the need for compliance and follow-up to minimize the risk of complications.

Complications

Common complications for patients with emphysema and hypertension include cardiomyopathy and arrhythmias.

Cardiomyopathy

In cardiomyopathy, the right or left ventricle enlarges over time in an attempt to overcome its own impaired pumping action and meet the body's need for oxygenated blood. Eventually, one of the ventricles fails. If the right ventricle fails, not enough blood will reach the left ventricle and the systemic circulation. The patient will then develop shock. If the left ventricle fails, the right ventricle usually fails as well.

Hypertension, which increases the left ventricle's workload as it pumps against increased systemic vascular resistance, may cause cardiomyopathy. And the pulmonary hypertension that occurs with emphysema contributes to the progression of cardiomyopathy by damaging the right ventricle. The increased workload of the right ventricle as it pumps against increased

DRUG ALERT

Drugs for emphysema and hypertension: Dangerous interactions

Emphysema drugs	Antihypertensives	Adverse effects	Nursing actions
• Theophylline and its salts (aminophylline, oxtriphylline, theophylline, sodium glycinate)	• Beta blockers (atenolol, metoprolol, nadolol, propranolol)	• Beta blocker may reduce theophylline's bronchodilating effect, causing bronchospasm. • Beta blocker may slow rate at which theophylline is metabolized, causing toxic serum levels.	• Expect to administer a cardioselective beta blocker (such as atenolol or metoprolol) to minimize risk of bronchospasm. • Monitor serum theophylline levels and be alert for signs and symptoms of toxicity, such as tachycardia and restlessness. • Auscultate breath sounds frequently and be alert for signs of bronchospasm, such as wheezing.
• Inhaled beta$_2$-agonist bronchodilators (albuterol, metaproterenol)	• Beta blockers (atenolol, metoprolol, nadolol, propranolol)	• Inhaled beta$_2$-agonist may reduce antihypertensive effect of beta blocker. • Inhaled beta$_2$-agonist may increase vagal tone and cause sinus bradycardia.	• Administer drugs several hours apart to reduce risk of adverse effects. • Monitor blood pressure frequently, checking for reduced response to antihypertensive. • Monitor heart rate frequently and be alert for dangerous slowing.
• Systemic corticosteroids (prednisone, methylprednisolone)	• All classes of antihypertensives	• Systemic corticosteroid may cause sodium retention and antagonize therapeutic effect of antihypertensive.	• Monitor blood pressure frequently. If it's elevated, expect to increase antihypertensive dose. • Assess patient for signs of fluid retention, such as ankle swelling and weight gain. • Restrict sodium and fluid intake, as appropriate.
	• Potassium-depleting diuretics (chlorothiazide, furosemide)	• Both drugs increase potassium excretion and may result in severe hypokalemia.	• Monitor serum potassium levels. • Monitor patient for signs and symptoms of hypokalemia, such as muscle weakness. • Administer prescribed potassium replacement agents.

pulmonary vascular resistance causes the right ventricle to fail and blood to back up into the peripheral venous system. Over time, right and left ventricular failure lead to decreased cardiac output and peripheral perfusion.

Confirming the complication

Signs and symptoms of cardiomyopathy vary depending on which ventricle is affected. In left ventricular cardiomyopathy, your patient may experience dyspnea when he exerts himself that eventually progresses to dyspnea when he's at rest. Emphysema can make the dyspnea even worse. You also may note your patient coughing and becoming easily fatigued. In right ventricular cardiomyopathy, you may detect jugular vein distention, pitting edema of dependent body parts, an enlarged liver, and tachycardia.

A physician may order several tests to help confirm the diagnosis of cardiomyopathy, including a chest X-ray, an echocardiogram, and an ECG. The chest X-ray will show an enlarged heart. The echocardiogram will reveal dilation and poor contraction of the left ventricle. And the ECG will show signs of left ventricular hypertrophy. Also, to evaluate the patient's cardiac filling pressures and pulmonary artery pressures, a physician may insert a cardiac catheter into the right side of the heart.

Nursing interventions

A patient with emphysema, hypertension, and cardiomyopathy requires close monitoring and frequent attention to help decrease his myocardial workload. If your patient needs complete or partial bed rest to decrease myocardial oxygen demand, make sure he's in an upright position that maximizes lung expansion. Reposition him frequently. Give supplemental oxygen and monitor his oxygen saturation levels with pulse oximetry and ABG measurements, as indicated.

Your patient may have a low tolerance for activity, so plan light activity and plenty of rest periods. Increase his activity level gradually. Obtain a physical therapy and occupational therapy consult to create a plan for maintaining your patient's activity levels after he's discharged.

Use cardiac monitoring to check for ischemic changes from increasing heart failure. Anticipate the insertion of a pulmonary artery catheter to evaluate your patient's hemodynamic status directly. Closely monitor his vital signs and LOC. Also, assess him for jugular vein distention and check his lungs for pulmonary congestion.

If your patient is receiving diuretic therapy, closely assess his fluid balance. Monitor his intake, output, and weight daily. And monitor his serum electrolyte levels and renal function test results. Check for hypokalemia and anticipate the need for potassium supplements.

If your patient has left ventricular failure and you need to restrict his fluids, remember that doing so can complicate his emphysema. Usually, emphysema patients need extra fluids to help loosen pulmonary secretions. To help avoid complications from fluid restrictions, encourage your patient to cough frequently, breathe deeply, and use the incentive spirometer. Give an oral mucolytic drug and a bronchodilator by nebulizer, as prescribed. Assess your patient closely after giving the bronchodilator because tachycardia, a common adverse effect,

can increase myocardial oxygen demand, worsening his condition. Give a vasodilator, as prescribed, to improve cardiac output and reduce afterload. Evaluate your patient's response.

If your patient has right ventricular failure, administer fluids as prescribed to maintain adequate cardiac output.

Usually, patients with cardiomyopathy who fail to respond to therapy are considered candidates for a heart transplant. However, patients with emphysema and hypertension typically don't qualify. Offer support to your patient and his family. Give them time to ask questions and expect them to begin grieving.

Arrhythmias

Arrhythmias, disruptions in the heart rate or rhythm, alter cardiac output and coronary artery perfusion, thus promoting myocardial ischemia. Emphysema patients are at increased risk because arrhythmias can be triggered by hypoxemia. And patients with hypertension are at increased risk because hypertension increases the myocardial workload and myocardial oxygen demand. Arrhythmias also may develop when antihypertensive drugs and bronchodilators are used together.

Confirming the complication

You may be able to feel an arrhythmia when taking your patient's pulse or hear one when you auscultate his chest. Arrhythmias are confirmed by an ECG.

Nursing interventions

The most important interventions are those intended to prevent arrhythmias, including controlling blood pressure and promoting ventilation and gas exchange. If your patient develops an arrhythmia, administer the prescribed antiarrhythmic drugs and begin continuous cardiac monitoring.

Monitor your patient's blood pressure and ECG to evaluate the effectiveness of therapy. Give supplemental oxygen as needed and monitor oxygen saturation levels using pulse oximetry and ABG measurements, as ordered. Urge your patient to tell you if he develops shortness of breath, chest pain, or palpitations. If your patient's arrhythmia doesn't respond to medication or his hemodynamic status declines, anticipate the need for cardioversion, defibrillation, or the application of an external pacemaker.

Before discharge, review all aspects of your patient's therapy, including any new medications. Reinforce all previous instructions about energy-conservation techniques, activity and exercise, respiratory care measures, diet, and lifestyle modifications. Remind your patient about the importance of compliance and follow-up. If appropriate, obtain a referral for home care visits to verify his compliance.

Emphysema and cirrhosis

Cirrhosis is a chronic degenerative liver disease. Initially, the liver enlarges because of changes to its parenchymatous cells. As the disease progresses, fibrosis spreads, and eventually the liver becomes small, hard, and nodular. Patients with emphysema and cirrhosis face an increased risk of complications linked to impaired gas exchange.

Pathophysiology

Patients with cirrhosis may develop a condition called hepatopulmonary syndrome—a condition characterized by low pulmonary vascular tone, a poor or absent hypoxic pressor response, a ventilation-perfusion mismatch, and mild to moderate hypoxemia. As the cirrhosis worsens, intrapulmonary shunting becomes severe, causing acute respiratory failure.

In a patient with emphysema and cirrhosis, the danger is great: his emphysema reduces gas exchange and increases the work of breathing, and his cirrhosis causes intrapulmonary shunting that leads to further hypoxemia.

To make matters worse, the progressive liver failure associated with cirrhosis leads to ascites, which causes even more trouble for the patient with emphysema. As ascites increases, it exerts more and more pressure on the diaphragm, further limiting chest expansion and gas exchange. The patient's dyspnea becomes worse than ever.

Adapting nursing care

Besides performing nursing care for emphysema, you'll need to take steps to prevent hypoxemia and minimize the effects of cirrhosis. For example, you'll need to ensure that your patient with cirrhosis limits his sodium and protein intake to help prevent fluid buildup, particularly in the peritoneum. Keep in mind that this treatment may work against the goals of emphysema therapy, which include maintaining a high-calorie diet. To help keep foods as appetizing as possible, work with the dietitian, the patient, and the patient's family to find ways to add flavor without adding excess protein and sodium. Offer smaller, more frequent meals.

If sodium and protein restriction doesn't control your patient's ascites, anticipate giving a diuretic, such as chlorothiazide or furosemide. Monitor your patient for signs and symptoms of electrolyte imbalances and obtain serum electrolyte levels. Give potassium supplements, as prescribed.

If ascites is severe and interferes with the patient's respiratory function, prepare him for paracentesis. During this procedure, the fluid, which contains large amounts of protein and electrolytes, will be removed over 30 to 90 minutes to prevent hypotension and syncope. Monitor your patient's serum electrolyte levels and watch for signs of fluid volume deficit caused by the removal of too much fluid. Then, monitor your patient's intake, output, and weight daily. Check abdominal girth at least every 8 hours. Keep in mind that fluid probably will accumulate again, and the patient may need paracentesis at regular intervals.

Monitor your patient's neurologic status closely. Changes in his LOC can result from hypoxemia or hepatic encephalopathy. To help determine the cause, check oxygen saturation and serum ammonia levels. If your patient develops hepatic encephalopathy, he'll probably require a protein restriction and lactulose or neomycin to help decrease serum ammonia levels.

The only treatment that can help most patients with advanced cirrhosis is a liver transplant.

PATHOPHYSIOLOGY

How emphysema and cirrhosis lead to right ventricular heart failure

This flowchart shows you at a glance how right ventricular heart failure can develop in a patient with emphysema and cirrhosis.

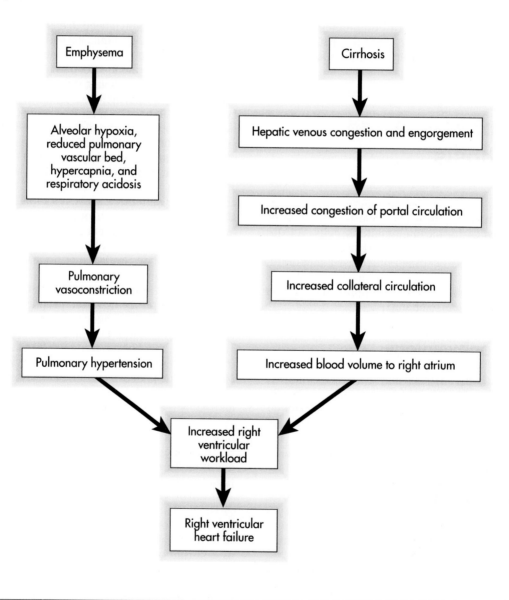

Unfortunately, patients with emphysema aren't considered good candidates for a liver transplant. For such a patient, provide emotional support and obtain a referral for home visits, as appropriate.

Complications

Patients with emphysema and cirrhosis are at risk for acute respiratory failure and other complications related to impaired gas exchange and fluid overload. But the most common complication for these patients is right ventricular heart failure.

Right ventricular heart failure

Patients with emphysema and cirrhosis have an increased risk of right ventricular heart failure because hypoxemia combines with the effects of cirrhosis on the heart. Cirrhosis obstructs blood flow, resulting in the formation of collateral circulation that returns more blood than normal to the right atrium, increasing its workload and thus raising the risk of heart failure. This risk is further increased by the pulmonary hypertension of emphysema, which adds to the workload of the right ventricle (see *How emphysema and cirrhosis lead to right ventricular heart failure*).

Confirming the complication

The patient may have distended neck veins, pitting edema in dependent body parts, tachycardia, dyspnea, and cyanosis. He may also be lethargic and use his accessory muscles during respirations.

An echocardiogram can confirm right ventricular heart failure by showing an enlarged, poorly functioning heart. An ECG and a chest X-ray can reveal hypertrophy of the right ventricle, common in right ventricular heart failure.

Nursing interventions

Nursing care focuses on balancing oxygen supply and demand while decreasing the heart's workload by eliminating excess fluid. Limit your patient's sodium, protein, and fluid intake to minimize fluid retention. But remember that fluid restrictions can thicken pulmonary secretions caused by emphysema.

Monitor your patient's oxygen saturation levels closely with pulse oximetry and ABG measurements. Give supplemental oxygen as needed, but use a low flow rate to avoid depressing his respiratory drive. If possible, have him sit upright to maximize lung expansion. Watch closely for signs of respiratory failure, such as increased lethargy, confusion, and ABG value changes.

Give the prescribed diuretic and bronchodilator to reduce systemic and pulmonary vascular resistance and improve cardiac contractility. Because of your patient's liver failure, the physician may prescribe reduced dosages of these drugs. Observe the patient closely for signs of drug toxicity.

Encourage your patient to cough, breathe deeply, and use his incentive spirometer frequently. Monitor him often and notify his physician if his condition changes significantly.

Suggested readings

Agusti AG, Roca J, Rodriguez-Roisin R. Mechanisms of gas exchange impairment in patients with liver cirrhosis. *Clin Chest Med.* 1996;17(1):49-66.

Anonymous. Standards for the diagnosis and care of patients with chronic obstructive pulmonary disease. American Thoracic Society. *Am J Respir Crit Care Med.* 1995;152(5Pt2):S77-S121.

Lewis S, Collier I, Heitkemper M. *Medical-surgical nursing: assessment and management of clinical problems.* 4th ed. St Louis, Mo: Mosby–Year Book, Inc; 1996.

Pierce LNB. *Guide to mechanical ventilation and intensive respiratory care.* Philadelphia, Pa: WB Saunders Co; 1995.

Raffy O, Sleiman C, Vachiery F, et al. Refractory hypoxemia during liver cirrhosis: hepatopulmonary syndrome or primary pulmonary syndrome. *Am J Respir Crit Care Med.* 1996; 153(3):1169-1171.

Szekely LA, Oelberg DA, Wright C, et al. Preoperative predictors of operative morbidity and mortality in COPD patients undergoing bilateral lung volume reduction surgery. *Chest.* 1997;111(3):550-558.

Thompson JM, McFarland GK, Hirsch JE, Tucker SM: *Mosby's clinical nursing.* 4th ed. St Louis, Mo: Mosby–Year Book, Inc; 1996.

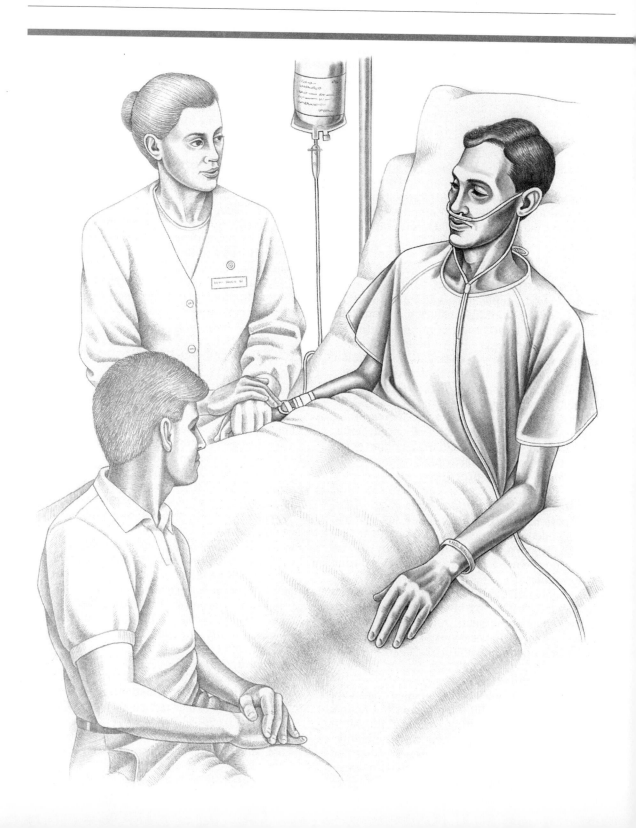

Pneumonia

An inflammatory disorder, pneumonia is the sixth most common cause of death in the United States and the leading cause of infection-related death.

Because pneumonia compromises the respiratory system, which is responsible for exchanging oxygen and carbon dioxide and regulating acid-base balance, it affects all other body systems. And changes in other body systems can affect the respiratory system's ability to provide adequate oxygenation.

Pneumonia commonly coexists with other serious disorders, such as chronic obstructive pulmonary disease (COPD), heart failure, and human immunodeficiency virus (HIV) infection.

A view of the gas-exchange airways

Collectively referred to as the acini, the gas-exchange airways include the respiratory bronchioles, alveolar ducts, and alveoli. Air enters through the terminal bronchiole, passes into the respiratory bronchioles, continues through the alveolar ducts, and eventually ends up in the alveoli. Through the thin walls of the alveoli, carbon dioxide and oxygen diffuse, allowing gas exchange to occur.

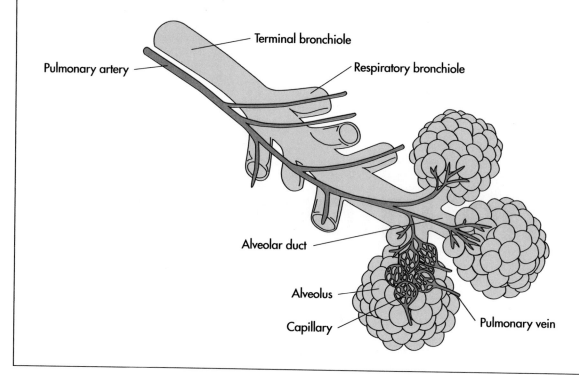

When pneumonia appears with one of these disorders, the patient can develop such serious complications as adult respiratory distress syndrome (ARDS), pulmonary edema, pleural effusion, respiratory failure, and HIV wasting syndrome.

Anatomy and physiology review

The respiratory system consists of the conducting airways (nose, mouth, nasopharynx, oropharynx, pharynx, larynx, trachea, and bronchi), gas-exchange airways (respiratory bronchioles, alveolar ducts, and alveoli), and the lungs. Chapter 7 gives a complete review of these structures.

Bronchi to alveoli

The right and left main bronchi branch from the trachea at the carina. The right bronchus is shorter, wider, and more vertically positioned than the left, making it more susceptible to aspiration of foreign bodies. The main bronchi further divide into two branches on the left and three on the right, with each branch supplying one lobe of the lungs. These branches subdivide into terminal bronchioles and then into small respiratory bronchioles. The main bronchi are made up of cartilage, smooth muscle, and epithelium. As they progressively divide into smaller structures, first cartilage then smooth muscle disappears. The smallest bronchioles contain only a single layer of epithelium.

The bronchial arteries that branch from the thoracic aorta and the intercostal arteries supply blood to the bronchi. Most of the blood is returned to the heart by the pulmonary veins.

The respiratory bronchioles end in alveolar ducts, which lead to alveolar sacs containing numerous alveoli. The alveoli are the site of gas exchange, the primary function of the respiratory system (see *A view of the gas-exchange airways*).

The thin alveolar walls contain two types of epithelial cells. The more abundant type I cells are thin, flat, and squamous. Across these cells, gas exchange occurs. Type II cells secrete surfactant, which coats the alveoli and facilitates gas exchange by decreasing surface tension and preventing the collapse of the alveoli. Both cell types—along with a minute interstitial space, capillary basement membrane, and endothelial cells in the capillary wall—make up the respiratory membrane that separates the alveoli and capillaries.

Gas exchange

In the lungs, gas exchange occurs by diffusion: Molecules of oxygen and carbon dioxide move between the alveoli and the capillaries, depending on the pressure of the gases. Because the partial pressure of arterial oxygen (PaO_2) is lower in the capillaries than in the alveoli, oxygen moves from the alveoli into the capillaries. And because the partial pressure of arterial carbon dioxide ($PaCO_2$) is lower in the alveoli than in the capillaries, carbon dioxide moves from the capillaries into the alveoli.

As long as the alveolocapillary membrane remains intact, oxygen and carbon dioxide move easily across it. After oxygen enters the capillary, it attaches itself to hemoglobin in the red blood cells (RBCs). Oxygen-laden RBCs then circulate to the tissues, where the oxygen diffuses across cell membranes to nourish the tissues. After carbon dioxide enters the alveoli, it's carried upward through the airways and exhaled (see *Gas exchange: How it works*, page 260).

For proper gas exchange to occur, two important processes must take place: ventilation and perfusion.

Ventilation

Ventilation, the process by which air is delivered to the terminal bronchioles and alveoli, consists of two phases: inspiration and expiration. Inspiration, the active phase, is accomplished by the contraction and downward movement of the diaphragm. The negative pressure that's created draws air in, causing the lungs to expand and fill with air. Usually, expiration is passive: As the muscles relax, air is expelled from the lungs and airways. However, expiration can be forced if a person uses his accessory muscles of respiration.

The central nervous system, specifically the medulla and pons, controls the rate and rhythm of respirations. Within the medulla lie the inspiratory and expiratory centers. The inspiratory center ensures spontaneous rhythmicity of inspiration; the expiratory center inhibits inspiration and triggers forced expiration during heavy breathing.

Within the pons lie the pneumotaxic and apneustic centers. The pneumotaxic center can inhibit the inspiratory center and thus control the rate and depth of inspiration. Stimulation of the pneumotaxic center produces rapid shallow inspirations, and suppression of this center produces the opposite effect. The role of the apneustic center isn't clear, but the center seems to cause prolonged inspiration.

Central and peripheral chemoreceptors also regulate ventilation. Changes in levels of carbon dioxide and hydrogen ions stimulate an area near the medulla. This, in turn, stimulates the inspiratory center to change the rate of inspiration. Peripheral chemoreceptors located in the aortic arch and carotid bodies respond to drops in oxygen levels by stimulating inspiration. They also respond to other factors, such as drops in blood pH and rises in temperature.

Perfusion

Perfusion is the process by which blood is delivered to the capillaries. Unoxygenated blood returns from the body tissues to the right atrium. Then it flows into the right ventricle, the

ANATOMY REVIEW

Gas exchange: How it works

Gases move from an area of higher concentration to an area of lower concentration. In the alveoli, the pressure of oxygen is higher than in the capillaries. Therefore, oxygen moves from the alveoli into the pulmonary capillaries, and eventually through the pulmonary vein back to the heart and then to the tissues. The pressure of carbon dioxide is higher in the capillaries than in the alveoli. Therefore, carbon dioxide moves from the pulmonary capillaries into the alveoli and is exhaled.

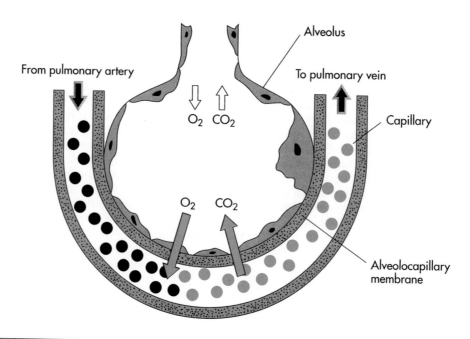

main pulmonary arteries, and progressively smaller blood vessels until it reaches the capillaries. After gas exchange occurs, the blood flows through progressively larger vessels and into the pulmonary veins. The left atrium receives this oxygenated blood from the pulmonary veins.

Normally, the pulmonary vasculature receives at least 5 liters of blood a minute. Anything that impedes this blood flow will reduce perfusion. Such impediments include increased blood viscosity (which occurs with increased hematocrit), increased pulmonary vascular resistance (which occurs with pulmonary disease), and reduced cardiac output (which occurs with heart failure). What's more, any mechanical obstruction, such as a pulmonary embolism, can reduce or stop blood flow to a specific area in the pulmonary vasculature. When this happens, blood can't receive oxygen molecules across the alveolocapillary membrane.

Ventilation-perfusion matching

Gravity pulls more unoxygenated blood to the lower and middle lung lobes than to the upper lobes, where most of the oxygen flows. As a result, ventilation and perfusion aren't equally matched throughout the lungs. In areas where perfusion and ventilation are well matched, gas exchange is more efficient. In areas where ventilation and perfusion aren't well matched, gas exchange is less efficient.

Pathophysiology

An inflammatory disorder, pneumonia is characterized by alveolitis and the accumulation of exudate and fluid, which leads to impaired gas exchange.

The lung is the largest epithelial surface of the body exposed to the external environment, and the airways are repeatedly subjected to airborne particles and pathogens during normal respiration. Generally, pathogens enter the lungs because they are directly inhaled, they are aspirated in secretions from the upper airways, or they spread from other sites of infection. The most common route is aspiration of secretions. For pneumonia to develop in the lower respiratory tract, the body must have a defect in the respiratory defense system, an overwhelming exposure to an organism, or exposure to a virulent organism.

Normally, pathogens deposited on the epithelium of the distal nasal surface are removed by sneezing. Those on the proximal ciliated surfaces are swept into the mucous lining to be swallowed or expectorated. The cough reflex and closure of the glottis protect the normally sterile lower respiratory tract. Pathogens deposited on the tracheobronchial surface are swept by ciliary motion toward the oropharynx. Pathogens that bypass the airway defenses and reach the alveolar surface are cleared by phagocytic cells and humoral factors.

Sources of pathogens

Healthy people may have common pulmonary pathogens—such as *Streptococcus pneumoniae*, *Streptococcus pyogenes*, *Mycoplasma pneumoniae*, and *Hemophilus influenzae*—in the nasopharynx. And anaerobic pulmonary pathogens—such as *Porphyromonas gingivalis*, *Prevotella melaninogenica*, *Fusobacterium*, and anaerobic streptococci—may reside in the gingival crevices and dental plaque. Other sources of infection include contaminated respiratory equipment, contaminated food or water, and the contaminated hands of health care workers.

In less than 2% of people, aerobic gram-negative bacilli colonize the oropharyngeal mucosa. Such colonization develops more commonly in people who are hospitalized; in those who have a severe underlying illness, a worsening debility, alcoholism, or diabetes mellitus; and in the elderly. Aerobic gram-negative bacilli can also colonize in a person's stomach if gastric pH increases. The pathogens may then be transferred to the respiratory tract during nasogastric (NG) intubation or by translocation.

About 50% of adults without physical problems aspirate oropharyngeal secretions into the lower respiratory tract during sleep. Also, such aspiration occurs frequently and is more severe in patients whose consciousness is impaired by substance abuse, seizures, a stroke, or general anesthesia. Plus, aspiration can result from mechanical impediments, such as NG and endotracheal (ET) tubes, neurologic dysfunction, and swallowing disorders. If the volume of aspirated material is large, if the material contains virulent flora or foreign bodies, or if the pathogens aren't held in check by the usual defense mechanisms, pneumonia may develop.

Sequence of events

If the patient's defense mechanisms are impaired, the invading pathogen will multiply when it reaches the distal airways, releasing damaging toxins. This stimulates a full-scale inflammatory and immune response, triggering the release of exudate and inflammatory cells. White blood cells (WBCs) attempt to phagocytize the organisms, releasing enzymes and immunologic mediators. These actions further increase the inflammation and trigger an antigen-antibody reaction. The pathogen releases endotoxins, damaging the bronchial mucous membranes and alveolocapillary membranes. This results in edema and inflammation, causing the acini and terminal bronchioles to fill with exudate and debris. As a portion of the lung fills with exudate and inflammatory cells, consolidation develops. Reduced lung volume, altered ventilation, and decreased perfusion lead to physiologic changes. Although the capillary blood flow continues normally, ventilation to the alveoli decreases because of the inflammation and exudate. The result: a ventilation-perfusion mismatch and impaired gas exchange. Further consolidation worsens the condition (see *How pneumonia develops*, page 262).

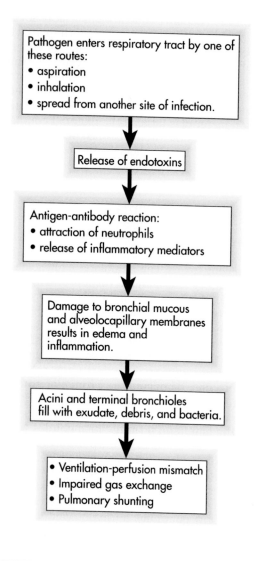

How pneumonia develops

Pneumonia begins when a pathogen enters the respiratory tract of a person with impaired defenses. This triggers a sequence of events that leads to a ventilation-perfusion mismatch, impaired gas exchange, and pulmonary shunting. The flowchart highlights this sequence.

Pathogen enters respiratory tract by one of these routes:
• aspiration
• inhalation
• spread from another site of infection.

↓

Release of endotoxins

↓

Antigen-antibody reaction:
• attraction of neutrophils
• release of inflammatory mediators

↓

Damage to bronchial mucous and alveolocapillary membranes results in edema and inflammation.

↓

Acini and terminal bronchioles fill with exudate, debris, and bacteria.

↓

• Ventilation-perfusion mismatch
• Impaired gas exchange
• Pulmonary shunting

Types of pneumonia

Pneumonia can be caused by many microorganisms, including bacteria, viruses, fungi, and parasites. Pneumonias are classified primarily by the microorganism. However, bacterial pneumonia, by far the most common type, is further classified as community acquired or hospital acquired (nosocomial). (Some community-acquired pneumonias stem from viral infections). Most patients who develop community-acquired pneumonia have a preexisting condition or impaired defense mechanisms.

More than 70% of all pneumonia cases result from *S. pneumoniae*. The second most common cause of community-acquired pneumonia is *M. pneumoniae*. Patients with other health problems, such as COPD or alcoholism, may develop community-acquired pneumonia from *Staphylococcus aureus* or *Klebsiella pneumoniae*.

Gram-negative bacteria—such as *Escherichia coli*, *K. pneumoniae*, and *Pseudomonas aeruginosa*—most frequently cause nosocomial pneumonia. These organisms cause more serious infections and may lead to lung necrosis, abscess, or empyema.

Influenza viruses usually cause viral pneumonia. Pneumonia also may be caused by fungi and *Legionella* species. Fungal pneumonia, which most commonly occurs in immunosuppressed people, is caused by *Candida*, *Mucor*, and *Aspergillus*. Histoplasmosis and coccidioidomycosis can infect both immunosuppressed and healthy people. Infections may occur in outbreaks or sporadically.

Parasitic pneumonias can be caused by protozoans, nematodes, and platyhelminths. The most common organism is *Pneumocystis carinii* (see *Pneumonia: Common causes*).

Assessment findings

Community-acquired pneumonia occurs as two distinct syndromes: typical and atypical. The typical syndrome, usually caused by *S. pneumoniae*, produces these signs and symptoms:
• sudden fever
• cough with purulent sputum
• decreased breath sounds
• crackles and wheezes

- signs of pulmonary consolidation, such as dullness, increased fremitus, egophony, and bronchial breath sounds
- pleuritic chest pain.

The atypical syndrome can result from bacterial pneumonia (especially in elderly, immunosuppressed, and chronically ill patients) or viral pneumonia. It develops more gradually. The patient may have a dry cough, fever, and chills. He also may experience a headache, fatigue, myalgias, sore throat, nausea, vomiting, and diarrhea.

Nosocomial pneumonia doesn't produce typical signs and symptoms. The patient may be hospitalized for a preexisting pulmonary disease that causes a fever and productive cough, or he may already have a systemic infection (see *Distinguishing among types of pneumonia,* page 264).

Diagnostic tests

No standard test exists for diagnosing pneumonia. Usually, the diagnosis is based on signs and symptoms, chest X-rays, sputum culture and sensitivity results, sputum Gram's stain, and blood tests.

Chest X-ray
A chest X-ray can confirm a diagnosis of pneumonia by showing the presence and location of pulmonary infiltrates. It can also show the extent of an infection, pleural involvement, pulmonary cavitation, and hilar lymphadenopathy.

Sputum culture and Gram's stain
A sputum culture and Gram's stain can rule out certain pathogens as the cause of pneumonia, and they can show sensitivity and resistance to certain antibiotics. If a sputum culture doesn't identify the pathogen, the physician may assume the pneumonia is viral.

Sputum cultures and Gram's stains are commonly contaminated with microorganisms from the upper respiratory tract and may be inconclusive. Pulmonary secretions obtained by protected-brush bronchoscopic techniques, transtracheal aspiration, and transthoracic lung puncture provide more accurate diagnostic

---

Pneumonia: Common causes

Pneumonia may result from bacteria, viruses, fungi, or parasites. The following pathogens are among the common causes of pneumonia.

Community-acquired bacterial pneumonia
- *Streptococcus pneumoniae*
- *Mycoplasma pneumoniae*
- *Staphylococcus aureus*
- *Hemophilus influenzae*
- *Legionella pneumophila*

Nosocomial bacterial pneumonia
- *Escherichia coli*
- *Klebsiella pneumoniae*
- *Pseudomonas aeruginosa*

Viral pneumonia
- Cytomegalovirus
- Varicella zoster

Fungal pneumonia
- *Candida albicans*
- *Aspergillus fumigatus*
- *Cryptococcus*

Parasitic pneumonia
- *Pneumocystis carinii*

---

information than sputum specimens. However, these invasive procedures aren't usually performed unless a diagnosis can't be made any other way.

If the patient has a pleural effusion, thoracentesis may be performed to obtain a specimen to identify the microorganism.

Blood studies
If the physician suspects bacteremia, blood cultures can be performed to diagnose pneumonia-causing organisms, such as *S. aureus.* Laboratory tests, including a complete blood count (CBC) and arterial blood gas (ABG) analysis, also may help. The CBC may reveal an elevated WBC count, indicating that the patient has an infection, but it won't, of course, help pinpoint its location. And a debilitated or

---

Distinguishing among types of pneumonia

Type of pneumonia	Assessment findings	Diagnostic findings
Bacterial	• Fever, chills, and diaphoresis • Cough with purulent sputum • Pleuritic chest pain • Crackles and wheezes • Egophony and bronchophony over consolidation • Hemoptysis	• Infiltrates and local consolidation on chest X-ray • Leukocytosis • Hypoxemia
Viral	• Abrupt onset and rapid progression • Fever • Dry cough with mucoid or blood-tinged sputum • Tachypnea • Dyspnea • Crackles and wheezes	• Normal white blood cell count • Absence of bacteria on Gram's stain • Diffuse infiltrates and absence of consolidation on chest X-ray • Hypoxemia
Fungal	• Acute onset • Fever • Chest pain • Dyspnea • Prostration • Weight loss	• Specific fungus identified in sputum sample
Parasitic	• Nonproductive cough • Dyspnea • Fever and night sweats • Tachycardia • Tachypnea • Crackles	• Interstitial and alveolar infiltrates on chest X-ray • Hypoxemia • Hypocapnia • Fluid for acid-fast staining and culture collected by bronchoscopy with bronchoalveolar lavage is positive for the parasite

---

immunosuppressed patient, even if he has pneumonia, may have a normal or low WBC count. An ABG analysis may reveal a low PaO_2 or high $PaCO_2$ because mucus and atelectasis interfere with gas exchange.

Medical interventions

Medical treatment of pneumonia—which depends on the patient's assessment findings and history, the severity of symptoms, and the cause of the pneumonia—usually begins with antibiotic therapy. The results of sputum cultures and Gram's stains determine the choice of drug. For example, if the Gram's stain demonstrates gram-positive diplococci, the patient may have pneumococcal pneumonia and should receive penicillin. If the patient is immunocompromised and develops a gram-negative bacillary pneumonia, a broad-spectrum penicillin, such as piperacillin, or a third-generation cephalosporin, such as cefotaxime, may be used. If no Gram's stain result is available, therapy should be based on the most likely pathogen. For example, patients with lung disease are likely to harbor an organism such as *H. influenzae*. Therefore, a physician may prescribe a second-generation cephalosporin.

Nosocomial pneumonias are difficult to treat, and typically require combinations of broad-spectrum antibiotics. Therapy should be based on Gram's stain results and a knowledge of the most common nosocomial pathogens. Commonly, the pathogen is a gram-negative bacillus, such as *P. aeruginosa* or *S. aureus*. *S. aureus* is generally resistant to methicillin and must be treated with vancomycin. When antibiotic resistance isn't a concern, gram-negative bacilli can be treated with a beta-lactam drug, such as ceftazidime, ticarcillin, or aztreonam. In severe cases, an aminoglycoside may be added.

A patient with atypical pneumonia caused by *M. pneumoniae* or *Legionella pneumophila* usually receives erythromycin. For patients who have *L. pneumophila*, a physician may add rifampin to the regimen. Used alone, rifampin increases the patient's risk of developing resistant organisms.

If a patient has viral pneumonia, treatment focuses on supportive care. If gas exchange is significantly impaired, ET intubation and mechanical ventilation may be needed to maintain oxygenation.

P. carinii is the most common organism causing pneumonia in immunosuppressed patients. It can lead to a life-threatening infection in patients with acquired immunodeficiency syndrome (AIDS). Medical treatment of pneumonia in these patients includes I.V. administration of trimethoprim-sulfamethoxazole, pentamidine, or dapsone-trimethoprim (see *Treating pneumonia with drug therapy*, page 266).

Nursing interventions

Key nursing interventions for your patient with pneumonia include recognizing hypoxemia and treating it with oxygen, promoting airway clearance, treating the infection with antibiotic therapy, maintaining adequate hydration and nutrition, and preventing cross-infection with infection-control measures. You'll also need to teach your patient about pneumonia and how to manage it at home.

Oxygen therapy

Hypoxemia may result from impaired gas exchange related to a ventilation-perfusion mismatch or ineffective airway clearance of tracheobronchial secretions. Be alert for changes in your patient's pulse rate and mental status. Commonly, the first signs of hypoxemia are tachycardia and restlessness. If hypoxemia is severe, an electrocardiogram (ECG) may be used to monitor your patient for arrhythmias.

To treat hypoxemia, you may administer supplemental oxygen by nasal prongs or mask, depending on the concentration required. If your patient has a severe intrapulmonary shunt, he may need positive-pressure mechanical ventilation. During therapy, continuously monitor your patient's oxygen saturation by pulse oximetry and maintain an oxygen saturation between 93% and 97%.

To help your patient breathe more easily, place him in an upright or semi-upright position. Place a pillow behind his head and one under each arm to help promote chest expansion and comfort. Place another pillow lengthwise behind his back. If your patient must be upright to sleep, he may be more comfortable resting his head and arms on pillows placed on an overbed table.

When your patient needs mechanical ventilation, you may have to use restraints to prevent him from removing his ET tube. If he's anxious, administer prescribed anxiolytics and analgesics. Remember, anxiety increases the work of breathing. Throughout mechanical ventilation, be alert for signs and symptoms of barotrauma. For instance, severe dyspnea, tracheal deviation toward the unaffected side, absent breath sounds, distended neck veins, and asymmetric chest expansion signal life-threatening tension pneumothorax.

Airway clearance

Fatigue, tracheobronchial inflammation, and dehydration may impair the patient's ability to clear airway secretions. To clear these secretions, perform the following interventions:
- Administer expectorants and fluids, as prescribed, to loosen secretions.
- Humidify supplemental oxygen to prevent dry mucous membranes.
- Monitor ABG levels for signs and symptoms of hypoventilation (PaO_2 less than 60 mm Hg, $PaCO_2$ greater than 45 mm Hg, and pH less than 7.35).
- Administer 100% oxygen and hyperinflate your patient's lungs before you suction him. Don't instill normal saline solution. (Lavaging doesn't thin secretions and may increase hypoxemia. It also may wash bacteria into the lungs.)

Treating pneumonia with drug therapy

The drug therapy prescibed for your patient will depend on the pathogen causing his pneumonia.

Pathogen	Drug therapy
Community-acquired bacterial infections	
Streptococcus pneumoniae	• Penicillin • First-generation cephalosporins
Pneumococcus	• Penicillin • Erythromycin, other macrolides • First-generation cephalosporins
Hemophilus influenzae	• Cefuroxime • Third-generation cephalosporins • Ampicillin • Chloramphenicol
Mycoplasma	• Erythromycin, other macrolides, possibly with rifampin • Tetracycline
Legionella	• Erythromycin, other macrolides • Trimethoprim-sulfamethoxazole • Tetracycline
Anaerobes	• Clindamycin • Penicillin • Metronidazole • Cefoxitin • Ticarcillin • Oxacillin • Vancomycin

Pathogen	Drug therapy
Nosocomial bacterial infections	
Staphyloccus aureus	• Aminoglycosides • Cephalosporins
Klebsiella pneumoniae	• Aminoglycosides • Piperacillin • Ceftazidime
Pseudomonas aeruginosa	• Aztreonam • Cefoperazone
Viral infections	
Cytomegalovirus	• Ganciclovir • Foscarnet
Varicella zoster	• Acyclovir
Fungal infections	
Cryptococcus neoformans	• Amphotericin B
Aspergillus	• Amphotericin B • Itraconazole
Parasitic infections	
Pneumocystis carinii	• Trimethoprim-sulfamethoxazole • Pentamidine • Dapsone-trimethoprim • Trimetrexate • Clindamycin • Primaquine • Atovaquone

- Provide chest physical therapy, including postural drainage and percussion.
- Turn your patient every 2 hours and encourage coughing and deep breathing.
- Teach your patient how to use incentive spirometry and offer assistance, as needed.
- Elevate the head of your patient's bed to 45 degrees.

Antibiotic therapy

Because antibiotics can cause allergies and other adverse reactions, obtain a thorough drug history from your patient. Consider the possibility of cross-sensitivity of different drugs. For example, a patient who's allergic to penicillin may also be allergic to cephalosporins.

Administer antibiotics at the scheduled times to maintain therapeutic blood levels.

Monitor peak and trough levels to determine the effectiveness of therapy.

Monitor your patient closely for adverse reactions, including anaphylaxis, rash, and renal or liver failure. If your patient has pneumonia caused by gram-negative bacteria and he's being treated with a beta-lactam antibiotic, such as aztreonam, monitor him closely when you give the first dose. It may stimulate his body's chemical mediators and begin the release of endotoxins, causing vasodilation and hypotension.

Hydration and nutrition

Dehydration, which leads to thick secretions, may be caused by a fever or inadequate fluid intake that results from fatigue, decreased energy, or poor appetite. Unless your patient has another condition that requires fluid restriction, maintain an I.V. or oral fluid intake of 2 to 4 liters per day to liquefy secretions. Monitor his intake and output carefully, and be alert for signs of fluid excess.

Your patient's hypermetabolic state may increase his nutritional needs, but he may be anorexic because of the infection. Encourage him to eat high-protein, high-carbohydrate meals. Provide small, frequent meals and supplemental liquid nutrition.

Infection control

To prevent cross-infection and nosocomial pneumonia, wash your hands meticulously and take these precautions:
- Use droplet precautions if your patient has mycoplasmal pneumonia (see *Standard precautions and droplet precautions*).
- Replace disposable respiratory equipment according to the manufacturers' recommendations and hospital policy.
- Clean all reusable equipment after patient use.
- Use only sterile water for humidifying oxygen.
- Drain and discard any condensate that accumulates in the tubing used for mechanical ventilation.
- Maintain sterile technique when performing invasive procedures.

Standard precautions and droplet precautions

Formerly known as universal precautions, standard precautions are designed to reduce the risk of transmitting infection during patient care. You should use these precautions for all patients, regardless of their diagnosis. That's because all patients and specimens are considered potential sources of infection.

Standard precautions consist of wearing gloves if you anticipate contact with a patient's blood, other body fluids, broken skin, or mucous membranes. Also, between patient encounters and after contact with blood or other body fluids, you should always wash your hands.

If your patient is diagnosed with *Mycoplasma pneumoniae,* you'll also need to implement droplet precautions. That's because the mycoplasma pathogen is transmitted by large droplets that become airborne when the patient sneezes or coughs. These droplets can travel as far as 3 feet. If an infected droplet contacts your conjunctiva or the mucous membranes of your nose or mouth, you may become a carrier of the disease, or you may contract it.

Droplet precautions call for wearing goggles and a face mask with a shield when entering your patient's isolation room. These barriers will protect your conjunctiva and the mucous membranes of your mouth and nose from contact with infected droplets.

- Instruct your patient to cover his nose and mouth with a tissue when he sneezes and to expectorate into an appropriate receptacle.
- Instruct your patient to wash his hands after coughing, sneezing, and expectorating.

Patient teaching

Focus your patient teaching on preventing infection and preparing your patient for discharge. Review with him what pneumonia is, how it spreads, and which risk factors he has. Teach him the proper techniques for hand washing and disposing of secretions. If your patient is at high risk for infection, encourage him to be immunized with the influenza virus vaccine and the pneumococcal polysaccharide vaccine.

Help your patient develop an activity regimen that balances rest and activity. Explain that weakness and fatigue can persist for several weeks after pneumonia resolves and that he should get extra rest and increase activity gradually.

If your patient will continue medication therapy after discharge, teach him the regimen and stress the need to finish all medications. Review possible adverse reactions and instruct him to notify his physician if any occur.

Teach your patient how to perform respiratory exercises, such as coughing, deep breathing, and incentive spirometry, at home. Ask him to repeat your demonstration of the proper techniques. If your patient will be using supplemental oxygen after discharge, teach him about home oxygen therapy, including safety measures. Refer him to a home care nurse for follow-up instruction and care.

Discuss with your patient the need for a proper diet and adequate fluid intake. Unless contraindicated, encourage him to drink 2 to 3 liters of fluids per day to thin secretions. Emphasize the need to eat foods high in protein and carbohydrates. If your patient smokes, advise him to stop.

Pneumonia and chronic obstructive pulmonary disease

Pneumonia causes mucosal irritation, increased mucus production, and an inflammatory response that increases the work of breathing. These effects can be life-threatening in a patient with chronic obstructive pulmonary disease (COPD). Such a patient already has excessive mucus production and small airway damage and requires extra effort to breathe. The additional burden imposed by pneumonia can lead to respiratory failure and death.

Pathophysiology

A disease process that obstructs airflow, COPD includes chronic bronchitis, pulmonary emphysema, and asthma. (For more information on asthma, see Chapter 10.) The pathophysiology of COPD doesn't necessarily follow a progressive order. A patient with COPD may have pure obstructive airway disease with bronchitis, severe emphysema without bronchitis, or some other combination of disorders. The disease process ranges from reversible abnormalities to end-stage cardiopulmonary insufficiency.

Patients with COPD are more susceptible to pulmonary infections because they tend to retain secretions and have altered defense mechanisms. The excessive secretion of thick mucus and the impaired ciliary function allow pathogens to enter the lower respiratory tract and become trapped. Even when these patients are stable, bacteria colonize their trachea and bronchi. The most common pathogens found in COPD are *H. influenzae* and *S. pneumoniae*.

Chronic bronchitis

Chronic bronchitis is characterized by hypertrophy and hypersecretion of bronchial mucous glands; structural changes of the bronchi and bronchioles, including a denuding of cilia along the epithelial surface; and a chronic cough. For bronchitis to be considered chronic, a patient must have it for 3 months of the year for 2 consecutive years. Inhalation of physical or chemical irritants, such as cigarette smoke, or viral or bacterial infections can cause chronic irritation.

Hypertrophy of the bronchial mucous glands causes excessive mucus production. The mucus is thick and tenacious, and ciliary clearance is impaired, making mucus clearance difficult. Thus, the defense mechanisms of the bronchi are compromised, resulting in increased susceptibility to infections and pneumonia.

Infection and injury further increase mucus production. The bronchial walls become inflamed and thickened from edema and the buildup of inflammatory cells. Eventually, all airways become affected, and the bronchial smooth muscle becomes hypertrophied. The combination of hypertrophied smooth muscle and thick mucus obstructs the airway, especially during expiration when it's already narrowed. This, in turn, leads to a ventilation-perfusion mismatch, hypoventilation, and hypoxemia.

Emphysema

In emphysema, the terminal bronchioles enlarge, and the alveoli become fragmented. Although the cause isn't known, emphysema probably results when connective tissue in the lungs is destroyed by proteases (enzymes released by polymorphonuclear leukocytes or alveolar macrophages).

The pathologic changes in emphysema lead to a loss of elastic recoil and airway support. Elastic recoil is lost because of the destruction of elastin and collagen in the lung parenchyma, and increased lung compliance results in a permanent overdistention of the lungs. The loss of parenchymal tissue causes the terminal airways to collapse or narrow, particularly during expiration. Air is trapped in the distal air spaces, causing further distention of the lungs. As the overdistended lungs press against the diaphragm, ventilation diminishes. Then as the patient works harder to force trapped air out of the lungs, intrapleural pressures increase, leading to more airway collapse.

The destruction of the alveolar and bronchiole walls decreases the alveolocapillary membrane surface area, causing impaired gas exchange. Also, pulmonary vasoconstriction reduces pulmonary diffusion. Hypoxemia, which causes generalized pulmonary artery constriction, and pressure from overdistended alveoli decrease the perfusion of normal alveoli, further impairing diffusion capacity. Diffusion abnormalities and airway obstruction may or may not lead to a retention of carbon dioxide.

Adapting nursing care

Pneumonia is a common complication of COPD. And a patient with this combination of diseases is at high risk for additional respiratory problems. For example, the pathophysiologic changes of both disorders worsen hypoxemia, airway obstruction, and air trapping, putting the patient at risk for possible respiratory failure.

Focus your nursing care on controlling hypoxemia, keeping the airway clear, relieving bronchoconstriction, preventing infection, and teaching your patient to perform breathing techniques. You'll also need to monitor the effects of certain drugs, maintain adequate nutrition, ensure safe exercise levels, and detect pulmonary hypertension and other complications.

Controlling hypoxemia

Your patient with pneumonia may need supplemental oxygen to correct hypoxemia. However, in the patient with COPD, hypoxemia triggers respiration—so oxygen therapy can interefere with the patient's stimulus to breathe. Oxygen therapy may also cause him to increase the frequency of respirations, thus shortening expiratory time and causing further hyperinflation. The increased work of breathing also may lead to respiratory muscle fatigue. Oxygen therapy can also worsen hypercapnia and produce respiratory acidosis. And administering oxygen at high flow rates can result in respiratory depression.

Before giving oxygen, check your patient's medical history to find out if he has a chronically elevated $PaCO_2$ level. If he does, he'll need to receive oxygen at a lower flow rate. Deliver oxygen at a rate that will maintain a PaO_2 of 60 mm Hg—usually 2 to 3 liters per minute given through a nasal cannula will do.

Throughout oxygen therapy, monitor your patient's oxygen saturation and PaO_2 levels. Evaluate your patient for signs and symptoms of hypoxemia and hypercapnia, such as a headache, irritability, confusion, increased somnolence, asterixis, tachycardia, and arrhythmias. Keep in mind that a patient who's chronically hypoxemic and hypercapnic may be asymptomatic because his body has adjusted to the abnormalities.

When oxygen therapy can't maintain an adequate PaO_2 level, ET intubation and mechanical ventilation may be necessary. Criteria for intubation vary but usually include a higher-than-normal $PaCO_2$, acidemia, hypoxemia, and altered consciousness.

Clearing the airways

For a patient with pneumonia and COPD, you need to keep the airways clear of secretions because they contribute to ventilation abnormalities. Retained secretions may also irritate the tracheobronchial mucosa, leading to increased bronchomotor tone and bronchospasm.

Postural drainage and percussion can help clear secretions. This procedure combines the force of gravity with the ciliary activity of the small bronchial airways to move secretions toward the main bronchi and the trachea, so the patient can expectorate them. You can use various postural drainage positions to help drain specific lung segments. Use pillows for positioning and support (see *Postural drainage positions*).

About 15 to 20 minutes before the procedure, administer the prescribed bronchodilator to aid the movement of secretions. Encourage the patient to breathe as deeply and cough as forcefully as possible during the procedure to help dislodge thickened secretions.

With the patient in the appropriate position, place your cupped hands over the area being drained and clap for about 1 minute to loosen secretions and stimulate coughing. Instruct the patient to take a deep breath. During the expiration of the deep breath, apply pressure using a short, repetitive, rapid, vibrating movement on the chest.

Postural drainage and percussion may be contraindicated in some patients. If your patient with pneumonia and COPD has severe dyspnea, he may not be able to tolerate the postural drainage positions. And if he has severe bronchospasm, percussion is contraindicated.

Relieving bronchoconstriction

To relieve bronchoconstriction, a physician may prescribe a bronchodilator, typically a beta blocker, theophylline, or a theophylline derivative.

Beta blockers

Beta$_1$ blockers, such as isoproterenol, act at beta$_1$-receptor sites in the myocardium. Beta$_2$ blockers, such as metaproterenol, act at beta$_2$-receptor sites located in smooth muscles of the airways.

Beta blockers are usually administered by metered-dose inhaler. Some drugs, such as albuterol and metaproterenol, may be given using a nebulizer. Regardless of the method, observe your patient while he takes the drug. Commonly, a patient with pneumonia and COPD is tired and has difficulty using a metered-dose inhaler correctly. If necessary, suggest that he use a spacer device. This molded plastic chamber fits onto the metered-dose inhaler and offers several advantages. Finer aerosol droplets can disperse more fully within the spacer, thus allowing them to be carried a greater distance into the airways. Also, the patient doesn't have to coordinate breathing and inhalation, so the medication can be inhaled more effectively. And spacers reduce the number and volume of puffs needed because doses are delivered and used more efficiently.

Alternatively, a physician may prescribe a breath-activated metered-dose inhaler. When positioned in the mouth, this device automatically releases a premeasured dose of the bronchodilator when the patient breathes.

If the patient uses a nebulizer, make sure the bronchodilator solution is properly diluted with saline solution or water. Whether your patient uses a metered-dose inhaler, nebulizer, or spacer, avoid placing him at risk for further infection by making sure the device he uses is cleaned according to the manufacturer's instructions and replaced as hospital policy directs.

Throughout therapy, monitor the patient's respiratory status, noting the use of accessory muscles, breath sounds, and the rate, depth, and character of respirations. Continuously assess oxygen saturation via pulse oximetry, and be alert for signs and symptoms of hypoxemia. Also, assess the patient for adverse reactions, especially if he's receiving beta$_1$ blockers. Report any complaints of palpitations, shakiness, tachycardia, and hypertension.

Theophylline

Traditionally, the xanthine compound theophylline has been used as a bronchodilator, although it's used less commonly today. Theophylline and its derivatives increase the force and rate of skeletal muscle contraction and increase the force generated by fatigued respiratory muscles. They also increase myocardial

Postural drainage positions

Postural drainage promotes the flow of secretions from different portions of the lung into the bronchi, trachea, and ultimately the throat, so they can be expectorated. These illustrations show how to position your patient to drain each area of the lung.

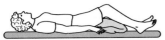

Upper anterior area of both lungs

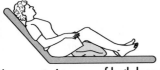

Upper anterior area of both lungs

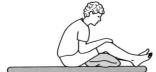

Upper posterior area of both lungs

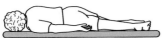

Upper posterior area of right lung

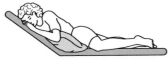

Upper posterior area of left lung

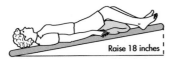

Middle anterior area of both lungs

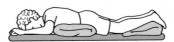

Middle posterior area of both lungs

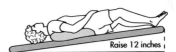

Raise 12 inches

Middle anterior area of right lung

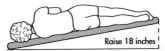

Raise 18 inches

Middle posterior area of right lung

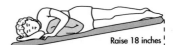

Raise 18 inches

Middle anterior area of left lung

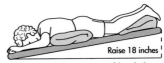

Raise 18 inches

Lower posterior area of both lungs

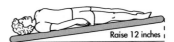

Raise 12 inches

Lower anterior area of left lung

contractility, provide diuresis, and stimulate the central respiratory drive.

When administering theophylline, keep in mind that some forms of the drug—such as extended-release or timed-release forms—must be taken on an empty stomach. Also, make sure the patient avoids a high-carbohydrate, low-protein diet, which decreases theophylline elimination.

Monitor theophylline blood levels routinely to evaluate the effectiveness of therapy. Therapeutic levels range from 10 µg/ml to 20 µg/ml. Advanced age, heart disease, liver disease, viral respiratory infections (such as viral pneumonia), and the use of concomitant drugs can decrease theophylline clearance, placing the patient at risk for theophylline toxicity. Signs and symptoms of theophylline toxicity include unexplained tachycardia and other arrhythmias, gastrointestinal (GI) symptoms, and central nervous system symptoms.

Controlling infection

Pneumonia usually requires antibiotic therapy I.V., at least until the patient begins to improve. If he doesn't respond to antibiotic therapy, the physician may order a Gram's stain and a sputum culture. If your patient is receiving antibiotic therapy and theophylline for COPD, be aware of drug interactions. Tetracycline and clarithromycin, for example, increase the risk of theophylline toxicity.

Teaching breathing techniques

Help your patient with pneumonia and COPD make his breathing more efficient by teaching techniques that prevent air trapping. Effective methods include controlling the inspiratory-expiratory rate, diaphragmatic breathing, pursed-lip breathing, and using incentive spirometry. Teach your patient how to perform these techniques, as indicated, and monitor their effectiveness.

If you're teaching a patient how to control his inspiratory-expiratory rate, tell him to slow the frequency of his respirations and breathe slowly and rhythmically, rather than trying to take in large amounts of air. Help him to concentrate on increasing the time he takes to inhale. Explain that this decreases the work of breathing and controls shortness of breath during stress and activity.

If your patient will be using diaphragmatic breathing, teach him how to use his diaphragm instead of his accessory muscles for breathing. Explain that the diaphragm, a large muscle, uses less oxygen than the smaller accessory muscles. It also increases the volume of air that's exchanged during a normal breath and enhances air distribution.

To demonstrate diaphragmatic breathing, have the patient lie down. Place a small pillow on his abdomen and tell him to raise the pillow on his abdomen as much as possible as he breathes in. Then tell him to pull in his abdomen as much as he can while he exhales. You can gently push down on his upper abdomen to help him exhale completely.

If you're teaching pursed-lip breathing, explain that it creates resistance to airflow, slowing expiration and increasing pressure in the airways. The airway pressure helps the alveoli stay open. As a result, less air is trapped and more inhaled air can enter. Demonstrate this breathing technique by having the patient inhale and then exhale as if he were trying to whistle.

If your patient will be using incentive spirometry, explain that it enhances deep breathing and strengthens the respiratory muscles. Then teach him how to use the spirometer and have him demonstrate his technique.

Monitoring drug therapy

To treat COPD, you may administer corticosteroids as well as other drugs, as prescribed. Remember that corticosteroids may compromise the patient's defenses against infection, including pneumonia. Also, be aware that corticosteroids may mask signs of infection. Closely monitor your patient for indications of an exacerbation of a current infection or a new infection. Signs include fever, tachypnea, and a change in color or an increase in the amount of sputum.

Providing nutrition therapy

Nutritional status may be markedly impaired in a patient with pneumonia and COPD. Typically, a patient experiences significant weight loss, primarily because of a 15% to 25% increase in resting energy expenditure resulting from the increased work of breathing. As body weight decreases, so do respiratory muscle size and strength. Because your patient's respiratory muscles are already stressed and fatigued, the work of breathing increases and respiratory status deteriorates.

Develop a nutritional plan that meets the patient's needs. Enlist the aid of a dietitian to help with meal planning. Offer small, frequent meals and high-protein snacks, which may be better tolerated and require less energy. Also, offer liquid, low-carbohydrate nutritional supplements between meals to provide additional protein and calories. If the patient is receiving oxygen, make sure therapy continues during mealtimes. If necessary, switch to a nasal cannula to avoid interfering with eating. Allow the patient to pace himself as he eats.

If the patient has advanced COPD, avoid a high-carbohydrate diet. A patient with advanced COPD already has high blood levels of carbon dioxide, and carbohydrate metabolism produces carbon dioxide as a by-product, further heightening blood levels.

Encouraging exercise

Most patients with pneumonia and COPD can't tolerate much activity, but your patient should exercise as much as he can. If his condition permits, he can perform leg-raising exercises to strengthen his abdominal muscles. Encourage your patient to walk, as appropriate.

Frequently monitor the patient's response to activity and exercise. And provide frequent rest periods. Position the patient comfortably to ease the work of breathing (see *Easing the work of breathing*, page 274).

Detecting pulmonary hypertension

Patients with long-standing COPD risk developing pulmonary hypertension because hypoxemia, a potent pulmonary vasoconstrictor, can lead to increased pulmonary artery pressure. Signs and symptoms of pulmonary hypertension are usually nonspecific but can include dyspnea, fatigue, dizziness, syncope, chest pain, palpitations, orthopnea, cough, and hoarseness.

If pulmonary hypertension is prolonged, the increased workload on the right ventricle results in cor pulmonale, a condition in which the right ventricle dilates, hypertrophies, or both in an attempt to overcome increasing pulmonary pressure. Eventually, cor pulmonale leads to right ventricular failure.

If your patient with pneumonia and COPD develops cor pulmonale, promote adequate ventilation and oxygenation. Monitor intake and output accurately, and weigh the patient at the same time and under the same conditions every day. Administer the prescribed diuretic and watch for adverse effects, such as volume depletion and electrolyte imbalances. Also, administer digitalis preparations, as prescribed. Assess your patient for complications, such as pleural effusions, characterized by decreased breath sounds and decreased fremitus.

Suspect right ventricular failure if your patient develops jugular vein distention, hepatomegaly, jaundice, and dependent peripheral edema. If he has a central line in place, you'll note elevated central venous pressure readings. If he has a pulmonary catheter in place, you'll note increased pulmonary artery pressure readings, including wedge pressure. If signs of right ventricular failure develop, notify the physician at once.

Patient teaching

Teach your patient with pneumonia and COPD about his disorders and their interrelationship. Reinforce teaching about medications, diet, energy conservation measures, activity, follow-up care, measures to reduce the risk of complications, and signs and symptoms of possible problems. Also, review the following teaching topics:

- measures to promote sleep, such as relaxation techniques and using pillows to maintain an upright position in bed to minimize dyspnea
- methods to decrease exposure to irritants and the risk of infection, including washing the hands properly, avoiding large crowds, and receiving influenza and pneumonia immunizations
- the need to seek medical help if the patient experiences a change in amount or color of sputum, increased cough or dyspnea, increased fatigue, or fever.

Easing the work of breathing

In a patient with pneumonia and chronic obstructive pulmonary disease, shortness of breath increases the work of breathing. By positioning your patient correctly, you can help him use less energy to breathe, reduce his oxygen demands, and make breathing easier, thus improving ventilation and gas exchange. These illustrations show two positions that can ease the work of breathing.

Place the patient in an upright or semi-upright position. Place a pillow behind his head and one under each arm to help promote chest expansion and comfort. Place another pillow lengthwise at the patient's back. This provides support and pushes the thorax forward slightly, making the diaphragm more available for use in breathing.

If your patient has severe dyspnea and must be upright to breathe, have him lean forward across his overbed table. Place a pillow on the table to support his head and arms. Place an additional pillow behind his back to offer support and help him maintain an upright position without expending energy.

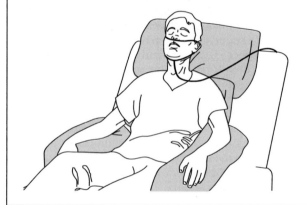

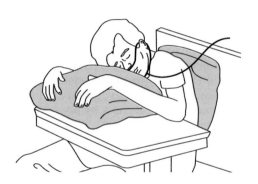

Complications

Common complications for patients with pneumonia and COPD include atelectasis and ARDS.

Atelectasis

Defined as the collapse of alveoli, atelectasis may develop because of an airway obstruction, ineffective ventilation, or compression from external pressure. In patients with pneumonia and COPD, airway obstruction and ineffective ventilation are the most likely causes.

In airway obstruction, a mucous plug or retained secretions decrease ventilation to the alveoli and lead to alveolar collapse. Ineffective ventilation may result from respiratory muscle fatigue. Atelectasis from compression may develop in a patient who has a pleural effusion. The external pressure exerted on the lung by the fluid can lead to alveolar collapse. Usually, draining the fluid relieves this type of atelectasis.

Confirming the complication

Because a patient with pneumonia and COPD already has impaired gas exchange and hypoxemia, physical assessment alone may not confirm the diagnosis of atelectasis. However, be alert for increased dyspnea, restlessness, and tachycardia. You may hear crackles on auscultation. You also may note decreased or absent breath sounds. An ABG analysis will reveal decreased Pao_2, but the extent of hypoxemia is related to the amount of shunting. Also, $Paco_2$ levels may be elevated.

A chest X-ray confirms atelectasis. Findings can range from a subtle decrease in lung volume without visible opacification to complete opacification of a segment, lobe, or lung. Patchy atelectasis appears as bilateral radiopaque areas; discoid atelectasis appears as linear bands of opacity. With an extensive volume loss, the X-ray may show a shift in the position of a lung fissure, a change in the position of the mediastinum, an elevation of the diaphragm on the affected side, or hyperexpansion of the uninvolved lung.

Nursing interventions
To prevent atelectasis, you'll need to take certain steps. If your patient is on bed rest, perform frequent position changes and chest physiotherapy. Encourage coughing, deep breathing, and incentive spirometry at regular intervals. When possible, increase and pace the patient's activities, providing adequate rest periods. Use humidification or mucolytic treatments to help the patient expectorate secretions. If he can't clear secretions by coughing, he may need ET suctioning or therapeutic bronchoscopy.

Untreated atelectasis places the patient at risk for further infection, fibrosis, and decreased lung function, possibly leading to respiratory failure. So if your patient has atelectasis, focus your interventions on improving ventilation and gas exchange. Auscultate breath sounds at least every 2 hours and report any decrease in breath sounds or increase in adventitious sounds. Continue to assess your patient for signs and symptoms of hypoxemia and hypercapnia, such as restlessness, agitation, a change in level of consciousness (LOC), and cyanosis.

Keep the airway clear of secretions and encourage the patient to use incentive spirometry to expand collapsed alveoli, thus improving gas exchange. Administer the prescribed medications to treat the pneumonia and COPD. Watch for signs and symptoms of worsening infection, a new infection, or respiratory failure. Monitor pulse oximetry continuously and obtain blood specimens for ABG analysis, as indicated, to evaluate oxygen saturation and PaO_2 levels.

Adult respiratory distress syndrome
A severe form of respiratory failure, ARDS results from diffuse pulmonary injury. It's characterized by a pattern of changes, including diffuse alveolocapillary wall injury, increased alveolocapillary permeability, noncardiogenic pulmonary edema, and atelectasis.

Pneumonia can lead to the development of ARDS. For a patient with COPD, the risk of developing ARDS increases when pneumonia accompanies the destruction in the alveolar and bronchial walls.

Confirming the complication
Recognizing and confirming ARDS is generally difficult in the early stages. A patient with pneumonia and COPD may already have the early signs and symptoms of ARDS, including tachypnea, restlessness, anxiety, and cough. In a patient who doesn't have existing pulmonary disease, ABG analysis reveals respiratory alkalosis and a normal to slightly low PaO_2. In a patient with pneumonia, however, these findings may not appear because of the existing ventilation-perfusion mismatch and impaired gas exchange.

If the patient is receiving supplemental oxygen, the first sign of ARDS may be decreased PaO_2 levels despite an increase in inspired oxygen, a condition called refractory hypoxemia. As the patient's condition worsens, pulmonary edema becomes evident. Auscultation of the lungs reveals crackles and wheezes. The patient may have cyanosis as ventilation-perfusion mismatching worsens and gas exchange is further impaired.

Other physical findings reflect the degree of hypoxemia. Increased carbon dioxide levels may cause changes in the patient's LOC, ranging from confusion to coma. As ARDS progresses and arterial oxygen content continues to decrease, signs and symptoms of decreased cardiac output appear. The patient may have hypotension, an increased or decreased heart rate, and decreased urine output. Inadequate cellular oxygenation leads to tissue hypoxia, anaerobic metabolism, and lactic acid production. The increase in lactic acid, which can be confirmed by direct measurement of serum lactate levels, leads to further damage of the lungs and other organ systems, especially the kidneys and liver.

A chest X-ray shows diffuse bilateral infiltrates that suggest pulmonary edema, and possibly focal infiltrates that indicate pneumonia. In the terminal stages of ARDS, the X-ray may appear completely white. At this point, ABG analysis will indicate metabolic and respiratory acidosis (a pH of less than 7.2 and a $Paco_2$ greater than 50 mm Hg) and refractory hypoxemia (a Pao_2 of less than 50 mm Hg despite oxygen therapy).

Nursing interventions

Your nursing goals include treating severe hypoxemia, correcting the underlying disease process, providing supportive care, and preventing complications. Usually, patients with ARDS are admitted to the intensive care unit, where they receive mechanical ventilation, invasive hemodynamic monitoring, medications, and nutritional support.

Mechanical ventilation: If your patient is receiving mechanical ventilation, administer the prescribed sedative to reduce discomfort, decrease anxiety, and reduce oxygen consumption. Anticipate giving a neuromuscular blocker to reduce skeletal muscle activity, decrease oxygen consumption, and help control metabolic acidosis. If a physician prescribes a paralytic drug, such as pancuronium, carefully monitor the patient for tachycardia and increased blood pressure, indications that he isn't properly sedated. Remember to explain all procedures because your patient can still hear you, even though he can't move.

While your patient is receiving mechanical ventilation, ensure adequate gas exchange, prevent secondary injury, and maintain adequate oxygenation. The physician will probably prescribe tidal volumes of 10 to 15 ml/kg and positive end-expiratory pressure (PEEP). Doing so improves gas exchange and allows you to deliver lower levels of oxygen. Be alert for complications of reduced cardiac output and barotrauma. A patient with COPD may be at a greater risk for these complications because he may have hyperinflated lungs and pulmonary hypertension.

PEEP reduces cardiac output in two ways. Positive pressure may compromise venous return, decreasing preload and thus cardiac output. Positive pressure may also increase right ventricular afterload, causing a mechanical displacement of the interventricular septum into the left ventricle. This displacement then decreases left ventricular stroke volume. You can treat reduced cardiac output by increasing vascular volume and by giving a prescribed vasopressor.

Barotrauma, such as tension pneumothorax, pneumomediastinum, and air emboli, can result from overdistension of nondiseased alveoli.

RAPID RESPONSE ▶ A tension pneumothorax is a medical emergency that requires immediate intervention. The increased intrapleural pressure on the affected side causes the mediastinum to shift to the opposite side. This exerts pressure on the heart and thoracic aorta, resulting in decreased venous return and decreased cardiac output. Tissue perfusion is compromised because the collapsed lung can't participate in ventilation. Be alert for these signs and symptoms:
• restlessness or agitation
• diaphoresis
• tachycardia
• tachypnea
• muffled heart sounds
• hyperresonance over the affected lung
• absent breath sounds over the affected lung
• midline tracheal shift
• asymmetric chest excursion
• increased airway pressures
• hypotension
• cardiac arrest.

If you detect tension pneumothorax, be ready to assist with a needle thoracotomy or chest tube insertion to relieve the increased pressure. Also, take these steps:
• Check the patient's pulse oximetry values and obtain blood specimens for ABG analysis to confirm hypoxemia. Administer supplemental oxygen as needed.
• Assess vital signs and cardiopulmonary status frequently for signs of respiratory distress. Monitor heart rate and blood pressure.
• Place the patient in the semi-Fowler position to allow for full lung expansion.
• Change the patient's position at least every 2 hours.
• Observe your patient for changes in his LOC and for signs of reduced cardiac output, such as hypotension and decreased urine output.
• Maintain closed chest drainage. ◀

Some patients with or at high risk for barotrauma may be placed on high-frequency jet ventilation. This type of mechanical ventilation can deliver from 100 to 600 breaths per minute at lower tidal volumes, helping to prevent further damage to bronchioles and alveoli while maintaining alveolar ventilation.

Fluid therapy: Your patient with ARDS may need a pulmonary artery catheter so you can administer fluid therapy and manage intravascular volume. The goal is to prevent further pulmonary edema while maintaining adequate circulation and perfusion. Monitor intake and output hourly, weigh the patient daily, and monitor and report hemodynamic measurements, such as pulmonary artery pressures, cardiac output, central venous pressure, pulmonary vascular resistance, and systemic vascular resistance, as necessary.

Drug therapy: Administer the prescribed antibiotics for pneumonia and monitor the patient's blood levels. You may also need to give bronchodilators to help reverse bronchoconstriction. Be alert for possible drug interactions.

Give the prescribed diuretic to decrease interstitial edema. Carefully measure and record the resulting urine output. A physician also may prescribe a corticosteroid to reduce pulmonary edema and stabilize pulmonary membranes. If you administer corticosteroid therapy, be aware that a patient with pneumonia and COPD is at high risk for complications, including sodium retention, potassium loss, muscle wasting, delayed healing, and increased susceptibility to infection.

Nutritional therapy: A patient with ARDS needs early, aggressive nutritional therapy because he's in a hypermetabolic state, which raises the risk of metabolic and infectious complications. Plus, a patient with pneumonia and COPD needs adequate nutrition to improve resistance to infection and increase respiratory muscle strength. Because of the patient's debilitated state, fatigue, and the need for increased nutrients, a physician may prescribe enteral or parenteral nutrition. Carefully monitor the rate of the infusion and routinely monitor electrolyte, glucose, blood urea nitrogen (BUN), and creatinine levels. Also, monitor the patient's weight for changes and assess hydration status.

Pneumonia and heart failure

When a patient has heart failure, his heart can't maintain a cardiac output sufficient to meet the metabolic and oxygen demands of his body and his heart. Heart failure usually results from changes in contractility, preload, afterload, or the ratio of oxygen supply to demand. If that same patient has pneumonia, his diminished ventilation, oxygenation, and gas exchange will further affect the available oxygen supply.

Pathophysiology

Hypoxemia and the increased metabolic demands associated with pneumonia can decrease myocardial oxygen supply. The altered ratio of oxygen supply and demand can precipitate or exacerbate heart failure (see *How pneumonia and heart failure affect myocardial oxygen supply,* page 278).

Right ventricular failure may develop from elevated pulmonary vascular resistance. When pulmonary vascular resistance increases, the right ventricle must work harder to maintain an adequate stroke volume, thereby increasing the oxygen demand.

If your patient with pneumonia develops sepsis, high-output heart failure can occur. The inflammatory process, the release of endotoxins, and the altered metabolism cause systemic vasodilation and fever. The lowered systemic vascular resistance and increased metabolic rate require increased cardiac output to maintain an adequate blood pressure and tissue perfusion. If the infection is overwhelming, the heart may not be able to compensate.

Adapting nursing care

Nursing care of a patient with pneumonia and heart failure focuses on enhancing cardiac output, identifying and correcting any precipitating causes, and relieving symptoms.

PATHOPHYSIOLOGY

How pneumonia and heart failure affect myocardial oxygen supply

In heart failure, the heart can't pump a sufficient amount of blood to the tissue—including the myocardial tissue. As a result, the myocardium doesn't receive enough oxygen.

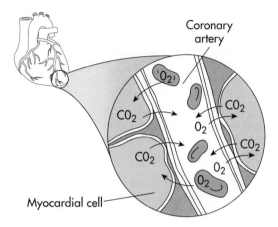

In pneumonia, the alveoli in the lungs become plugged with exudate. As a result, less oxygen moves across the alveolocapillary membrane into the blood and less carbon dioxide moves into the alveoli.

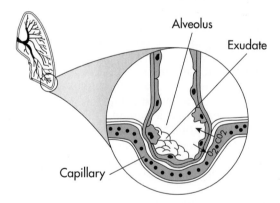

In a patient with pneumonia and heart failure, the supply of oxygen to the myocardium is insufficient for two reasons. Not only is the heart pumping less blood to the myocardium, but the blood it's pumping is carrying less oxygen.

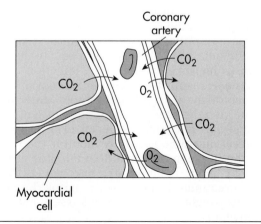

Improving cardiac output

Administer prescribed medications, such as diuretics, inotropic drugs, and vasodilators. Diuretics enhance sodium and water excretion, thus reducing preload and symptoms of systemic and pulmonary venous congestion. Among the most commonly used diuretics are loop diuretics, such as furosemide. However, diuretic therapy can lead to electrolyte imbalance and excessive diuresis. Monitor your patient's serum electrolyte levels and report any changes. Keep in mind that hypokalemia can result from diuretic therapy and may predispose the patient to cardiac arrhythmias. If your patient is also receiving digoxin to improve myocardial contractility, his risk for arrhythmias increases. Evaluate his ECG for any arrhythmias that may result from drug toxicity or electrolyte imbalance (see *Drugs for pneumonia and heart failure: Dangerous interactions*, page 280).

Although adequate hydration helps clear secretions and lower the risk of dehydration, too much fluid can increase preload and overwhelm the patient with heart failure. Also, be alert for excessive diuresis, which can lead to intravascular volume depletion. Monitor intake and output carefully and weigh your patient daily. Check his skin turgor and mucous membranes for signs of dehydration. Assess him for signs of fluid overload, such as increasing dyspnea and crackles. Continuously monitor his oxygen saturation, using pulse oximetry. Continue to assess him for signs of worsening heart failure, such as S_3 and S_4 heart sounds, wheezing, peripheral edema, and jugular vein distention.

During acute heart failure, your patient may require a pulmonary artery catheter. Use the pulmonary catheter readings to monitor his fluid balance. If fluid volume is depleted, central venous pressure and pulmonary artery wedge pressures will be low, and the patient may need additional fluids. Conversely, if fluid overload occurs, these values will be elevated, and the patient may need additional diuretic therapy.

If indicated, also use the pulmonary artery catheter to monitor your patient's cardiac output, cardiac index, and systemic vascular resistance. A decreased cardiac output and index indicate that heart failure is worsening. If the patient's systemic vascular resistance increases, the left ventricle must exert more force to eject blood during systole. This, in turn, increases myocardial oxygen demand. As prescribed, administer digoxin and inotropic drugs, such as dopamine and dobutamine, to improve contractility. Watch for the hemodynamic effects of these drugs and be prepared to titrate dosages based on your patient's response.

You may also need to administer a vasodilator to decrease afterload and limit venous return. Some drugs, such as nitroprusside and hydralazine, act on arterial smooth muscle to decrease impedance to left ventricular ejection. Other drugs, such as nitroglycerin, act on the vascular smooth muscle to reduce elevated preload and limit venous return.

A physician may prescribe morphine to cause peripheral pooling, redistributing blood away from the congested pulmonary circulation. Morphine not only reduces preload but also decreases the patient's anxiety and tachypnea. Plus, it helps relax airway smooth muscle and facilitate gas exchange. However, because morphine also depresses the respiratory center, you'll need to administer it cautiously. As prescribed, give small, intermittent doses. Closely monitor your patient's respiratory status.

Providing supportive care

Your patient with pneumonia and heart failure may have impaired gas exchange. And he may have other respiratory problems, such as dyspnea resulting from pulmonary congestion and left ventricular failure. Expect to administer supplemental oxygen to reduce the workload of the heart and support adequate tissue oxygenation. Auscultate his breath sounds frequently to detect increased congestion. Encourage the patient to cough, breathe deeply, and use incentive spirometry.

Teach your patient to pace his activities according to his tolerance level and the severity of symptoms. Provide for adequate rest periods to reduce demands on the heart, oxygen demand, and fatigue. If your patient is receiving a vasodilator, check for postural hypotension. Monitor his blood pressure while he's sitting, lying, and standing. Instruct him to dangle his legs before getting out of bed, and stay with him when he stands up and walks. Be alert for complaints of dizziness and light-headedness when he sits up or stands.

DRUG ALERT

Drugs for pneumonia and heart failure: Dangerous interactions

Antibiotics	Drugs for heart failure	Adverse effects	Nursing actions
• Broad-spectrum penicillins	• Digoxin	• The combination causes hypo-kalemia, and broad-spectrum penicillins increase risk of digoxin toxicity.	• Monitor serum potassium levels closely. • Watch for signs and symptoms of hypokalemia such as drowsiness, weakness, anorexia, depressed reflexes, orthostatic hypotension, and polyuria. • Administer potassium supplements, as prescribed. • Encourage intake of high-potassium foods. Watch for signs of hyperkalemia resulting from increased intake of high-potassium foods. • Assess apical pulse before administering each dose of digoxin. • Monitor your patient for signs and symptoms of digoxin toxicity, such as nausea, vomiting, and halo vision. • Begin cardiac monitoring to detect arrhythmias.
• Macrolide antibiotics (azithromycin, clarithromycin, erythromycin)	• Digoxin	• Macrolide antibiotics slow metabolism of digoxin in GI tract, increase serum digoxin levels, and increase risk of toxicity.	• Assess apical pulse before administering each dose of digoxin. • Monitor serum digoxin levels. • Monitor your patient for signs and symptoms of digoxin toxicity, such as nausea, vomiting, and halo vision.
• Tetracyclines	• Digoxin	• Tetracyclines increase the risk of digoxin toxicity.	• Assess apical pulse before administering each dose of digoxin. • Monitor your patient for signs and symptoms of digoxin toxicity, such as nausea, vomiting, and halo vision. • Begin cardiac monitoring to detect arrhythmias.
• Aminoglycosides	• Loop diuretics	• Loop diuretics increase the risk of ototoxicity.	• Obtain baseline audiometric testing. • Monitor serum peak and trough levels of antibiotic. • Assess patient's hearing; note any changes indicating hearing loss. • Anticipate a change in the antibiotic prescription.

Your patient needs adequate nutrition to meet his body's increased metabolic demands. Enlist the aid of a dietitian to help with planning meals. Offer frequent, small meals to minimize exertion and reduce GI blood requirements, which can overwork the heart. If your patient is retaining sodium and water, restrict his intake of dietary sodium. Encourage high-protein foods to meet the increased metabolic demands imposed by pneumonia and heart failure. If necessary, administer liquid oral supplements or provide enteral or parenteral nutrition.

Patient teaching

When teaching your patient about his condition and its treatment, emphasize the importance of monitoring fluid balance. Instruct him to watch for signs of fluid overload, such as weight gain, shortness of breath, swelling of the feet and ankles, fever, and a persistent cough. At the same time, explain the need for adequate hydration. Teach the patient to recognize and report the symptoms of dehydration, such as dizziness, decreased urine output, rapid heart rate, and dry mucous membranes. Stress the importance of eating low-sodium meals and maintaining an adequate fluid intake.

Teach your patient about his prescribed medications, their doses, and possible adverse effects. Reinforce the need for compliance with his medication plan and the importance of completing the prescribed course of treatment.

Complications

Common complications for patients with pneumonia and heart failure include pulmonary edema, pleural effusion, and respiratory failure.

Pulmonary edema

Pulmonary edema, an excess of water in the extravascular space of the lung, may result from a condition such as heart failure. And if a patient also has pneumonia, gas exchange can be severely impaired.

In left ventricular failure, the filling pressures on the left side of the heart increase, causing a simultaneous increase in the pulmonary hydrostatic pressure. If the hydrostatic pressure exceeds the capillary oncotic pressure, which holds fluid in the capillaries, fluid moves into the interstitial space. Initially, the lymphatic system removes the fluid from the lungs. When the movement of fluid from the capillaries exceeds the lymphatic system's ability to remove it, pulmonary edema develops.

This usually occurs when the left atrial pressure or the pulmonary capillary wedge pressure exceeds 20 mm Hg. However, pulmonary edema can develop at lower hydrostatic pressures if capillary oncotic pressure is decreased. This may occur in pneumonia because the patient is in a hypermetabolic state and may have impaired nutrition and lowered plasma protein levels.

Pulmonary edema may also be caused by capillary injury that increases capillary permeability. In a patient with pneumonia, endotoxins released by the pulmonary pathogens damage the alveolocapillary membrane, leading to the accumulation of exudate and debris in the acini and terminal bronchioles. When capillary permeability increases, water and plasma proteins can leak into the interstitial space, increasing the interstitial oncotic pressure. When this pressure equals or exceeds capillary oncotic pressure, water moves out of the capillary into the interstitial space. As pulmonary edema progresses, the impaired diffusion between the capillaries and alveoli inhibits gas exchange, which is already impaired in the patient with pneumonia and heart failure.

Confirming the complication

With acute pulmonary edema, the patient feels extremely breathless and anxious. His respiratory rate is elevated, and you may see nasal flaring and signs of accessory muscle use, such as intercostal muscle movement and bulging neck muscles. The patient will expectorate pink, frothy secretions; have loud inspiratory and expiratory gurgling sounds; and be diaphoretic. As respiratory distress worsens, he may feel that he's suffocating, which further increases his anxiety and heart rate. The increased heart rate reduces ventricular filling time and further depresses cardiac function. Hypoxemia from impaired gas exchange and decreased cardiac output lead to tissue hypoxia.

Analysis of ABG levels may reveal hypoxemia and acidemia. A chest X-ray usually shows an enlarged cardiac shadow, pulmonary venous congestion, and interstitial edema. In the early stages, an X-ray may show dilation and redistribution of pulmonary blood flow to the upper lobes. On an X-ray, interstitial edema appears as characteristic lines, called Kerley's lines, that represent thickened interlobular septa.

Nursing interventions

Nursing care measures for your patient with pneumonia and heart failure who develops pulmonary edema include promoting oxygenation, improving cardiac output, and decreasing pulmonary congestion. The treatments are similar to those used for heart failure; however, they're applied more vigorously.

RAPID RESPONSE ▶ Acute pulmonary edema is a medical emergency that requires prompt intervention.

- Immediately place your patient in the high Fowler position, or have him sit upright supported by an overbed table to decrease the work of breathing and enhance gas exchange.
- Administer morphine I.V., as prescribed, to decrease anxiety, slow the respiratory rate, and reduce venous return.
- Provide supplemental oxygen and be prepared for intubation if your patient experiences increasing hypoxemia, acidemia, and changes in mental status.
- Monitor your patient's ABG levels and oxygen saturation for changes.
- Auscultate his breath sounds and be alert for crackles, which may signal alveolar fluid congestion.
- Begin cardiac monitoring and evaluate your patient's ECG for arrhythmias.
- Monitor your patient's vital signs (including pulse, heart rate, and blood pressure) every 15 to 30 minutes, or more frequently if necessary. Note a decrease in blood pressure of more than 20 mm Hg. Monitor your patient for irregular or increased heart rate or skipped beats. Also, monitor him for signs and symptoms of decreased cardiac output, such as hypotension and tachycardia.
- Administer prescribed medications, such as inotropic drugs, to improve myocardial contractility.
- Administer bronchodilators, as prescribed, to relieve bronchospasm and wheezing.
- Administer diuretics, as prescribed, and carefully monitor your patient's response. Monitor intake and output hourly.
- Obtain serum electrolyte levels and be alert for signs and symptoms of electrolyte imbalance.
- Throughout your patient's care, be alert for signs and symptoms of increasing respiratory distress. Have emergency equipment readily available.
- After your patient's condition has stabilized, continue to institute measures to support cardiac output, maximize gas exchange, and promote rest. ◂

Pleural effusion

An accumulation of fluid in the pleural space, pleural effusion may result from the pathophysiologic changes caused by pneumonia and heart failure. The pleura is a permeable membrane that allows fluids in the lung to cross into the pleural space. The migration of fluids and blood components through the walls of intact capillaries bordering the pleura is the most common mechanism of pleural effusion.

The fluid can be transudative or exudative. Transudative effusion is watery and diffuses from the capillaries as a result of increased hydrostatic pressure or decreased capillary oncotic pressure. Heart failure can lead to transudative effusion.

Exudative effusion results from inflammation or infection and the inflammatory response that damages the alveolocapillary membrane and increases capillary permeability. This fluid is less watery and contains plasma proteins and WBCs. Pneumonia can lead to exudative effusion.

Confirming the complication

A small pleural effusion may produce no signs and symptoms, and the lymphatic system may drain the fluid. A large pleural effusion may produce signs and symptoms related to how fast and how much fluid accumulates. The patient may have dyspnea, compression atelectasis, and impaired ventilation. You may observe decreased chest expansion on the affected side and tracheal deviation toward the unaffected side. Auscultation may reveal decreased or absent breath sounds over the affected area. You may note dullness to flatness when percussing over the area, and sometimes you may hear a pleural friction rub.

A chest X-ray shows blunting of the lateral costophrenic angle (meniscus sign). If the pleural effusion is subpulmonic, the diaphragm will appear elevated. If the effusion is on the left side, the distance between the gastric air bubble and the pseudodiaphragm will be greater.

Nursing interventions

Your care measures depend on what's causing your patient's pleural effusion and how severe the symptoms are. Watch for signs and symptoms of impaired ventilation (dyspnea, tachypnea, hypoxemia, and acidemia) and decreased cardiac output (hypotension and changes in mental status). Place your patient in the semi-Fowler to high Fowler position. If he needs to remain supine, reposition him every 2 hours.

If the effusion is small, keep the unaffected lung below the affected lung to help match ventilation to perfusion. However, if the effusion is large, this positioning could place pressure on the unaffected lung, causing reduced expansion and possibly worsening the ventilation-perfusion mismatch. In this case, be prepared to assist with thoracentesis, a needle aspiration of the pleural fluid, or placement of a thoracotomy tube.

Respiratory failure

Respiratory failure develops when the pulmonary system fails to maintain adequate gas exchange. Based on ABG results, respiratory failure is classified as hypoxemic normocapnic (type I) or hypoxemic hypercapnic (type II). Respiratory failure usually stems from another disorder, such as pneumonia or heart failure. When the two disorders occur together, the risk of respiratory failure greatly increases.

Hypoxemia, the most common sign of acute respiratory failure, occurs because of impaired gas exchange. Hypoxemia can be caused by alveolar hypoventilation, right-to-left intrapulmonary shunting, ventilation-perfusion mismatch, and diffusion abnormalities. When the amount of oxygen being brought into the alveoli is inadequate to meet the body's metabolic needs, alveolar hypoventilation develops.

Right-to-left intrapulmonary shunting occurs when blood goes to the arterial system without passing through ventilated areas of the lung. When a portion of the lung isn't ventilated, such as occurs with alveolar collapse or consolidation, the blood perfusing that area does not participate in gas exchange.

Ventilation-perfusion mismatch, the most common cause of hypoxemia, occurs when blood passes through alveoli that are under-ventilated in relation to the amount of perfusion. Such mismatching may result from pulmonary edema associated with heart failure.

Diffusion abnormalities occur when the equilibrium between oxygen pressure in alveoli and pulmonary capillaries is impaired. It may result from pulmonary edema.

Regardless of the cause, the process of respiratory failure is the same. Untreated hypoxemia can lead to cellular hypoxia. An imbalance between oxygen demand and supply leads to tissue hypoxia, anaerobic metabolism, and the development of lactic acidosis. Cerebral tissue hypoxia stimulates the sympathetic nervous system, leading to an increase in respiratory rate and cardiac output to compensate for the decreased tissue perfusion.

Confirming the complication

Assessment findings that indicate hypoxemia and hypercapnia are subtle, but ABG analysis helps to confirm respiratory failure. In type I respiratory failure, the Pao_2 is less than 50 mm Hg with the patient breathing room air, and the $Paco_2$ is normal. Type II respiratory failure is characterized by a Pao_2 of less than 50 mm Hg with the patient breathing room air and a $Paco_2$ of more than 50 mm Hg. In both types, the respiratory rate may be more than 30 breaths per minute or less than 8 breaths per minute. The vital capacity is less than 15 ml/kg.

Other signs and symptoms depend on the underlying cause of the heart failure and the degree of tissue hypoxia. The patient may be restless, anxious, and confused and have a decreased LOC. Cardiovascular signs may include tachycardia, hypertension or hypotension, and arrhythmias.

Nursing interventions

Focus your nursing interventions on improving oxygenation and ventilation, preventing complications, facilitating nutritional support, and providing comfort and emotional support.

Continuously monitor oxygen saturation levels using pulse oximetry, and obtain blood specimens for ABG analysis. Note any changes that indicate deterioration in your patient's respiratory status. Observe the effect of your interventions and your patient's activities on his oxygen saturation. Administer supplemental oxygen, as prescribed, and position your patient to facilitate ventilation. Determine the best position based on oxygen saturation values.

Institute cardiac monitoring and evaluate your patient's ECG for the effects of hypoxemia, such as increased heart rate, arrhythmias, and ischemic changes. Watch your patient for evidence of worsening heart failure, such as jugular vein distention, peripheral edema, cough, and crackles. Also, look for signs of increasing respiratory distress.

If your patient's respiratory distress worsens—as indicated by intercostal retractions, a respiratory rate of more than 30 breaths per minute, paradoxical breathing, and changes in his LOC—anticipate the need for mechanical ventilation. If ET intubation and mechanical ventilation are required, give a sedative and a neuromuscular blocker, as prescribed, to provide comfort and decrease the work of breathing. Explain the effects of neuromuscular blockers to your patient and offer reassurance. Take measures to prevent skin breakdown, atelectasis, and deep vein thrombosis. Frequent turning, repositioning, coughing, deep-breathing exercises, incentive spirometry, and isometric leg exercises help to minimize these risks of immobility.

Carefully monitor your patient's fluid balance. Hypovolemia can impair tissue perfusion, but volume overload can tax the heart, further compromising cardiac output and, ultimately, tissue perfusion. Maintain adequate nutrition with enteral feedings, if possible, or parenteral feedings, if necessary. Remember that nutritional support can also contribute to volume overload and increased carbon dioxide production.

Monitor your patient closely. Weight him daily and check intake and output. Monitor electrolyte, BUN, glucose, and creatinine levels. As appropriate, tailor your care according to your patient's underlying condition and the specific cause of the respiratory failure.

Pneumonia and HIV infection

Patients infected with the human immunodeficiency virus (HIV) may be at risk for lung pathogens that cause many types of pneumonia, including community-acquired bacterial pneumonia, nosocomial pneumonia with and without neutropenia, fungal pneumonia, viral pneumonia, and parasitic pneumonia. *P. carinii*

pneumonia is the most common pulmonary infection in patients with AIDS.

Pathophysiology

A retrovirus, HIV consists of a ribonucleic acid (RNA) core and a protective protein coat. To replicate, the virus incorporates itself into a host cell's RNA, which causes production of viral cells rather than host cells. Specifically, the virus cell binds to a CD4+ receptor on the surface of a T cell and injects its RNA into the T cell. The virus destroys the T_4 lymphocyte cells, which regulate the body's immune responses. This destruction causes widespread immunodeficiency and places the patient at risk for developing opportunistic infections.

If a patient has an HIV infection, his lungs are a main target of opportunistic infections because the HIV infection compromises the pulmonary defenses. And *P. carinii* pneumonia may be life-threatening in an immunocompromised patient. A patient may report a history of a fever greater than 101° F, fatigue, and weight loss for several weeks to months before developing respiratory symptoms, such as shortness of breath and a nonproductive cough. As the pneumonia worsens, the patient may develop a productive cough. His immunocompromised state also increases his risk of developing other types of nosocomial and community-acquired pneumonia.

Adapting nursing care

The care you give your patient with an HIV infection and pneumonia is similar to that for a patient with pneumonia, but you'll need to adapt your care to accommodate his immunosuppressed state. Your nursing goals should focus on maintaining optimal ventilation and oxygenation, preventing further infection, maintaining adequate hydration, promoting nutrition, promoting skin integrity, and educating and counseling the patient and his family.

Monitor your patient for changes in respiratory status. Check vital signs, skin color, breath sounds, and sputum production. Monitor pulse oximetry and ABG levels, as necessary. Encourage coughing, deep breathing, and incentive spirometry. And administer supplemental oxygen, as necessary. Anticipate the possibility of mechanical ventilation. Throughout your patient's care, explain all procedures and treatments and provide support and counseling.

As you care for your patient, use standard precautions to protect yourself from infection, which may be transmitted through increased exposure to secretions, such as sputum, and to body fluids, such as blood samples. If your patient develops *M. pneumoniae*, follow droplet precautions for the duration of his illness.

If your patient has *P. carinii* pneumonia, he may require treatment with trimethoprim-sulfamethoxazole or pentamidine isethionate. Trimethoprim-sulfamethoxazole therapy is preferred because of the risk of adverse effects with pentamidine. However, trimethoprim-sulfamethoxazole may cause hypersensitivity reactions in patients who are allergic to sulfa drugs. Other drugs used to treat *P. carinii* pneumonia include dapsone-trimethoprim, trimetrexate, clindamycin, primaquine, and atovaquone.

Your patient with pneumonia and an HIV infection needs thorough teaching about his condition, its treatment, and the prevention of complications. Before he's discharged from the hospital, make sure he understands all aspects of home care (see *Preventing infection at home*).

Complications

Common complications for patients with pneumonia and an HIV infection include HIV wasting syndrome and tuberculosis.

HIV wasting syndrome
Characterized by anorexia, weight loss, diarrhea, and fever, HIV wasting syndrome helps in the diagnosis of AIDS. For a patient who has pneumonia, the risk of developing this complication is increased because of the difficulty of maintaining adequate nutrition. For example, sputum production may interfere with taste sensations. And fatigue, weakness, and shortness of breath may interfere with the patient's ability to eat. Eating requires considerable energy, which can tire a patient who has impaired

 GOING HOME

Preventing infection at home

For a patient with pneumonia who's also infected with human immunodeficiency virus (HIV), the risk of developing other infections increases because of his immunocompromised status. The risk of complications also rises because pneumonia exacerbates an already compromised state. To minimize these risks, teach your patient how to prevent infection when he goes home.

Emphasize the importance of using standard precautions at all times to reduce the risk of transmitting the HIV infection to others. Also, explain specific measures to protect the patient from exposure to infections. Advise your patient to follow these guidelines.
- Maintain good hygiene. Bathe regularly with soap and water.
- Wash your hands regularly with soap and water, especially before, during, or after any activity.
- Cover any cuts or broken skin with a bandage.
- Monitor your temperature regularly. Call your physician if it rises above 100° F (37.7° C).
- Report a new cough or shortness of breath.
- Call your physician if you notice a change in the color of your sputum.
- Clean all your respiratory equipment—such as holding chambers, tubing, and mouthpieces—after each use.
- Dispose of all tissues and secretions promptly in an appropriate receptacle.
- Avoid crowds and people with infections, including upper respiratory tract infections. If this isn't possible, wear a mask that covers your nose and mouth.

gas exchange. Plus, the fever associated with pneumonia increases metabolism.

Confirming the complication
The Centers for Disease Control and Prevention define *HIV wasting syndrome* as an involuntary weight loss of more than 10% of baseline body weight, two or more loose stools every day, and a chronic weakness with intermittent or constant fever for more than 30 days. Typically, the patient appears cachectic and malnourished. A diagnosis requires ruling out other conditions that could cause these findings.

Nursing interventions

Perform a comprehensive nutritional and dietary assessment to find out why your patient isn't consuming enough fluids and food. If your patient experiences nausea, vomiting, and diarrhea, his physician may order an antiemetic and an antidiarrheal. If your patient is severely ill, he may need continuous enteral or parenteral nutrition.

Monitor and record your patient's daily weight and his food and fluid intake. Check his oxygen saturation for changes that may indicate hypoxemia. Encourage your patient to consume 2 to 3 liters of fluids daily to liquefy secretions if appropriate. To aid your patient's digestion and decrease the risk of aspiration, encourage him to eat his meals out of bed. Offer him small, frequent meals, which he may tolerate better than three large meals. And provide high-protein foods that are textured and easy to swallow—such as yogurt, pudding, and instant breakfast drinks—to minimize energy expenditure during eating. Encourage your patient to brush his teeth frequently, including before meals, to stimulate digestive juices and enhance the taste of food.

Encourage your patient's family and friends to visit during mealtimes. Ask them to bring home-prepared foods that the patient prefers, but instruct them to avoid foods with naturally occurring microbes, such as raw fruits and vegetables or rare meat, which could expose the patient to further infection.

To treat fever, cautiously administer antipyretics. But don't give your patient aspirin; the HIV infection may have already altered his blood's ability to coagulate, and aspirin could exacerbate the situation. Tepid sponge baths and frequent linen changes can help the patient feel more comfortable. If he's dehydrated from fever and sweating and can't take in at least 2,500 ml of fluid each day, anticipate starting I.V. therapy to promote hydration.

Tuberculosis

HIV infection causes a progressive depletion of the patient's T cells and affects his macrophage and monocyte functions, which raises his risk of developing tuberculosis. When pneumonia compromises his immune system even more than the HIV infection alone, the patient faces an even greater risk.

Confirming the complication

A patient with tuberculosis may have few or no symptoms, or he may report fever, a productive cough, shortness of breath, night sweats, and weight loss.

Depending on the patient's level of cellular immunity, a chest X-ray may show anything from cavitation in the lung parenchyma to a diffuse interstitial or nodular pattern. Lymphadenopathy as well as diffuse and focal infiltrates also may appear on a chest X-ray.

Most patients with an HIV infection don't react to a tuberculin skin test, so a negative result doesn't rule out tuberculosis. Acid-fast bacilli may appear on a Gram's stain, and sputum cultures may show mycobacteria.

In a patient with a disseminated infection, elevated alkaline phosphatase and lactic dehydrogenase levels indicate liver involvement. If the bone marrow is affected, the patient may have anemia and pancytopenia.

Fiberoptic bronchoscopy may help in diagnosing some patients. If your patient is scheduled to undergo a bronchoscopy with bronchoalveolar lavage, the lavage fluid should be sent for acid-fast staining and mycobacterial culture. Because tubercle bacilli may spread during bronchoscopy, you need to follow standard precautions for HIV and tuberculosis. Using high-efficiency particulate air masks, ultraviolet lights, and proper air ventilation and filtration can reduce the risk of transmission.

Nursing interventions

Focus your care on relieving symptoms and observing your patient for complications. Help him relieve fatigue and shortness of breath by pacing his activities, providing frequent rest periods, and administering supplemental oxygen.

Carefully monitor his oxygenation and ventilation. Also, monitor and report the results of ABG analysis and continuously monitor oxygen saturation. Control your patient's fever by administering an antipyretic (not aspirin), encouraging him to drink fluids, and promoting rest. If your patient has night sweats, provide clean, dry linens and skin care.

Drug therapy for tuberculosis in patients with pneumonia and an HIV infection includes a 2-month regimen of isoniazid, rifampin, and pyrazinamide. If your patient develops a disseminated infection or resistance to isoniazid, his physician may also prescribe ethambutol. Treatment with isoniazid and rifampin continues for at least 9 months, including 6 months after a culture no longer shows infection. Pyrazinamide therapy continues for 2 months. Because liver function may already be altered, watch for hepatic complications when administering these drugs.

If your patient also has a fungal infection, he may be receiving ketoconazole and fluconazole. Interactions between these antifungal drugs and isoniazid and rifampin may cause both types of drugs to be ineffective.

Explain to your patient that if he doesn't take his medications properly he may develop drug-resistant strains of tuberculosis, resulting in multiple drug-resistant tuberculosis. A patient with multiple drug-resistant tuberculosis must be treated with several drugs, placing him at greater risk for adverse effects. Some effects, such as nausea and vomiting, threaten his nutritional status and contribute to fatigue and weakness, thus increasing the patient's risk for further complications.

Until your patient responds satifactorily to drug therapy, follow these infection-control guidelines:
- Place the patient in a private room with the door closed.
- Ensure that the room has 6 to 12 air exchanges each hour. Recirculate air through a high-efficiency filter.
- Make sure everyone who enters the room wears a personal respirator. Take special care to avoid exposure during procedures, such as bronchoscopy, endotracheal suctioning, sputum induction, and aerosolization of medication.
- Instruct your patient to cover his mouth and nose with a tissue when coughing or sneezing.

- Have your patient wear a mask or personal respirator if he must be transported outside the room.

Your patient may feel isolated during his illness. Be sensitive to his feelings and allow him to express his fears. Explain the need and rationale for instituting infection control precautions.

Suggested readings

Bone RC, ed. *Pulmonary and critical care medicine.* Vol 2. St Louis, Mo: Mosby–Year Book; 1997.

Bongard FS. *Critical care diagnosis and treatment.* New York, NY: Prentice Hall; 1997.

Greenbaum D. Critical care clinics: management of the AIDS patient in the ICU. 9(1) Philadelphia, Pa: WB Saunders Co; Jan 1993.

Handbook of critical care nursing. Springhouse, Pa: Springhouse Corp; 1996.

Hudak CM, Gallo B. *Critical care nursing: a holistic approach.* Philadelphia, Pa: Lippincott-Raven Pubs; 1994.

Kinney MR, Packa D, Dunbar S. *AACN's clinical reference for critical care nursing.* St Louis, Mo: Mosby–Year Book; 1993.

Long BC, Phipps WJ, Cassmeyer VL. *Medical-surgical nursing: a nursing process approach.* 3rd ed. St Louis, Mo: Mosby–Year Book; 1993.

McCance KL, Huether SE. *Pathophysiology: the biological basis for disease in adults and children.* 2nd ed. St Louis, Mo: Mosby–Year Book; 1994.

Murray JF, Nadel JA. *Textbook of respiratory medicine.* 2nd ed. Philadelphia, Pa: WB Saunders; 1994.

Seidel HM, Dains JE, Ball JW, Benedict W. *Mosby's guide to physical examination.* 3rd ed. St Louis, Mo: Mosby–Year Book; 1995.

Stillwell S. *Mosby's critical care nursing reference.* 2nd ed. St Louis, Mo: Mosby–Year Book; 1996.

Thelan LA, Davies JK, Urden LD, Lough ME. *Critical care nursing: diagnosis and management.* 2nd ed. St Louis, Mo: Mosby–Year Book; 1994.

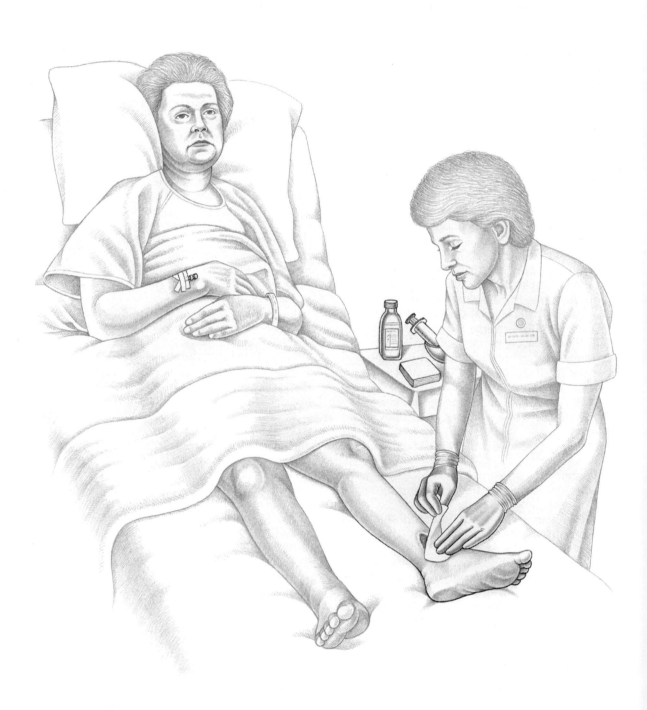

9

Peripheral Vascular Disease

When a patient develops peripheral vascular disease, life-threatening or limb-threatening complications can result. If the patient has chronic peripheral vascular disease, those complications may take years to develop. If she has acute peripheral vascular disease, however, complications can develop in minutes or hours.

Commonly, peripheral vascular disease appears in patients who are elderly and who have other disorders—hypertension or pulmonary embolism, for example. Therefore, caring for a patient with peripheral vascular disease can present quite a nursing challenge, especially when the patient develops multisystem complications, such as cardiogenic shock, respiratory failure, arterial occlusion, and heart failure.

Anatomy and physiology review

By definition, the peripheral vasculature includes all arteries and veins not involved in myocardial circulation. As you know, arteries and veins are distinctly different types of vessels that perform distinctly different functions (see *Major arteries and veins*, pages 292 and 293).

Arteries

Arteries transport oxygenated blood from the heart to the cells. They also circulate blood through the liver and kidneys to remove metabolic wastes. Arteries also help regulate body temperature by directing blood toward or away from the skin surface. Because arteries are innervated by the autonomic nervous system, they constrict and dilate in response to cell and tissue needs.

Arteries can be classified as conductive or distributive. Conductive arteries follow a relatively straight course and have few branches. They include the aorta, the common and external iliac arteries, the common and superficial femoral arteries, and the popliteal arteries. Atherosclerosis tends to affect them most at their points of bifurcation.

Distributive arteries arise from conductive arteries and divide into many branches. They include the internal iliac arteries and the deep femoral arteries. A few arteries have features of both conductive and distributive vessels, such as the anterior and posterior tibial arteries and the peroneal artery.

All arteries consist of three layers: tunica intima, tunica media, and tunica adventitia. The innermost tunica intima has a single layer of endothelial cells that rests on a layer of connective tissue. The tunica media is a relatively thick layer containing smooth-muscle cells, collagen, and elastic fibers. The outermost tunica adventitia contains connective tissue with collagen and some elastic fibers; it provides most of the strength of the arterial wall.

With normal aging, the tunica intima becomes thicker and its collagen content increases, decreasing its elasticity and inhibiting diffusion of nutrients from the arterial lumen. The internal elastic membrane calcifies and degenerates, and smooth-muscle cells in the tunica media degenerate.

Usually, arterial blood flow parallels the vessel walls. It typically becomes turbulent where the arteries branch, curve, narrow, or taper. Arterial blood flow depends on the force with which blood is ejected from the heart, blood viscosity, friction levels against arterial walls, and peripheral vascular resistance.

Veins

The veins carry blood from the capillaries to the right side of the heart and thus are subjected to less pressure from pulsing blood. Consequently, though they consist of the same three layers as the arteries, the layers tend to be thinner. The venous system can accommodate large volumes of blood without experiencing significant pressure changes.

Veins also differ from arteries in that they have internal, one-way valves (see *How venous valves work*). Each valve consists of two thin-walled cusps that arise at opposite sides of the vein wall and overlap in the middle. When pressure above a valve exceeds that below it, it closes, and the overlapping cusps prevent backward blood flow. In general, valves are more numerous and closer together in smaller, more distal veins. Closer to the heart, the veins increase in diameter and wall thickness, decrease in number, and contain fewer valves. For example, the femoral veins contain only a few valves; the vena cava and common iliac veins have none.

Like arteries, veins help to regulate body temperature and blood pressure. Here's how: The superficial veins are richly supplied with sympathetic nerves. In response to cold, for example, the thermoregulatory center in the hypothalamus stimulates these nerves, causing the veins to constrict. This redirects venous blood to the deep veins, thus reducing heat loss.

Pathophysiology

When blood can't flow normally through the arteries and veins, peripheral tissues receive a reduced amount of oxygen and other nutrients. Plus, cellular wastes build up instead of being carried away in the bloodstream.

Any condition that narrows, obstructs, or damages blood vessels can impede blood flow. Common causes include atherosclerosis, cardiac disorders, and hypertension. Smoking contributes as well. Other factors may include injury to the vessel epithelium, hypercoagulability, high cholesterol levels, and prolonged immobility, which promotes venous stasis. Some congenital disorders, such as an arteriovenous fistula and varicose veins, also can impede blood flow. Over time, acute occlusion, ulceration, or gangrene may develop, depending on whether the problem affects arterial or venous circulation.

Arterial problems

When you think of atherosclerosis, you probably think of its effect on the coronary arteries. But it also affects the peripheral arteries. In fact, atherosclerosis—which alters the structure and function of arterial walls and reduces the arterial lumen—is the most common cause of peripheral arterial disease. Atherosclerosis primarily affects the aorta and large and medium arteries, which contain more elastin than smooth muscle. Other peripheral arterial disorders include Raynaud's phenomenon and Buerger's disease.

Venous problems

Normal venous function depends on continuous blood flow, competent valves, and regular contractions of surrounding muscles to help pump blood toward the heart. A problem involving any of these factors can result in peripheral venous disease.

Thrombus formation is the most common cause of obstructed venous blood flow. Usually, a thrombus develops in a deep vein as a result of venous stasis, hypercoagulability, and injury to the endothelial layer of the vessel wall. These three factors are called Virchow's triad; the resulting condition is called deep

 ANATOMY REVIEW

How venous valves work

When muscles around the venous circulation contract, they force blood through one-way valves positioned along the veins. When those muscles relax, the valves close, thus preventing blood from flowing backward.

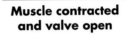

Muscle contracted and valve open **Muscle relaxed and valve closed**

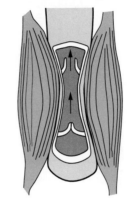 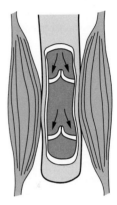

vein thrombosis (DVT). When surrounding tissues become inflamed and the vein wall thickens in response to a thrombus, the condition is called thrombophlebitis. It may occur in superficial or deep veins, usually in the calf.

If a piece of the thrombus breaks off, it will travel in the bloodstream until it becomes lodged in a smaller vessel, possibly in the lung. If a thrombus or embolus blocks peripheral blood flow completely, blood will back up behind the occlusion unless collateral circulation can take over. With complete occlusion, venous pressure increases and fluid can leak into surrounding tissues. Over time, this leakage can cause edema and a brownish skin discoloration. If blood backs up for too long, the patient will develop edema, and possibly gangrene. What's more, formation of a thrombus can destroy the valve cusps.

(Text continues on page 294.)

ANATOMY REVIEW

Major arteries and veins

Use these illustrations to refresh your memory of the major arteries and veins and to compare the structures of the two vessels. Note the extra thickness of arteries, which allows them to withstand higher blood pressures. And note the valves that prevent venous blood from flowing backward.

Major arteries

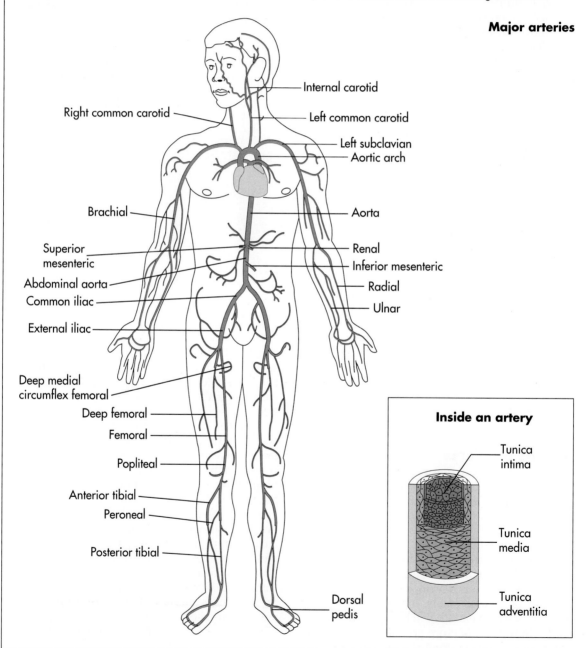

Internal carotid

Right common carotid

Left common carotid

Left subclavian
Aortic arch

Brachial

Aorta

Superior mesenteric

Renal
Inferior mesenteric

Abdominal aorta

Radial

Common iliac

Ulnar

External iliac

Deep medial circumflex femoral

Deep femoral

Femoral

Popliteal

Anterior tibial

Peroneal

Posterior tibial

Dorsal pedis

Inside an artery

Tunica intima

Tunica media

Tunica adventitia

Major veins

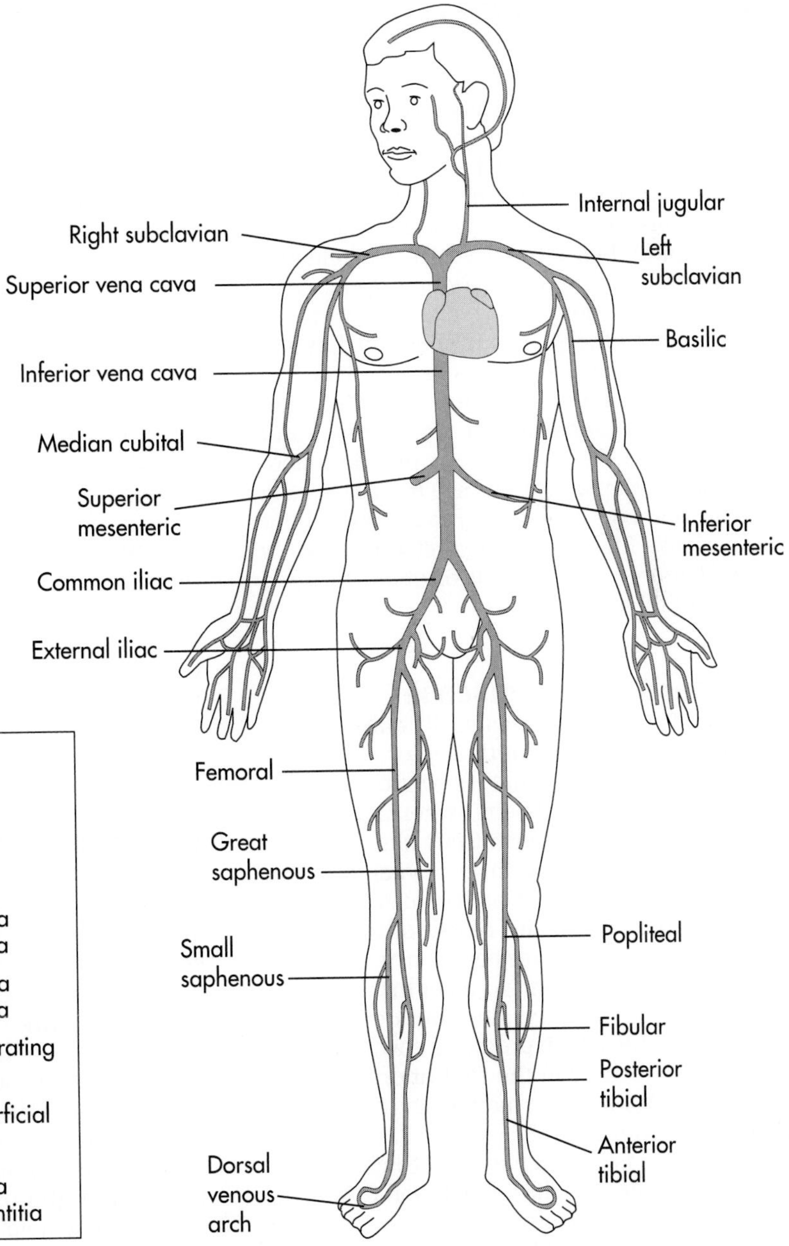

Internal jugular

Right subclavian

Superior vena cava

Left subclavian

Inferior vena cava

Basilic

Median cubital

Superior mesenteric

Inferior mesenteric

Common iliac

External iliac

Femoral

Great saphenous

Small saphenous

Popliteal

Fibular

Posterior tibial

Anterior tibial

Dorsal venous arch

Inside a deep vein

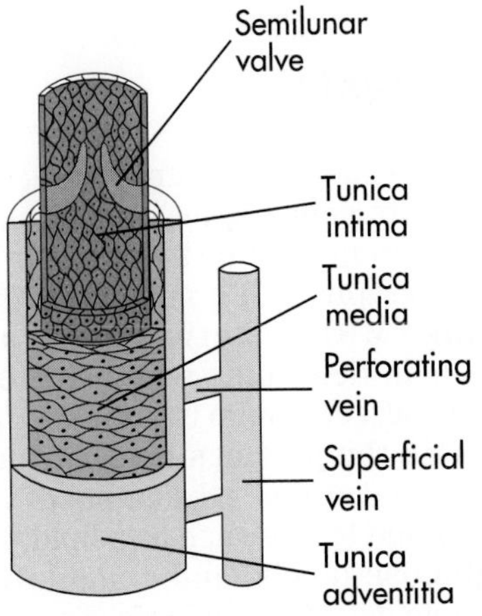

Semilunar valve

Tunica intima

Tunica media

Perforating vein

Superficial vein

Tunica adventitia

Venous valve insufficiency is another common cause of peripheral venous disease. It may result from local injury, inflammation, stretching, or a defective vein wall. Valve insufficiency can occur in patients who stand or sit for prolonged periods of time. It can also result from obesity and pregnancy.

Assessment findings

To accurately assess a patient who may have peripheral vascular disease, start with a thorough health history that covers pertinent risk factors. For example, ask the patient if she has had circulatory problems in the past. If so, ask for a detailed description. Also, find out if she or her family has a history of hypertension, phlebitis, thrombi, pulmonary embolism, cerebrovascular accident (CVA), diabetes, varicose veins, or leg ulcers. Ask if she ever has leg cramps. Find out if her arms or legs ever feel cool and look pale. Ask about her diet, too. Does she eat foods high in cholesterol and sodium? Does she use tobacco or drink alcohol? Ask which medications she uses. Does she take an oral contraceptive? Finally, ask about the patient's lifestyle and exercise routine. Is she sedentary? Must she sit or stand for long periods of time in her job?

Peripheral arterial disease

Peripheral arterial disease usually causes intermittent, cramping pain in the leg or calf. A patient will probably say that it's worse when she walks or exercises and better when she rests—a condition called intermittent claudication, which results from too little oxygen and too much metabolic waste in active muscle tissue.

If the patient complains of calf or leg pain at rest, especially if it wakes her up, arterial blood flow isn't even sufficient to meet her basic tissue needs. Eventually, she may develop ischemic neuritis, which produces severe, shooting pain, especially in the foot and toes. This pain may subside if she moves her leg to a dependent position.

Progressive ischemia may lead to changes in skin color. Pallor results when blood flow is directed to an active muscle and away from the skin. Redness or a reddish blue color indicates reactive hyperemia or capillary and venular responses to anoxia.

You may note that an affected limb feels cool and dry. Over time, the skin may become thin, shiny, and devoid of hair. Toenails may become hard, brittle, thickened, and deformed. And the affected limb may seem thinner and less toned than the unaffected one. You may have trouble palpating peripheral pulses distal to the occlusion. You also may notice a prolonged capillary refill in the affected limb.

Over time, inadequate arterial blood flow without effective collateral circulation can lead to ischemic ulceration and to gangrene and tissue necrosis. With gangrene, the affected area typically is deep purple. When necrosis sets in, the affected area turns black and may eventually shrivel and harden.

Peripheral venous disease

Peripheral venous disease produces more of an aching pain, especially when the limb is dependent. The limb also may become cyanotic. Peripheral pulses usually are normal, although they may be difficult to palpate if the patient's limb is edematous. Skin temperature will probably be normal, or it may be elevated in areas of venous congestion.

In acute venous occlusion, petechiae may develop. In chronic disease and valvular disease, the patient may develop the brown pigmentation of stasis dermatitis around her ankles. Over time, the skin thickens and may eventually ulcerate. Gangrene rarely occurs.

Diagnostic tests

Diagnostic tests—such as the ankle-brachial index, Doppler ultrasonography, duplex ultrasonography, impedance plethysmography, computed tomography (CT), magnetic resonance imaging (MRI), arteriography, and venography—help determine whether blood flow through the affected limb is normal or abnormal, estimate the patient's level of functional limitation, and evaluate the extent of vascular disease. Blood tests—such as a lipid profile, blood glucose levels, and coagulation studies—can help detect possible risk factors.

Ankle-brachial index

The most common test for peripheral arterial disease, the ankle-brachial index compares systolic blood pressure in ankle arteries with systolic blood pressure in the brachial artery. A normal index is 1.0 to 1.2. An index of 0.8 to 1.0 suggests a mild obstruction. An index of 0.5 to 0.8 reveals a moderate obstruction. An index below 0.5 indicates a severe obstruction. And an index below 0.25 indicates severe ischemia and impending gangrene.

Doppler ultrasonography

This test uses high-frequency sound waves to evaluate blood flow directly. As the transducer moves across the skin, sound waves bounce back from red blood cells, producing an audible tone that correlates directly with blood velocity.

Duplex ultrasonography

This highly sensitive test, which uses ultrasound imaging and Doppler ultrasonography, identifies the site of peripheral vascular disease and the extent to which blood flow is compromised. It can evaluate venous blood flow in the legs and detect DVT. It also can assess arterial blood flow and determine the presence, amount, and location of plaques. Plus, it helps determine the cause of claudication.

Impedance plethysmography

Impedance plethysmography measures the change in blood volume that results from a temporary venous occlusion in the calf. A pneumatic cuff is applied to the thigh and electrodes are applied to the calf. Measurements are then taken with the cuff inflated and deflated. These measurements correspond to changes in blood volume that result from decreased circulation distal to the affected area.

Scanning

CT and MRI can show changes in blood vessels and arterial blood flow. In peripheral vascular disease, the tests typically reveal vessel changes, decreased blood flow, decreased perfusion pressure, or obstruction.

Arteriography and venography

During arteriography or venography, a radiologist instills a dye to help visualize the arteries or veins on X-ray film. Vessel wall changes, obstructions, and aneurysms appear, and abnormal blood flow can be identified. Characteristics of arterial circulation proximal and distal to an obstruction can be determined. Venography also detects valvular incompetence.

Medical interventions

Treatments for peripheral vascular disease depend largely on whether the patient has an arterial or a venous disorder. In general, however, interventions include reducing risk factors, prescribing medications, and performing invasive or surgical procedures.

Arterial disease

Initial interventions focus on controlling the disease for as long as possible. They include weight control, smoking cessation, and daily exercise (especially walking) with planned rest periods. Dietary management includes reducing serum lipid levels, if needed, and reducing fat intake to 30% or less of daily calories.

Medications include antiplatelet drugs, such as aspirin and ticlopidine, and anticoagulants, such as warfarin. If an occlusion develops in a critical area, such as the femoral artery, the patient probably will undergo one of these invasive or surgical procedures:

- bypass grafting
- endarterectomy, which involves removing plaque
- balloon angioplasty, in which a balloon opens the lumen by being inflated in the occluded area
- laser angioplasty, in which a laser opens the lumen by destroying the plaque
- atherectomy, in which plaque is stripped away with a specialized catheter

How the Greenfield filter works

The Greenfield filter allows blood to flow relatively freely while still catching emboli before they reach the lungs. Usually, the filter is positioned in the inferior vena cava above the common iliac vein but below the renal vein. Hooks at the ends of the filter's legs hold it in place.

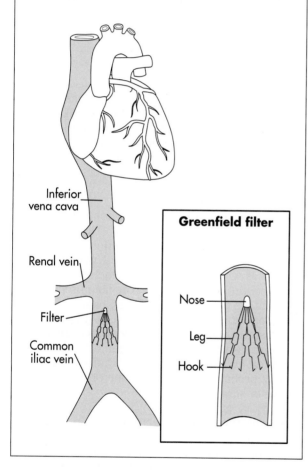

Venous disease

Anticoagulants and thrombolytics are used to treat an acute venous occlusion caused by thromboembolism. Heparin, the most common treatment for venous occlusion, prevents the formation of new thrombi and greatly reduces the risk of pulmonary embolism. Usually, a patient receives heparin I.V. for 5 to 10 days. About 4 to 5 days before the I.V. heparin therapy stops, oral anticoagulant therapy, typically with warfarin, begins. Warfarin then maintains a prolonged anticoagulation state, usually for 3 months. Typically, the physician tries to maintain the patient's international normalized ratio (INR) at 1.5 to 2.0 times the control level.

Thrombolytic drugs—including streptokinase, urokinase, and tissue plasminogen activator—may be used for an acute venous occlusion as well. These drugs actually dissolve thrombi by accelerating the formation of plasmin from plasminogen.

A physician also may prescribe analgesics, bed rest with the affected limb elevated, elastic support stockings, sequential pneumatic compression, and optimal hydration. Bed rest usually lasts 5 to 7 days, so the thrombus has time to adhere to the vein wall rather than embolizing. Then, progressive ambulation can start. To minimize risk factors and prevent venous stasis, the patient should avoid prolonged standing or sitting, avoid wearing constrictive clothing, and, if appropriate, stop smoking, lose weight, and reduce her intake of fat and sodium.

If the patient develops emboli during anticoagulant therapy or if anticoagulant therapy is contraindicated, a surgeon may place a filter in her vena cava to help prevent pulmonary embolism. Usually, it's a Greenfield filter (see *How the Greenfield filter works*). Other indications for a vena cava filter include major trauma, a recent hemorrhage, a recent CVA, gastrointestinal bleeding, and chronic liver disease.

Another option for patients who don't respond to anticoagulants or thrombolytics is a thrombectomy, but thrombosis commonly recurs after this surgery.

- intravascular stent placement, in which a flexible, cagelike device is expanded in the occluded area.

A patient with severe tissue destruction may need to have a limb amputated at the level of well-perfused tissue.

Nursing interventions

When caring for a patient with peripheral vascular disease, your top priorities include promoting

Signs and symptoms of vascular occlusion

Signs and symptoms	Arterial occlusion	Venous occlusion
Pain	• Sudden, excruciating, constant pain in affected limb	• Sharp, constant, localized pain
Related complaints	• Paresthesia of affected limb	• Feeling of fullness in affected limb
Skin color	• Pale, then mottled	• Slight reddening
Skin temperature	• Affected limb becomes cool to touch	• Slight increase in limb temperature
Other findings	• No pulses in affected limb • Paralysis of affected limb	• Edema of affected limb • Venous pattern becomes more prominent in affected limb

tissue oxygenation, maintaining skin integrity, and teaching the patient how to manage her condition at home.

Promoting tissue oxygenation

If the patient has arterial occlusive disease, place her legs in a slightly dependent position, so gravity can enhance tissue perfusion. Minimize pressure on the legs. Check her peripheral pulses (using a Doppler device, if necessary) and the color and temperature of her skin at least every 4 hours. Also, check capillary refill. Normally, it's 3 seconds or less. Keep in mind, however, that environmental factors can alter it. Report changes in pulses, color, and temperature to the physician right away; a sudden change could warn of an acute occlusion that needs immediate attention (see *Signs and symptoms of vascular occlusion*).

If your patient has venous disease, raise her legs above the level of her heart when she's lying down or sitting, except during mealtimes. Avoid flexing her knees or hips, however, to keep venous blood from pooling below her waist. You can raise the foot of her bed, but be sure the head stays flat. You can also use pillows to help support the affected limb. Keep antiembolism stockings on the patient while she's awake to promote venous return and decrease leg swelling. Dorsiflex her foot; if she feels calf pain, she has a positive Homans' sign. Although not conclusive, a positive Homans' sign may indicate thrombophlebitis.

If the patient has edema, check for pitting. Also, measure calf circumference for each leg and compare your findings. Make sure you mark the place where you measured, so you can repeat the measurements later.

Ask the patient if her affected limb feels cold, numb, or tingly. Encourage her to tell you about any pain she feels, including its type, location, severity, onset, and duration. Ask too what relieves the pain. Note any changes in her pain.

Administer anticoagulant and thrombolytic therapy, as prescribed. Monitor the patient's coagulation studies closely to evaluate the effectiveness of the therapy. Watch for signs of bleeding, including bruising, petechiae, and frank or occult blood in the stool, urine, vomitus, or saliva.

If possible, perform active and passive range-of-motion (ROM) exercises to improve circulation. Also, encourage the patient to walk, as tolerated. Increase her exercise levels gradually. Obtain a physical therapy consult to help plan an appropriate exercise regimen.

Maintaining skin integrity

Because patients with peripheral vascular disease face an increased risk of skin breakdown,

Characteristics of leg ulcers

Arterial and venous leg ulcers have different characteristics, as this table shows.

Characteristic	Arterial (ischemic) ulcer	Venous (stasis) ulcer
Onset	• May be spontaneous, but ulcer usually results from pressure or slight trauma	• May be spontaneous or ulcer may result from trauma • Commonly follows deep vein thrombosis
Location	• Toe, heel, dorsum of foot • Common over bony prominences	• Common around ankles, especially medial malleoli
Pain	• Severe, worst at night • Relieved by dangling leg	• Mild when patient walks or ulcer is infected • Relieved by elevation
Surrounding skin	• Atrophic • Cool or cold to touch • Gangrene may develop	• Dry and scaly, possibly leathery • Stasis dermatitis, including ankle edema, brown pigmentation, patchy erythema, petechiae, and induration
Appearance of ulcer	• Deep, punched-out look • Pale base, possibly with eschar • Little granulation tissue • Even, definite edge	• Superficial • Broad and flat • Pink base • Granulation tissue • Uneven edge

inspect the skin for redness and irritation at least every 8 hours. Keep the room warm and humidified to help prevent vasoconstriction and dry, cracked skin. And pad any affected areas of the skin.

To bathe the patient, use tepid water and neutral soap. Wash the skin gently; don't rub or scratch. Then pat the skin to dry it. Avoid using alcohol because of its drying effect. Instead, use lotions or emollients. Also, consider adding oil to the bath water.

Keep in mind that decreased circulation decreases the patient's ability to feel, so she may not sense a developing problem or injury. Assess her sensory function, comparing one limb to the other. Provide frequent, meticulous foot care, and urge the patient to wear cotton socks and well-fitted footwear when out of bed.

Unfortunately, even with the best care, a patient may develop a vascular ulcer. If she does, document its location, size, characteristics, and drainage (see *Characteristics of leg ulcers*).

Ulcer treatment may include wet-to-dry saline dressings, bed rest, topical or systemic antibiotics, and immobilization of the limb. Each time you perform wound care, document the size and appearance of the ulcer, the color and amount of drainage, and any changes. Monitor the patient's vital signs. In particular, be alert for fever, which may signal an infection. Obtain a wound culture, as indicated.

Immobilizing the limb minimizes oxygen demands and preserves new tissue growth. Bed rest also helps decrease the limb's metabolic demands. However, you should perform ROM exercises with the unaffected limb, as tolerated.

Patient teaching
Before the patient goes home, you'll need to provide teaching aimed at helping her minimize the risk of problems. For example, if the

patient smokes, help her to stop. Explain that smoking is strongly related to vascular problems. Tell her that nicotine constricts her vessels and that the carbon monoxide in smoke reduces the blood's ability to carry oxygen.

Urge the patient to inspect her legs and feet every day and to care for her feet properly. Warn her to avoid constrictive clothing, such as tight knee-high stockings or boots, girdles, or tight pantyhose or waistbands.

Show the patient how to use antiembolism stockings (see *When your patient needs antiembolism stockings*, page 300). Tell her not to sit or stand for long periods of time and to avoid crossing her legs. Also, tell her to avoid exposure to cold temperatures.

Review the patient's diet plan, emphasizing the appropriate cholesterol, fat, caffeine, and sodium restrictions. Enlist the aid of a dietitian to help with meal planning and food selection.

If the patient will be using heparin at home, show her how to prepare and inject it. If she'll be taking warfarin, tell her to eat consistent amounts of foods that are high in vitamin K. Emphasize that ingesting too much vitamin K may reduce the effectiveness of her warfarin. Reinforce the need for safety measures to prevent bleeding. And review with her the signs and symptoms of bleeding that she should watch for. Also, urge the patient to keep follow-up appointments to check the effectiveness of her therapy.

If the patient needs wound care, show her and her caregiver what to do. Emphasize that they must use aseptic technique, and make sure they're familiar with the signs and symptoms of infection. If necessary, obtain a home care referral for follow-up and evaluation.

Peripheral vascular disease and pulmonary embolism

An acute, possibly life-threatening disorder, pulmonary embolism typically occurs when a piece of a thrombus detaches from a deep leg vein, floats into the pulmonary circulation, and partially or completely obstructs the pulmonary artery or one of its branches.

Pathophysiology

In peripheral vascular disease, a thrombus may form in a deep vein because of venous stasis, hypercoagulability, and injury to the endothelial layer of the vessel wall. Inflammation and vein wall thickening may lead to thrombophlebitis. If a piece of a thrombus breaks off, it may travel in the bloodstream until it becomes lodged. When it lodges in the pulmonary circulation, blood flow is obstructed to some portion of a lung. The injury draws platelets, which release vasoactive substances, causing vasoconstriction. Histamine, serotonin, and prostaglandins are also released, resulting in bronchoconstriction. These substances are largely responsible for the increase in pulmonary vascular resistance.

If the obstruction persists, vasoconstriction and bronchoconstriction act together to produce a ventilation-perfusion imbalance. Typically, ventilation is adequate but perfusion isn't, an imbalance that eventually leads to hypoxemia. In an attempt to compensate for this imbalance, the patient typically breathes faster, which blows off carbon dioxide and worsens the bronchoconstriction and vasoconstriction.

The hemodynamic consequences of pulmonary embolism can be severe. Decreased arterial blood flow through the lungs causes pulmonary pressures to rise, which may cause right ventricular hypertrophy and failure. Cardiac output eventually decreases from right ventricular failure and decreased left ventricular preload. Systemic hypotension and shock typically follow. Occasionally, the embolus may lead to pulmonary infarction, which can cause lung-tissue necrosis, infection, and abscess formation.

Adapting nursing care

Ideally, your nursing care should focus on prevention. If your patient has peripheral venous disease, check her frequently for unilateral

When your patient needs antiembolism stockings

For patients with increased venous leg pressure, antiembolism stockings can reduce discomfort by compressing distended veins and preventing blood pooling. The stockings also help prevent tiny tears in the vein walls that can result from overdistention.

To get the maximum benefit from these stockings, a patient must wear them correctly.

Making measurements

Stockings that are too tight or too loose can do more harm than good, so be sure to assess your patient's legs carefully before choosing a size. Measure the patient's leg circumference at the ankle and the calf. Also, measure from the bottom of her foot to 1 inch below the knee (for knee-high stockings) or 1 inch below the groin (for thigh-high stockings).

For most patients, you'll use knee-high stockings because they're more comfortable and less expensive, and they prevent deep vein thrombosis as well as the thigh-high version. Plus, stockings that reach above the knee can bind the popliteal space and act as a tourniquet, especially when the patient bends her knee.

Remember to remeasure leg sizes if the patient gains or loses weight or if edema increases or decreases.

Applying the stockings

Apply the stockings by walking them up the legs, and teach your patient to do the same. Use a little powder, if necessary, to ease the process. Teach the patient not to pull antiembolism stockings onto her legs because she'll create too much friction and shear.

When the stockings are in place, make sure the heels and gussets stay in their proper positions. If the heel migrates above or below its intended spot, the stockings' pressure gradient could change.

Wearing the stockings

Urge the patient not to sit or stand for long periods of time because doing so will increase pressure in the small blood vessels of her legs, possibly worsening swelling. When the patient sits, make sure her legs are elevated to promote venous blood return.

Urge the patient to wear her stockings every time she gets up to walk. Explain that the elastic compression can help return venous blood to her heart while minimizing venous pressure in her legs.

Be sure the patient knows how long to wear the stockings. Usually, the physician will prescribe them for the entire hospitalization and then for 6 to 8 weeks after discharge. Some patients need the stockings permanently. Others wear them only at night.

Some patients remove their stockings for significant periods of time because they think the skin needs to breathe. Warn your patient not to do that. Explain that removing the stockings for too long reduces their effectiveness. Be sure to teach your patient how often she should assess her skin and which signs she should look for.

Performing ongoing care

Remove the patient's stockings every 8 hours to assess the skin, especially the heels and ankles, and provide skin care. Then reapply the stockings and document your findings. If your patient has signs or symptoms of tissue damage, you may need to inspect the skin more frequently. Don't massage reddened skin areas because you could increase the tissue damage.

Teach your patient to keep her stockings clean by washing and drying them together with other light clothing items. Warn her not to wash the stockings in water that exceeds 160° F (71° C) or dry them at temperatures over 250° F (121° C). Advise her not to use excessive amounts of bleach.

edema, pain, deep or generalized muscle tenderness, a low-grade fever, cyanosis of an arm or leg, or vein distention. If she's bedridden or recovering from surgery, urge her to perform deep-breathing exercises to increase ventilation and promote venous return. Also, help her walk as soon as possible. When she's sitting up, advise her to sit so the balls of her feet can touch the floor. That way, she won't put excess pressure on her popliteal spaces by dangling her legs.

Using sequential compression therapy

A physician may order sequential compression therapy as one way to prevent deep vein thrombosis (DVT), possibly in addition to using antiembolism stockings. The idea is simple: Cuffs wrapped around the patient's legs inflate and deflate repeatedly. With each inflation, they push venous blood out of the legs and toward the patient's heart.

Contraindications

If your patient has DVT or has had it in the last 6 months, a physician won't order sequential compression therapy because it can break up a thrombus, creating emboli. Also, a physician should avoid sequential compression therapy if your patient has any of these conditions:
• severe atherosclerosis
• ischemic vascular disease
• massive leg edema
• significant leg injury
• dermatitis
• gangrene
• a recent skin graft.

Using the device

Start by explaining the device—and the concept behind it—to the patient and his family. Then measure the patient's upper thigh circumference to determine the appropriate cuff size. As you're measuring,

inspect the skin for swelling, redness, irritation, and breakdown. If you note skin problems, notify the physician.

Check the lower legs for color, temperature, capillary refill, and pedal pulses. If you have trouble palpating pulses, use a Doppler ultrasound device and mark the site with a permanent marker, so you can listen at the same place next time.

Apply antiembolism stockings, if indicated. Then apply the compression sleeves. To do so, start by placing each leg on a sleeve. Make sure the back of the knee aligns with the popliteal opening, and the back of the ankle aligns with the ankle mark. Then, wrap a sleeve snugly around each leg and fasten the sleeve.

Double-check the tightness of the sleeves. You should be able to fit two fingers between the sleeve and the patient's leg.

Connect each sleeve to the tubing of the controller and operate the device according to the instructions.

Check skin color, temperature, pulses, and capillary refill at least every 2 hours. Evaluate the patient for pain and swelling. Check the skin around the sleeve edges and under the sleeve every shift. If you find problems, stop the compression therapy and notify the physician right away.

If you need to raise the patient's lower legs or feet, raise the whole leg rather than bending her knees. Use elastic support stockings or, if appropriate, sequential pneumatic compression (see *Using sequential compression therapy*). Remember that compression sleeves can be cumbersome and uncomfortable; be sure you explain their purpose and benefits to the patient.

If pulmonary embolism develops despite your preventive efforts, your nursing care may consist of administering drug therapy, promoting oxygenation, and providing postoperative care. Also, of course, you'll need to teach the patient to take steps to prevent a recurrence (see *Patient teaching after pulmonary embolism*, page 302).

Medications

If the patient needs thrombolytic therapy, obtain baseline coagulation studies, as ordered, and watch for signs and symptoms of bleeding.

Give the prescribed anticoagulant, such as low-dose, subcutaneous heparin two to three times a day or warfarin daily. Be sure to monitor the patient's platelet count, prothrombin time (PT), activated partial thromboplastin time (APTT), and INR.

Also, give prescribed antiplatelet drugs, such as aspirin or dipyridamole. Aspirin works against platelet aggregation by inhibiting the release of adenosine diphosphate (ADP) from platelets and by blocking the adhesion of platelets to collagen fibers. It also helps avoid DVT by blocking the adhesion of platelets to

GOING HOME

Patient teaching after pulmonary embolism

After your patient with peripheral vascular disease has recovered from pulmonary embolism, you'll need to teach her how to care for herself at home and how to reduce her risk of a recurrence.

Venous return
- Urge your patient to avoid sitting or standing for long periods of time, crossing her legs, and wearing constrictive clothing.
- Stress the need for a regular exercise program. Walking is one of the easiest and best ways to promote venous return. Also, suggest ankle flexion, extension, and rotation exercises, which contract the leg muscles and enhance venous return.
- Encourage her to wear antiembolism stockings. Make sure she has the right size and knows how to put them on properly. Tell her not to roll the tops down because doing so reduces venous flow.

Skin care
- Tell the patient to inspect her legs and feet for redness, irritation, and breakdown every day.
- Advise her to use lotions and emollients to prevent dry, cracked skin.
- Suggest that she wear cotton clothing and socks to allow perspiration to evaporate.
- Tell her to wear properly fitted shoes and to avoid going barefoot.

Drug therapy
- Review the patient's drugs and their adverse effects. If she goes home taking an anticoagulant, make sure she knows how and when to take it. Suggest that she take it at the same time every day to help maintain her blood levels.
- Teach safety measures to help her reduce her risk of bleeding. For example, tell her to use a soft toothbrush and an electric razor.
- Urge her to keep follow-up laboratory appointments to evaluate her anticoagulation status.

Other precautions
- Encourage her to wear a medical alert bracelet or carry an identification card in case of emergency.
- Tell her to report signs and symptoms of deep vein thrombosis right away. They include leg swelling, pain or tenderness in a calf or thigh, cramping, local warmth, changes in skin color, a heavy feeling in the leg, one leg that's bigger than the other, and fever.
- Tell her to report signs and symptoms of pulmonary embolism immediately. They include shortness of breath, sudden chest pain with breathing, abnormally rapid breathing, coughing, coughing up blood, sweating, and a feeling of apprehension or doom.

---

the fibrin mesh. A single dose of aspirin can alter platelet function for 7 days. Dipyridamole also inhibits the release of ADP.

Finally, give dextran, as prescribed. This volume expander interferes with clotting in several ways. It coats the surface of platelets and blocks the platelet-phospholipid coagulation factor. It also coats the inner surfaces of blood vessels and decreases surface contact with coagulation factors. The resulting increased fluid volume in the vascular space decreases blood viscosity and increases venous return. Be sure to monitor the patient for adverse effects of dextran therapy, including fluid overload, sensitivity reactions, and renal failure.

Oxygenation
If possible, raise the head of the bed to promote chest expansion. Give supplemental oxygen by nasal cannula or face mask to help decrease hypoxemia. Monitor oxygen saturation levels with pulse oximetry and arterial blood gas (ABG) measurements. If oxygen saturation continues to fall, anticipate endotracheal (ET) intubation and mechanical ventilation.

Assess the patient's vital signs at least hourly, including her respiratory rate, heart rate, and blood pressure. Anticipate the insertion of a central venous or pulmonary artery catheter to evaluate the patient's hemodynamic status.

Administer the prescribed analgesic and sedative to help reduce the patient's anxiety and discomfort. These drugs not only decrease the respiratory rate, but also ease vasoconstriction and bronchoconstriction.

Postoperative care

If anticoagulant or thrombolytic therapy isn't effective, a patient may need an embolectomy or vena cava filter. Indications for pulmonary embolectomy include massive emboli documented by an arteriogram, hemodynamic instability despite maximal resuscitation and anticoagulant therapy, a failure of thrombolytic therapy, or a contraindication to thrombolytic therapy.

After an embolectomy, monitor the patient for bleeding and signs and symptoms of emboli distal to the embolectomy. Monitor her vital signs, skin color, capillary refill, temperature, and peripheral pulses. Closely monitor her respiratory status and encourage her to use incentive spirometry to enhance ventilation and gas exchange.

If your patient receives a vena cava filter, monitor the femoral vein insertion site for bleeding. Watch for complications, such as recurrent pulmonary emboli, venous insufficiency, air embolism, and migration of the filter.

Complications

Common complications for patients with peripheral vascular disease and pulmonary embolism include cardiogenic shock and respiratory failure.

Cardiogenic shock

Cardiogenic shock, the main cause of death in patients with pulmonary embolism, results from a failure of the right ventricle. This happens when pulmonary artery occlusion and the subsequent vasoconstriction and bronchoconstriction reduce the available pulmonary vascular surface for gas exchange. Pulmonary vascular resistance rises, causing right ventricular afterload to increase. In response, right ventricular wall tension and myocardial oxygen consumption increase in an attempt to overcome the pulmonary vascular resistance. Right atrial and ventricular pressures rise, and right ventricular

heart failure develops. Cardiac output drops and blood backs up into the systemic circulation. Consequently, the patient develops profound hypotension and shock.

Confirming the complication

A patient with pulmonary embolism resulting from peripheral vascular disease and DVT may have a painful, red, warm area on her leg, indicating phlebitis. She'll also probably have signs and symptoms typical of pulmonary embolism, such as acute dyspnea and chest pain.

Keep in mind, however, that cardiogenic shock typically results from massive pulmonary emboli. Therefore, assess the patient's chest pain carefully. In many cases, it's severe, similar to the pain of angina pectoris or a dissecting thoracic aortic aneurysm. In fact, the patient may have anginal pain in addition to pleuritic pain because of the right ventricular ischemia. As pulmonary hypertension and right ventricular failure develop, the patient may develop tachycardia, a more intense S_2 heart sound, syncope, jugular vein distention, an S_3 and S_4 gallop, and a paradoxical pulse.

A 12-lead electrocardiogram (ECG) may reveal arrhythmias and signs of right ventricular strain, such as right axis deviation, tall peaked T waves, and ST-segment changes. ABG studies reveal hypoxemia and, as shock progresses, metabolic acidosis.

As shock continues, the patient may develop hypotension, cyanosis, diminished peripheral pulses, a sense of impending doom, diaphoresis, decreased urine output, and a decreased level of consciousness (LOC). If she has a pulmonary artery catheter, you'll see her cardiac output and cardiac index drop, usually abruptly, and her pulmonary vascular resistance rise. She may develop sudden cardiopulmonary arrest, usually from arrhythmias, such as severe bradycardia and electromechanical dissociation. Efforts to resuscitate the patient at this stage typically are unsuccessful because the right ventricle can't overcome pulmonary vascular resistance and maintain peripheral perfusion.

Nursing interventions

RAPID RESPONSE ▸ The focus of nursing care is to swiftly stabilize the patient's hemodynamic status and correct her ventilation-perfusion mismatch. Take the following steps:

- Assess the patient's vital signs and other hemodynamic measurements.
- If a pulmonary artery catheter isn't in place, anticipate its insertion. After it's inserted, assess the readings and their trends, particularly pulmonary artery pressures, cardiac output, cardiac index, and pulmonary vascular resistance.
- Begin continuous cardiac monitoring and evaluate the ECG waveforms for changes. Watch for life-threatening arrhythmias, such as ventricular tachycardia, and prepare to intervene with cardioversion. Restoring a normal sinus rhythm may correct the patient's shock.
- Give supplemental oxygen, as prescribed.
- If the patient's respiratory status declines and hypoxia develops, prepare for ET intubation and mechanical ventilation.
- Monitor oxygen saturation levels continuously with pulse oximetry and serial ABG studies, as indicated.
- If the patient has metabolic acidosis, give sodium bicarbonate I.V., as prescribed.
- If the patient is hypotensive, doesn't have pulmonary edema, and does have right ventricular failure, prepare to give the prescribed I.V. fluid challenges. Giving such fluids helps increase right ventricular end-diastolic pressure and helps the right ventricle overcome increased pulmonary vascular resistance.
- If shock persists despite adequate cardiac filling pressures, give the prescribed systemic arterial vasoconstrictor, such as epinephrine, to raise the patient's blood pressure and combat shock.
- If the patient isn't hypotensive, give morphine sulfate, as prescribed, for acute chest pain and anxiety. Morphine also dilates coronary arteries, thus improving myocardial circulation and oxygenation. ◄

A patient with cardiogenic shock from massive pulmonary emboli may respond favorably to prompt treatment. However, if treatment is unsuccessful, the patient may require further intervention, such as thrombolytic therapy or pulmonary embolectomy.

Respiratory failure

A patient who develops pulmonary embolism from peripheral vascular disease and DVT faces a high risk of respiratory failure—a complication that results when the lungs can't meet the body's oxygen needs because of a lack of perfusion, ventilation, or both.

Because the embolus blocks blood flow to some alveoli, they can't take part in gas exchange even though air can fill them. Oxygen diffuses across the alveolocapillary membrane, but sits in the capillary—a dead-space area. Consequently, ventilation may be normal, but perfusion isn't, creating a ventilation-perfusion mismatch.

Also, alveoli tend to collapse in areas of lung tissue not blocked by the embolus. That's because the chemicals released by bronchoconstriction—such as histamine, serotonin, and prostaglandins—reduce alveolar surfactant, which decreases surface tension and causes alveoli to collapse. This leads to a loss of ventilation in the collapsed area. Thus, even if perfusion is normal, ventilation is not.

Eventually, if a ventilation-perfusion mismatch isn't corrected, hypoxemia and hypercapnia develop, and respiratory failure ensues.

Confirming the complication

Signs and symptoms of respiratory failure include severe dyspnea, orthopnea, anxiety, restlessness, tachycardia, confusion, and pale or ashen skin. Because some of these signs, such as anxiety, may accompany pulmonary embolism, you'll need to monitor your patient's respiratory status carefully to determine if she's developing respiratory failure.

The results of ABG studies help confirm the diagnosis by revealing profound hypoxemia. Typically, partial pressure of arterial oxygen (PaO_2) levels are below 50 mm Hg, partial pressure of arterial carbon dioxide ($PaCO_2$) levels exceed 50 mm Hg, pH is below 7.35, and oxygen saturation is below 90%. As hypoxemia and respiratory failure progress, the patient may lose consciousness.

Nursing interventions

RAPID RESPONSE ► If you suspect that your patient is developing respiratory failure, you'll need to intervene quickly. Take these steps to help normalize gas exchange and minimize ventilation-perfusion mismatching:

- If the patient's blood pressure is stable, sit her in an upright position to promote lung expansion.
- Monitor oxygen saturation levels continuously, using pulse oximetry and ABG studies, as indicated.
- Begin continuous cardiac monitoring and evaluate the patient's ECG for arrhythmias, especially life-threatening ventricular arrhythmias. Also, watch for signs of ischemic changes.
- Monitor the patient's vital signs and check for indications that her condition is worsening, such as hypotension, decreasing heart and respiratory rates, decreasing respiratory effort, and decreasing LOC.
- Give supplemental oxygen, as indicated. If the patient can't maintain optimal Pao_2 or $Paco_2$ levels despite receiving supplemental oxygen, prepare for ET intubation and mechanical ventilation.
- Prepare for the insertion of a central venous catheter or pulmonary artery catheter if one isn't already in place. ◂

As you care for the patient, be sure to explain to her what you're doing and why you're doing it. She's probably extremely anxious, and anxiety further interferes with adequate ventilation. Provide support and stay calm. Try to minimize distractions. And urge the patient to take slow deep breaths to improve ventilation and to relax. Be sure to include the patient's family in your care.

After the patient's condition stabilizes, review all aspects of the treatment plan for her peripheral vascular disease. Stress the importance of sticking to the plan to prevent a recurrence of respiratory failure.

Peripheral vascular disease and hypertension

The high-pressure blood flow characteristic of hypertension can damage vessel walls. And, of course, peripheral vascular disease, especially atherosclerotic peripheral vascular disease, damages vessel walls as well. Consequently, a patient with both atherosclerotic peripheral vascular disease and hypertension faces an increased risk of complications from both conditions—and an increased risk that complications will develop more quickly.

Pathophysiology

In hypertension, prolonged vasoconstriction and increased arterial pressures cause the smooth-muscle cells of the tunica media and tunica intima to enlarge and multiply. Eventually these overcrowded cells narrow the arterial lumen.

In atherosclerosis, the endothelial lining of the artery is disrupted, and plasma proteins move into the tunica intima, causing plaques to develop. Later, the lipid-rich plaques calcify, ulcerate, and form thrombi. Eventually, the arterial wall weakens and the plaque ruptures, possibly leading to a partial or complete occlusion of the affected artery.

When a patient has hypertension, atherosclerotic plaques progress more rapidly because of the increased pressure against the endothelial cells of the arterial wall. The increased pressure increases endothelial permeability, leading to increased cholesterol uptake and increased platelet adhesion. This, in turn, releases growth factors that further promote the proliferation of smooth-muscle cells.

Adapting nursing care

Throughout the patient's care, monitor her blood pressure and other vital signs carefully. Take readings with the patient lying down, sitting up, and standing up. Note any changes in blood pressure of 10 mm Hg or more, which indicate orthostatic hypotension.

Administer antihypertensive medications, as prescribed. Typically, a physician will prescribe a beta blocker, an alpha blocker, a peripherally acting adrenergic blocker, a vasodilator, an angiotensin-converting enzyme (ACE) inhibitor, or a calcium channel blocker.

Some patients may need more than one of these drugs to achieve the desired effect.

A physician also may prescribe an antiplatelet drug, such as aspirin or ticlopidine, to prevent arterial thrombus formation. If the patient has hyperlipidemia, the physician is likely to prescribe an antilipemic as well, such as gemfibrozil, cholestyramine, or lovastatin.

Continue measures to enhance the patient's peripheral perfusion. Encourage frequent position changes while the patient is in bed. Urge her to walk, as tolerated. But monitor her for complaints of dizziness or light-headedness when she gets out of bed. Keep in mind that many antihypertensive drugs cause orthostatic hypotension. Advise the patient to dangle her legs before she gets out of bed and to change positions slowly.

Be sure to inspect the patient's arms and legs for changes in color, temperature, and pulses. Watch for complaints of increased pain, paresthesia, or decreased movement.

During your assessment, find out if the patient was ever diagnosed with hypertension before. If so, find out how it was treated, whether it responded, and whether the patient complied with her regimen. Whether she has been diagnosed before or not, assess her knowledge of hypertension and the prescribed treatment. Make sure she understands the importance of controlling her weight, quitting smoking, limiting her alcohol intake, and exercising as well as taking her prescribed medications. Also, note her willingness and ability to comply.

Weight control

Explain to the patient that even a minor weight loss can reduce blood pressure and promote tissue perfusion, especially if the patient has venous valve disease. Help her set up an appropriate diet and exercise program. Outline a low-fat, low-cholesterol, low-sodium diet, as prescribed, and give the patient a specific daily calorie allotment. Enlist the aid of a dietitian for meal planning, as necessary.

Smoking cessation

If your patient smokes, urge her to stop. Refer her to support groups or community programs to help her stop smoking. And, if appropriate, discuss with her physician the advisability of a transdermal nicotine patch. Remember, however, that nicotine patches may be contraindicated for a patient with peripheral vascular disease and hypertension. That's because a patient receives nicotine from a patch, even though she isn't smoking.

Alcohol limitation

If your patient drinks too much alcohol, talk with her about its dangers. Tell her that it increases her heart rate and blood pressure and interferes with the metabolism of many antihypertensive and anticoagulant medications. Provide counseling and support group information.

Exercise

Consult with the physician and a physical therapist to create a helpful exercise program for your patient. Explain that she should start slowly and build her tolerance gradually. Tell her to rest if she begins to feel pain in her calf (intermittent claudication). Also, mention that the proper footwear and clothing can help prevent skin irritation and injury.

Self-care

Before discharge, make sure the patient understands the treatment plan. Review all medications, including the name, dosage, and possible adverse effects.

Review the signs and symptoms of complications, including increased pain, changes in the appearance of any wound, and changes in the color, temperature, and size of the limbs. Reinforce the need for follow-up appointments with the physician to evaluate blood pressure and vascular status. If appropriate, teach the patient how to monitor her blood pressure at home. Obtain a referral for home follow-up to help promote compliance and provide postdischarge education and assessment.

Complications

Common complications for patients with peripheral vascular disease and hypertension include arterial occlusion and heart failure.

Arterial occlusion

Because peripheral vascular disease and hypertension raise the risk of vascular damage, they also raise the risk of arterial occlusion. It can be a chronic narrowing or an acute obstruction. Usually, it affects the legs.

Confirming the complication

A patient with chronic arterial occlusion typically complains of tightening pressure or a sharp, cramping sensation in the calves, thighs, or gluteal muscles. At first, this symptom occurs while walking and disappears within a minute or two of rest. Over time, the pain appears with less and less exertion. Eventually, it occurs even at rest. It may awaken the patient from sleep because lying supine decreases blood flow and increases ischemic pain. Dangling a foot over the side of the bed or getting up to walk around may make the pain go away. The patient also may experience a dull aching in the toes or forefoot from nerve ischemia.

With an acute occlusion, the patient typically has pain, pallor, pulselessness, paresthesia, and paralysis in the affected limb. The limb feels cool or cold. Muscle necrosis may develop within 2 to 3 hours after the occlusion. Complete paralysis, with stiff muscles and joints, indicates irreversible damage.

To confirm arterial occlusion, a physician may order Doppler ultrasonography and plethysmography, digital subtraction angiography, or segmental limb pressures and pulse volume measurements.

Nursing interventions

For a patient with peripheral vascular disease and hypertension who develops a chronic arterial occlusion, you'll need to focus on maximizing tissue perfusion and controlling blood pressure. Carefully assess the patient's blood pressure and peripheral pulses. Measure arterial blood pressure in the legs with a Doppler ultrasound device.

Also, take steps to promote skin integrity, prevent infection, relieve pain, and reduce the risk of injury. Keep the skin clean, dry, and free from pressure. If the patient has a leg ulcer from diminished arterial blood flow, evaluate the tissue around it for edema, capillary refill, pallor, dependent rubor, and skin temperature. Anticipate the need for dressing changes and wound debridement.

RAPID RESPONSE ▶ If the patient has an acute arterial occlusion, act swiftly:

- Place the patient on bed rest and protect the affected limb from pressure and trauma.
- Closely assess the limb for further deterioration, such as stiffening muscles and joints. These signs may indicate the need for surgery, such as an embolectomy, to prevent further damage.
- Begin thrombolytic or anticoagulant therapy, as prescribed. Anticoagulant therapy may begin with heparin; later, the patient may receive an oral anticoagulant, such as warfarin. During therapy, monitor the patient's PT, APTT, and INR.
- Watch for indications of hemorrhage, including hematuria, epistaxis, bruising, petechiae, hematoma, and bleeding from the gums or rectum.
- Continue to assess the patient's condition frequently and report any significant changes. ◀

If the patient undergoes surgery, such as an embolectomy for an acute arterial occlusion or peripheral revascularization for a chronic occlusion, provide routine postoperative care and closely monitor her blood pressure. Anticipate the need for I.V. antihypertensive therapy if the patient is allowed nothing by mouth or if her blood pressure is difficult to control. Remember that the stress of surgery, fluid volume replacement, and anesthetics can disrupt blood pressure control.

After revascularization surgery, check pedal pulses at least every hour for the first 24 hours, then at least every 4 hours, as indicated. Evaluate sensory and motor function, capillary refill, temperature, and color. Compare your findings bilaterally. Report any bleeding immediately.

If the patient develops irreversible damage and she's scheduled for amputation, prepare her for surgery, as indicated. Do your best to prepare her physiologically and psychologically and to provide support and comfort (see *Helping your patient adjust to amputation,* page 308).

COMFORT MEASURES

Helping your patient adjust to amputation

When a patient with peripheral vascular disease and hypertension develops an arterial occlusion, she may require a limb amputation. Why? Primarily because of the unrelenting pain from ischemia, necrosis, or gangrene. In fact, she may have such severe burning pain in her toes and forefoot that it wakes her up, leading eventually to sleeplessness, exhaustion, a lack of appetite, and debilitation.

If your patient is scheduled for an amputation, she'll naturally be anxious and upset, despite the prospect of relief from this severe pain. In addition to providing sound physical care, you'll need to respond to her psychological needs as well.

Before surgery

Throughout the preoperative period, maintain a calm voice and demeanor. By doing so, you'll soothe the patient and help her control her anxiety.

Help manage the patient's pain by keeping her affected limb in a slightly dependent position. Elevating the limb will make the pain worse.

Reducing pain and stress helps control blood pressure, so carefully assess your patient's need for a sedative or anxiolytic agent. Also, assess the effectiveness of her antihypertensive therapy.

Support the patient and her family through the decision-making process. Encourage the patient to talk about her fears over losing her limb. Talk with her about her ability to walk after the surgery, and help her figure out how to manage daily functions. Remember that the patient may feel guilty or angry if she didn't comply with her prescribed therapy.

Even though the patient may feel strong fear, anger, or guilt, she probably also feels some relief when she thinks about being pain-free. Help her concentrate on the positive aspects of the upcoming surgery and the abilities she'll still have afterward.

Tell the patient that after surgery she may feel as though her limb is still there. Tell her that she may even feel pain that seems to be coming from the missing limb. Assure her that these phantom limb sensations are normal and that they typically disappear within hours after surgery. Do mention, however, that a few patients experience them for months or years after surgery.

After surgery

Your patient may express relief after surgery and be ready to rebuild her independence. However, some patients will be angry and depressed. If your patient is angry, remember that she's angry over the loss of her limb and her independence. To help defuse her anger, give her opportunities to restore a sense of control over daily functions. Offer her choices, whenever possible.

If your patient is depressed, she may cry easily, eat little, sleep too much or too little, and withdraw from interaction. If she has lost a leg, she may believe she'll never walk again, so early mobilization can be a highly effective therapeutic intervention. Also, encourage the patient and her family to talk about their feelings and concerns.

Throughout the postoperative period, assess the patient for pain. Give an analgesic, as prescribed. Assess the patient for phantom limb sensations and reiterate that they're normal.

When possible, use nondrug measures to relieve the patient's anxiety. Try deep breathing, relaxation, guided imagery, and distraction. Such measures not only promote physical and psychological comfort but also help control the patient's blood pressure.

Remember, promoting independence is the ultimate goal of rehabilitation. You play an essential role in helping the patient with activities of daily living, teaching her new ways of doing tasks, and reinforcing the exercises and techniques taught by her physical therapists. A patient who feels nurtured, cared for, and encouraged will gradually increase her participation in self care. As she does, her self-esteem and comfort level will improve.

After an amputation, elevate the stump for the first 24 hours, then lay it flat to prevent hip flexion contracture. Check the dressing for bleeding and drainage. Inspect the incision at least every 8 hours to detect infection and monitor healing. Also, check the color, temperature, and pulses of the other limb. Protect it from trauma, provide meticulous skin care, and maintain its ROM.

Before discharge, review the patient's medications, exercise plan, and skin and foot care. Help her plan for lifestyle changes needed to control her blood pressure. If she had an amputation, reinforce stump-care measures. Obtain a referral for rehabilitation and home care follow-up, as appropriate.

Heart failure

In patients with prolonged, uncontrolled hypertension, the left ventricle must pump with increased force to open the aortic valve against elevated systemic arterial pressure. The heart's muscle fibers compensate by thickening and enlarging the ventricle wall. As a result of this compensatory hypertrophy, myocardial workload and oxygen consumption increase. Eventually, the heart can no longer meet the demands for increased blood supply and oxygen; that is, the left ventricle fails.

Early in heart failure, the body tries to compensate using the adrenergic and renin-angiotensin-aldosterone systems, mechanisms that may sustain cardiac function briefly. However, as heart failure progresses, they may actually worsen the degree of failure and the underlying peripheral vascular disease. That's because adrenergic stimulation releases epinephrine and norepinephrine, which cause peripheral vasoconstriction and shunt blood from nonvital organs and peripheral tissues to vital organs, such as the heart and brain. The patient with compromised peripheral blood flow now faces a substantial risk of limb ischemia. What's more, vasoconstriction increases systemic vascular resistance, worsening hypertension. If not promptly recognized and treated, vasoconstriction will continue, and the patient may lose a limb or go into shock.

Confirming the complication

A patient with left ventricular heart failure may have dyspnea on exertion, orthopnea, paroxysmal nocturnal dyspnea, nocturia, tachycardia, and tachypnea. She may gasp for air and thrash about as if suffocating. She also may complain of fatigue and describe a feeling of impending doom. On auscultation, you may hear crackles and wheezes in her lungs and an S_3 heart sound.

A chest X-ray may reveal an enlarged cardiac silhouette, pulmonary venous congestion, and interstitial edema. Echocardiography may show ventricular hypertrophy, decreased contractility, and a decreased ejection fraction. An ECG may reveal signs of left ventricular hypertrophy or myocardial ischemia.

Pulmonary artery catheterization may indicate decreased cardiac output and cardiac index and elevated pulmonary artery diastolic, systolic, and wedge pressures. Early in heart failure, hyperventilation may lead to respiratory alkalosis. Later, the patient may develop respiratory acidosis and hypoxemia.

Liver function test results as well as bilirubin, blood urea nitrogen (BUN), and creatinine levels may be elevated. Elevated BUN and creatinine levels reflect renal hypoperfusion. Urine output is typically low, and urine is concentrated.

Nursing interventions

Focus your care on decreasing the patient's cardiac workload, optimizing cardiac function, and promoting emotional and physical rest. During periods of breathlessness, restrict her activity or keep her on bed rest, as indicated. Raise the head of the bed to allow maximum respiratory excursion. However, don't raise it high enough to risk pooling blood in the patient's hips or legs.

Auscultate breath sounds frequently to assess respiratory effort and detect improvement or worsening of congestion. Give supplemental oxygen as indicated to alleviate hypoxemia. Monitor oxygen saturation levels using pulse oximetry and ABG studies. If the patient's ventilatory status worsens, prepare for ET intubation and mechanical ventilation.

Give the prescribed vasodilator to decrease preload and dilate the peripheral vessels. Also, give the prescribed diuretic to decrease preload by stimulating the excretion of excess fluid. Monitor the patient's hemodynamic response closely and observe her for signs of drug interactions (see *Drugs for heart failure and hypertension: Dangerous interactions*, page 310). Begin continuous ECG monitoring, as appropriate, to evaluate for arrhythmias and signs of ischemic changes.

DRUG ALERT

Drugs for heart failure and hypertension: Dangerous interactions

Drugs for heart failure	Drugs for hypertension	Adverse effects	Nursing actions
• Cardiac glyco-sides	• Beta blockers	• Excessive bradycardia and other arrhythmias	• Monitor pulse and heart rate and rhythm; note pulse rate less than 60 beats/minute. • Evaluate ECG for arrhythmias. • Begin safety precautions. • Anticipate reducing dosages of both drugs or switching the antihypertensive.
	• Loop and thiazide diuretics	• Increased excretion of potassium with subsequent increased risk of digoxin toxicity	• Monitor serum digoxin level. • Evaluate ECG for arrhythmias. • Assess pulse and heart rate and rhythm. Notify physician if rate goes below 60 or above 100 beats/minute.
	• Hydralazine, calcium channel blockers	• Increased risk of digoxin toxicity	• Expect to switch the antihypertensive. • Teach the patient how to monitor pulse.
• Diuretics	• Angiotensin-converting enzyme inhibitors	• Increased hypotensive effects	• Monitor blood pressure with patient lying, sitting, and standing. • Note drop in blood pressure with position changes. • Begin safety precautions. • Tell patient to change positions slowly. • Anticipate reducing dosage of one or both drugs.
• Hydralazine	• Beta blockers	• Increased effect of beta blocker	• Monitor blood pressure with patient lying, sitting, and standing. • Note drop in blood pressure with position changes. • Begin safety precautions. • Tell patient to change positions slowly. • Anticipate reducing dosage of beta blocker.

Monitor the patient's daily weight and intake and output closely. Check her serum creatinine and BUN levels to evaluate renal function. If she's receiving a diuretic, monitor her serum electrolyte levels for imbalances. Note a weight increase of 2 pounds or more.

Provide meticulous skin care and take measures to prevent skin breakdown. Patients with peripheral vascular disease, hypertension, and heart failure risk severe skin breakdown from such factors as immobility, inadequate nutrition, edema, and decreased perfusion to the skin and subcutaneous tissue. Reposition the patient at least every 2 hours and pad dependent areas. Closely inspect all skin areas for redness, irritation, and breakdown.

Help conserve the patient's energy by separating activities and procedures with rest periods. Check her oxygen saturation levels to evaluate the effect of activity. Encourage active ROM exercises to promote circulation and minimize the risk of stasis. Or perform passive ROM exercises, as appropriate. Then increase activity levels in gradual steps. As needed, obtain a physical therapy consult to help devise an appropriate exercise program.

As with all patients who have peripheral vascular disease, use antiembolism stockings and avoid flexing the hips and knees. Keep in mind that diuretics used to enhance fluid excretion may also make the blood more viscous and raise the patient's risk of thrombus formation.

Before discharge, teach the patient and her family about her disease and the underlying cause. Also, explain how heart failure can develop. Instruct the patient to weigh herself each morning after voiding and before breakfast. Tell her to report a weight gain of more than 2 pounds in 24 hours. Also, tell her to report shortness of breath.

Teach the patient energy conservation measures. Advise her to limit salt in her diet and avoid foods high in sodium, such as luncheon meats, fast foods, and canned foods. And be sure to review her medication regimen, including dosages, administration times, and adverse effects.

Suggested readings

Cantwell-Gab K. Identifying chronic peripheral arterial disease. *Am J Nurs.* 1996;96(7):40-46.

Capeheart JK. Chronic venous insufficiency: a focus on prevention of venous ulceration. *J Wound Ostomy Continence Nurs.* 1996;23(4):227-234.

Fahey VA. *Vascular nursing.* 2nd ed. Philadelphia, Pa: WB Saunders Co; 1994.

Gefter WB, Hatabu H, Holland GA, Gupta KB, Henschke CI, Palevsky HI. Pulmonary thromboembolism: recent developments in diagnosis with CT and MR imaging. *Radiology.* 1995;197(3):561-574.

Goldhaber SZ. Contemporary pulmonary embolism thrombolysis. *Chest.* 1995;107(1 Suppl):45S-51S.

Guiliani ER, Gersh BJ, McGoon MD, et al. *Mayo Clinic practice of cardiology.* 3rd ed. St Louis, Mo: Mosby–Year Book; 1996.

Handler JA, Feied CF. Acute pulmonary embolism: aggressive therapy with anticoagulants and thrombolytics. *Postgrad Med.* 1995;97(1):61-62.

Karch AM. Pain, pills, and possibilities: drug therapy in peripheral vascular disease. *AACN Clin Issues.* 1995;6(4):614-630.

Layish DT, Tapson VF. Pharmacologic hemodynamic support in massive pulmonary embolism. *Chest.* 1997;111(1):218-224.

Lualdi JC, Goldhaber SZ. Right ventricular dysfunction after acute pulmonary embolism: pathophysiologic factors, detection, and therapeutic implications. *Am Heart J.* 1995;130(6):1276-1282.

Majoros KA, Moccia JM. Embolism: targeting an elusive enemy. *Nursing.* 1996;26(4):26-31.

Manganelli D, Palla A, Donnamaria V, Giuntini C. Clinical features of pulmonary embolism: doubts and certainties. *Chest.* 1995;107(1 Suppl):25S-32S.

Phipps WJ, Sands JK, Lehman MK, Cassmeyer V. *Medical-surgical nursing: concepts and clinical practice.* 5th ed. St Louis, Mo: Mosby–Year Book; 1995.

Regensteiner JG, Hiatt WR. Medical management of peripheral arterial disease. *J Vasc Interv Radiol.* 1994;5(5):669-677.

Thelan LA, Davie JK, Urden LD, Lough ME. *Critical care nursing: diagnosis and management.* 2nd ed. St Louis, Mo: Mosby–Year Book; 1994.

Thompson JM, McFarland GK, Hirsch JE, Tucker SM. *Mosby's clinical nursing.* 4th ed. St Louis, Mo: Mosby–Year Book; 1997.

Wheeler EC, Brenner ZR. Peripheral vascular anatomy, physiology, and pathophysiology. *AACN Clin Issues.* 1995;6(4):505-514.

Woods SL, Sivarkian Froelicher ES, Halpenny CJ, Underhill Motzer S. *Cardiac nursing.* 3rd ed. Philadelphia, Pa: Lippincott-Raven Pubs; 1995.

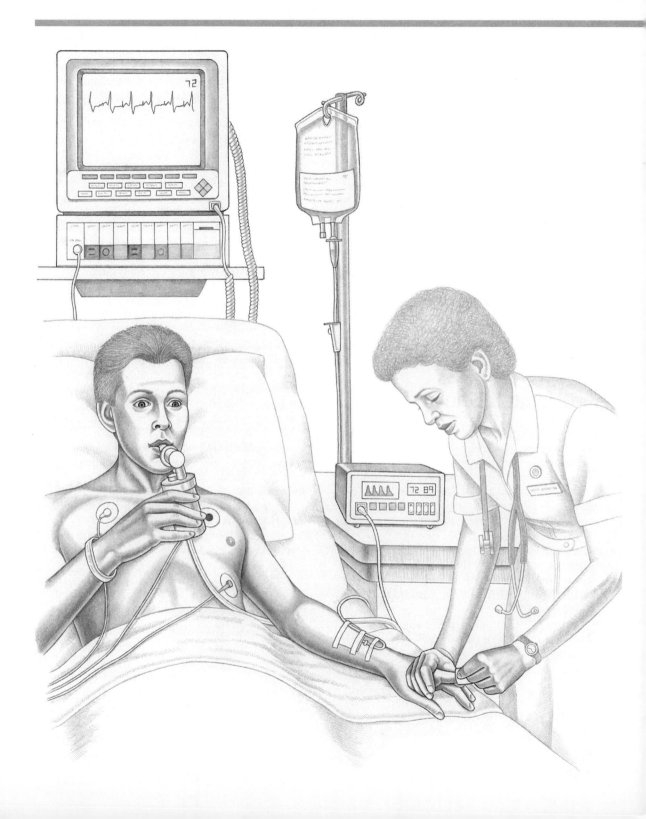

10

Asthma

O ver the last decade or so, asthma has become the most common disorder of chronic respiratory obstruction in the United States. Currently, about 13 million Americans have asthma, a third or more of them younger than age 18.

Not everyone shares an equal risk of developing asthma. Before puberty, twice as many boys are affected as girls. And Hispanic (especially Puerto Rican) and African-American children have a higher risk of asthma than white children. Of those who die from asthma, about 21% are African-Americans, even though African-Americans make up only about 12% of the U.S. population.

In most people, asthma can be controlled with proper treatment. However, an asthma attack can turn deadly if status asthmaticus develops. And when complicated by other disorders, asthma and its treatment can contribute to such serious problems as atelectasis, respiratory acidosis, acute respiratory failure, heart failure, and cardiac arrest.

Anatomy and physiology review

As described in detail in Chapter 7, the respiratory system includes the upper and lower airways and the lungs. The effects of asthma take place in the lower airways, primarily in the bronchioles but occasionally in the bronchi. Those effects alter the airways' mucosal lining and the lungs' ability to exchange oxygen and carbon dioxide.

Lower airways

As you know, the lower airways include the trachea, the mainstem bronchi, segmental and subsegmental bronchi, bronchioles, and alveoli. The bronchi and larger bronchioles are supported by cartilaginous rings and sheathed in a fibroelastic membrane. In contrast, the respiratory bronchioles, located just proximal to the alveolar ducts, contain no cartilage. Instead, they're formed by two complete, concentric rings of smooth-muscle fibers. When these muscles constrict, as in asthma, the airways narrow.

The terminal respiratory units, called the acini, consist of the respiratory bronchioles, the alveolar ducts, and the alveoli. Oxygen and carbon dioxide diffuse across the alveolocapillary membrane that separates the alveoli from the surrounding pulmonary capillary beds.

Mucosal lining

As air moves deep into the respiratory tree, particles of debris not trapped in the nose and trachea get lodged in the mucus produced by the bronchial mucosal lining. Then, constantly beating cilia propel them to the pharynx so they can be expelled by coughing, swallowing, or sneezing.

The mucosal lining has three layers: the epithelial layer, the lamina propria, and the basement membrane (see *Inside the bronchi and bronchioles*).

The epithelial layer contains several cell types. The three most important are the ciliated cells, the goblet cells, and the Clara cells. Ciliated cells, which propel secretions out of the respiratory tract, appear in the larger airways on the columnar epithelium and in the smaller airways on the cuboidal epithelium. Goblet cells, which synthesize and secrete mucus, are located between ciliated cells in the larger airways. And Clara cells, which probably produce fluid, are located in the cuboidal epithelium of the smaller airways.

The lamina propria contains lymphoid nodules, lymphocytes, plasma cells, mast cells, and a few polymorphonuclear leukocytes embedded in elastic fibers. The mast cells release inflammatory mediators, such as histamine and leukotrienes, during asthma attacks or allergic reactions. Lymphoid nodules help trigger immune responses in the lungs.

The basement membrane is a thin, noncellular layer of adhesive, permeable material that separates the epithelial layer from the lamina propria.

Airway secretions contain two immunoglobulin antibodies: immunoglobulin G (IgG) and immunoglobulin A (IgA). IgG helps defend the body against bacterial infections. IgA, made in part by the lymphoid nodules, probably helps protect against viral infections.

Ventilation

Ventilation, the process by which air is delivered to the alveoli, consists of inspiration and expiration. When respiratory muscles contract, the thoracic cavity expands. Cohesion between the visceral and parietal pleura then expands the lungs as well, creating negative intrapleural pressure. In response, air moves into the lungs.

When respiratory muscles relax, the lungs' natural elastic recoil returns them to their normal resting state, pushing air out. This tendency to recoil results from the interstitial elastin fibers and surfactant.

A certain amount of pressure (or force) is required to expand the lungs to overcome their natural tendency to recoil. This force is called

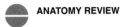

Inside the bronchi and bronchioles

Asthma typically affects the mucosal lining of the bronchi and bronchioles. The illustrations below show cross sections of the mucosal lining in these airways.

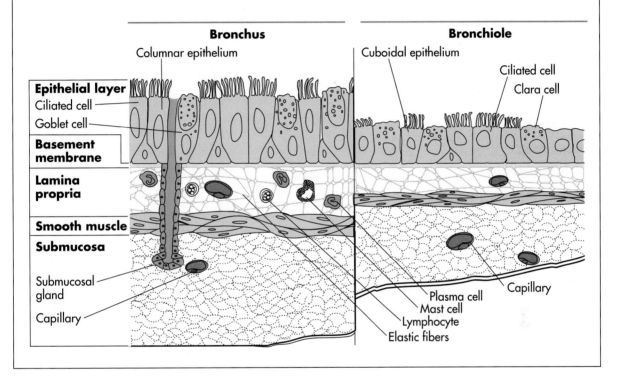

compliance, and it's the reciprocal of elasticity. High compliance means that the lungs have little elastic force working to keep them in their resting state. Poor compliance means that the lungs have excessive elastic force working to keep them in their resting state. Consequently, expanding them requires more force. Lung compliance decreases with any condition that interferes with lung expansion (such as asthma), blocks the airways, or makes lung tissue fibrotic or edematous.

Another factor that affects the smooth flow of air in and out of the lungs is pulmonary resistance. As the lungs expand, tissues move against each other, creating tissue resistance. Likewise, as air flows through the airways, friction develops between gas molecules and the sides of the airways, creating airway resistance. When airway diameters shrink, as in bronchoconstriction or inflammation, airway resistance rises.

Diffusion

When air reaches the alveoli, oxygen crosses the alveolocapillary membrane into the blood because the partial pressure of arterial oxygen (Pao_2) in alveoli exceeds that in venous blood. Conversely, carbon dioxide diffuses in the opposite direction because the partial pressure of arterial carbon dioxide ($Paco_2$) in venous blood exceeds that in alveoli. This process, known as diffusion, may be altered by several factors, including the thickness of the alveolocapillary membrane, the surface area available

Characteristics of extrinsic and intrinsic asthma

Characteristic	Extrinsic asthma	Intrinsic asthma
Family history of allergies	Common	Uncommon
Childhood onset	Common	Uncommon
Childhood allergies	Common	Uncommon
Allergens as precipitants	Yes	No
Elevated immunoglobulin E	Common	Uncommon
Positive skin test	Yes	No
Eosinophilia	Yes	Yes
Typical attack	Acute and self-limiting	Usually severe and difficult to treat

for gas exchange, and the difference in partial pressures of the gases being diffused.

Ventilation-perfusion matching

Normally, the amount of air flow (ventilation) closely matches the amount of blood flow (perfusion), a balance that ensures an adequate exchange of oxygen and carbon dioxide—and healthy arterial blood gas (ABG) values. However, several clinical conditions can alter the ventilation-perfusion ratio, resulting in abnormal ABG values. For example, when bronchioles are blocked by mucous plugs, as in asthma, ventilation to the alveoli declines. Perfusion remains normal, however, which means that a portion of blood in the pulmonary circulation doesn't get oxygenated. This ventilation-perfusion mismatch results in a low PaO_2 level.

Pathophysiology

Asthma is a frightening disorder marked by sudden attacks of widespread bronchoconstriction in a patient whose airways are hypersensitive to certain substances. If the hypersensitivity stems from allergies, the patient has extrinsic asthma. Otherwise, the patient has

intrinsic asthma (see *Characteristics of extrinsic and intrinsic asthma*).

Extrinsic asthma usually develops in childhood and is associated with other allergies, such as skin and nasal allergies. Three asthmatic children in four have a family history of allergies and evidence of allergic reactions mediated by immunoglobulin E (IgE), such as hay fever. Extrinsic asthma attacks tend to be caused by such allergens as pollen, mold, animal dander, and aspirin.

Intrinsic asthma usually develops later in life. Typically, the patient has no family history of asthma, no history of allergies, and no evidence of IgE-mediated reactions. Attacks can be triggered by a wide range of factors, including respiratory infections, cigarette smoke, exercise, cold air, environmental pollutants, and strong emotions.

In many cases, asthma attacks probably result from a combination of allergic and nonallergic triggers, a condition called mixed asthma.

Another way to classify asthma is by its precipitating factors. Thus, a patient may have occupational asthma, exercise-induced asthma, asthmatic bronchitis (chronic bronchitis with bronchospasm), or aspirin-induced asthma.

Keep in mind that although the underlying causes of asthma attacks may differ, the principle remains the same. In an asthmatic patient, hypersensitive airways react strongly to certain triggers, which is why you'll hear asthma called a reactive airway disease. Smooth muscles surrounding the bronchi and bronchioles constrict, leading to a host of other respiratory consequences.

Mechanism of an attack

When one or more trigger factors invade the small airways, a number of responses work together to create an asthma attack. Early on, eosinophils, neutrophils, mast cells, macrophages, and activated T lymphocytes infiltrate the bronchial mucosa. Mast cells and T lymphocytes release cytokines that promote the production of abnormally large amounts of IgE antibodies. These antibodies, in turn, increase vascular permeability, disrupt the epithelium, stimulate neural reflexes and mucus production, and cause mucus-secreting glands to proliferate.

Other chemical mediators are released as well, including histamines, bradykinins, and leukotrienes. These substances cause bronchial smooth-muscle spasms that narrow the airways. They also increase vascular permeability, leading to vascular congestion and edema, further narrowing the airways. Plus, these mediators increase mucus production. The overall effect of these actions: the patient's airways become constricted, inflamed, and filled with mucus (see *An inside look at asthma*, page 318).

To make matters worse, the mucus produced by this inflammatory process is typically viscous and tough to clear. It tends to form plugs that block parts of the airway, trapping air in the alveolar sacs. Some alveoli collapse, and others hyperinflate to maintain oxygenation. The patient has increased airway resistance, decreased lung compliance, and impaired mucociliary clearance. Eventually, the smooth-muscle layer enlarges to as much as three times its normal size.

As lung volumes increase from trapped air, intrapleural and alveolar gas pressures rise, reducing alveolar perfusion and causing a ventilation-perfusion mismatch. As a result, the patient develops hypoxemia without retaining carbon dioxide. The hypoxemia stimulates the respiratory centers in the brain, and this stimulation makes the patient hyperventilate, further decreasing his carbon dioxide levels and increasing his pH.

This process leads to mild respiratory alkalosis. As the obstruction progresses, however, the number of affected alveoli increases, gas exchange decreases, carbon dioxide levels rise, and the patient develops respiratory acidosis.

Assessment findings

Depending on the severity, asthma can cause a wide range of signs and symptoms. Patients with mild asthma may report little more than slight wheezing and weakness, occasional shortness of breath, and a minor cough. Patients with severe asthma, on the other hand, may have almost unrelenting shortness of breath, a nearly continuous cough, chest wall retractions, and a greatly diminished ability to carry out daily activities (see *Assessing the severity of asthma*, page 319).

If you're assessing a child who has respiratory problems, remember that asthma typically begins between ages 3 and 8. Signs that a child may have asthma include rapid or labored breathing, frequent or unusually severe colds, a chronic cough or wheezing, and an inability to be as active as other children his age.

Keep in mind that in children, asthma may be commonly misdiagnosed as a middle or lower respiratory tract infection, a blocked or compressed trachea or bronchus, congenital laryngeal stridor, or cystic fibrosis.

When assessing a child or an adult, find out about allergy-related signs and symptoms, such as eczema, nasal polyps, hay fever, and sensitivity to pollens, plants, mold, or animal dander. Be sure to determine whether any other family members have a history of allergies or asthma.

Also, find out if the patient's respiratory problem seems to be associated with another condition or an activity. For example, ask if it tends to occur during exercise. Also, ask if it occurs after a sinus infection, a cold, or another viral infection. Find out if it develops during certain seasons, in a cold environment, or after the person experiences great excitement or another strong emotion. Ask, too, if the patient

An inside look at asthma

Asthma causes bronchial smooth-muscle constriction, inflammation of the mucosa, excessive mucus production, mucous plugs, and hyperinflated alveoli.

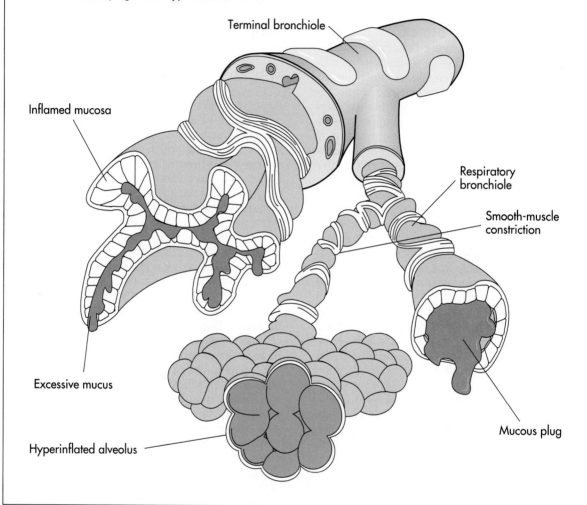

Terminal bronchiole

Inflamed mucosa

Respiratory bronchiole

Smooth-muscle constriction

Excessive mucus

Mucous plug

Hyperinflated alveolus

has trouble sleeping. Is he exposed to irritants or allergic triggers in the bedroom?

When you auscultate the patient's lungs, you may hear wheezing, especially on expiration. But don't rely too heavily on wheezing as an indicator: it can diminish as asthma worsens and the airways grow smaller.

Asthma attack

During an attack, a patient typically has trouble breathing. He may say that his chest feels tight, that he can't sleep, that he wheezes, or that he can't catch his breath. If he's already taking an asthma medication, he may need more of it than usual to control his symptoms.

A patient may say that his symptoms arise in minutes or that they develop over days or

Assessing the severity of asthma

Findings	Mild asthma	Moderate asthma	Severe asthma
Assessment	• Attacks once a week or less • No restrictions on daily activities • Effective response to bronchodilator in 24 hours • No signs of asthma between attacks • No sleep disruption • No hyperventilation • Mild dyspnea on exertion • Cough • Slight wheezing • Weakness • Adequate air exchange	• Attacks more than once a week and lasting several days • Some restrictions on daily activities • Decreased activity and exercise tolerance • Coughing and wheezing between attacks • Some sleep disruption • Occasional emergency care • Dyspnea at rest • Hyperpnea • Marked coughing and wheezing • Air exchange normal or slightly obstructed	• Frequent severe attacks • Major restrictions on daily activities • Poor exercise and activity tolerance • Incomplete response to bronchodilators • Continuous symptoms • Frequent sleep disruption • Occasional hospitalization and emergency care • Marked dyspnea at rest • Marked wheezing or absent breath sounds • Chest wall retractions • Paradoxical pulse greater than 25 mm Hg • Obstructed air exchange
Diagnostic tests	• Chest X-ray normal • Forced expiratory volume (FEV) or peak expiratory flow rate (PEFR) 80% or more than predicted value; slight variability between morning and evening readings • Lung volumes normal or mildly increased • pH normal or increased • Partial pressure of arterial oxygen (Pao_2) normal or decreased • Partial pressure of arterial carbon dioxide ($Paco_2$) normal or decreased • Oxygen saturation normal or decreased	• Hyperinflation on chest X-ray • FEV or PEFR 60% to 80% of predicted value; 20% variability between morning and evening readings • Lung volumes increased • pH usually increased • Pao_2 decreased • $Paco_2$ usually decreased • Oxygen saturation decreased	• Hyperinflation on chest X-ray • FEV or PEFR less than 60% of predicted value; great variability between morning and evening readings • Lung volumes markedly increased • pH normal or decreased • Pao_2 decreased • $Paco_2$ normal or increased • Oxygen saturation decreased

weeks. Either way, your assessment will likely reveal an increased respiratory rate resulting from several factors, including anxiety, hypoxic stimulation of peripheral chemoreceptors, and decreased lung compliance. You may see the patient using his trapezius and sternocleidomastoid muscles during inspiration and his abdominal and external and internal oblique muscles during expiration. Also, expect to see substernal, supraclavicular, and intercostal retractions during inspiration, as the patient struggles to overcome his reduced compliance. Because he must create a higher-than-normal negative intrapleural pressure to inhale, the muscles between the ribs and in the substernal area retract with each breath.

The patient probably will have prolonged expirations. And he may be wheezing audibly. If he's hypoxic, you may see evidence of peripheral and central cyanosis, such as nail bed and mucosal changes, as well as confusion and lethargy.

Expect the patient's blood pressure and pulse rate to be elevated. These changes stem from hypoxic stimulation of peripheral chemoreceptors. The patient's heart rate, blood pressure, and cardiac output increase to counteract the hypoxemia produced by pulmonary shunting.

The patient probably also will have a paradoxical pulse, a condition in which systolic blood pressure is usually greater by more than 10 mm Hg during expiration than it is during inspiration. In asthmatic patients, this probably results from the large difference in intrapleural pressure between inspiration and expiration.

The patient will be coughing and most likely producing increased amounts of thick sputum. If the sputum contains large numbers of eosinophils and other white blood cells (WBCs), it may look purulent. It probably also will contain large numbers of eosinophil fragments, called Charcot-Leyden crystals.

If the patient has a fever, assume that he also has an infection. Asthmatic patients are prone to developing such infections as bacterial and viral pneumonia.

During chest palpation, expect decreased tactile and vocal fremitus from lung consolidation interfering with sound transmission. During percussion, expect hyperresonance from hyperinflated alveoli. During auscultation, expect to hear diminished breath sounds from alveolar hyperinflation and diminished air flow from bronchospasm and increased airway resistance.

Status asthmaticus

If your asthma patient has a severe, prolonged asthma attack, keep in mind that he could be in status asthmaticus. If so, you'll note that his respiratory efforts increase despite treatment. He'll probably be highly anxious. And he'll probably have an almost continuous nonproductive cough. He may stop wheezing. If the attack continues, the patient may develop hypoxia and cyanosis. Eventually, he may lose consciousness.

Diagnostic tests

Several tests can be used to diagnose and evaluate asthma. Pulmonary function and bronchial provocation tests typically provide the most information. Other tests may include

ABG analysis, chest X-ray, electrocardiogram (ECG), sputum culture, and blood tests.

Pulmonary function tests

Pulmonary function tests can help confirm a diagnosis of asthma, determine the degree of airway obstruction, and measure the patient's response to bronchodilator therapy. Keep in mind that during an asthma attack, the patient's expiratory flow rate will be sharply reduced. Specific tests used to evaluate a patient's pulmonary function include the following:

- forced vital capacity (FVC), the total amount of air exhaled as forcefully as possible after a patient takes a maximal inhalation. In a patient with asthma, FVC may be normal or slightly decreased because of airway obstruction.
- forced expiratory volume in 1 second (FEV_1), the volume of air exhaled during the first second of a forced exhalation. In a patient with asthma, FEV_1 may be decreased because the airways are obstructed; after the patient inhales a bronchodilator, FEV_1 may return to normal.
- residual volume (RV), the amount of air remaining in the lungs after a maximal exhalation. In a patient with asthma, RV may be increased because of trapped air.
- forced expiratory flow, the average flow rate during the middle half of the FVC. This test offers the most accurate estimate of airway resistance. In a patient with asthma, forced expiratory flow may be decreased because the small airways are obstructed; after the patient inhales a bronchodilator, forced expiratory flow may return to normal.
- peak flow, the maximal flow rate during a forced exhalation. This measurement helps detect early signs of airway obstruction and evaluate the effectiveness of treatment.

Bronchial provocation test

The bronchial provocation test can help when a physician still suspects asthma, even after a patient's pulmonary function test results are normal. It is not used, however, for patients known to be asthmatic or for those whose flow rates are abnormal.

During the test, the patient receives increasing doses of a bronchoconstrictor, such as methacholine or histamine. After each dose, his expiratory flow rate is measured. In patients who have normal airways, the flow rate remains the same. In patients who have asthma, the flow rate decreases. This test can also be performed using exercise or cold air to provoke a response.

ABG analysis
Between attacks, early in an attack, or during a mild attack, an asthma patient's ABG values may be normal. In general, however, changes in ABG values provide the most reliable guide to the severity of an asthma attack.

In a mild asthma attack, the patient's $Paco_2$ declines, and his pH may rise. That's because airway obstruction, anxiety, and dyspnea tend to make the patient hyperventilate. Consequently, he blows off increased amounts of carbon dioxide, which leads to hypocapnia and respiratory alkalosis.

If the attack becomes severe, hypoxemia may develop because of a ventilation-perfusion mismatch. When that happens, the patient's Pao_2 level drops, sometimes down to 40 mm Hg. As airway resistance increases, his $Paco_2$ rises, possibly above normal. Cerebral dilation develops as a result, and the patient may complain of a headache. He also may grow drowsy. These are important signals that the patient can no longer hyperventilate.

As $Paco_2$ continues to increase, the patient's pH falls. As hypoxia progresses, his body begins to produce lactic acid, and bicarbonate levels fall. If an attack of this severity isn't reversed, the patient will need endotracheal (ET) intubation and mechanical ventilation.

Chest X-ray
Usually, chest X-rays are normal in asymptomatic asthma patients. During an attack, however, residual lung volume increases, and density decreases as the alveoli enlarge. Thus, the chest X-ray looks more translucent, or darker, than normal. Also, the patient's diaphragm is depressed and flattened. A chest X-ray also helps rule out such complications as pneumonia, pneumothorax, pneumomediastinum, and cardiomegaly.

Electrocardiogram
During an asthma attack, a patient may develop sinus tachycardia, ventricular ectopic beats, or other arrhythmias. Also, you may observe prominent P waves. These changes usually resolve within a few hours after treatment.

Sputum culture
Thick or purulent-looking mucoid sputum doesn't necessarily indicate a bacterial infection in a patient who has asthma. Instead, it may result from increased levels of eosinophils in the patient's airway secretions. Nevertheless, because asthma patients have an increased risk of pulmonary infections, a physician may order a sputum specimen for culture and sensitivity testing to rule out infection as a cause of the asthma attack.

Blood studies
Blood tests can help you evaluate your patient's status and detect associated complications. The differential WBC count, for example, may reveal mild eosinophilia. The patient's leukocyte count may be elevated if he takes high doses of a corticosteroid or if he has an infection. A serum potassium test can detect hypokalemia from corticosteroid therapy, high-dose $beta_2$-agonist therapy, or respiratory alkalosis. And a blood glucose test may reveal hyperglycemia from corticosteroid therapy.

Medical interventions

Medical interventions can't cure asthma, but they can help control its symptoms. In fact, a variety of options exist for easing the effects of chronic asthma and for managing an attack, even if it turns into status asthmaticus.

Controlling chronic asthma
The most common elements in a management plan for chronic asthma are medications and environmental adjustments. Usually, the patient tries to eliminate asthma triggers from his environment. And his physician prescribes an inhaled or oral bronchodilator to start. Later, the physician may add anti-inflammatory or

How drug therapy fights asthma

This flowchart shows how various asthma drugs work to stop an asthma attack.

other drugs, as necessary (see *How drug therapy fights asthma*).

Bronchodilators

Bronchodilators include beta$_2$ agonists, theophylline, and anticholinergic drugs.

Beta$_2$ agonists: The most commonly used asthma drugs and usually the first choice in treating asthma, beta$_2$ agonists dilate bronchial smooth muscle, increase ciliary action, prevent bronchospasm, and increase the effect of corticosteroids. They can be given parenterally, but the short-acting beta$_2$ agonists albuterol and terbutaline are inhaled. In recommended dosages—two to four puffs three to four times a day—they're well tolerated and cause few adverse effects. Plus, they bring rapid relief of symptoms.

Long-acting beta$_2$ agonists, such as salmeterol, provide effective bronchodilation over a 12-hour period, making them especially useful for patients with nocturnal asthma. Because of their slow onset of action, they can't be used to relieve immediate symptoms.

Theophylline: A methylxanthine derivative, theophylline has been used to treat asthma for more than 50 years. However, it's less effective than beta$_2$ agonists. It commonly causes adverse effects, and it requires close monitoring of plasma levels. Thus, today it's most commonly used when treating severe or nocturnal asthma. The I.V. form of theophylline is aminophylline, which can be used during an asthma attack.

Anticholinergics: Acetylcholine contracts smooth muscle and increases mucus production. That's why inhaled anticholinergic drugs, such as ipratropium, which work against acetylcholine, can be effective in treating asthma. However, they have a slower onset than beta$_2$ agonists, so they're typically used as adjunctive therapy or for cardiac patients who can't take beta$_2$ agonists or theophylline.

Anti-inflammatory drugs

Anti-inflammatory drugs, such as corticosteroids and mast-cell stabilizers, can help ease a patient's asthma symptoms.

Corticosteroids: These drugs (including beclomethasone, fluticasone propionate, budesonide, triamcinolone acetonide, and flunisolide) are inhaled, but some forms can be given I.V. (methylprednisolone sodium succinate) or orally (prednisone). Corticosteroids work by suppressing macrophages and eosinophils, reducing microvascular permeability, and decreasing the action of inflammatory cells in the airways. They have a relatively slow onset; it takes several days for an inhaled corticosteroid to take effect.

Dosages range from two to six puffs two to four times daily. Although inhaled corticosteroids don't cause many systemic adverse effects, they do cause local effects, such as a sore throat, dry mouth, coughing, and oral fungal infections.

Mast-cell stabilizers: Mast-cell stabilizers, such as cromolyn and nedocromil, are especially helpful in preventing seasonal, exercise-induced, or cold-air-induced asthma. The usual dose is two puffs four times daily.

Antileukotriene drugs

Leukotrienes are bronchoconstrictors with 100 to 1,000 times the power of histamines. These substances also mobilize WBCs (especially neutrophils, eosinophils, and monocytes) and increase capillary permeability. The result is increased edema and mucus, bronchospasm, and decreased ciliary action. The antileukotriene drugs zafirlukast and zileuton block these effects.

Zafirlukast, a leukotriene-receptor antagonist, is used as adjunctive treatment for chronic asthma. It isn't a bronchodilator and shouldn't be used to reverse bronchospasm or asthma attacks. The typical dosage is 20 mg orally twice a day; the patient should take the drug on an empty stomach. The most common adverse effects include headache, infection, nausea, and diarrhea.

Zileuton, a leukotriene-pathway inhibitor, is used as adjunctive treatment of chronic asthma in patients age 12 and older. The typical dosage is 600 mg orally four times daily. The most common adverse effects include dyspepsia and elevated liver function test results.

Environmental adjustments

A majority of asthma patients have allergies to inhaled substances that can trigger asthma attacks. So for most patients, asthma treatment involves not only medications but also environmental awareness and adjustment. Depending on the allergy, a patient may need to stay indoors during allergy season. He may need to try to eliminate indoor allergens, such as dust mites, animal dander, and mold. Or he may need to avoid indoor irritants, such as smoke from tobacco and wood-burning stoves, strong odors, and sprays.

If a patient can't eliminate these asthma triggers or if drugs can't control his symptoms, he may benefit from immunotherapy. If it helps control his symptoms, he'll receive it monthly for 3 to 5 years. If not, a physician typically stops immunotherapy after two allergy seasons.

Treating an asthma attack

A patient having an asthma attack usually needs to inhale large doses of a beta$_2$ agonist. The doses may be inhaled every 15 to 60 minutes or continuously until the symptoms subside. For added effect, an anticholinergic may be inhaled with or after the beta$_2$ agonist. The patient also may receive another bronchodilator I.V., such as aminophylline.

A systemic corticosteroid, such as methylprednisone, can be given I.V. to help reduce airway inflammation, but it takes several hours to produce a measurable improvement. The typical dosage is 60 to 80 mg every 6 to 8 hours.

Most patients also need supplemental oxygen to correct hypoxemia during an asthma attack.

Stopping status asthmaticus

Status asthmaticus, a severe asthma attack that doesn't respond to usual bronchodilator therapy and lasts longer than 24 hours, can quickly develop into respiratory failure. Treatment aims to correct the patient's hypoxemia and improve his ventilation by giving larger drug doses, giving them more often, or both. Depending on the patient's condition and response to treatment, he may need ET intubation and mechanical ventilation.

Nursing interventions

Asthmatic patients require a wide variety of nursing interventions. Over the long term, your most important contribution may be teaching the patient about his condition and its treatment. But during an asthma attack, you'll need to perform several key interventions quickly and accurately to improve the patient's condition.

If your patient has an asthma attack, ask him which asthma medications he takes. Then find out when he last used his inhaler or nebulizer and how many puffs he inhaled.

Obtain his baseline vital signs, then monitor them often. Remember that certain signs warn of a severe attack, including a heart rate above

110 beats per minute, a respiratory rate above 25 breaths per minute, and a paradoxical pulse.

As you assess the patient's respiratory rate, depth, and character, note whether he's using his accessory muscles to breathe. Auscultate his lungs for inspiratory or expiratory wheezes. Remember, diminishing wheezes may signal an improvement or worsening of your patient's condition.

Ask the patient about his cough—specifically, when it started, how severe it is, and how much mucus he's coughing up. Then, observe how often the patient coughs, how severe it is, and how productive it is. Obtain a sputum specimen for culture and Gram's stain, as ordered.

As you assess your patient, remember that he's probably anxious. Stay with him and reassure him to help reduce his anxiety. Speak in a calm, soothing voice. To promote ventilation, place him in the high Fowler position with his arms supported and encourage him to perform pursed-lip breathing.

Check his oxygen saturation levels using pulse oximetry and ABG studies. Give supplemental oxygen and adjust it to keep his oxygen saturation level above 92%. Consider using a Venturi mask to deliver more precise oxygen concentrations.

Administer I.V. fluids and the prescribed medications, such as a bronchodilator and a corticosteroid. Depending on the patient's condition, you may need to give his medications I.V.; if you give aminophylline or terbutaline I.V., use an infusion pump. Obtain baseline serum levels and monitor them, as ordered. Be especially alert for aminophylline toxicity, which can develop when serum levels exceed 20 mg/ml. Signs and symptoms of toxicity include vomiting, diarrhea, headache, and arrhythmias.

Anticipate administering aerosolized nebulizer treatments, even if the patient normally uses a metered-dose inhaler.

Be sure to monitor the patient's response to his aerosolized medications. Measure his peak flow rate before and 15 to 30 minutes after each treatment. A decrease in peak flow rate could warn of a deterioration.

Responding to status asthmaticus

RAPID RESPONSE ▶ If your patient goes into status asthmaticus, the health care team must act

COMFORT MEASURES

Easing the fear of status asthmaticus

Every nurse knows that a patient in status asthmaticus needs immediate, intensive respiratory care to halt this potentially life-threatening complication. Harder to remember, perhaps, is the equally important need to manage the patient's fears and anxiety.

Status asthmaticus typically produces a profound sense of doom and agitation. Not only do these feelings frighten the patient, they also worsen his hypoxemia by increasing dyspnea and restlessness. Plus, the patient may be so severely distressed that he can't speak to express his feelings. By taking steps to ease your patient's fears, you can increase the effectiveness of his treatment and help him cope with his condition. To start, try the steps outlined below.

Be there
Being alone—or feeling alone—can make a frightening situation even worse. Help calm your patient by staying with him throughout his ordeal. If you must leave, assign someone to stay with him until he's out of status asthmaticus. If your patient is a child, bringing a parent to the bedside may do wonders. Pay attention, though, because not all parents are good at providing comfort in stressful situations.

Be clear
In clear and simple terms, explain everything that's happening, as it happens, even if you've explained it before. Don't assume that the patient remembers earlier conversations or that he knows medical terms or physiology. In fact, hearing detailed explanations that he doesn't understand in a flurry of activity can make his anxiety—and hypoxemia—worse.

Also, tell the patient that the treatments he's receiving may make him feel jumpy or feel as though his heart is racing. Assure him that these feelings are temporary.

Be brief
If you need information from your patient, ask him simple questions that require only yes or no answers. If he doesn't answer you, don't assume he doesn't want to talk. In fact, he may be too short of breath to speak. Tell him that you understand and that he can nod or shake his head to communicate. Above all, try to devise a means of communication that lets him express his feelings without interfering with his attempts to breathe.

Be calm
Finally, help the patient and his family stay calm by being calm and organized yourself. Organize your care to minimize disruptions. And help the patient use relaxation techniques. Ask him to think of a peaceful scene to distract him from his anxiety. Have him concentrate on breathing slowly and deeply. Besides helping the patient feel better emotionally, you'll also help his treatment succeed.

quickly to save his life (see *Easing the fear of status asthmaticus*). Treatment will be similar to that for an asthma attack, though you may give larger drug doses and give them more often. Specifically, you may be directed to do some or all of the following:
- If the patient doesn't respond to a beta$_2$ agonist, administer aminophylline I.V.
- Prepare for administration of continuous nebulizer treatments. If so, perform continuous cardiac monitoring to detect developing arrhythmias. Even without continuous treatments, the combined use of inhaled and I.V. bronchodilators increases the risk of arrhythmias.

- Administer a corticosteroid I.V., although it won't take effect for up to 12 hours. Give this drug every 4 to 6 hours.
- Administer sodium bicarbonate, as ordered, to correct acidosis.
- Continuously monitor the patient's ABG values, using an arterial catheter.
- Give supplemental oxygen by Venturi mask or nasal prongs to maintain the ordered oxygen saturation level.
- Give I.V. fluids to maintain the patient's hydration.

If the patient doesn't respond and risks progressive hypoxemia, hypercapnia, and respiratory acidosis or arrest, anticipate ET intubation and mechanical ventilation. ◄

Even when your patient is out of danger, keep checking his respiratory status to make sure he's responding to treatment and not developing complications. Auscultate his lungs frequently; note wheezing and check the amount of air movement. Look for muscle retractions. Also, observe the frequency and nature of the patient's cough. Determine the amount, color, and tenacity of his sputum, and report any increase in the amount or change in the color.

Review the patient's ABG values, complete blood count, and serum electrolyte and theophylline levels. Also, evaluate the patient's pulmonary function test results and check his oxygen saturation level, using pulse oximetry.

Long-term care

Make sure your patient knows how to use his metered-dose inhaler correctly. If he has trouble with it, suggest that he use a spacer. If he inhales a corticosteroid, inspect his mouth and tongue for white patches that could indicate a *Candida* infection. Remind him to rinse, gargle, and expectorate each time he inhales the corticosteroid.

Assess the patient's hydration status because hyperventilation increases insensible fluid loss. Also, systemic corticosteroids given during attacks can alter his fluid and electrolyte balance. Encourage him to drink up to 2,600 ml daily, unless such intake is contraindicated. Monitor his intake and output and his daily weights. Check his serum electrolyte levels for signs of an imbalance.

Many asthma patients have trouble carrying out their daily activities, so be sure to determine if your patient needs help. Space his activities, so he can rest between demanding tasks. And urge him to use pursed-lip breathing to help control his shortness of breath and decrease the work of breathing. Be sure to monitor his oxygen saturation levels in response to activity.

If the patient needs allergy testing and desensitization, help with the testing, as ordered. During and after the tests, monitor him for adverse systemic allergic responses, such as increased wheezing and tachycardia.

Finally, assess your patient's level of anxiety and his ability to cope with episodes of shortness of breath. Remember that strong emotions can trigger attacks. Discuss using appropriate measures to reduce anxiety, such as massage, progressive muscle relaxation, and deep breathing. Avoid giving anxiolytic and hypnotic drugs because they can cause respiratory depression.

Patient teaching

To help your patient manage his asthma successfully, you'll need to teach him or his caregiver about the disease, the measures needed to monitor it, and the steps needed to prevent complications. You'll also need to teach him how to avoid known triggers. And you'll need to teach your patient about his prescribed plan of care.

Explain that, even though we don't know exactly what causes asthma, we do know what happens in the lungs, what causes attacks, and how to minimize the severity of attacks. Above all, stress that knowing what causes attacks can help the patient avoid them. Talk about triggers and help the patient identify the ones that precipitate his attacks. Mention that the same trigger may affect him differently at different times and that all triggers may be more troublesome just after he's had a cold. If the patient can identify specific allergens, help him make a realistic plan to avoid them. Also, stress the importance of avoiding factors known to harm everyone's lungs, such as tobacco smoke and heavy air pollution (see *Avoiding asthma triggers*).

Next, help the patient recognize the warning signs of an impending asthma attack. Explain that they differ for each person. Tell him to seek immediate medical care if any of the following occurs:
- His breathing worsens after he takes his medication and waits for it to work.
- His peak flow rate drops to below half of his best level.
- His peak flow rate stays the same or declines after he uses a bronchodilator.
- His lips or fingernails turn blue or gray.
- He struggles to breathe, he hunches over or lifts his shoulders to breathe, or his chest and neck muscles suck inward with each breath.
- He has trouble walking or talking.

Review the patient's medications, including their names, dosages, actions, and adverse effects. Teach your patient how to use and clean his metered-dose inhaler, spacer, or nebulizer. If

Avoiding asthma triggers

Use this table to teach your patient how to prevent asthma attacks caused by these triggers.

Trigger	Preventive action
Allergens, such as animal dander, mites, other household insects, pollen, mold, foods, and aspirin	• Comply with allergy testing and desensitization. • Avoid animals. If that's not possible, keep cats, dogs, and birds outside the house. Have someone bathe cats and dogs weekly to reduce allergens. Consider placing pets in new homes. • Avoid foods that contain sulfites, such as wine, beer, and shellfish. • Avoid all products containing aspirin. Read the labels of all over-the-counter drugs and check with your physician before using them.
Air pollutants, such as car exhaust, smog, and tobacco smoke	• Avoid going out during rush hour, particularly during hot, humid weather when air pollution tends to be worse. • Check radio or television news for air pollution alerts. • If you smoke, stop. Get help if you need it. • Avoid smoke-filled rooms. Ask smokers to respect your need for clean air. • Use an air conditioner instead of opening the windows in your home or car.
Household dust	• Dust frequently with a damp cloth, so heavy dust can't accumulate. • Mop floors instead of sweeping them. • Wear a mask when dusting or vacuuming. • Change filters on hot-air furnaces and air conditioners frequently. • Keep few knickknacks and other dust collectors. • Use shades instead of blinds and washable curtains instead of heavy drapes. • Cover your mattress and pillow with plastic or vinyl cases. • Consider using a high-energy particulate air filter.
Household vapors and aerosol sprays	• Avoid breathing vapors or using cleaning solvents, liquid chlorine bleach, paint, and paint thinner. • Use baking-soda–based and vinegar-based cleaning products. • Choose nonaerosol furniture polish, starch, cleaners, deodorants, and hair products. • Avoid talcum powder, heavy perfumes, and scented cosmetics.
Respiratory tract and sinus infections	• Get flu and pneumonia vaccinations. • Keep your immune system strong with exercise, nourishing food, and adequate sleep. • Avoid close contact with people who have colds or flu, especially in the early stages. • Call your physician at the first sign or symptom of infection: a fever, chills, increased cough, shortness of breath, wheezing, a change in mucus, or a loss of appetite.
Exercise	• Use your short-acting bronchodilator before you exercise. • Warm up before you exercise. • Start slowly and gradually build intensity. • Avoid exercising outdoors when the environment is very cold, hot and dry, or hot and humid.
Nighttime activities	• Eat small meals and don't eat within 2 hours of going to bed. • Avoid excess alcohol intake. • Raise the head of your bed. • Talk with your physician about taking an antacid or long-acting bronchodilator at night.
Strong emotions	• Remember that emotions can change the way you breathe and tighten muscles in your airways. • Learn and practice breathing and relaxation techniques to control breathing. • Ask your physician about taking extra medication when you're under severe stress.

Teaching your patient to use a peak flow meter

If the physician wants your asthma patient to use a peak flow meter, spend some time teaching him how to use and care for it. Start by explaining that there are more than a dozen peak flow meters on the market but that they all perform the same function: measuring how forcefully a person can expel air from his lungs. By providing this measurement, a peak flow meter can help your patient detect changes in his airways even before he can feel them. Then he can respond to the changes before an emergency develops.

Using the meter
Give your patient the following instructions and walk him through the procedure, so he knows how to use his meter correctly.
- Make sure the indicator is at the bottom of the scale.
- Stand up straight.
- Take the deepest breath you can, close your lips around the mouthpiece, and exhale as hard and as fast as you can in one forceful blast.
- Watch how far the indicator moves up the scale in response to air flowing through the meter.
- Repeat this process two more times. If the results are nearly the same, you'll know you've used the meter correctly.
- Record your highest reading, not an average of the three.

Some people take peak flow measurements once in the morning and once in the evening. Others do it before and after taking their medication. Tell your patient that he can use either method, as long as he uses it consistently. That way, he can track the results over time.

Besides recording his meter readings and the times he obtained them, your patient should note how he felt at the time and if he changed his medication dose. Remind him to take his records with him to his medical appointments.

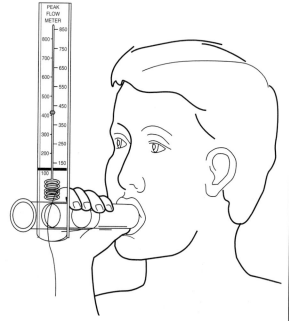

Urge the patient to clean his meter regularly with mild soap and hot water. Some meters can withstand a dishwasher. Warn the patient not to stick anything (a bottle washer, for example) into the meter or to stand it on a prong in the dishwasher.

Responding to readings
Tell your patient that his peak flow meter readings can vary by about 20% from his baseline reading and still be considered normal. However, if the reading drops to 50% to 80% of his baseline, he may need extra medication or an accelerated dosing schedule. And if his reading drops below 50% of his baseline, he may need immediate medical attention.

he uses a spacer, tell the patient it helps him by making sure he gets all his medication. If he inhales a bronchodilator and a corticosteroid, remind him to take the bronchodilator first, then the corticosteroid. That way, his airways will be open enough to receive the corticosteroid.

Show the patient how to use and clean his peak flow meter. Tell him to keep a record of his peak flow readings and to bring it to his medical appointments. And teach him what to do to avoid an asthma attack if his peak flow readings drop (see *Teaching your patient to use a peak flow meter*).

Review pursed-lip breathing, diaphragmatic breathing, and controlled coughing. Urge the patient to perform them often. Also, urge him to exercise in the manner prescribed by his physician. Show him some simple relaxation techniques and encourage him to practice them every day.

Remind the patient to drink six to eight glasses of fluid daily to keep his mucus thin. And encourage him to eat a balanced diet to help prevent fatigue and respiratory infection. Caution him about foods that may trigger asthma. For additional support and education, refer him to a local pulmonary support group.

Asthma and pneumonia

Pneumonia, an inflammatory disorder affecting the respiratory bronchioles and alveoli, usually results from an infection with *Streptococcus pneumoniae*. Pneumonia may cause asthma attacks, or it may develop partly in response to worsening asthma. Either way, the combination can open the door to potentially serious complications.

Pathophysiology

Asthma raises the risk of pneumonia for many reasons. An asthma patient produces an excessive amount of thick mucus that's difficult to cough up. These retained secretions provide an ideal medium for the growth of pneumonia-causing organisms.

Also, many asthma patients need long-term corticosteroid therapy. Corticosteroids suppress the immune system, raising the patient's risk of infections, including pneumonia.

Inhalers and nebulizers can also raise the risk of pneumonia if a patient doesn't clean them properly. And a patient who needs ET intubation and mechanical ventilation has an increased risk of nosocomial pneumonia from the colonization of microorganisms.

No matter how the pathogens reach the airways of an asthma patient, they cause similar results. Acute inflammation of the lung tissue worsens the inflammatory process already created by asthma. The airways narrow even further. And the body's defenses have difficulty destroying and removing the pathogens. Consequently, they multiply quickly. The patient's lungs produce even more mucus, which leads to more blockage, air trapping, and infection. The result: an overwhelming lower respiratory tract infection that rapidly develops into pneumonia.

Adapting nursing care

If an asthma patient develops pneumonia, you need not only to treat the pneumonia but also to minimize its aggravating effects on the patient's asthma. Priorities include maintaining the patient's airway, providing oxygen, treating the infection, and ensuring hydration and nutrition.

Airway and oxygen

Clearly, your top priority is to establish and maintain a patent airway. You'll probably be giving the patient supplemental oxygen by nasal cannula or Venturi mask to prevent or correct hypoxemia. Give up to 6 liters per minute, as ordered, and monitor the patient's response using pulse oximetry and ABG studies.

To loosen mucus and make expectoration or suctioning easier, make sure you're giving humidified oxygen. Also, give aerosolized bronchodilators, as prescribed, to open the patient's airways and make secretion removal easier. Urge the patient to deep-breathe, cough, and use an incentive spirometer at least every 2 hours. Auscultate his lungs before and after these measures to detect any improvement.

When monitoring your patient for complications, remember that some signs that seem to indicate hypoxemia can actually result from other causes, including the therapy itself. Tachycardia, for example, can result from bronchodilator therapy, a fever caused by the pneumonia, or anxiety related to respiratory distress. Some signs of hypercapnia, such as flushing or sweating, may also result from fever. However, if your patient's $Paco_2$ continues to rise and his pH drops, he's facing impending respiratory failure. Report these changes to the physician immediately and prepare to assist with ET intubation and mechanical ventilation.

Antibiotic therapy

Successful treatment of pneumonia depends on accurate identification of the infecting organism. To identify it, obtain sputum specimens for culture and sensitivity testing, as ordered. If your patient can't produce a specimen, try giving him hypertonic saline aerosol mist to stimulate a cough and loosen secretions.

Collect sputum specimens in sterile containers and have them delivered promptly to the laboratory. Expect to start giving the patient an oral or I.V. antibiotic while the physician awaits the laboratory results. After you get the results, the physician may switch the patient to another antibiotic.

Hydration and nutrition

Patients with asthma and pneumonia face a serious risk of dehydration. That's because several factors—including an increased respiratory rate and effort, fever, infection, and diaphoresis—increase insensible fluid loss. Once dehydration develops, mucus becomes even more difficult to remove.

Monitor the patient closely for poor skin turgor and dry mucous membranes. Unless contraindicated, administer at least 3,000 ml of oral fluids, parenteral fluids, or both each day. Take the patient's temperature every 4 hours and give an antipyretic to control the fever and reduce insensible fluid loss.

Because of shortness of breath, many patients with asthma and pneumonia have difficulty eating enough to replace the calories and amino acids needed to fight the infection. To help maintain nutrition, give your patient soft foods that are high in calories and protein. Offer small meals up to six times daily to help avoid abdominal distention that can worsen the patient's feelings of breathlessness.

Patient teaching

As your patient's pneumonia resolves, provide discharge instructions to aid his recovery at home and prevent another respiratory infection.

- Tell him that any kind of respiratory infection, especially pneumonia, can make his airways more irritable for a few weeks. Urge him to use extra caution to avoid triggers that could cause an asthma attack.
- Advise him to avoid visitors who are sick or smoking.
- Instruct him to take his temperature daily and call his physician if it goes higher than 99.5° F (37.5° C).
- Tell him to ask his physician if he should get an annual flu vaccination.
- If he took part in an exercise program before he contracted pneumonia, tell him to check with his physician before resuming it.
- Tell him to use white, unscented, disposable tissues and to check his sputum for changes in color, consistency, amount, and odor. Urge him to promptly report any such changes as well as any increase in coughing, shortness of breath, or wheezing.
- If he goes home while taking an oral antibiotic, stress the importance of taking all of the prescribed medication, even if he starts to feel better before he completes it.
- Make sure he knows how to use and clean his respiratory devices, such as his peak flow meter, metered-dose inhaler, spacer, or nebulizer. Explain that unclean equipment can make his pneumonia recur.
- Remind him to rinse his mouth and expectorate after each time he uses his inhaler, especially if he inhales a corticosteroid, to reduce unwanted effects. Some bronchodilators leave a metallic taste in the mouth.
- Urge him to keep a diary of his symptoms and his peak expiratory flow rate readings.
- If he needs medical equipment at home, such as supplemental oxygen equipment or a handheld nebulizer, contact the discharge planner, social services, or respiratory care department for help with the arrangements. A social worker also can evaluate whether the patient needs financial aid or other assistance at home.
- If your patient will need further instruction in his home, obtain a home care consultation.
- If he needs an I.V. antibiotic at home, a home health nurse can administer it or teach him to administer it.

- If the patient needs continued education and support in managing his asthma, obtain a referral for a nearby pulmonary rehabilitation program, or refer him to his local lung association or an asthma support group.

Complications

Common complications for patients with asthma and pneumonia include atelectasis, respiratory acidosis, and acute respiratory failure.

Atelectasis
In atelectasis, some alveoli can't inflate properly. When a patient has asthma and pneumonia, atelectasis may develop because excess mucus blocks the airways, causing some alveoli to collapse. Venous blood passes through those regions without picking up oxygen, eventually resulting in hypoxemia.

Confirming the complication
Evidence of atelectasis depends largely on the extent of the problem. Small areas of collapsed tissue scattered throughout the lungs may produce no evidence at all. Large collapsed areas can cause severe dyspnea and pleuritic chest pain. The patient probably will have tachycardia, cyanosis, and diaphoresis. And mediastinal structures will be shifted toward the affected side. The patient may have flaring nostrils and use his accessory muscles to breathe. Plus, he'll be highly anxious.

On palpation, you'll note decreased movement and increased fremitus over the affected areas. Percussion sounds will be dull or flat over those areas. And auscultation may reveal decreased or absent breath sounds as well as end-inspiratory crackles that disappear when the patient takes a deep breath.

Atelectasis can be confirmed by chest X-ray, ABG studies, and pulse oximetry. Typically, X-rays show horizontal lines in the lower lung fields, dense shadows in areas of segmental or lobar collapse, an elevated diaphragm on the affected side, and deviation of the trachea, heart, and mediastinum toward the affected side. Pulse oximetry and ABG studies indicate hypoxemia and respiratory acidosis.

Nursing interventions
Because atelectasis typically results from increased secretions, your priority is to help the patient remove them. Begin by reassessing his ability to remove them on his own. Urge him to cough, deep-breathe, and use an incentive spirometer every hour or two while he's awake. Remember that these steps will be more effective if he receives an aerosolized bronchodilator first.

Assess the patient's respiratory status every 2 hours. If it doesn't improve, you may need to perform postural drainage and percussion or suction the patient's nasopharynx to help him remove secretions (see *Performing postural drainage and percussion*, page 332). Be prepared to assist with therapeutic bronchoscopy to remove mucus, if necessary.

Also, monitor your patient's hydration status. Unless contraindicated, encourage him to drink at least 3,000 ml a day to help liquefy his secretions.

Have the patient change positions and walk as much as possible to promote lung expansion and deeper breathing. Tell him to use pursed-lip breathing if the increased activity makes him short of breath. Be sure to balance periods of rest with periods of activity.

You'll also need to monitor your patient's pulse oximetry and ABG studies more frequently, as ordered, including during activities. Report $Paco_2$ increases of 10 to 15 mm Hg and Pao_2 decreases of 10 to 15 mm Hg. Correct hypoxemia by adjusting oxygen flow rates or concentrations according to the physician's order or the oxygen therapy protocol.

Before discharge, reinforce all aspects of the patient's regimen. Above all, stress the importance of removing secretions from the lungs by staying active, coughing, and deep breathing.

Respiratory acidosis
Patients with asthma and pneumonia have a high risk of developing respiratory acidosis, an acid-base imbalance characterized by hypercapnia and acidemia. It may develop as an acute condition in status asthmaticus. But more commonly, it results from progressive exhaustion caused by airway obstruction. Either way, a patient who develops respiratory acidosis from asthma and pneumonia has a life-threatening problem that requires immediate attention.

Performing postural drainage and percussion

When a patient with asthma and pneumonia develops atelectasis, you may need to perform postural drainage and percussion to clear tenacious mucous plugs from his airways.

Before the procedure

- Schedule the procedure before or at least 2 hours after meals or tube feedings to prevent nausea and aspiration.
- Assess your patient's respiratory status. Auscultate his lungs and note areas where you find absent, diminished, or adventitious sounds. As you assess, remember that moving air out of the bronchioles takes longer in a patient with asthma.
- If your patient is in severe respiratory distress because of the thick secretions produced by asthma and pneumonia and the decreased air exchange caused by atelectasis, don't perform the procedure. Instead, notify the physician right away. If your patient's respiratory status is stable, continue to prepare him for the procedure.
- About 10 to 15 minutes before the procedure, have the patient inhale the prescribed bronchodilator to dilate his narrowed airways as much as possible and prevent shortness of breath during the procedure.
- Have tissues available to catch secretions and a sputum cup to obtain a specimen.
- Explain to your patient that the procedure helps move mucus from very small airways into larger airways, so they can be coughed up or suctioned out.
- Explain that he'll need to lie flat or with his head lower than his feet for a short time so that gravity can help move mucus toward his larger airways. This news may make him anxious because patients with asthma and pneumonia usually sit upright or lean slightly forward, so they can use their accessory muscles to breathe. Reassure him by telling him that both the bronchodilator and the procedure itself will help him breathe more easily. Also, explain that as part of the procedure you'll be thumping on his chest and back to create rhythmic waves that help dislodge the mucus.

During the procedure

- If the patient can tolerate having his head lower than his feet, raise the foot of the bed 15 to 30 degrees. Then place him in a position that will drain the affected lung segment. Use pillows to help support and maintain the position. Because of the combination of airway narrowing and increased tenacious secretions, the patient may feel as though he's suffocating, even if you don't raise the foot of the bed. If he simply can't tolerate lying flat, discuss alternative positions with his physician.
- Place a gown or a towel over areas to be percussed.
- Using cupped hands to create air pockets, clap rhythmically for about 1 minute over each area. Don't percuss over the spine or scapulae or over a woman's breasts.
- Ask the patient to inhale through his nose and exhale in three short huffs. Then have him inhale again and cough two or three times with his mouth slightly open. Remind him to cover his mouth with a tissue to prevent organisms from becoming airborne. Ask him to expectorate any sputum into the sputum cup. If ordered, obtain a sputum specimen at this time.
- Repeat this clapping and coughing sequence two or three times.
- Encourage the patient to use pursed-lip breathing, and let him rest a little while before changing positions to treat another area of his lungs.
- If your patient complains of a headache, nausea, or severe shortness of breath, stop the treatment.

After the procedure

- Return your patient to a comfortable position.
- Note the amount, color, and consistency of secretions expectorated during the procedure. If sputum was obtained, send it to the laboratory promptly.
- Auscultate the patient's lungs to check the effectiveness of treatment.
- If the treatment doesn't relieve his airway obstruction and the collapsed area involves a lung lobe, he may need bronchoscopy or bronchial lavage.

That's because the increased secretions and inflammation associated with asthma and pneumonia only worsen the airway obstruction—and the respiratory acidosis.

Confirming the complication

The patient may have signs and symptoms of central nervous system problems, such as a headache, restlessness, confusion, apprehension, somnolence, flapping hand tremors (asterixis), or even coma. If he has a severe airway obstruction, the patient may be unable to speak and may have an increased paradoxical pulse.

If hyperkalemia has developed, the patient may have ventricular or other arrhythmias. Other signs of respiratory acidosis include depressed reflexes and hypertension. In severe acidosis, the patient may have vasodilation; thus, you may detect full, bounding peripheral pulses and warm, flushed, sweaty skin.

Respiratory acidosis is confirmed by a Pa_{CO_2} greater than 45 mm Hg, a pH less than 7.35, and a bicarbonate level that's normal in the acute stage and elevated in the chronic stage.

Nursing interventions

RAPID RESPONSE ▶ To reverse respiratory acidosis, you need to improve the patient's alveolar ventilation. Usually, when a patient with asthma and pneumonia develops respiratory acidosis, you can reverse the hypercapnia within a few hours by giving large doses of I.V. and aerosolized bronchodilators together with a corticosteroid. Be sure to closely monitor your patient's reaction to these drugs. Many complain of jitteriness, palpitations, or a racing sensation. Reassure the patient that these feelings will subside when he stops receiving the drugs. You may need to perform cardiac monitoring to check for arrhythmias caused by the drugs.

Also, perform these interventions:
- To help thin the patient's tenacious respiratory secretions, administer the prescribed mucolytic.
- Maintain hydration with I.V. and oral fluids.
- Monitor the patient's intake and output carefully and watch for signs of fluid volume excess or deficit.
- Check for electrolyte imbalances from high-dose $beta_2$-agonist therapy and a decreasing pH.
- Give supplemental oxygen as prescribed to promote gas exchange.
- Monitor the patient's oxygen saturation levels frequently, using pulse oximetry and ABG measurements. Report significant changes promptly.
- If the patient's Pa_{CO_2} doesn't start going down and his pH continues to drop, he may need ET intubation and mechanical ventilation.

Intubation and mechanical ventilation also may be needed if the patient becomes exhausted during therapy.

Throughout therapy, watch for changes in central nervous system function. Report such changes immediately. If the patient's level of consciousness declines, be sure to keep him safe. If possible, try not to use restraints because they may make him agitated and thereby increase his oxygen demand. Instead, reduce his anxiety by maintaining a quiet, restful environment and giving him short, simple explanations of care procedures. Provide emotional support for the patient and his family. And try to allay the family's fears by keeping them informed. ◀

Acute respiratory failure

A patient who has asthma and pneumonia must struggle constantly to move air through his narrowed, partially blocked airways. Over a long period of time, maintaining the struggle may require more energy from the patient than he's able to expend. If that happens, he may develop acute respiratory failure.

Confirming the complication

Acute respiratory failure isn't always easy to detect because it looks different in different patients. However, a patient who develops respiratory failure on top of asthma and pneumonia will have one characteristic symptom: increasing dyspnea. You'll want to watch for clues that your patient is having a hard time breathing; for example, you may notice your patient begin to sit in a more upright position because it allows him to breathe more easily.

Because the patient's respiratory function is already compromised from asthma and pneumonia, even mildly increased dyspnea can cause him severe gas-exchange problems. Thus, he may exhibit nasal flaring and use his accessory muscles to breathe. He also may have shallow or deep respirations, or he may alternate between the two. He may show signs and symptoms of hypoxemia, such as central cyanosis (bluish discoloration of the oral mucosa and lips), tachycardia, tachypnea, restlessness, anxiety, and lack of coordination.

As hypercapnia and acidemia worsen, the patient becomes increasingly lethargic. He develops flapping, fine tremors, or jerky motions.

He may have full, bounding peripheral pulses and warm, flushed, sweaty skin caused by vasodilation. His reflexes may be depressed, and he may have papilledema. Plus, his breath sounds may be markedly diminished or absent, and he may not be able to speak.

Typically, acute respiratory failure is confirmed by a PaO_2 less than 50 mm Hg or a $PaCO_2$ greater than 50 mm Hg, coupled with a pH below 7.25.

Nursing interventions

A patient with asthma, pneumonia, and acute respiratory failure is critically ill and may slide into respiratory arrest with little or no warning. That's why he'll probably need ET intubation and mechanical ventilation. And he'll need close monitoring and intensive management.

Intubation can worsen your patient's airway obstruction by stimulating irritant receptors in his trachea. To minimize this response, give him 1 to 2 mg of atropine by nebulizer or 0.5 mg parenterally, as prescribed.

After the ET tube has been inserted, tape it securely and mark its position at the patient's nares or mouth. Auscultate the patient's lungs for equal breath sounds and obtain a chest X-ray to confirm that the tube has been placed correctly. After the placement has been confirmed, continue auscultating the patient's breath sounds and checking the tube's position frequently. Measure ET cuff pressure every 8 hours.

Before suctioning the ET tube, hyperoxygenate the patient to avoid hypoxia during suctioning. To avoid introducing pathogens that could worsen his pneumonia, always use aseptic technique when suctioning. After suctioning, note the quantity, color, and consistency of the patient's sputum.

Administer humidified oxygen to maintain the patient's oxygen saturation level at 90% to 92% and his PaO_2 at 55 mm Hg or more. Use pulse oximetry and ABG measurements to track his oxygenation status, and be sure to report any significant changes to his physician.

Remember that the patient may continue to have a somewhat increased $PaCO_2$ and a somewhat decreased pH. That's because a patient with asthma, pneumonia, and respiratory failure has severely narrowed airways, air trapping, and increased dead space, which means that he needs high airway pressures to achieve adequate ventilation. To avoid excessively high pressures, the physician may accept a higher-than-normal $PaCO_2$ (called permissive hypercapnia) and some level of respiratory acidosis.

Make sure the patient's ventilator is on the correct settings, then check them often. Observe the patient for complications from the high peak pressures commonly used to treat respiratory failure. They include barotrauma (lung injury caused by positive pressure) and pneumothorax (see *Barotrauma: Detection and intervention*).

The combination of positive-pressure ventilation and sedatives given to help the patient relax may produce hypotension, so monitor his blood pressure closely. If hypotension develops, notify the physician.

Also, check the patient's ventilator tubing frequently. Make sure condensed water, which provides an ideal medium for microorganisms, isn't draining into the patient's airways. Empty accumulated water into a collection bag.

During all procedures, avoid excessive movement of the ET tube to reduce the risk of tube displacement, extubation, and tissue necrosis. Also, regularly check for other complications, such as sinusitis, atelectasis, pneumothorax, and stress ulcers. If the patient has an oral tube, perform mouth care regularly and check for thrush and ulceration.

Reposition the patient every 1 to 2 hours to prevent pooling of respiratory secretions and complications of immobility. Use postural drainage and percussion to help loosen secretions and aid in their removal.

Explain to the patient and his family that he won't be able to talk with an ET tube in place. Help him communicate with pen and paper, a picture or word chart, or an alphabet board. When he no longer needs mechanical ventilation, help him understand what happened and why. Before discharge, help him develop a plan to control his asthma, prevent pneumonia, and recognize the early signs of respiratory failure.

Barotrauma: Detection and intervention

Patients with asthma and pneumonia who develop respiratory failure are particularly susceptible to barotrauma, a serious complication that can lead to cardiopulmonary arrest. These patients are susceptible because they require mechanical ventilation with high peak pressures to achieve adequate oxygenation, and such high pressures can traumatize delicate lung tissue, causing the alveoli to rupture. Air then leaks from the alveoli into the surrounding tissues.

The result can be interstitial or subcutaneous emphysema or subpleural air cysts. Or the air can leak into the pleural space, causing pneumothorax; into the mediastinum, causing pneumomediastinum; into the pericardium, causing pneumopericardium; or into the peritoneum, causing pneumoperitoneum.

Assessment

When your patient with asthma and pneumonia requires mechanical ventilation, monitor him closely. Suspect barotrauma if you detect any of the following:
- a sudden loss of breath sounds
- hyperresonance on percussion
- decreased chest excursion on one side
- crepitation on palpation or auscultation
- a crunching sound on mediastinal palpation
- signs and symptoms of noncardiogenic pulmonary edema
- signs of decreased cardiac output, such as increased heart rate and decreased blood pressure
- a sudden increase in peak inspiratory pressure on the ventilator pressure manometer
- decreased oxygen saturation levels.

If you suspect barotrauma, notify the patient's physician at once. Then prepare the patient for a chest X-ray, which will be used to confirm barotrauma.

Interventions

When caring for a patient with barotrauma, perform these interventions:
- Monitor his vital signs and breath sounds at least every 4 hours to detect complications of barotrauma. Be on the lookout for a sudden rise in heart rate or a drop in blood pressure, which may indicate cardiac tamponade. Also, note an absence of breath sounds, which may indicate an inadvertent intubation of the right bronchus or a spontaneous pneumothorax.
- Make sure the positive-pressure ventilator setting is as prescribed. Excessive positive pressure can worsen barotrauma. Regularly check the settings for tidal volume, peak pressure, plateau pressure, and positive end-expiratory pressure, as well.
- If your patient has a spontaneous pneumothorax, prepare for emergency air aspiration using a chest tube, percutaneous pneumothorax catheter, or a thoracic vent.
- If air aspiration doesn't resolve the pneumothorax, expect to assist with pleurodesis, a procedure in which doxycycline or talc is injected into the pleural space to cause adhesion of the pleural surfaces.
- If air has entered the pericardial or peritoneal space, an air-aspiration catheter will be inserted. Monitor the patient closely. Arrhythmias or pericardial friction rubs may indicate pericardial inflammation. Muffled heart sounds may indicate cardiac tamponade. Auscultate the abdomen at least every 4 hours for bowel sounds.
- Prepare the patient for diagnostic tests, especially frequent X-rays, to monitor the effectiveness of treatment.

Asthma and arrhythmias

Arrhythmias commonly result from decreased oxygenation of myocardial tissue. And because asthma and its treatment can reduce oxygenation, asthma patients face an increased risk of arrhythmias. What's more, patients with asthma and arrhythmias face an increased risk of potentially life-threatening complications.

Pathophysiology

The hypoxemia caused by asthma affects cardiac tissue just as it does the body's other tissues. And the respiratory acidosis caused by asthma attacks can delay electrical conduction and cause bradycardia, heart block, and other arrhythmias.

To make matters worse, drugs used to treat asthma—beta$_2$ agonists and aminophylline, for example—can induce arrhythmias, such as sinus tachycardia and atrial tachyarrhythmias. Beta$_2$ agonists also can create an intracellular potassium shift that causes hypokalemia, a condition that can lead to atrial and life-threatening ventricular arrhythmias.

Adapting nursing care

Expect to begin ECG monitoring for a patient with asthma and an arrhythmia. Treat the arrhythmia as you would for any patient.

Before and after giving a beta$_2$ agonist, assess your patient's heart rate and rhythm. After an inhaled beta$_2$ agonist is given through the ventilator circuit of an intubated patient, be sure to check for adverse cardiac effects. Expect to withhold the next dose if a beta$_2$ agonist triggers an arrhythmia.

If you need to give large doses of terbutaline, monitor your patient's potassium levels carefully. Report decreased levels promptly and expect to withhold or decrease the next dose.

Use pulse oximetry and ABG measurements to assess your patient's oxygen saturation levels. Try to correct asthma-induced hypoxemia as quickly as possible to prevent it from causing or worsening arrhythmias.

Make sure your patient has a patent I.V. line with an access port at or near the catheter hub, so you can administer antiarrhythmic drugs if they become necessary. Also, have solution for flushing the I.V. line and emergency equipment readily available. Monitor the patient's blood pressure frequently and watch for signs of decreased cardiac output if he develops a tachyarrhythmia.

Before discharge, make sure the patient understands his regimen. Make special note of asthma medications that tend to cause adverse cardiac effects and tell him to report palpitations or an increased heart rate to his physician. Make sure the patient knows how to take his pulse.

Complications

Common complications for patients with asthma and arrhythmias include heart failure and cardiac arrest.

Heart failure

Arrhythmias can cause or aggravate heart failure, especially in an asthmatic patient, because they reduce cardiac output by altering filling times in the heart chambers. Initially, the heart tries to compensate for the reduced cardiac output by increasing left ventricular end-diastolic pressure. This action eventually raises pulmonary vascular pressures in the lung, creating congestion and possibly worsening the patient's asthma.

The falling cardiac output also causes a compensatory rise in peripheral vascular resistance, which initially raises blood pressure. Although this change works to maintain perfusion, it eventually leads to increased afterload, which makes the heart work harder. Over time, the constant need to pump blood against increased resistance causes the heart to weaken and become less effective. The result is reduced contractility, which leads to heart failure.

Confirming the complication

A diagnosis of heart failure usually is based on assessment findings and such diagnostic tests as a chest X-ray and echocardiogram.

Signs and symptoms vary, depending on whether the patient has left ventricular or right ventricular heart failure. Left ventricular failure makes the patient's dyspnea and orthopnea worse. He may report waking up suddenly, short of breath—a condition called paroxysmal nocturnal dyspnea. Decreased cardiac output and increased pulmonary congestion also may cause tachycardia, tachypnea, coughing, cyanosis, confusion, dizziness, and postural hypotension. Auscultation may reveal an S$_3$ heart sound, crackles, and decreased breath sounds.

With right ventricular failure, a patient probably will have jugular vein distention, an enlarged liver and spleen, and dependent edema. He may complain of anorexia, nausea, or abdominal pain.

DRUG ALERT

Drugs for asthma and heart failure: Dangerous interactions

Asthma drugs	Heart failure drugs	Adverse effects	Nursing actions
• Beta₂ agonists (albuterol, terbutaline)	• Digoxin	• Both drugs may alter blood pressure and cause hypokalemia, precipitating tachyarrhythmias.	• Monitor electrocardiogram (ECG) for tachyarrhythmias. • Check blood pressure frequently. • Observe patient for signs of hypokalemia, such as muscle weakness. • Monitor serum potassium levels and give prescribed potassium replacement.
• Anticholinergics (ipatropium)	• Digoxin	• Anticholinergic may increase digoxin blood level.	• Observe patient for signs and symptoms of digoxin toxicity, such as anorexia, nausea, vomiting, arrhythmias, hypotension, and atrioventricular block. • Monitor digoxin and serum potassium levels.
• Theophylline and aminophylline	• Dobutamine	• Drugs are incompatible in solution. • Drugs may cause tachyarrhythmias.	• If drugs must be given at the same time, use separate I.V. lines. • With I.V. administration, monitor ECG and blood pressure every 5 minutes. • Closely monitor serum theophylline levels. • Observe patient for tachyarrhythmias and worsening heart failure.
• Systemic corticosteroids	• Potassium-depleting diuretics (chlorothiazide, furosemide)	• Both drugs increase potassium excretion.	• Observe patient for signs of hypokalemia, such as muscle weakness. • Monitor serum potassium levels and give prescribed potassium replacement.

In a patient with left ventricular failure, chest X-rays reveal an enlarged heart. A pleural effusion suggests biventricular heart failure.

An echocardiogram can detect the structural changes of heart failure, such as enlarged chambers and ventricular hypertrophy.

Nursing interventions
If your asthma patient has an arrhythmia and is experiencing acute heart failure, place him in the Fowler position to maximize chest expansion and gas exchange. Give supplemental oxygen as indicated and be sure to monitor his vital signs and cardiac rhythm closely. Anticipate the insertion of a pulmonary artery catheter to monitor hemodynamic measurements, such as cardiac output, pulmonary artery pressure, and pulmonary capillary wedge pressure. Auscultate the patient's heart for abnormal sounds, such as an S_3 heart sound, and the lungs for increased crackles or wheezes.

Maintain a patent I.V. line and administer morphine, antiarrhythmic drugs, and a rapid-acting diuretic, as prescribed. Monitor the patient for signs of drug interactions (see *Drugs for asthma and heart failure: Dangerous interactions*).

Ordinarily, you'd want to increase fluid intake in a patient with asthma to help liquefy secretions. But extra fluids are contraindicated for patients with left ventricular failure, so anticipate the potential need to give a mucolytic drug, as prescribed, to help loosen secretions. Also, emphasize the importance of coughing and deep breathing.

Monitor intake and output carefully. If the patient has an indwelling catheter, report an output of less than 30 ml per hour (or less than 240 ml per shift), which may indicate fluid retention. Also, weigh the patient daily at the same time and on the same scale. Report a rapid gain of 2 pounds or more; this too can signal fluid retention. Assess the patient daily for dependent edema.

Monitor the patient's serum potassium levels for hypokalemia, which can further aggravate his arrhythmia and heart failure. If he has hypokalemia, notify his physician and expect to administer supplemental potassium therapy.

Use pulse oximetry and ABG measurements to monitor oxygen saturation levels, as indicated. Increasing hypoxemia may signal worsening heart failure, asthma, or both.

Note any changes in the patient's mental status, such as restlessness, confusion, and somnolence. If respiratory failure develops because of left ventricular heart failure, prepare the patient for ET intubation and mechanical ventilation.

When the patient's condition stabilizes, make sure he understands all aspects of the treatment plan, including taking his medications for asthma, arrhythmias, and heart failure. Urge the patient to keep follow-up appointments so that the physician can check his progress. If the patient is taking a loop or thiazide diuretic for his heart failure, teach him to watch for signs and symptoms of hypokalemia. Also, encourage him to eat foods high in potassium. Tell him to weigh himself two to three times a week and to report a rapid gain of 2 pounds or more. Finally, obtain a referral for home care so that a nurse can assess the patient's progress in his own environment.

Cardiac arrest

If an asthma attack is severe enough, it can produce profound hypoxia that prevents the heart from beating. When asthma is complicated by arrhythmias, the risk of cardiac arrest increases even further because the arrhythmias reduce cardiac output, which decreases blood flow to the myocardium.

Confirming the complication

If your patient has a cardiac arrest, he'll become unresponsive and stop breathing. He'll have no pulse, no heart beat, and no blood pressure. His ECG will show ventricular fibrillation or asystole.

Nursing interventions

RAPID RESPONSE ▶ If your patient develops cardiac arrest, summon help and initiate cardiopulmonary resuscitation (CPR). You must act quickly to prevent hypoxic brain damage.

- Assess the patient's airway and open it if necessary, using the head-tilt or chin-lift maneuver.
- Look, listen, and feel for breathing. If the patient isn't breathing, ventilate him. If possible, insert an oropharyngeal airway and give two slow breaths with a pocket face mask. Between breaths, allow him 1 to 2 seconds to exhale. Make sure his head is tilted back so that he can exhale.
- Quickly check for a pulse at the carotid artery on the side closer to you. Palpate for 5 to 10 seconds because the pulse may be difficult to detect if it's slow, irregular, weak, or rapid.
- If you don't detect a pulse, perform closed-chest compressions following basic life support (BLS) guidelines.
- Assess the quality and effectiveness of chest compressions and ventilations repeatedly throughout the resuscitative effort.
- If the patient has ventricular fibrillation or pulseless ventricular tachycardia, prepare to defibrillate him. (Within 2 minutes of your call for help, trained personnel should arrive with a defibrillator and other equipment.)
- Follow advanced cardiac life support (ACLS) guidelines when performing defibrillation. Deliver up to three countershocks immediately.
- Perform the following secondary survey:
  Airway. Verify that someone is preparing to perform ET intubation. Select the proper-sized tube, check the laryngoscope, and prepare for suctioning.
  Breathing. Observe the patient's chest and note if it's rising and falling bilaterally. Also, auscultate his lungs for bilateral breath sounds with ventilations. Assist with intubation and obtain a chest X-ray immediately to confirm that the tube is placed correctly.
  Circulation. Obtain I.V. access and begin infusing normal saline solution. Be prepared to administer emergency medications I.V. or endotracheally. To enhance parenteral delivery of medications, administer a 20-ml to 30-ml bolus of I.V. fluid and elevate the patient's

arm after giving each medication. Follow each ET injection with a 10-ml flush of normal saline solution, then immediately attach the ventilation bag and forcefully ventilate the patient three or four times. ◄

After resuscitation, make sure your patient has oxygen, an ECG monitor, resuscitation equipment, and trained personnel nearby. Monitor him closely. When his condition is stable, explain what happened and which changes have been made to his treatment plan.

Suggested readings

Anonymous. Asthma inhalation therapy. *Medical Sciences Bulletin.* 1 January 1994;19(3).

Anonymous. Zafinlukast approved for asthma, *Medical Sciences Bulletin.* 1 November 1996; 19(3).

Barnes PJ. Current therapies for asthma: promise and limitations. *Chest.* 1997;111(2):17S-26S.

Bellomo R, McLaughlin P, Tai E, Parkin G. Asthma requiring mechanical ventilation: a low morbidity approach. *Chest.* 1994;105(3):891-896.

Bhatia T. Pulse oximetry: the fifth vital sign. *RT.* 1996;55-60.

Centers for Disease Control and Prevention. Asthma-United States, 1982-1992. *MMWR Morb Mortal Wkly Rep.* 1995;43:952-954.

Corbridge TC, Hall JB. The assessment and management of adults with status asthmaticus. *Am J Respir Crit Care Med.* 1995;151(5):1296-1316.

Cummins R, ed. *Textbook of advanced cardiac life support.* American Heart Association. 1994.

Davies RJ, Wang J, Abdelaziz MM, et al. New insights into the understanding of asthma. *Chest.* 1997;111(2Suppl):2S-10S.

Des Jardins T. *Clinical manifestations and assessment of respiratory disease.* 3rd ed. St Louis, Mo: Mosby–Year Book, Inc; 1995.

Enright PL, Ward BJ, Tracy RP, Lasser EC. Asthma and its association with cardiovascular disease in the elderly. The Cardiovascular Health Study Research Group. *Asthma.* 1996;33(1):45-53.

Expert Panel Report II. *Guidelines for the diagnosis and management of asthma.* National Asthma Education and Prevention Program; February 1997.

George RB. *Current pulmonology.* Vol. 17. St Louis, Mo: Mosby–Year Book, Inc; 1996.

Grossman J. One airway, one disease. *Chest.* 1997;111(2Suppl):11S-16S.

Hay DW. Pharmacology of leukotriene receptor antagonists: more than inhibitors of bronchoconstriction. *Chest.* 1997;111(2Suppl):35S-45S.

Huether SE, McCance KL. *Understanding pathophysiology.* St Louis, Mo: Mosby–Year Book, Inc; 1996

Hunt LH, Swedlund HA, Gleich GJ. Effect of nebulized lidocaine on severe glucocorticoid-dependent asthma. *Mayo Clin Proc.* 1996;71(4):361-368.

Karpel JP, Schacter EN, Fanta C, et al. A comparison of ipratropium and albuterol vs albuterol alone for the treatment of acute asthma. *Chest.* 1996;110(3):611-616.

Leff AR. Future directions in asthma therapy: is a cure possible? *Chest.* 1997;111(2Suppl):61S-68S.

Meduri GU, Cook TR, Turner RE, Leeper KV. Noninvasive positive pressure ventilation in status asthmaticus. *Chest.* 1996;110(31):767-74.

Murray J, Nadel J. *Textbook of respiratory medicine.* 2nd ed. Philadelphia, Pa: WB Saunders Co; 1994.

Reisner C, Kotch A, Duorkin G. Continuous versus frequent intermittent nebulization of albuterol in acute asthma: a randomized, prospective study. *Ann Allergy Asthma Immunol.* 1995;75(1):41-47.

Sandford A, Weir T, Pare P. The genetics of asthma. *Am J Respir Crit Care Med.* 1996;153(6Pt1):1749-1765.

Teach your patients about asthma: a clinician's guide. Bethesda, Md: US Department of Health and Human Services; October 1992. National Institutes of Health Publication No. 92-2737.

Warner DO, Warner MA, Barnes RD, et al. Perioperative respiratory complications in patients with asthma. *Anesthesiology.* 1996;85(3):460-467.

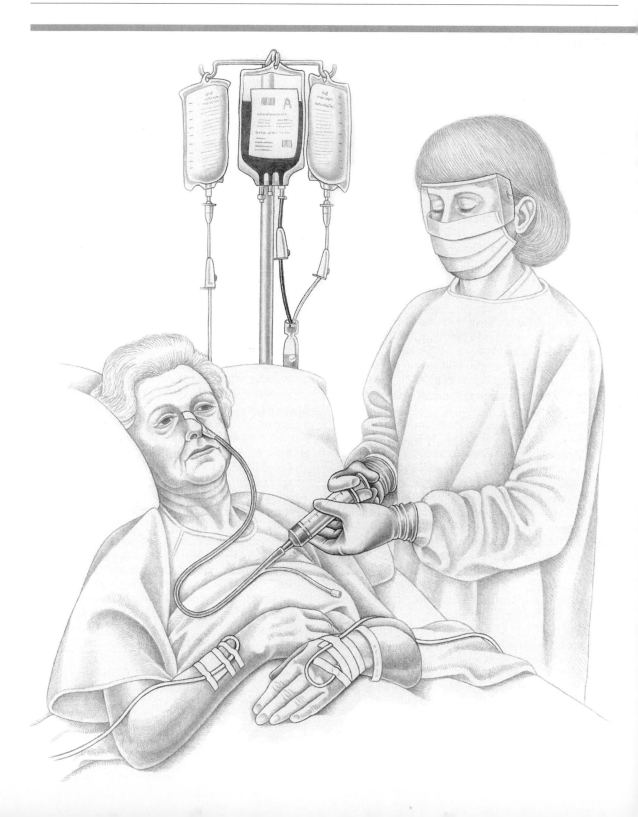

11

Peptic Ulcer Disease

Buffeted by highly acidic secretions and strong, churning muscular movements, the upper gastrointestinal (GI) tract has developed certain adaptations to prevent or quickly repair injuries to its mucosal layer. In about 10% of the population, however, damage occurs despite these mucosal adaptations, and peptic ulcer disease develops.

Peptic ulcer disease is a term used to describe acute or chronic mucosal erosion (or ulceration) in an area of the GI tract exposed to acid and pepsin. Typically, peptic ulcer disease isn't life threatening. In fact, some peptic ulcers produce no apparent illness at all. With proper treatment, most heal in 4 to 6 weeks.

When complicated by other disorders, however, peptic ulcer disease may develop into a serious problem, possibly leading to hemorrhage, peritonitis, or recurrent myocardial infarction. By detecting and responding to peptic ulcer disease appropriately and by minimizing the influence of other disorders and their treatments, you can help your patient avoid these dangerous complications.

Anatomy and physiology review

As you know, different facets of digestion and absorption take place in different areas of the GI tract. In the mouth, for example, food is moistened, chewed, and broken down for easy passage. Swallowing and peristalsis force the food bolus through the esophagus to the lower esophageal sphincter, which permits passage to the stomach. Most of the mechanical breakdown of food occurs in the stomach and duodenum. Because of the strongly acidic secretions used to liquefy ingested foods and kill most microorganisms, the stomach and duodenum have the greatest risk of mucosal erosion. The small and large intestines serve primarily to absorb nutrients and water and to prepare undigested substances for elimination.

Stomach

Tucked behind and between the liver and the spleen, the stomach lies just under the diaphragm and slightly left of the midline. The stomach's size varies greatly with the volume of its contents. A typical stomach has a capacity approaching 1,500 ml (see *Stomach and duodenum*).

The stomach stores food and mechanically digests it by mixing and liquefying the food bolus into a loose, semisolid substance called chyme. To accomplish this purpose, cells lining the stomach secrete 1,500 to 3,000 ml of gastric juice each day.

Little chemical digestion occurs in the stomach, although an enzyme called pepsin performs some chemical digestion by breaking proteins into polypeptides, proteases, and peptones. Minimal fat digestion takes place in the stomach, and little absorption takes place across the stomach wall. Only small amounts of water, alcohol, glucose, and weak acids cross the stomach's mucosal lining.

Controlling sphincters

Two sphincters block the stomach's proximal and distal openings to prevent acidic stomach contents from leaking back into the esophagus or moving too quickly into the duodenum. The lower esophageal sphincter, also called the cardiac sphincter, connects the esophagus to the cardia of the stomach. The lower esophageal sphincter doesn't contain specialized tissue. Rather, the pressure difference between the thoracic cavity and the abdominal cavity (negative pressure above the diaphragm and positive pressure below) holds the lower esophageal sphincter closed, thus preventing reflux of stomach contents into the esophagus.

The pyloric sphincter, at the stomach's distal end, acts like an anatomic valve. Composed of ringlike muscle, the pyloric sphincter remains closed at rest, preventing a constant flow of stomach contents into the duodenum. The pyloric sphincter opens in rhythm with stomach contractions, allowing only a small amount of chyme to enter the duodenum with each wave.

Stomach wall

The stomach wall is composed of several layers. The outermost, called the serosa, is visceral peritoneum. Beneath the serosa are three layers of smooth muscle, each oriented in a different direction. In addition to the circular and longitudinal muscle layers throughout most of the GI tract, the stomach also has an oblique smooth-muscle layer. This extra layer means that stomach contents are not only propelled forward but are also churned vigorously while inside the stomach, effectively liquefying the food bolus by mixing it with gastric juices. This additional muscle layer also contributes to the stomach's considerable distensibility.

Beneath the three muscle layers lies the submucosa, which contains blood vessels, lymph vessels, and nerves. The innermost layer, the mucosa, has a host of secretory cells and a thick gel covering produced by those epithelial cells. The mucosal epithelial cells also secrete bicarbonate, which helps to neutralize acidic secretions at the mucosal surface.

ANATOMY REVIEW

Stomach and duodenum

The stomach forms a pouch bounded on each end by a sphincter. As the illustration on the left shows, the stomach is divided into four anatomic regions. The illustration on the right shows the layers of the stomach wall, including the three layers of smooth muscle, which run in different directions. Both illustrations show the duodenum, the portion of the small intestine just below the stomach.

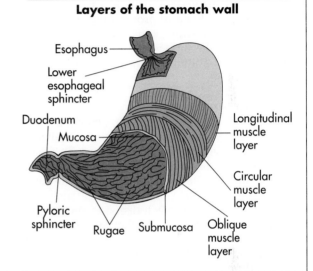

Anatomic regions of the stomach

Fundus

Cardia

Body

Pylorus

Layers of the stomach wall

Esophagus

Lower esophageal sphincter

Duodenum

Mucosa

Longitudinal muscle layer

Circular muscle layer

Pyloric sphincter

Rugae

Submucosa

Oblique muscle layer

The mucosa is almost totally impervious to hydrogen ions. Together, hydrogen impermeability and bicarbonate secretion protect the mucosal layer from gastric secretions that have a pH of less than 2. In fact, despite these acidic secretions, the mucosa's intraluminal pH remains near 7.

Secretory cells

The stomach lining contains four major types of secretory cells:

- Chief cells, also called peptic or zygomatic cells, secrete mucus and pepsinogen. Pepsinogen is the precursor of the protein-digesting enzyme pepsin.
- Parietal cells, also called oxyntic cells, secrete hydrochloric acid and water. The amount of acid the stomach can secrete depends largely on the number of parietal cells the mucosa contains. Parietal cells also produce intrinsic factor, which is essential for vitamin B_{12} absorption in the terminal ileum.
- Mucous cells secrete a sticky, alkaline mucus that adheres to the epithelial surface and helps protect the gastric wall from acid.
- Enteroendocrine cells secrete a variety of hormone and hormonelike substances, including gastrin, histamine, and serotonin.

The combined secretions of all these cells is called gastric juice. It's produced at a steady basal rate throughout the day, with temporary increases prompted by hormonal, neural, and local stimuli.

Hormones that stimulate secretion of gastric juice include acetylcholine (a cholinergic transmitter), histamine released by the enteroendocrine cells, and gastrin. These three substances bind with receptors on the secretory cells themselves. The receptors then activate the secretory process. Acetylcholine stimulates all secretory cells. Histamine and gastrin stimulate mainly acid secretion. Working in concert, these three substances prompt the secretion of much more gastric juice than any of them working alone.

Some nervous system control of gastric secretion originates in the brain and travels along the vagus nerve and its branches, which pass through nervous system structures in the stomach wall to reach the gastric glands. Additional nervous system control comes from within the enteric nervous system itself as a response to local reflexes. Factors prompting these local reflexes include stomach distention, mechanical stimuli on the surface of the stomach lining, and chemical stimuli from amino acids, peptides, and acid.

Digestive process

When food enters the stomach, protein in the food mixes with gastric acid and neutralizes the acid, raising the pH to as high as 6. The rise in pH as well as the rise in peptides and amino acids stimulate the release of the hormone gastrin, which is a potent stimulator of gastric acid secretion. As the stomach distends, mechanoreceptors in the mucosa further stimulate gastrin release.

About an hour after a meal, the food's buffering ability is exhausted and acid secretion peaks. By then, however, a significant portion of the meal has moved into the small intestine. Maximum acid secretion combined with a decreasing food load causes the stomach's acid concentration to rise. As it rises, the dropping pH inhibits gastrin release, which in turn causes acid secretion in the stomach to decline.

As chyme moves from the stomach to the duodenum, digested protein products prompt gastrin release in the duodenum. However, intestinal stimuli produce a much smaller amount of acid than the amount secreted in the stomach.

Duodenum

The duodenum, the shortest portion of the small intestine, begins at the stomach's pyloric sphincter and stretches for about 10 inches until it merges with the jejunum. The ligament of Treitz suspends this junction from the posterior abdominal wall. The pancreatic and common bile ducts empty their secretions into the duodenum.

In the duodenum, enzymes from the pancreas, bile from the liver and gallbladder, and intestinal enzymes complete the digestion of chyme. Brunner's glands secrete an alkaline mucus that protects the wall of the small intestine from digestive enzymes and helps neutralize the acid in chyme as it enters from the stomach. Other intestinal epithelial cells secrete bicarbonate, which, together with the mucus, maintains the gastric mucosal pH at about 7. Mucosal cells also produce the hormones secretin and cholecystokinin, which stimulate pancreatic enzymes and bile.

Pathophysiology

Cells lining the stomach and duodenum replace themselves rapidly, about every 3 days, which makes the GI tract well equipped to repair minor erosions and mucosal injuries. But despite the host of adaptations that protect the stomach and duodenum from their own byproducts, the protective process can sometimes break down. When it does, the outcome is peptic ulcer disease.

In a general sense, peptic ulcer disease results when, for whatever reason, the erosive power of gastric juice overcomes the defenses of the gastric and duodenal mucosa. Consequently, any condition that boosts the secretion of gastric juices, increases stimulation of the vagus nerve, decreases inhibition of gastric secretion, increases the number or secretory capacity of parietal cells, or increases parietal cell response to stimulation can cause peptic ulcer disease. Obviously, the erosive power of gastric juice emanates directly from gastric acid. In fact, some level of gastric acid must be present for peptic ulcer disease to develop, leading to wide professional acceptance of the phrase, "No acid, no ulcer." The fact that even normal levels of gastric acid can lead to ulcer formation attests to the importance of a competent mucosa.

Usually, ulcers form in the stomach or duodenum. Duodenal ulcers are more common than gastric ulcers and usually form close to the pylorus. Gastric and duodenal ulcers differ markedly. In fact, some experts consider them separate disorders (see *Comparing gastric and duodenal ulcers*).

Comparing gastric and duodenal ulcers

Characteristic	Gastric ulcer	Duodenal ulcer
Most common location	• Junction of fundus and antrum	• Up to 1.5 cm from pylorus
Age at onset	• Most common between ages 50 and 70	• Most common between ages 20 and 50
Sex	• Almost equal in men and women	• More common in men than women
Acid secretion	• Normal or decreased	• Increased
Parietal cell mass	• Normal or decreased	• Increased
Gastrin levels	• Increased	• Normal
Pepsinogen levels	• Normal	• Increased
***Helicobacter pylori* infection**	• 60% to 80% of cases	• 95% to 100% of cases
Pain	• Variable pattern • 1 to 2 hours after meals • Relief or exacerbation with food or antacids	• 2 to 4 hours after meals and at night • Relieved by food and antacids
Nutritional status	• Possible malnutrition • Weight loss	• Normal nutrition • Possible weight gain

Many factors can play a role in creating or aggravating peptic ulcer disease. These factors either increase gastric acid secretion or decrease the ability of gastric mucosa to protect itself against its acid environment.

Helicobacter pylori infection
A corkscrew-shaped bacterium, *H. pylori* infects the mucosal layer of the stomach and duodenum. Virtually all patients with duodenal ulcers and most patients with gastric ulcers have an *H. pylori* infection.

In 1994, a consensus panel of the National Institutes of Health suggested that this organism plays a major role in the development of peptic ulcer disease not caused by nonsteroidal anti-inflammatory drugs (NSAIDs). Recently, studies have found *H. pylori* infection to be the most powerful predictor of ulcer recurrence. They've also found that curing the infection through antibiotic treatment can reduce the chance of recurrence from about 75% to about 10%.

No one knows exactly how *H. pylori* influences ulcer formation. But it almost certainly does so by secreting an enzyme called urease. Urease breaks down urea into ammonia, carbon dioxide, and water. Ammonia initiates an inflammatory response, leading to mucosal irritation.

Nonsteroidal anti-inflammatory drugs
Drugs such as aspirin, indomethacin, naproxen, and ibuprofen injure the mucosa by inhibiting the enzyme cyclooxygenase. This enzyme is required for the synthesis of prostaglandins, which help prevent the corrosive effects of acid and pepsin on the mucosa. Prostaglandins protect the stomach by:
• suppressing the secretion of gastric acid
• promoting the secretion of bicarbonate and mucus
• promoting vasodilation, which maintains submucosal blood flow.

By inhibiting the synthesis of these important protective substances, NSAIDs therapy, especially long-term NSAIDs therapy, increases the risk of peptic ulcer disease considerably. Another effect of NSAIDs, especially aspirin, is the suppression of platelet aggregation needed to promote healing.

Contributing factors

At one time, health care professionals thought that peptic ulcers resulted from a stress-filled life, an aggressive or anxious personality, and a diet filled with spicy foods. Few professionals believe that any more. However, these and other lifestyle and environmental factors do have an effect on peptic ulcer disease.

For example, stressful events can increase gastric acid secretion, thereby aggravating existing ulcers. Certain foods can intensify the pain of existing ulcers. Cigarette smoke and nicotine may accelerate the emptying of gastric acid into the duodenum, promoting mucosal breakdown. Also, cigarette smoke and nicotine inhibit pancreatic secretion of bicarbonate, thereby increasing gastric acid concentration. And alcohol and caffeine can damage the mucosa directly.

Medications other than NSAIDs can contribute to the pathophysiology of peptic ulcers as well. By inhibiting prostaglandin synthesis, glucocorticoids increase gastric acid and pepsin secretion, reduce gastric mucosal blood flow, and decrease the protective mucus. To complicate matters, glucocorticoids may mask the signs of ulcer formation. That means the patient may not seek treatment until hemorrhage or perforation develops.

Certain illnesses are also associated with ulcer formation. These include pancreatitis, liver disease, Crohn's disease, and Zollinger-Ellison syndrome.

Other predisposing factors include:
- Blood type. Gastric ulcers are more common in patients with type A blood. Duodenal ulcers are more common in patients with type O blood.
- Genetic factors. Duodenal ulcers are more common in first-degree relatives of patients with duodenal ulcers than in the general population.

- Trauma. Stress ulcers may develop after severe trauma, such as burns, multisystem injury, an intense hypotensive incident, cardiac arrest, lengthy cranial surgery, mechanical ventilation, or massive infection. They result from mucosal ischemia from the massive sympathetic nervous stimulation that occurs during the physiologic stress response.
- Aging. Weakening of the pyloric sphincter with age allows bile reflux into the stomach, contributing to gastric ulcer formation.

Assessment findings

The most common history and physical examination findings for a patient with peptic ulcer disease are epigastric pain, appetite changes, weight changes, and signs and symptoms of complications. Signs and symptoms may differ somewhat depending on whether the patient has a duodenal or gastric ulcer.

A patient with a duodenal ulcer usually reports a specific pain-food-relief pattern. The typical patient experiences a pain pattern directly related to food, which acts as a buffer for the increased amount of acid. Pain usually occurs 1 to 2 hours after meals and at night. This patient usually doesn't experience anorexia or lose a significant amount of weight. Because food may alleviate the ulcer pain, the patient may even gain weight.

A patient with a gastric ulcer usually reports a variable pain pattern based on an individual response to the presence of acid. Food may relieve pain, or it may cause or worsen pain. This patient is more likely to eat poorly because food sometimes causes pain. Consequently, the patient may report weight loss.

Remember that assessment findings for an elderly patient with peptic ulcer disease may not be the same as those for a younger patient. For instance, the weakened abdominal muscles and diminished pain perception that can occur with aging may mask early symptoms. The patient may have only nonspecific indications, such as mental confusion, or none at all. Later signs and symptoms—such as pain, bleeding, and perforation—may be the only indications of peptic ulcer disease in an elderly patient.

If your examination reveals fatigue, pallor, and activity intolerance, your patient may have anemia from chronic GI bleeding. In fact, bleeding is the most common complication of peptic ulcer disease, especially gastric ulcers. Your goal is to assess the severity of the problem.

Small areas of erosion may produce only slight capillary bleeding. Over time, however, the slow leak can result in signs and symptoms of anemia. You may also be able to detect digested blood in the patient's stool, either by using an occult blood test or by observing that the stool is dark and tarry.

Acute GI bleeding may develop if the erosion extends through the wall of a large blood vessel or if granulation tissue begins to bleed. A patient with acute bleeding may report vomiting bright red blood or a substance that looks like coffee grounds.

Also, watch for indications of less common complications of ulcer disease, which include obstruction and perforation. Obstruction usually develops gradually and produces abdominal distention, gastric fullness, early satiety, and, if the obstruction becomes complete, emesis.

Perforation produces acute abdominal pain, large amounts of red or coffee-ground vomitus, or both. Perforation is the most life-threatening complication of peptic ulcer disease because the escape of hydrochloric acid, pepsin, bile, and pancreatic fluid causes a chemical peritonitis. Bacterial peritonitis develops 6 to 12 hours later. If your patient reports vomiting red blood or coffee-ground vomitus, quickly assess her for common signs and symptoms of peritonitis: severe abdominal pain that may radiate to the shoulder, a rigid boardlike abdomen, and absent bowel sounds. You may also observe signs of shock.

Diagnostic tests

A diagnosis of peptic ulcer disease typically is based on the patient's signs and symptoms and endoscopy and X-ray findings. Additional tests may be performed to check the patient's hematologic status and detect bleeding.

Endoscopy

Fiberoptic endoscopy is the standard test for diagnosing ulcers, monitoring progress, and determining ulcer recurrence. It provides direct

Viewing the stomach lining

To diagnose peptic ulcers, a physician will use a flexible, fiberoptic endoscope, as shown. The endoscope not only provides light and visualization but also has ports through which an examiner can use biopsy forceps and cytology brushes. Video imaging may be used to view stomach motility.

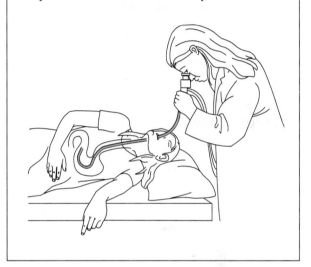

visualization of the ulcer and can be used to determine the ulcer's precise location and stage of healing. A biopsy can be performed through the endoscope to check for *H. pylori* infection and cancerous changes (see *Viewing the stomach lining*).

However, a physician may postpone an endoscopy for patients who are at high risk for complications. These patients include those with the following:
- respiratory decompensation that requires endotracheal (ET) intubation and mechanical ventilation
- hypotension or syncope less than 12 hours before endoscopy
- life-threatening arrhythmias less than 24 hours before endoscopy
- massive bleeding that requires more than 8 units of transfused packed red blood cells (RBCs)
- severe, uncorrected coagulopathy

- recurrent angina less than 12 hours before endoscopy
- acute renal failure
- severe sepsis
- cerebrovascular accident less than 24 hours before endoscopy.

X-rays

An upper GI X-ray series using a contrast agent (usually barium swallowed before and during the test) may reveal the duodenal or gastric deformity caused by the ulcer. Although X-rays are less useful than endoscopy, they may be performed first for patients whose symptoms aren't severe.

Gastric analysis

Gastric analysis allows you to determine the amount of gastric acid secreted over time. You perform the test by collecting gastric secretions through a nasogastric (NG) tube for a specified period of time and measuring their volume. This test can be used to identify or rule out hyperchlorhydria. However, because endoscopy is much more definitive for diagnosing ulcers, gastric analysis is an uncommon choice.

Other tests

Other diagnostic tests, especially a complete blood count (CBC) with hemoglobin level and hematocrit, can be used to evaluate the patient's hematologic condition. You also may check the patient's stool for frank or occult blood. Other laboratory studies include measurements of serum gastrin levels and albumin levels. Low albumin levels may indicate malnutrition. White and differential blood cell counts can be performed to evaluate the possibility of infection.

Medical interventions

Treatment for peptic ulcer disease aims to alleviate symptoms, promote healing by decreasing or neutralizing hydrochloric acid and strengthening the mucosa, and prevent recurrences and complications.

Treatment options include diet therapy and lifestyle modification, drug therapy, and surgery.

Diet therapy and lifestyle modification

Historically, dietary restrictions formed the foundation of ulcer treatment. Today, dietary therapy focuses only on foods that cause pain for an individual patient. Pain indicates that gastric acid is irritating the ulcer. If the patient feels no pain, the ulcer isn't being irritated. Each patient must determine which foods are safe to eat and which foods cause pain. The patient can then avoid the offending foods. Obviously, this process is highly individualized. Some ulcer patients may tolerate even spicy foods; others may tolerate only bland foods.

Some substances are not acceptable even when assessed individually. For example, all patients with peptic ulcers should avoid coffee. Even decaffeinated coffee has an acid-stimulating effect. In fact, ulcer patients should avoid all sources of caffeine, including chocolate, tea, and soft drinks. Most patients should avoid alcohol (one of the few substances absorbed across the stomach mucosa) as well, although some patients can have small amounts of alcohol when they eat a full meal.

Nicotine is another substance best avoided by ulcer patients because it has been associated with increased ulcer formation. If your ulcer patient wants to quit smoking, remember to weigh the benefits of using a transdermal nicotine patch against the possible aggravation of the ulcer disease.

Dispel the myth that milk provides the best relief for ulcer pain. Although it may provide transient relief for some patients, the amino acids and calcium in milk tend to increase gastric acid production. Most patients can continue to drink milk if they wish, but urge them to do so only when they eat a full meal.

Meal frequency may have an effect on ulcers as well. Some patients benefit from small, frequent meals; others do not. The key is to assemble a list of well-tolerated foods and a meal schedule that minimizes pain for each patient.

Because stress increases gastric acid secretion, lifestyle modifications may form an important aspect of treatment for some patients with ulcer disease. Urge these patients to schedule rest periods and to find relaxing ways to reduce stress. Some patients benefit from medications that help alleviate the effects of stress on acid production. Keep in mind, however, that the perception of stress is highly individualized. Like dietary changes, stress reduction measures must suit the particular patient.

Drug therapy

Drug therapy continues to be the mainstay of treatment for peptic ulcer disease—to relieve symptoms, promote healing, and prevent recurrence. Medications may be given to neutralize gastric acid, inhibit acid secretion, reinforce the mucosal surface, eradicate *H. pylori* infection, and control GI motility.

Neutralizing gastric acid

Antacids relieve pain by reacting chemically with gastric secretions to neutralize or buffer stomach contents without affecting the rate of gastric emptying. The goal of antacid therapy is to raise gastric pH above 4 and thus inhibit the proteolytic activity of pepsin. Except for sodium bicarbonate, antacids are poorly absorbed and therefore don't alter systemic pH.

An antacid's onset of action depends on its solubility. For example, magnesium trisilicate is poorly soluble and thus has a delayed onset. The duration of action is determined by the rate of gastric emptying. If a patient is fasting, the duration of action could be 20 to 60 minutes. If a patient has eaten an hour before taking an antacid, the duration of action could last 1 to 3 hours.

Antacids are most beneficial when the concentration of acid is high and the gastric emptying rate is low. Both of these factors are present 1 to 3 hours after a meal. Thus, giving an antacid 1 hour after a meal buffers the acid concentration and relieves acid-induced pain. Giving an antacid at bedtime is less beneficial because the stomach is empty and the gastric emptying rate is fairly rapid, about 20 to 30 minutes.

Although antacids are effective for brief periods and relatively safe to use, they aren't without problems. Some patients may switch among the variety of antacids on the market because of cost or taste. The problem is that antacids aren't necessarily interchangeable. They may contain aluminum hydroxide, magnesium hydroxide, calcium, or sodium. Taken imprecisely, these substances can interfere with the absorption rates of prescribed drugs. They may even be contraindicated in patients with some chronic disorders.

Suppressing gastric acid secretion

Several drugs are available for suppressing gastric acid secretion. The introduction of H_2 blockers in the 1970s revolutionized the treatment of peptic ulcer disease and created standard prophylaxis against stress ulceration. These drugs provide effective, safe, sustained control of gastric acid secretion by inhibiting the action of histamine at H_2-receptor sites on gastric parietal cells. H_2 blockers include cimetidine, ranitidine, famotidine, and nizatidine.

Although adverse effects are uncommon for most of these drugs (except cimetidine), patients should be monitored for headache, confusion, dizziness, and drowsiness. Cimetidine interferes with the liver's metabolism of some drugs, including warfarin, phenytoin, and theophylline, so lower doses of these medications may need to be prescribed.

More recently, drugs have been developed that inhibit hydrogen-potassium adenosine triphosphatase. Called proton-pump inhibitors, these drugs reduce gastric aid by blocking the final common pathway of hydrogen ion secretion in the parietal cell. Proton-pump inhibitors are much more potent than H_2 blockers, and many are capable of suppressing 90% of acid secretion for up to 24 hours. Proton-pump inhibitors also help to eradicate *H. pylori* by increasing gastric pH. These drugs include omeprazole and lansoprazole.

Omeprazole has been approved for short-term therapy of ulcers and reflux disorders and for long-term therapy of hypersecretory disorders. Like cimetidine, this drug decreases liver metabolism of warfarin, phenytoin, and theophylline. Lansoprazole, a newer proton-pump inhibitor, is more potent and longer lasting, and it eradicates *H. pylori* more effectively. It's well tolerated and has minimal interaction with other drugs. Remember, however, that any drug that raises gastric pH or prevents gastric absorption may alter absorption of other medications.

Pirenzepine, an anticholinergic drug, has been used to treat duodenal ulcer disease in recent years because it blocks the muscarinic receptors that regulate gastric acid secretion. Typical anticholinergic side effects—dry mouth and blurred vision—are minimal with pirenzepine.

Protecting the mucosa

Drugs that act by enhancing the mucosal protective mechanisms include sucralfate and misoprostol. Sucralfate reacts with gastric acid to form a thick paste complex that selectively adheres to ulcer surfaces, protecting them from the effects of gastric acid, pepsin, and bile salts. Sucralfate has been approved for acute and maintenance therapy for duodenal ulcers. It also has been used to treat gastric ulcers. This drug requires an acid medium to form the paste complex, so it must be taken on an empty stomach.

Sucralfate has little systemic absorption and no known serious adverse effects. However, it does bind with some drugs, such as cimetidine, digoxin, warfarin, phenytoin, and tetracycline, causing reduced bioavailability. Sucralfate contains aluminum hydroxide, which may cause constipation.

Misoprostol acts as a prostaglandin analog, decreasing gastric acid secretion and increasing production of protective mucus. Originally used to prevent ulcers that resulted from long-term NSAID use, misoprostol has also been used to treat ulcers unrelated to NSAIDs. Common adverse effects of misoprostol include diarrhea, abdominal pain, dysmenorrhea, and vaginal spotting. Because misoprostol stimulates uterine contractions, it should be used with caution in women of childbearing age. It should not be used during pregnancy.

Eradicating H. pylori

No drug combination has achieved complete success in eradicating *H. pylori*, and no specific regimen has been approved by the Food and Drug Administration. Many physicians choose a multidrug regimen that includes a bismuth compound and two antibiotics, usually metronidazole and either amoxicillin or clarithromycin.

Bismuth-containing compounds, such as bismuth subsalicylate, can also promote ulcer healing. Mechanisms of action include formation of a protective barrier over the ulcer, promotion of bicarbonate and prostaglandin secretion, and suppression of *H. pylori* growth. These drugs are essentially harmless. The most striking adverse effect is black stool, which may confound a diagnosis of GI bleeding. Bismuth is only available in the United States as Pepto-Bismol. Other regimens substitute a proton-pump inhibitor for bismuth.

The major concerns with these multidrug regimens are cost and compliance with the treatment plan. Most patients must take 15 to 20 pills per day for 7 to 14 days for the regimen to be effective.

Controlling GI motility

Prokinetic drugs, such as cisapride, stimulate motility in the GI tract, thus preventing acid from remaining in the stomach or duodenum for too long. The most common side effects of these drugs are headache, abdominal pain, and diarrhea.

Surgery

When peptic ulcer disease doesn't respond to conservative therapy or complications develop, the patient may require surgery. Surgical procedures vary from a relatively simple vagotomy, in which nerves that stimulate gastric secretion are selectively severed, to gastric resection, in which the ulcerated area of the stomach is removed. If the patient experiences GI bleeding uncontrolled by medical interventions, emergency surgery may be necessary (see *Emergency surgery for bleeding peptic ulcers*).

Nursing interventions

Nursing interventions for your patient with peptic ulcer disease include managing pain, promoting good nutrition and diet therapy, monitoring complications, and patient teaching.

Emergency surgery for bleeding peptic ulcers

Gastrointestinal bleeding caused by peptic ulcers sometimes can be controlled by medical interventions, such as gastric lavage. When medical interventions can't control bleeding, a surgeon may perform one of the following four types of emergency surgery.

Suture ligation of a duodenal ulcer with vagotomy and pyloroplasty

In this procedure, a surgeon sutures a bleeding duodenal ulcer to control the bleeding and resects the vagus nerves to decrease acid production. To improve gastric emptying, the surgeon widens the pyloric opening.

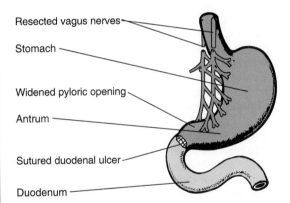

Resected vagus nerves

Stomach

Widened pyloric opening

Antrum

Sutured duodenal ulcer

Duodenum

Vagotomy and gastrectomy of the antrum with gastroduodenostomy

To perform this procedure (also called Bilroth I), a surgeon resects the vagus nerves and removes the antrum. Then he sutures the remaining portion of the stomach to the duodenum.

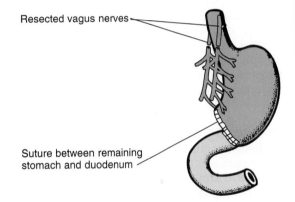

Resected vagus nerves

Suture between remaining stomach and duodenum

Vagotomy and gastrectomy of antrum with gastrojejunostomy

To perform this procedure (also called Bilroth II), a surgeon resects the vagus nerves and removes the antrum. Then he sutures the remaining portion of the stomach to the jejunum and closes off the duodenal stump with sutures.

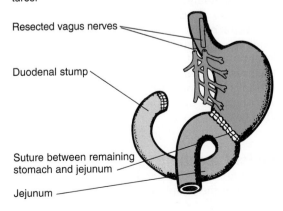

Resected vagus nerves

Duodenal stump

Suture between remaining stomach and jejunum

Jejunum

Distal gastrectomy with Roux-en-Y anastomosis

A surgeon removes the lower two-thirds to three-quarters of the stomach and sutures the remaining stomach to the side of the jejunum. The surgeon then sutures a short segment of small intestine to the jejunum below the anastomosis to provide drainage and prevent reflux, creating the shape of the letter *Y*.

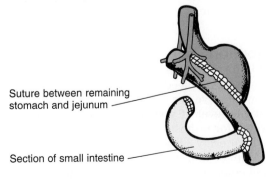

Suture between remaining stomach and jejunum

Section of small intestine

Managing pain

Obtain a pain history from your patient. Ask her specifically about the relationship between pain and food intake. When your patient reports pain, administer antacids or other ulcer medications as prescribed. Provide physical care to keep your patient comfortable. Maintain a quiet environment, which may mean limiting visitors and telephone calls. Consider not only how much activity your patient can tolerate but the effect of inactivity as well. Explore relaxation techniques to help her reduce stress and anxiety.

Monitor your patient carefully for pain that increases in intensity, radiates to the back, is associated with abdominal rigidity or rebound tenderness, or isn't relieved by prescribed medications. These symptoms may warn of a serious complication, such as perforation. Usually, perforation and the resulting peritonitis cause the sudden onset of sharp, localized, abdominal pain along with abdominal rigidity.

Promoting diet therapy

Help your patient make a list of foods that cause pain and foods that don't. Naturally, advise her to avoid foods that cause pain. Ensure that appropriate foods are available at all times. Consult with a dietitian if appropriate.

Encourage your patient to eat slowly and chew food thoroughly to prevent overdistention and reflux. To prevent increased nighttime acid secretion, discourage snacking at night. Evaluate your patient's eating patterns. If it helps reduce your patient's pain, provide small, frequent meals rather than three large meals. Don't give your patient coffee, tea, cola drinks, or chocolate.

Monitoring complications

Monitor your patient carefully for signs and symptoms of bleeding, obstruction, or perforation. Observe her color, activity tolerance, and fatigue level. If your patient is hospitalized, watch for orthostatic blood pressure changes at least every 8 hours.

Monitor your patient's vital signs for changes that could indicate bleeding, including systolic blood pressure under 100 mm Hg, a pulse rate over 100 beats per minute, or a 10 mm Hg or more drop in blood pressure with position changes.

Monitor laboratory test results, including RBC counts, hemoglobin level, and hematocrit. Decreases in these counts and values may indicate anemia from chronic or acute blood loss. Check stool color and test for occult blood. Note any bloody or coffee-ground vomitus or NG tube drainage. If you're not sure, test your patient's NG drainage for occult blood.

Obstruction usually results from edema or scarring. Warning signs and symptoms of obstruction include abdominal distention, nausea, complaints of fullness, and vomiting of partially digested food. Check for bowel sounds, and anticipate the need for NG decompression. Withhold food and fluids by mouth and administer prescribed fluids I.V. to maintain fluid and electrolyte balance.

Perforation occurs when an ulcer erodes through the gastric or duodenal wall, creating an opening between the GI tract and the peritoneal cavity. GI contents spill through the opening, resulting in peritonitis. If your patient complains of sudden, sharp, severe, midepigastric pain that spreads over the abdomen, she may have developed peritonitis. Irritation of the phrenic nerve may cause referred shoulder pain. The abdomen becomes rigid and boardlike. Respirations become rapid and shallow, and the patient develops tachycardia, pallor, cold and clammy skin, and hypotension. Peritonitis progresses rapidly and may cause death within 72 hours.

RAPID RESPONSE ▶ If your patient has a perforation, immediately institute NG decompression, administer fluids and electrolytes I.V. as ordered for replacement, and administer antibiotics as ordered to treat the infection. Place your patient in the low Fowler position to limit the area of the abdomen involved. If the perforation is large, prepare your patient for surgery. Throughout, monitor her status closely for changes. ◀

Patient teaching

Most patients with peptic ulcer disease aren't treated in the hospital. Only those with severe symptoms or complications are admitted. Therefore, the need for patient teaching about diet, medications, and signs of complications is critical.

Teach your patient how to take the prescribed medications. Stress the importance of adhering strictly to the medication schedule. Warn her to check with her physician before taking any over-the-counter (OTC) drugs. This includes OTC H_2 blockers, such as cimetidine, which can interact with such drugs as warfarin, theophylline, and phenytoin. Review other medications your patient may be taking. Discuss interactions that could occur when ulcer medications are taken with other agents— NSAIDs, for example—for treatment of chronic disorders.

Instruct your patient to take antacids 1 hour after a meal to provide longer pain relief. If she's taking both an antacid and an H_2 blocker, tell her not to take the drugs within 1 hour of each other.

Explain that food tolerance varies from person to person. Suggest that your patient keep a daily record of foods eaten and the amount of pain experienced. Urge her to avoid foods that have caused pain in the past. Encourage your patient to avoid cigarettes, alcohol, coffee (even decaffeinated), and other sources of caffeine. If needed, enlist a dietitian to help your patient and her family select and plan a balanced diet based on tolerated foods.

Stress the importance of physical and mental rest. Individualize your patient's activity and rest program. If appropriate, encourage your patient to take planned rest periods throughout the day and to avoid strenuous work around the house.

Instruct your patient in the importance of follow-up care and the need to report promptly severe abdominal pain, nausea, vomiting, abdominal distention, or persistence of her original symptoms despite compliance with treatment.

Allow your patient to express her feelings about the changes needed to promote healing and reduce the risk of recurrence. Help her identify factors that interfere with compliance, and explore ways of handling them. Involve your patient's family in planning for self-care, and recommend counseling or support groups as needed.

Peptic ulcer disease and myocardial infarction

Patients with peptic ulcer disease are at an increased risk for problems if they also have a myocardial infarction (MI). In some cases, peptic ulcer disease with severe GI bleeding can precipitate an MI. In other cases, patients with an MI may face an increased risk of ulceration because of the effects of physiologic stress.

Pathophysiology

MI results from prolonged myocardial ischemia, caused in most cases by an occlusive coronary thrombus secondary to atherosclerotic stenosis. Rarely, an infarction may result from hypoperfusion, anemia, or excessive metabolic demand. Ischemia from reduced blood flow to the myocardium causes cells to die and release myocardial lysosomal enzymes, particularly creatine kinase and lactic dehydrogenase. Because cardiac cells can't regenerate, nonfunctioning scar tissue replaces the infarcted area.

More than 1% of all MI patients develop acute GI bleeding. An additional smaller percentage develops occult bleeding within 3 weeks of an MI. The infarction itself may precede the bleeding or result from the bleeding. For example, an MI may develop because of severe anemia and hemodynamic compromise that result from GI bleeding. Or treatment of an MI with an anticoagulant or thrombolytic drug may result in GI bleeding. A patient with a healed ulcer faces a higher risk of bleeding if she receives thrombolytic therapy for an acute MI or anticoagulant therapy after an MI (see *How GI bleeding leads to an MI*, page 354).

Another complication is the development of stress ulcers after an MI. Stress places the patient at moderate risk for ulcer development, and mechanical ventilation that lasts more than 5 days raises the risk even more. Gastric mucosal lesions develop rapidly in critically ill

How GI bleeding leads to an MI

If a patient with peptic ulcer disease has an episode of severe gastrointestinal bleeding, the resulting volume depletion and ischemia could lead to a potentially devastating complication: myocardial infarction. This flowchart depicts the chain of events.

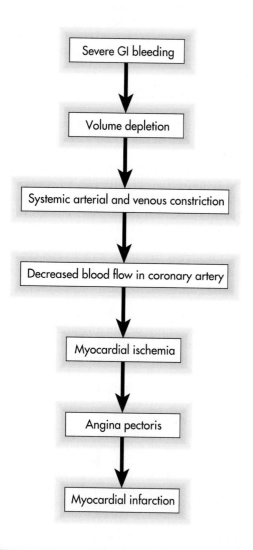

Severe GI bleeding

↓

Volume depletion

↓

Systemic arterial and venous constriction

↓

Decreased blood flow in coronary artery

↓

Myocardial ischemia

↓

Angina pectoris

↓

Myocardial infarction

patients. In fact, hyperemia of the gastric mucosa may develop within 24 hours of a traumatic event.

Adapting nursing care

If your patient has had an MI, ask about previous medical conditions, especially peptic ulcer disease, and the use of antacids. Many patients who have been treated for peptic ulcer disease in the past may have forgotten or not realize the importance of telling you about their condition. Ask your patient for the name of the physician who treats her peptic ulcer disease. If possible, notify this physician about the patient's MI and admission.

Pain and activity

Assess your patient's pain carefully. The difference between cardiac and noncardiac pain may be very subtle. Ask about the location, quality, and severity of the pain as well as factors that precipitate or alleviate it. Patients may describe acid reflux pain and ischemic cardiac pain in the same way, locating it in the substernal area. Both can be described as squeezing, tight, or pressurelike. Nitroglycerin may relieve both types of pain, so it isn't reliable for determining what's causing the pain. Pain that radiates to the arms and results from exertion is probably cardiac. Pain that lasts several hours, wakes the patient at night, or worsens when the patient lies down, is probably upper GI. Heartburn is usually identified by its relationship with meals.

Evaluate your patient's activity tolerance, so you can avoid setting unrealistic or potentially harmful activity goals. For example, if your patient with myocardial ischemia has had surgery for peptic ulcer disease, plan for a less aggressive activity routine than you would for a patient with no cardiac compromise.

Laboratory values

Pay close attention to laboratory values specific to both conditions. In addition to laboratory studies to monitor the effects of peptic ulcer disease, such as a CBC, monitor typical laboratory and diagnostic studies for an MI, such as electrocardiogram (ECG), serum cardiac enzyme levels, and coagulation studies. Notify a physician of any changes indicating ischemia. Give special consideration to values related to anemia.

Drugs

After an MI, patients may be taking many medications, including antiarrhythmics, positive inotropic drugs (such as digoxin), beta blockers, calcium channel blockers, angiotensin-converting enzyme (ACE) inhibitors, and antihypertensives. If even routine ulcer medications are added to the regimen (such as an H_2 blocker and an antacid), the number of medications may increase the risk of noncompliance. Check all medications for the possibility of drug interactions, which can place your patient at risk for serious problems. Remember that cimetidine and omeprazole alter the metabolism of warfarin (see *Drugs for peptic ulcer disease and MI: Dangerous interactions*, page 356).

Diet

Dietary modifications may be significant. Patients with peptic ulcer disease must adhere to a diet that works for them, avoiding foods that cause pain. MI patients typically must restrict fat, cholesterol, and sodium. Patients with both conditions may be overwhelmed by all the food restrictions. Work with your patient to develop appropriate food choices that address both conditions. Take into consideration any possible food–drug interactions that might occur. For example, a patient receiving warfarin should eat foods that allow her to maintain a consistent amount of vitamin K. Provide the patient with a written list of food choices, so that after discharge she can use it to help plan appropriate meals.

Surgery

For your patient with peptic ulcer disease and an MI, surgery can exacerbate either or both conditions and place her at high risk for complications.

Take special care when preparing your patient for surgery. A baseline ECG is essential because persistent arrhythmias increase the risk of complications. Also, obtain baseline vital signs, serum cardiac enzyme values, CBC, and coagulation studies, along with a careful history of the ischemic event. This information may influence decisions about premedications, anesthesia, surgical approaches, and postoperative care.

Patient teaching

Educate your patient about medication therapy. She must know all the drugs involved and their doses, actions, frequencies, and possible adverse effects and interactions. Your patient may feel overwhelmed about how and when to take her drugs. Help her develop a plan that fits her lifestyle.

Also, instruct your patient about signs and symptoms that should prompt a call to her physician. Caution her to check with her physician before taking any OTC medications because they could interfere with her prescribed medications.

Educate your patient about lifestyle modifications, such as diet, smoking cessation, activity, and rest. Include your patient's family in these discussions as appropriate (see *Teaching a patient with peptic ulcer disease and an MI*, page 357).

Complications

Common complications for patients with peptic ulcer disease and an MI include hemorrhage, reinfarction, and peritonitis.

Hemorrhage

If a peptic ulcer erodes the wall of an artery, the patient's GI tract will begin to bleed. If the ulcer erodes a relatively large artery, the bleeding may be rapid, heavy, and difficult to control. Ulcers along the posterior wall of the proximal duodenum may erode into branches of the gastroduodenal artery. Ulcers high in the gastric body may involve branches of the left gastric artery.

The relationship between an episode of profound GI bleeding and a simultaneous or subsequent MI is clear. The massive and commonly rapid loss of blood from a large artery causes

DRUG ALERT

Drugs for peptic ulcer disease and MI: Dangerous interactions

Drugs for peptic ulcer disease	Drugs for myocardial infarction (MI)	Adverse effects	Nursing actions
• Cimetidine	• Oral anticoagulants (warfarin)	• Cimetidine may inhibit hepatic metabolism of warfarin, thus increasing serum warfarin levels and increasing the risk of bleeding.	• Monitor prothrombin time (PT). • Check for signs of bleeding. • Protect patient from injury. • Ask physician about changing to another H_2 blocker. • Anticipate reducing warfarin dosage.
	• Antiarrhythmics (lidocaine, procainamide, propranolol, verapamil)	• Cimetidine may inhibit hepatic metabolism of antiarrhythmic, thus causing toxic serum antiarrhythmic levels.	• Monitor serum antiarrhythmic levels. • Watch for signs and symptoms of toxicity, such as confusion, restlessness, bradycardia, and respiratory distress. • Monitor electrocardiogram (ECG) for changes. • Ask physician about changing to another H_2 blocker.
• Gastric mucosal protectants (sucralfate)	• Oral anticoagulants (warfarin)	• Gastric mucosal protectant may interfere with warfarin absorption by binding with warfarin in gastrointestinal (GI) tract.	• Monitor PT. • Anticipate increasing warfarin dosage. • Separate administration of two drugs by at least 2 hours.
	• Inotropic drugs (digoxin)	• Gastric mucosal protectant may interfere with inotropic drug absorption by binding with inotropic drug in GI tract.	• Monitor heart rate and pulse. • Evaluate ECG for changes. • Anticipate increasing digoxin dosage. • Administer two drugs at least 2 hours apart.
• Proton-pump inhibitors (omeprazole)	• Oral anticoagulants (warfarin)	• Proton-pump inhibitor may inhibit hepatic metabolism of warfarin, thus increasing serum warfarin levels and increasing the risk of bleeding.	• Monitor PT. • Check for signs of bleeding. • Protect patient from injury. • Anticipate reducing warfarin dosage.
• Antacids	• All oral drugs used to treat MI	• Antacid may decrease rate and extent of absorption of oral drugs.	• Administer two drugs at least 2 hours apart. • Check for signs and symptoms of decreased drug effectiveness. • Monitor serum drug levels, as appropriate.

volume depletion, myocardial ischemia, and subsequent infarction. In addition, if a patient with peptic ulcer disease has an MI, she faces an increased risk of hemorrhage caused by the erosive effects of excess gastric acid produced by the physiologic stress of the MI. Thrombolytics and anticoagulants for treating the MI also place the patient at a higher risk for bleeding.

Bleeding dominates the signs and symptoms of simultaneous GI bleeding and MI. The patient is usually hypotensive and tachycardic, with hematemesis or bloody aspirate from an NG tube. Only about half of these patients have chest pain.

Consider the possibility of an MI any time a patient has bleeding massive enough to produce hypotension or severe tachycardia. Neurologic symptoms—such as syncope, dizziness, and confusion—may develop as well. These symptoms result from cerebral hypoperfusion, not arrhythmias. Neurologic complications are rare.

The mortality rate is much higher in patients who experience a GI hemorrhage and an MI than it is in patients who experience only one of these disorders. This high rate results from cardiovascular failure and multisystem failure.

Patients who don't have chest pain but do have upper GI bleeding and signs and symptoms of hypoperfusion (syncope, confusion, dizziness, hypotension) should be monitored in an intensive care setting. An MI should be ruled out.

Confirming the complication

Bright red vomitus or drainage from an NG tube confirms an acute GI hemorrhage. The drainage may at first resemble coffee grounds before escalating to frank bleeding.

If bleeding is less severe, the first indications may be a pulse above 100 beats per minute, systolic blood pressure below 100 mm Hg, hyperactive bowel sounds, tarry stools, dyspnea, dizziness, or signs of shock. A drop in blood pressure of 10 mm Hg or more when the patient sits up or stands up after lying down and a heart rate over 120 beats per minute suggest that she may have lost 20% to 25% of her blood volume. Systolic pressure that drops below 90 mm Hg when the patient sits up or stands up may mean that she's lost 25% to 50% of her blood volume. If the patient is in shock—as evidenced by a systolic blood pressure below 90 mm Hg, tachycardia, and cold, clammy skin—she may have already lost up to half of her blood volume.

With a GI hemorrhage, RBC counts and hemoglobin levels will be decreased, but the mean corpuscular volume will be normal, indicating RBCs of normal size. A drop in hemoglobin levels of 1 gm/dl indicates a blood loss of 500 ml. During an acute bleeding episode, plasma and RBCs are lost equally, so the hematocrit won't change. However, over the next 24 to 72 hours, the patient's body will try to compensate for volume lost from the extracellular space by shifting fluid out of the intracellular space. This fluid shift, plus the addition of I.V. fluids, ultimately will result in a decreased hematocrit from hemodilution.

GOING HOME

Teaching a patient with peptic ulcer disease and an MI

If your patient has peptic ulcer disease and also is recovering from an acute myocardial infarction (MI), your discharge teaching should emphasize three important areas: medications, diet, and stress.

- Review with your patient the possible interactions between her ulcer medications and the drugs prescribed as a result of her MI. Help her devise a medication schedule to minimize potential confusion and maximize compliance.
- Review the patient's dietary habits. Make a list of foods that typically relieve or prevent ulcer pain but that are now contraindicated because of the patient's post-MI diet.
- Review the effect of stress on both disorders and help the patient identify methods to reduce stress. Point out the value of exercise for both the cardiovascular and gastrointestinal systems.
- Include the patient's caregiver in your discharge teaching. Doing so will help avoid compliance problems caused by a caregiver's misunderstandings. If necessary, request additional assistance and follow-up support from a home care agency.

Changes in serum electrolyte levels point to fluid and electrolyte imbalances. These changes result from fluid loss caused by hemorrhage.

Abnormal coagulation studies and platelet counts may also suggest a bleeding disorder. If the patient has received thrombolytic drugs or anticoagulants, anticipate that coagulation values will increase. For example, if the patient is receiving heparin, expect the partial thromboplastin time (PTT) to be 1.5 to 2 times normal. Although this result indicates the drug's effectiveness, it also warns of an increased risk of hemorrhage. Decreases in coagulation study values and platelet counts also may result from blood loss.

Changes in serum creatinine levels indicate decreased renal function related to decreased perfusion. Blood urea nitrogen (BUN) levels will rise with upper GI bleeding as a result of

ADAPTING YOUR CARE

When a patient with peptic ulcer disease and an MI needs gastroduodenoscopy

If your patient with peptic ulcer disease and myocardial infarction (MI) develops acute gastrointestinal (GI) bleeding, a physician may perform endoscopy to assess the problem and try to stop the bleeding. Because of the patient's underlying disorders, special adaptations will be needed to ensure her safety.

Before the procedure
- Ideally, you should make sure the patient takes nothing by mouth for at least 8 hours before the test. Ask a physician if your patient should take her cardiac medications with a small amount of water.
- If the patient's endoscopy will take place in a separate department, she'll probably receive her preprocedure medication there. However, you should check to see which medication she's scheduled to receive. Many patients receive midazolam for conscious sedation during endoscopy—a drug that can cause dangerous cardiopulmonary side effects, including arrhythmias, cardiac arrest, and respiratory arrest. Therefore, be sure the gastroenterologist knows about your patient's underlying cardiac status.
- If the procedure will be done at the bedside, make sure a cardiac monitor and pulse oximetry device are in place for continuous evaluation.
- Have a nasal cannula and oxygen source on hand. In addition, keep resuscitation equipment

available in case the patient develops severe respiratory depression or cardiac arrest.
- Explain to the patient that she'll receive conscious sedation and that although she'll be awake and able to respond to her physician, she won't remember the procedure after it's over.
- Tell the patient that a local anesthetic will be sprayed on the back of her throat.
- Obtain a signed consent.

During the procedure
- Monitor the patient's blood pressure, pulse, pulse oximetry, and cardiac status throughout the procedure. Be especially vigilant for arrhythmias and decreasing oxygen saturation. Notify the gastroenterologist of any changes.
- Be prepared to administer supplemental oxygen, as indicated.

After the procedure
- Don't give the patient anything by mouth until her gag reflex returns. If her throat is sore, suggest that she gargle with warm saline solution.
- Monitor her vital signs, especially her temperature. A sudden rise in temperature can indicate perforation.
- Report a chest pain complaint immediately because it could indicate cardiac ischemia or GI perforation.

transient hypovolemia and the absorption of blood proteins by the upper portion of the small intestine.

Endoscopy is used to diagnose the location and severity of upper GI bleeding. Keep in mind, however, that patients undergoing endoscopy are especially susceptible to cardiopulmonary complications. If your patient has a history of MI and requires endoscopy, monitor her ECG and pulse oximetry measurements.

For patients with severe active bleeding and a recent MI who are hemodynamically stable and would otherwise require surgery for the bleeding, the benefits of endoscopy outweigh

the risks. Sometimes the bleeding can be arrested during endoscopy through electrocautery or sclerosing of the bleeding vessels.

Nursing interventions
If your patient develops acute upper GI bleeding, you'll need to intervene quickly and efficiently to prevent hypovolemic shock from massive fluid loss, extension of the MI from hypoperfusion of the already compromised coronary arteries, and death. During the acute phase of bleeding, focus on maintaining an adequate intravascular volume, stabilizing your patient's hemodynamic status, and preventing further myocardial ischemia or damage.

RAPID RESPONSE ▶ Notify a physician as soon as you suspect GI bleeding. Then take these measures:

- Check your patient's vital signs for indications of hypovolemic shock, such as hypotension and a weak, rapid pulse. Check orthostatic blood pressure.
- Don't give your patient any food or fluid by mouth. Insert an NG tube, if indicated. The tube can be used to assess the severity of bleeding, maintain gastric decompression, and prevent vomiting. Perform gastric lavage, if indicated.
- Check laboratory test results for serum hemoglobin, glucose, creatinine, and electrolyte levels; BUN levels; platelet count; PT; and activated PTT.
- Obtain blood for typing and crossmatching, as needed. Make sure several units of packed RBCs are available for transfusion.
- Establish at least one I.V. line with a large-bore catheter so that you can administer fluids and blood products.
- Administer fluids I.V. (such as lactated Ringer's solution or normal saline solution) to maintain plasma volume and promote renal perfusion.
- Administer prescribed blood and blood products to replace RBCs and platelets. Closely monitor the patient for signs and symptoms of heart failure and pulmonary edema, such as dyspnea, orthopnea, and pink, frothy sputum.
- If indicated, insert an indwelling urinary catheter and monitor urine output. If it drops below 30 ml per hour, notify a physician. Maintain accurate intake and output records, including vomitus and stool.
- Administer oxygen by nasal cannula or mask, if indicated. Monitor your patient's oxygen saturation levels and arterial blood gas values for signs of hypoxemia. If your patient's breathing becomes severely compromised, prepare for ET intubation and mechanical ventilation.
- Monitor your patient's ECG for signs of further myocardial ischemia or damage, such as flattening of the T wave and depression of the ST segment. Also, look for arrhythmias, such as premature ventricular contractions.
- If your patient develops chest pain or significant ECG changes, notify her physician and obtain a 12-lead ECG. If appropriate, also obtain serial cardiac enzyme levels. If the patient's blood pressure is stable, administer the prescribed nitrate for chest pain. ◀

If endoscopy is necessary, obtain baseline vital signs, pulse oximetry measurements, and a 12-lead ECG. If the procedure is performed at the bedside, monitor these findings continually and notify the gastroenterologist of any changes (see *When a patient with peptic ulcer disease and an MI needs gastroduodenoscopy*).

Being treated for massive GI bleeding can be a frightening experience. And the level of stress can be harmful, especially for a patient with ischemia. Try to maintain a calm environment. Reassure your patient that the health care team knows just what to do in this situation (see *Easing the anxiety of GI bleeding*, page 360).

Reinfarction

Reinfarction is a term used to describe further necrosis of myocardial tissue already affected by an infarction. Reinfarction that occurs within the first 10 days of the original MI is called early reinfarction. In early reinfarction, the amount of necrotic myocardium increases; usually, the necrosis penetrates more deeply into the affected muscle. Late reinfarction occurs after the immediate post-MI period. It causes necrosis in areas either adjacent to or remote from the first infarction.

Factors that increase a patient's risk for early reinfarction include subendocardial infarction, female gender, previous infarction, and a large infarction associated with cardiogenic shock. Other risk factors include an episode of hypotension preceding the onset of early reinfarction and post-MI angina or ECG changes. Patients with early infarction have a greater incidence of heart failure, arrhythmias, cardiogenic shock, and sudden death. Late reinfarction occurs in 10% to 20% of patients who've experienced an MI. The risk increases for patients who've had any type of surgery within 6 months after the MI.

Thrombolytic therapy—the treatment of choice for acute MI—increases the risk for both early and late reinfarction. This treatment uses

COMFORT MEASURES

Easing the anxiety of GI bleeding

A patient with peptic ulcer disease and a myocardial infarction who experiences massive upper gastrointestinal (GI) bleeding may be alert and conscious through much of the event. The sudden appearance of bright red blood, either in vomitus or nasogastric tube drainage, and the obvious concern of physicians and nurses can be terrifying.

Increased anxiety and the stress associated with it increases your patient's myocardial oxygen demands, further compromising heart function. Plus, the stress increases GI acid secretion, setting the stage for even more mucosal damage.

Although you must hurry to meet the patient's physiologic needs, don't forget to address her psychologic needs as well. Calmly tell her what's happening. Explain what the procedures are and why they're being done. For example, when performing gastric lavage, explain that the irrigation solution is cool because it helps slow or stop the bleeding.

Reassure and calm the patient during other procedures, such as blood drawing, I.V. line insertion, and X-rays. Doing so helps to allay the patient's fears and anxieties and diminish her stress, thereby decreasing myocardial oxygen demands and acid secretion.

Besides explaining procedures to the patient to keep her calm, take the following steps:
- Keep the patient covered. Provide extra blankets to prevent chilling and added stress. Doing so will help minimize the heart's demand for oxygen.
- Check for symptoms of hypoperfusion, such as dizziness, confusion, hypotension, chest pain, or shortness of breath.
- Continuously monitor the patient's electrocardiogram for changes indicating ischemia.
- Maintain a normal environment in the room as much as possible by discarding used equipment and washing away blood.
- And don't forget about family and significant others who may be waiting for information. Keep them as informed about the patient's progress as possible. Keeping them calm may help you keep the patient calm.

the thrombus. But if the drug doesn't completely dissolve the thrombus, residual thrombi or strands of thrombi can cause reinfarction. In fact, early and late reinfarction account for 25% of deaths that follow thrombolytic therapy.

Thrombolytic therapy poses a further risk for patients who also have peptic ulcer disease by greatly increasing the risk of life-threatening GI bleeding. If aspirin, heparin, beta blockers, or ACE inhibitors are given along with the thrombolytic drug, the risk of reinfarction drops. However, the use of aspirin in patients with peptic ulcer disease may increase the risk of bleeding.

Paradoxically, thrombolysis is also the treatment of choice for early and late reinfarction. If streptokinase or anisoylated plasminogen streptokinase activator complex (APSAC) was used previously, then TPA should be used as the new therapy; TPA can be repeated if it was the original drug. Other treatment may involve revascularization by percutaneous transluminal coronary angioplasty or coronary bypass surgery. The oxygen demand of these reinfarction patients can be lowered with beta blockers to reduce heart rate and nitroglycerin to increase coronary blood flow. Calcium channel blockers also may be used.

Confirming the complication

Diagnosis of early or late reinfarction may be difficult depending on the time elapsed since the acute MI. Changes in the ECG and cardiac enzyme levels may not be noticeable when compared with alterations from the original infarction. Additionally, ventricular remodeling—healing and scar tissue formation that alter appearance—may have occurred.

Post-MI angina and changes in the ECG (such as premature ventricular contraction, ventricular tachycardia, ventricular fibrillation, and accelerated idioventricular rhythm) suggest that reinfarction may be occurring.

Nursing interventions

Carefully monitor your post-MI patient for angina and ECG changes. Any recent episode of hemorrhage places this patient at high risk of developing reinfarction. At the same time,

such drugs as streptokinase, urokinase, and tissue plasminogen activator (TPA) to reestablish coronary artery blood flow by dissolving use of thrombolytic drugs or anticoagulants to treat either the original infarction or a reinfarction places a patient with peptic ulcer disease at risk for bleeding.

Assess this patient closely for signs and symptoms of GI bleeding. Monitor all physiologic measurements and laboratory studies. Provide supportive care.

After the patient's condition has stabilized, educate her about the potential complications of GI bleeding and reinfarction, any contributing factors, and steps she can take to reduce the risk of occurrence.

Peritonitis

The peritoneum covers most of the GI organs in the abdominal cavity. Only the pancreas, duodenum, ascending and descending colon, kidneys, and bladder lie outside the peritoneum. They're called retroperitoneal organs.

The peritoneum is made up of two layers: the parietal layer, which lines the walls of the abdominal cavity, and the visceral layer, which covers most of the organs within the cavity. Between the two layers is a potential space that contains about 100 ml of serous fluid. This fluid allows organs within the abdominal cavity to move without friction.

Peritonitis, an inflammation of the peritoneum, occurs when a breach in the GI wall—as from a perforated ulcer—allows GI contents to spill into the abdominal cavity. This original spillage is called chemical peritonitis. Once bacteria from the GI tract enter the abdominal cavity, however, chemical peritonitis quickly develops into bacterial peritonitis. Bacterial peritonitis commonly results from *Escherichia coli*, alpha-hemolytic and beta-hemolytic streptococci, *Staphylococcus aureus*, enterococci, and gram-negative rods. These organisms spread easily throughout the abdominal cavity. They also may enter the bloodstream from the peritoneum, causing life-threatening septicemia.

Peritonitis is treated with antimicrobial therapy, symptom management, and correction of the original cause. The original cause typically requires immediate surgical repair, even though a patient who has had an MI within the previous 6 months typically isn't a good surgical risk. However, this risk needs to be carefully weighed against the potential for death if the cause of acute peritonitis can't be resolved in any other way. The rapid development of shock from peritonitis can severely diminish blood flow to a heart with already compromised function.

Confirming the complication

If peritonitis results from GI perforation, the patient probably has a history of dyspepsia or peptic ulcer disease. The onset of pain is sudden and incapacitating, and you may observe signs of shock, such as hypotension, weak and rapid pulse, sweating, and stupor. The patient's abdomen will be rigid, with marked guarding, rebound tenderness, and possibly absent bowel sounds. Definitive diagnosis of peritonitis is by symptoms, abdominal X-rays, and an elevated white blood cell count. Peritonitis is difficult to recognize in elderly or immunosuppressed patients. And patients who take NSAIDs may have no previous complaints of dyspepsia.

Nursing interventions

In addition to attending to the rapidly advancing needs of your patient with peritonitis, you'll need to pay careful attention to her cardiac function. Begin cardiac monitoring during the critical period of the peritonitis. Look for typical ECG changes associated with ischemia. Monitor your patient's blood pressure, pulse, and respiratory status frequently.

Assess her for chest pain, including location, type, and duration. This may be difficult because the abdominal pain associated with peritonitis is usually severe, and your patient may find it difficult to discern abdominal pain from chest pain. In addition, pain from peritonitis can be referred to the shoulder, further confusing the patient. To make matters worse, your patient may have an altered level of consciousness and be unable to communicate.

Provide supportive care, and administer antimicrobial therapy as prescribed. If necessary, prepare your patient for surgery.

After your patient's condition has stabilized, educate her about the complication, any contributing factors, and steps she can take to reduce the risk of recurrence.

Peptic ulcer disease and rheumatoid arthritis

Rheumatoid arthritis—a systemic, chronic inflammatory disease—causes progressive, unremitting, and irreversible destruction of synovial tissue in the joints. It affects 6.5 million Americans, about half of whom have progressive disease. More common in women than men, rheumatoid arthritis typically begins between ages 20 and 30 and ages 60 and 70. Smoking may increase a patient's susceptibility to the disease.

Signs and symptoms of rheumatoid arthritis include redness, swelling, and pain in the joints, especially the small joints of the hands and feet. Because rheumatoid arthritis is a systemic disorder, the patient also may experience weakness, malaise, a low-grade fever, anemia, vasculitis, and skin nodules.

If your patient with rheumatoid arthritis has or risks developing peptic ulcer disease, using NSAIDs to treat pain and inflammation can cause further harm to the patient's GI tract and mucosa. (see *Using NSAIDs in a patient with rheumatoid arthritis and peptic ulcer disease*).

Pathophysiology

Rheumatoid arthritis begins as a nonspecific inflammatory synovitis characterized by swelling and hypertrophy of the synoviocytes and underlying connective tissues. As the inflammation continues, lymphocytic and plasma cells proliferate and infiltrate the synovium, sometimes forming nodules. The inflamed synovium that covers the articular cartilage surface is called the pannus (mantle). Eventually, the pannus fills the joint space. Subsequent fibrosis, connective tissue proliferation, and calcification can cause permanent ankylosis (loss of movement of the joint) and deformities that severely impair function.

The cause of rheumatoid arthritis isn't known, but the most common pathologic theory involves the activation of helper T cells and B cells. When activated, helper T cells produce a number of mediators. In turn, these mediators release tissue-destructive enzymes that perpetuate inflammation. At the same time, B-cell activation causes the production of antibodies, some of which fail to recognize the body's own tissue. This autoimmune reaction may cause the disease to progress because the body constantly produces the autoantibody.

Although peptic ulcer disease has many possible causes, the patient with rheumatoid arthritis usually develops it from using NSAIDs. What's more, the use of aspirin and other NSAIDs has been identified in nearly 80% of all cases of GI bleeding, whether the patient has rheumatoid arthritis or not. By interfering with blood platelet function, aspirin impairs clotting. Ingestion of 300 mg per day increases the risk of bleeding by a factor of eight. Ingestion of 1,200 mg per day doubles the risk again.

Antiarthritis medications not only induce ulcers and impair clotting by inhibiting platelet function, but they also increase the likelihood of bleeding from existing ulcers. The risk of bleeding during NSAID therapy is greater if a previous GI problem exists.

Aspirin is considered the prototype NSAID. In an attempt to find other drugs with fewer adverse effects, pharmaceutical companies have developed many drugs. In the United States, more than 20 NSAIDs are available. Although they all inhibit prostaglandin synthesis, some nonaspirin NSAIDs have more side effects than others. The risk of GI complications appears to be lower with ibuprofen and diclofenac, higher with indomethacin and piroxicam, and most common with ketoprofen.

Adapting nursing care

Your main concern when caring for a patient with peptic ulcer disease who also has rheumatoid arthritis is the effect of the antiarthritis medications on her ulcer disease. Ask your patient if she takes an NSAID or a corticosteroid. These drugs suppress prostaglandins and irritate the GI mucosa. Find out which medications your patient takes regularly, the dosages, and

Using NSAIDs in a patient with rheumatoid arthritis and peptic ulcer disease

For many patients with rheumatoid arthritis, non-steroidal anti-inflammatory drugs (NSAIDs) form the foundation of treatment. For patients who also have peptic ulcer disease, however, NSAIDs can worsen the ulcer and lead to gastrointestinal bleeding. This flowchart shows the mixed results of using NSAIDs for a patient with rheumatoid arthritis and peptic ulcer disease.

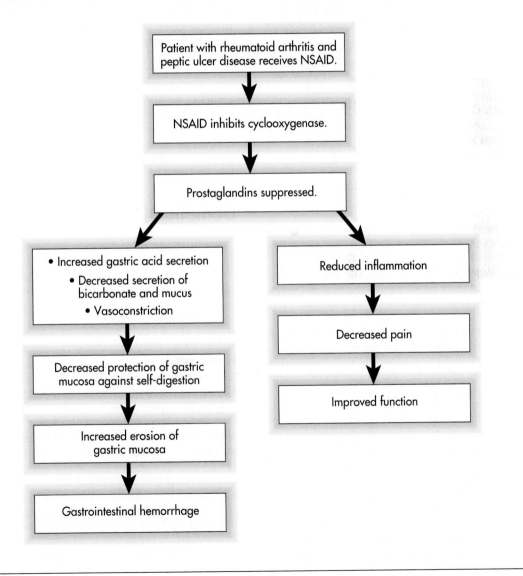

DRUG ALERT

Rheumatoid arthritis drugs that exacerbate peptic ulcer disease

Many drugs used to treat rheumatoid arthritis can affect the gastrointestinal (GI) tract, placing the patient with peptic ulcer disease at increased risk. If your patient is taking any of these medications, be alert for increased complaints of pain and signs of GI bleeding.
- Salicylates (aspirin, choline salicylates)
- Other nonsteroidal anti-inflammatory drugs (diclofenac, diflunisal, ibuprofen, indomethacin, ketoprofen, naproxen, piroxicam, sulindac, tolmetin)
- Corticosteroids (prednisone)
- Antimalarials (chloroquine, hydroxychloroquine, quinacrine)
- Methotrexate
- Sulfasalazine

the schedule. Watch for drugs known to aggravate ulcers (see *Rheumatoid arthritis drugs that exacerbate peptic ulcer disease*).

Discuss with your patient the potential adverse effects of these medications, and review the signs and symptoms of GI bleeding, anemia, and other bleeding problems. Remember that your patient is probably receiving antiulcer drugs in addition to antiarthritis drugs. Help her establish a schedule that maximizes absorption of all prescribed medications and minimizes danger to the gastric mucosa.

When administering any of these drugs, be alert for increased complaints of GI pain. Many of the drugs used for rheumatoid arthritis can be taken with food to minimize GI irritation. However, avoid giving them with milk because milk can increase acid secretion, causing more pain.

Antacids commonly used in peptic ulcer disease can affect the absorption of some oral drugs, including some antiarthritis drugs, thus decreasing their effectiveness. Give antacids 1 to 2 hours after giving other oral drugs. Sucralfate must be administered on an empty stomach, so administer this drug 1 hour before or 2 hours after meals.

Because rheumatoid arthritis can be painful, your patient may be reluctant to cut back or switch medications that relieve her pain. She may avoid telling you about darkened stools, ulcer pain, or even bloody vomitus if she thinks that her pain-relieving medication might be taken away.

If your patient takes aspirin, give her information about the various formulations of the drug. Buffered aspirin is no different from plain aspirin in its effect on the gastric mucosa. Enteric-coated preparations are commonly used by patients with rheumatoid arthritis, but their absorption rate is delayed because they're not absorbed until they reach the intestine. Aspirin suppositories also have varied absorption, and rectal irritation can occur.

Teach your patient about nonpharmacologic measures that she can use to treat her rheumatoid arthritis, such as rest and heat and cold therapy on the affected joints. Also, discuss exercise and lifestyle modifications.

Complications

Complications of patients with peptic ulcer disease and rheumatoid arthritis include penetration of the ulcer to an attached structure, such as the pancreas, and perforation. However, the most common complication for these patients is hemorrhage.

Hemorrhage

GI bleeding that results from the ingestion of NSAIDs or other antiarthritis medications probably won't appear as an acute bleeding episode. Consequently, you'll want to monitor patients with peptic ulcer disease and rheumatoid arthritis for signs of chronic bleeding.

Confirming the complication

Any signs or symptoms of anemia, which are commonly vague and nonspecific, should be followed up with laboratory assessments. An RBC count, hemoglobin level, and hematocrit can provide data about hemodynamic status. A positive stool test for occult blood indicates bleeding. Stools may appear dark or tarry. Endoscopy may be necessary to confirm the site and severity of the bleeding.

Nursing interventions

To help counteract GI bleeding caused by antiarthritis medications, administer an antacid and other GI medications (such as an H_2 blocker) by mouth or I.V. as ordered. Don't administer antiarthritis medications until the source and severity of the bleeding can be determined. Consult with your patient's physician about other medications that can be used to alleviate pain during this time.

Monitor your patient carefully for escalation of the bleeding: check stools for blood and, if an NG tube is present, consistently watch for bloody or coffee-ground drainage. Monitor your patient's vital signs, especially her blood pressure and pulse.

Suggested readings

Bellamy N, Bradley LA. Workshop on chronic pain, pain control and patient outcomes in rheumatoid arthritis and osteoarthritis. *Arthritis Rheum.* 1996;39(3):357-362.

Brozenec S. Ulcer therapy update. *RN.* 1996;59(9):48-53.

Cappell MS. A study of the syndrome of simultaneous acute upper gastrointestinal bleeding and myocardial infarction in 36 patients. *Am J Gastroenterol.* 1995;90(9):1444-1449.

Cave DR, Hoffman JJ. Management of *Helicobacter pylori* infection in ulcer disease. *Hosp Pract.* 1996;31(1):63-75.

Fabius D. Identifying infarctions: how you can use the ECG. *Nursing.* 1994;24(12):32L-32P.

Fisher RL, Pipken GA, Wood JR. Stress-related mucosal disease: pathophysiology, prevention, and treatment. *Crit Care Clin.* 1995;11(2):323-345.

Fries JF, Williams CA, Morfeld D, Singh G, Sibley J. Reduction in long-term disability in patients with rheumatoid arthritis by disease-modifying antirheumatic drug-based treatment strategies. *Arthritis Rheum.* 1996;39(4):616-622.

Handerhan B. Investigating peritoneal irritation. *RN.* 1994;57(4):71-73.

Heigh RI. Use of NSAIDs: an assault on the upper gastrointestinal tract. *Postgrad Med.* 1994;96(6):63-68.

NIH Consensus Conference. *Helicobacter pylori* in peptic ulcer disease. NIH Consensus Development Panel on *Heliobacter pylori* in peptic ulcer disease. *JAMA.* 1994;272(1):65-69.

Pope RM. Rheumatoid arthritis: pathogenesis and early recognition. *Am J Med.* 1996;100(2A):3S-9S.

Rourk RM, Caldwell SH, Barritt AS 3rd, McCallum RW. Endoscopy for gastrointestinal bleeding after acute myocardial infarction. *Va Med Q.* 1994;121(4):246-248.

Rush C. Gastrointestinal bleeding: preventing hypovolemic shock. *Nursing.* 1995;25(8):33.

Schlant RC, Alexander W, eds. *Hurst's the heart: arteries and veins.* 8th ed. New York, NY: McGraw-Hill Book Co; 1994.

Silman AJ, Newman J, MacGregor AJ. Cigarette smoking increases the risk of rheumatoid arthritis. *Arthritis Rheum.* 1996;39(5):732-735.

Thompson WG. *The ulcer story: the authoritative guide to ulcers, dyspepsia, and heartburn.* New York, NY: Plenum Publishing Corp; 1996.

Tsunoda D. Clinical snapshot: acute myocardial infarction. *Am J Nursing.* 1996;96(5):38-39.

Winalski CS, Palmer WE, Rosenthal DI, Weissman BV. Magnetic resonance imaging of rheumatoid arthritis. *Radiol Clin North Am.* 1996;34(2):243-258.

Yamada T, Alpers DH, Powell DW, Owyang C, Silverstein FE, eds. *Textbook of gastroenterology: self-assessment review.* 2nd ed. Philadelphia, Pa: Lippincott-Raven Pubs; 1995.

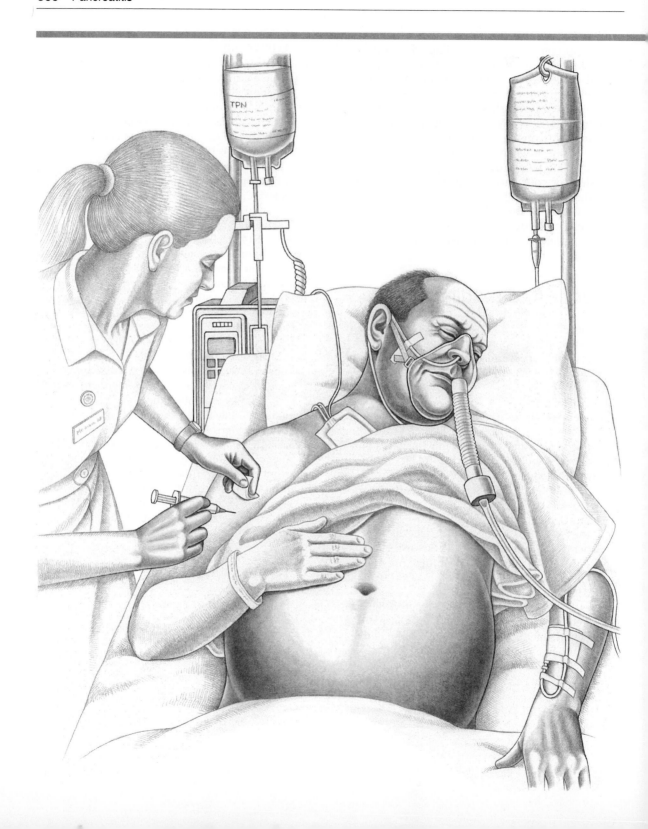

12

Pancreatitis

An acute or chronic inflammation of the pancreas, pancreatitis affects both men and women, usually in the fifth decade of life.

Acute pancreatitis may occur as a single episode or as repeated attacks. With early treatment, the pancreas usually returns to normal. However, repeated attacks can result in scarring and calcification of the pancreatic tissue and, ultimately, in chronic pancreatitis.

Chronic pancreatitis involves progressive damage to the pancreatic tissue. Eventually, the tissue becomes fibrotic, and irreversible damage results.

Anatomy and physiology review

A slender glandular organ, the pancreas lies at the level of the second lumbar vertebra. It's positioned behind the stomach in the curvature of the duodenum, near the spleen and left kidney in the retroperitoneal space. Consisting of a head, neck, body, and tail, the pancreas is about 12 to 20 inches long. Unlike the liver and other organs, the pancreas isn't covered by a tight connective-tissue capsule. Instead, it has a loose connective-tissue covering that invaginates into the gland, dividing it into lobules. Because of this covering, inflammation can spread freely and affect the surrounding organs.

The rich arterial blood supply of the pancreas comes primarily from the splenic artery (which branches from the celiac artery), the superior mesenteric artery, and the gastroduodenal artery (which branches from the common hepatic artery). Venous blood leaves the head and neck of the pancreas through the portal vein, with the body and tail being drained through the splenic vein. All hormonal pancreatic secretions pass through the portal vein into the liver. Sympathetic nerves from the celiac plexus and parasympathetic fibers from the vagus nerve innervate the organ.

The pancreas functions as both an endocrine and an exocrine gland. The endocrine function takes place in the islets of Langerhans. Within the islets, alpha cells secrete glucagon, and beta cells secrete insulin, both of which regulate serum glucose levels. Also within the islets, delta cells secrete somatostatin, which inhibits glucagon secretion from alpha cells and insulin secretion from beta cells. Somatostatin also inhibits the pituitary secretion of growth hormone.

Exocrine function

Pancreatitis primarily affects the exocrine function of the pancreas, which takes place in the acinar cells. These cells secrete enzymes to digest proteins, fats, and carbohydrates. They also produce sodium, bicarbonate, and water, which help neutralize the highly acidic chyme as it enters the duodenum from the stomach. The clear alkaline fluid that contains the enzymes and other substances is called pancreatic juice. Normally, the pancreas produces 1,200 to 3,000 ml of pancreatic juice daily.

The acinar cells empty into ductules. In turn, these ductules empty into the main pancreatic duct (also called the duct of Wirsung), which empties into the duodenum. In most people, the common bile duct and the pancreatic duct join at a small area called the ampulla of Vater before emptying into the duodenum.

The flow of pancreatic juice is controlled by the sphincter of Oddi, located between the ampulla of Vater and the duodenum. In some people, an accessory pancreatic duct (also called the duct of Santorini) enters the duodenum at an opening called the minor duodenal papilla (see *Inside the pancreas*).

Enzyme secretion

In their inactive form, the pancreatic enzymes are stored in the acinar cells. When a person smells, tastes, chews, and swallows food, the vagus nerve stimulates the secretion of the still-inactive enzymes. The vagus nerve also increases the activity of the stomach contents and stimulates the release of gastrin from the stomach, which also causes the pancreas to secrete these enzymes.

Acidic chyme in the duodenum stimulates the secretion of secretin and cholecystokinin from the mucosa of the small intestine. Secretin is secreted when the pH of the duodenum is 4.5 or lower. Cholecystokinin is primarily secreted in the presence of free fatty acids in the duodenum. Secretin stimulates the pancreas to release water and bicarbonate, whereas cholecystokinin acts as yet another stimulant that causes the pancreas to secrete its enzymes.

The release of bicarbonate increases the pH of chyme, promoting an alkaline environment necessary for pancreatic enzyme function. In the duodenum, the enzymes are converted to their active state.

The enzymes that break down proteins include trypsin, chymotrypsin, carboxypolypeptidase, ribonuclease, and deoxyribonuclease. Trypsin, the most abundant enzyme, is converted from its inactive form, trypsinogen, by enterokinase, which is secreted by the intestinal lining.

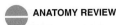
Inside the pancreas

This cross-sectional view shows the major structures of the pancreas and the portion of the duodenum that receives digestive juices from the pancreas.

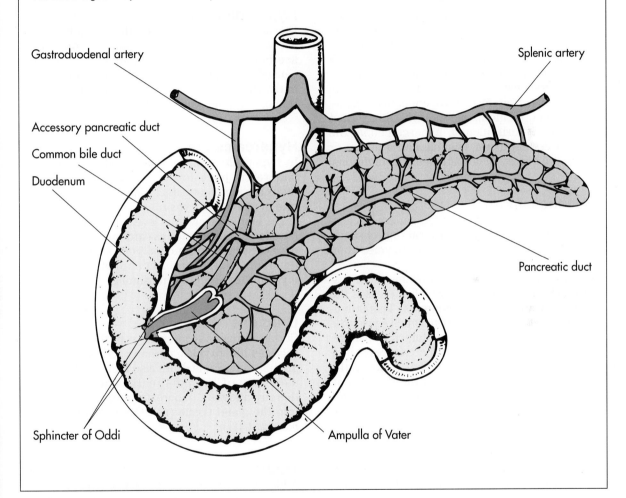

Pathophysiology

Acute pancreatitis is an autodigestive disease in which the pancreas is damaged by the enzymes it produces. The disease probably occurs when ductal obstruction, spasm, or inflammation causes the pancreas to distend. This leads to the retention and activation of pancreatic enzymes, which then extravasate into the surrounding tissue. The activated enzymes then begin the process of autodigestion and destruction of the surrounding tissues and cellular membranes. Edema, interstitial hemorrhage, vascular damage, and necrosis may develop. Tissue injury causes the release of histamine and bradykinin, which increase vascular permeability and vasodilation and worsen the edema.

In chronic pancreatitis, progressive destruction of the pancreas leads to exocrine insufficiency. Most commonly found in patients with alcoholism, chronic pancreatitis causes protein precipitates to occlude the pancreatic ducts, which leads to ductal obstruction, atrophy, dilation, and, eventually, fibrosis. This fibrosis may cause common bile duct strictures, which can lead to common bile duct obstruction.

The exact cause of pancreatitis isn't known. However, certain factors are linked with its development, including alcoholism, biliary tract disease, hyperlipidemia, hypercalcemia, the use of certain drugs, trauma, and a family or personal history of certain medical conditions.

Alcoholism

Alcohol appears to irritate the pancreas, causing protein precipitates to form and obstruct the acinar ductules. Trapped enzymes then begin to digest the pancreas.

Alcohol may also increase the amount of gastric acid in the stomach, which increases the acidity of the duodenal contents. This stimulates the secretion of secretin, which causes the pancreas to produce large volumes of pancreatic juice. Plus, alcohol may increase resistance at the sphincter of Oddi, which controls the flow of pancreatic juice into the duodenum. The resulting obstruction of pancreatic juice causes increased pancreatic duct permeability, extravasation of pancreatic juice into the pancreatic tissue, and tissue destruction.

Alcoholic pancreatitis may develop after an alcohol binge, although it more commonly affects patients who've been drinking large quantities of alcohol for 7 to 10 years. Typically, the patient is a man between ages 30 and 45.

Biliary tract disease

Biliary tract disease, especially gallstones, is commonly a precursor to pancreatitis. Bile reflux irritates the pancreas, and pancreatic outflow is blocked. As a result, enzymes become activated within the gland, leading to autodigestion.

In many cases, gallstones don't appear on X-rays, but they're excreted in the patient's stool when symptoms subside. Biliary tract disease linked with pancreatitis usually occurs in women over age 50.

Hyperlipidemia

Elevated lipid levels increase the amount of lipase within the pancreatic capillaries. And lipase begins hydrolyzing triglycerides, which causes the release of free fatty acids. Apparently, these acids irritate the capillary membrane, initiating pancreatitis.

Hypercalcemia

In hypercalcemia, increased calcium in the pancreatic juice forms calcium stones that block the pancreatic duct. Calcium also plays a role in activating trypsin.

The increased calcium levels may result from iatrogenic causes, such as cardiopulmonary bypass surgery, or from conditions such as T-cell leukemia, parathyroid adenomas, multiple myeloma, or vitamin D poisoning.

Drug use

Certain drugs may alter the way the pancreas secretes its enzymes, perhaps activating them prematurely. Some drugs also increase the permeability of the pancreatic duct mucosa, thereby allowing pancreatic enzymes to leak into the gland tissue (see *Drugs linked with pancreatitis*).

Trauma

A history of abdominal surgery or trauma may precede acute pancreatitis. The disease process is initiated by pancreatic duct trauma or vascular compromise, both of which stimulate an inflammatory response. Endoscopic retrograde cholangiopancreatography may also trigger acute pancreatitis.

Other medical conditions

Patients with a family history of pancreatitis or an autoimmune disease, such as Crohn's disease, are at a higher risk for developing pancreatitis. Infections—such as mumps, rubella, scarlet fever, coxsackievirus, Epstein-Barr virus, mycoplasmal infection, and hepatitis A, B, and C—may cause acute pancreatitis. Other possible causes include human immunodeficiency virus infection and migration into the pancreatic duct by the parasitic roundworm ascaris.

Assessment findings

A patient with pancreatitis usually has acute abdominal pain, rebound tenderness, and other signs and symptoms similar to those caused by acute appendicitis, acute cholecystitis, a perforated ulcer, or an intestinal obstruction. In pancreatitis caused by alcohol use, symptoms may develop 12 to 48 hours after the patient drinks an excessive amount.

Typically, a patient with acute pancreatitis experiences unrelenting abdominal pain. The specific location of the pain roughly corresponds with the position of the pancreatic lesion. For example, lesions in the pancreas tail typically produce left upper quadrant pain, whereas lesions in the pancreas head result in right upper quadrant pain, which may be referred to the back. The patient may describe the pain as severe and deep, knifelike, twisting, bandlike, or, rarely, burning. The pain may worsen after a heavy meal. Usually, the patient is most comfortable in the knee-chest, or fetal, position. He may also experience nausea and persistent vomiting, which may result from reflux irritation caused by the inflamed pancreas. Vomiting doesn't relieve the pain.

A patient with chronic pancreatitis experiences intense gnawing, burning, relentless abdominal pain. Typically, other signs and symptoms include clay-colored or frothy, foul-smelling stool; weight loss; and dark yellow or cola-colored urine.

Upon physical examination, a patient with acute pancreatitis may have abdominal rigidity, and his bowel sounds may be decreased as a result of paralytic ileus. Grey Turner's sign (bluish discoloration of the flanks) or Cullen's sign (bluish discoloration around the umbilicus) are late indicators of necrotizing pancreatitis.

The patient may have slight jaundice from obstruction caused by edema of the pancreas and

---

Drugs linked with pancreatitis

Some drugs are strongly linked with the development of pancreatitis; others are suspected of playing a part in its development. This list classifies drugs as known, probable, and possible factors in the development of pancreatitis.

Known factors
- Aminosalicylates
- Anticholinesterase drugs
- Calcium
- Didanosine
- Estrogen
- Valproic acid

Probable factors
- Angiotensin-converting enyzme inhibitors
- Asparaginase
- Clozapine
- Analgesics, including nonsteroidal anti-inflammatory drugs
- Thiazides and related diuretics
- Vinca alkaloids

Possible factors
- Antibiotics
- Antitubercular drugs
- Azathioprine
- Cisplatin
- Cyclosporine
- Furosemide
- Mercaptopurine
- Metronidazole

---

compression of the extrahepatic biliary tree. He may also have a fever of 101° F (38.3° C) or higher, dyspnea caused by diaphragmatic irritability, and tachycardia. If shock is developing, he may be diaphoretic and have tachycardia and hypotension. He also may have abdominal rigidity caused by pooling of fluid in the retroperitoneal area and peritoneal cavity.

The patient may have a pleural friction rub from a pleural effusion. The pleural effusion may develop from the passage of pancreatic exudate through lymph channels into the chest or from extravasation of pancreatic exudate through the diaphragm. Pseudoaneurysms or abscesses may form fistulas into the chest cavity. The patient

Calculating the amylase-creatinine ratio

To calculate the amylase-creatinine ratio, multiply the patient's serum amylase level by his urine creatinine concentration. Divide this result by the product of his urine amylase level and his serum creatinine concentration. Then multiply the result by 100%. Here's the formula:

$$\frac{\text{Serum amylase} \times \text{urine creatinine}}{\text{Urine amylase} \times \text{serum creatinine}} \times 100\% = \text{Amylase-creatinine ratio}$$

Normally, the amylase-creatinine ratio is less than 3%. If it's greater than 5%, the patient has pancreatitis.

---

may have diminished breath sounds because abdominal distention and pain have produced hypoventilation, which in turn has caused atelectasis. Also, he may have crackles from pulmonary edema if circulating toxins have caused an alveolocapillary leak.

A patient with chronic pancreatitis may have jaundice, ascites, and abdominal tenderness. If he has a pancreatic pseudocyst or abscess, he may have a mass in his left upper abdominal quadrant. Because respiratory complications, such as pleural effusion, commonly accompany chronic pancreatitis, you may auscultate a pleural friction rub. Also, the patient may experience dyspnea and orthopnea. Other assessment findings may include muscle wasting, weight loss, and signs and symptoms of diabetes, such as polyuria, polydipsia, and polyphagia from extensive pancreatic endocrine dysfunction.

Diagnostic tests

Serum and urine amylase and serum lipase levels help confirm the diagnosis of pancreatitis. Other blood tests, including a white blood cell (WBC) count, a red blood cell (RBC) count, and serum electrolyte levels, provide further information. Radiography, ultrasonography, computed tomography (CT), and certain other tests may also be used.

Amylase levels

Amylase is manufactured not only in the pancreas but also in the salivary glands, lungs, and fallopian tubes. Normally, serum amylase levels range from 35 to 115 units/liter. In patients with acute and chronic relapsing pancreatitis, the serum amylase level is typically twice the normal value. A value over 300 units/liter usually indicates pancreatitis. However, because of numerous sources of amylase, such an elevation isn't a definitive indicator of the disease. Elevated amylase levels can also reflect pancreatic cancer, salivary lesions, peritonitis, a perforated ulcer, an intestinal obstruction, macroamylasemia, acute cholecystitis, an ectopic pregnancy, renal failure, mesenteric thrombosis, or mumps. Plus, amylase levels may rise with the administration of meperidine.

In patients with pancreatitis, serum amylase levels typically rise 2 to 12 hours after the onset of symptoms, peak within 20 to 30 hours, and return to normal in 5 to 7 days. The rapid decline is caused by the short half-life of amylase: 90 to 120 minutes.

Amylase is excreted in the urine, and urine amylase levels may remain elevated for 3 to 5 days after the onset of symptoms. Because of the many other causes of elevated serum and urine amylase levels, they should be used along with the serum and urine creatinine concentrations to confirm pancreatitis (see *Calculating the amylase-creatinine ratio*).

Lipase levels

A patient's serum lipase levels rise only with pancreatic disease. Normal levels range from 32 to 80 units/liter. Elevated serum lipase levels may indicate acute pancreatitis or a pancreatic duct obstruction. Levels remain elevated for 5 to 7 days.

Additional blood tests

Usually in pancreatitis, a patient's WBC count is elevated because of the acute inflammatory process. The RBC count is elevated from the hemoconcentration that occurs with the leakage of plasma and pancreatic juice into the interstitial spaces. A rapid drop in the RBC count may indicate necrotizing pancreatitis.

Arterial blood gas (ABG) studies may reveal hypoxemia and carbon dioxide retention secondary to respiratory complications, such as a pleural effusion or pneumonia.

Serum electrolyte levels may be used to evaluate fluid and electrolyte balance. Hypokalemia may appear if the patient has been vomiting or has received nasogastric (NG) suction. Hypocalcemia, common with fulminant pancreatitis, usually indicates pancreatic fat necrosis.

Serum glucose levels may be elevated if the beta cells have been damaged, especially in chronic pancreatitis.

Serum triglyceride levels may be measured because hypertriglyceridemia is associated with the development of pancreatitis. Triglyceride levels may be extremely high.

The physician may order measurements of bilirubin, alkaline phosphatase, alanine aminotransferase, and aspartate aminotransferase levels. Usually, these levels are elevated if the pancreatitis results from biliary tract disease.

Radiography

Radiologic evaluation confirms a diagnosis of pancreatitis and excludes other possible causes of abdominal pain. Plain abdominal and chest X-rays may reveal pleural effusions and a hazy epigastric region. In almost half the patients with acute pancreatitis, an ileus appears as a distended loop of intestine in the left upper quadrant of the abdomen.

Ultrasonography

Abdominal ultrasonography may show pancreatic edema, peripancreatic fluid collections, or gallstones. It also may show increased thickening of the gallbladder, pericholecystic fluid, marked gallbladder distention, or Murphy's sign (pain on deep inspiration during palpation of the gallbladder), which may indicate cholecystitis. The bile duct may be dilated, which suggests obstruction. Ultrasonography can also identify pancreatic abscesses, pseudocysts, and, less reliably, areas of pancreatic necrosis.

Computed tomography

A CT scan may show an enlarged, irregular pancreas. Usually, pancreatic inflammation, biliary obstruction, and complications of acute pancreatitis, such as pancreatic pseudocysts or abscesses, can be identified, although mild edematous changes may not be visible.

Because a CT scan provides more accurate anatomic definition than an ultrasound scan, it can be used to grade the severity of acute pancreatitis. A CT scan using an I.V. contrast medium can identify underperfused portions of the pancreas that may be necrotic. Such a scan allows for more accurate grading of the severity of the disease.

If the patient has renal failure and the use of a contrast medium is contraindicated, magnetic resonance imaging can also allow for accurate grading of the disease.

Endoscopic retrograde cholangiopancreatography

This endoscopic-radiographic test allows a physician to visualize the biliary tract and pancreatic duct directly. After an acute pancreatitis attack subsides, a physician may order this procedure to look for biliary stones or duct stenosis. It also helps distinguish pancreatic cancer from biliary stones.

Secretin-pancreozymin test

A secretin-pancreozymin test assesses pancreatic exocrine function to confirm a diagnosis of chronic pancreatitis. During this 3-hour procedure, a physician inserts a double-lumen gastrointestinal (GI) tube; one lumen is inserted into the duodenum to aspirate duodenal secretions, and the other lumen is inserted into the stomach to drain stomach contents so they don't contaminate the duodenum. Duodenal samples are obtained before and after I.V. administration of secretin and pancreozymin. The secretin triggers the pancreas to release water and bicarbonate; the pancreozymin stimulates pancreatic enzyme release. Low levels of enzymes and bicarbonate in the duodenal secretions indicate chronic pancreatitis.

Medical interventions

Therapeutic objectives for treating a patient with pancreatitis include minimizing pancreatic secretory activity, maintaining adequate circulatory volume, and preventing or treating complications as they arise. Treatment focuses on resting the pancreas and intestine, replacing fluid and electrolytes, controlling glucose levels, alleviating pain, providing nutrition, controlling infection, and, if necessary, performing surgery.

Pancreas and bowel rest

The pancreas and intestine are rested by having the patient receive nothing by mouth and undergo GI decompression. An NG tube attached to intermittent suction is used to control nausea and vomiting, prevent gastric stimulation of pancreatic secretions, and relieve abdominal distention and discomfort if the patient has an ileus. Also, these drugs may be prescribed:

- an anticholinergic, such as atropine, to decrease GI motility
- an antacid to neutralize hydrochloric acid and thus decrease pancreatic stimulation
- an H_2 blocker, such as cimetidine, to inhibit gastric acid secretion
- 5-fluorouracil to reduce the metabolic rate of the pancreatic cells and the production of enzymes.

Somatostatin may be used to decrease intestinal motility and reduce endocrine and exocrine secretions. As a result, the risk of local complications—such as the formation of pseudocysts and abscesses, pancreatic ascites, and upper GI tract bleeding—may be reduced.

Fluid and electrolyte replacement

With pancreatitis, massive amounts of fluid may be lost into the retroperitoneal space, the peritoneal cavity, and the intestines. Because these areas aren't easily visible, the extent of the volume depletion may not be easy to assess. Also, serum albumin levels may be reduced because of altered capillary permeability and exudate formation from pancreatic autodigestion.

Plasma expanders, such as plasma or albumin, and I.V. fluids, such as lactated Ringer's solution or saline solution, may be used with blood products to correct hypovolemia and maintain fluid balance. A patient's fluid needs are calculated based on his heart rate, blood pressure, urine output, serum hematocrit, and central venous pressure (CVP) or cardiac ouput and cardiac filling pressures. A patient with persistent hypotension despite adequate volume replacement may receive a vasopressor, such as dopamine or norepinephrine.

Electrolyte replacement may consist of administering sodium, potassium, chloride, calcium, magnesium, and phosphorus. Typically, these electrolytes are infused through a central venous catheter to avoid causing tissue necrosis from infiltration into subcutaneous tissue. Plus, if the patient is in shock, peripheral absorption would be limited.

Glucose control

In pancreatitis, hyperglycemia commonly results from the catecholamine-mediated stress response, increased glucagon secretion, and insulin insufficiency. To treat hyperglycemia, a physician may prescribe insulin.

Pain relief

Pain may result from edema and distention of the pancreatic capsule, biliary obstruction, and peritoneal inflammation. Because analgesics can elevate serum amylase and lipase levels, they're usually withheld until the initial blood samples are drawn. Meperidine is the drug of choice for pain control because it relaxes the sphincter of Oddi. Morphine and codeine aren't used because they produce contractions and spasm of the sphincter of Oddi.

When a patient has chronic pancreatitis, a physician may perform a nerve block to achieve long-term pain management. Either a bilateral splanchnic or left celiac ganglion block may be done.

Nutritional support

The patient doesn't resume taking food and fluids by mouth until the abdominal pain subsides and serum amylase levels return to normal. Giving oral feedings prematurely may stimulate the autodigestive process, thus aggravating pancreatic inflammation and raising the risk of pancreatic abscess formation.

Typically, a physician orders nutritional support if the patient has taken nothing by mouth for 2 days. Initially, the patient receives total parenteral nutrition (TPN), consisting of hypertonic glucose, amino acids, and fat emulsions. Usually, fat emulsions don't exacerbate acute pancreatitis and are given to prevent fatty-acid deficiency. If the patient has hypertriglyceridemia, however, fat emulsions are given with extreme caution or withheld.

As soon as the acute inflammatory episode begins to resolve, the patient may receive enteral feedings. Stimulation of the pancreas can be minimized by instilling elemental, neutral-pH liquid nutrition into the proximal portion of the jejunum.

After bowel sounds return to normal, oral feedings can begin. The patient is usually given 100 to 300 ml of clear liquids every 4 hours for the first 24 hours. If he tolerates these liquids, he progresses to a full liquid diet. If he tolerates that, his diet is advanced gradually over 3 or 4 days to include soft foods and, eventually, solid foods. Typically, a physician prescribes a moderate-carbohydrate to high-carbohydrate, high-protein, low-fat diet. The total caloric content is gradually increased from 160 to 640 calories per meal.

Infection control

Antibiotics aren't routinely prescribed for patients with mild or moderate pancreatitis. However, patients with severe acute pancreatitis may be given ceftazidime, amikacin, or metronidazole to prevent infections.

A patient with pancreatitis and gallstones may receive a broad-spectrum antibiotic for a biliary tract infection. Antibiotics are also used to treat necrotizing pancreatitis.

A patient with a pancreatic abscess, a walled-off collection of purulent material within or around the pancreas, may receive antibiotic therapy. A pancreatic abscess may result from liquefaction of an area of pancreatic necrosis or from an acute pseudocyst, a walled-off collection of purulent fluid outside the pancreas.

Pathogens include *Escherichia coli*, *Klebsiella proteus*, *Enterobacter*, and *Pseudomonas enterococcus*.

Drainage, needle aspiration, or peritoneal lavage also may be used to treat a patient with an infection. Internal or external drainage or needle aspiration may be used to treat a pseudocyst, which can be life-threatening if it obstructs neighboring structures or if it ruptures and bleeds, triggering hemorrhagic shock. However, not all pseudocysts are treated; some resolve spontaneously.

For a patient with severe peritonitis, peritoneal lavage may be performed to remove toxins released from the peritoneal cavity before they're systemically absorbed. In this procedure, a physician places a dialysis catheter percutaneously into the peritoneum and starts a continuous infusion of 1 to 2 liters of isotonic solution. Usually, the fluid is drained immediately. If peritoneal lavage is effective, the patient's condition usually improves immediately. Commonly, peritoneal lavage is reserved for patients who have failed to respond to other medical interventions during the first 48 to 72 hours of hospitalization.

Surgery

When a definitive diagnosis hasn't been made and the patient doesn't improve, experiences a setback, has positive blood culture results, or develops sepsis, he may undergo surgery. Usually, drains are inserted during surgery to prevent fluid accumulation and to provide access for continuous postoperative irrigation.

If necessary, the surgeon may debride obviously necrotic tissue. The surgeon also may perform pancreatic resection to remove necrotic or infected tissue or to prevent systemic complications of acute necrotizing pancreatitis, such as septic shock. In some patients, pancreatectomy is performed. If pancreatitis results from biliary tract disease, surgery may be performed to alleviate an obstruction by a gallstone.

In chronic pancreatitis, persistent inflammation, calcification, and duct obstruction in the pancreatic head completely block the flow of pancreatic juice from the body and tail. The surgeon may decompress the ducts and remove the head of the pancreas.

Nursing interventions

Your patient with acute pancreatitis may be extremely ill and need critical care monitoring. Nursing interventions focus on restoring fluid and electrolyte balance, maintaining cardiac and respiratory function, providing comfort, promoting nutrition, and providing patient teaching.

Fluid and electrolyte balance

Evaluate your patient for signs of hypovolemic shock, such as decreasing blood pressure with a rapidly rising pulse rate. To assess fluid balance, monitor his intake and output frequently, about every 2 to 4 hours. During the acute phase, assess his body weight daily. At least every 8 hours, check skin turgor to assess hydration, and check capillary refill to assess peripheral blood flow. Inspect the mucous membranes for dryness. Monitor his vital signs, especially his pulse and blood pressure. Also, check his CVP. If your patient doesn't have a CVP line, check orthostatic blood pressure and pulse rates. If his blood pressure decreases and pulse rate increases when he sits or stands, he may be hypovolemic. Notify the physician of orthostatic changes.

Check the patient's urine, stool, and NG tube drainage for frank or occult bleeding. Inspect his umbilical and flank areas for Cullen's and Grey Turner's signs (see *Recognizing Cullen's sign and Grey Turner's sign*). Measure abdominal girth at least every 8 hours, or as indicated, to check for increasing abdominal distention. Keep in mind that fluid replacement is adequate when urine output reaches 40 to 60 ml per hour. A fall in urine output to less than 30 ml per hour is an early sign of hypovolemia and kidney hypoperfusion.

In patients who are hemodynamically unstable, a pulmonary artery catheter may be inserted to assess hemodynamic status and monitor cardiac filling pressures. The pulmonary capillary wedge pressure is the most sensitive measure of the patient's fluid volume status and left ventricular filling pressure.

Administer fluid replacement, as prescribed. Anticipate giving I.V. solutions and colloids to expand the patient's fluid volume. Prepare to administer blood or blood products to a patient with necrotizing pancreatitis.

Monitor the patient's serum electrolyte levels closely. Be especially alert for signs and symptoms of hypocalcemia, such as tetany, positive Chvostek's and Trousseau's signs, and muscle twitching and irritability. Administer the prescribed electrolyte replacements, such as potassium and calcium.

Cardiac function

A patient with acute pancreatitis may experience decreased cardiac output and impaired cardiac function. That's because kinins, which decrease myocardial contractility, are released during acute pancreatitis. Also, the electrolyte imbalances that may result from acute or chronic pancreatitis may affect the electrical activity of the heart.

Assess the patient's level of consciousness (LOC) for signs of restlessness, irritability, or agitation. Evaluate the skin color and circulation to the arms and legs, being alert for cyanosis and edema. Check pedal pulses, too. Monitor vital signs closely, at least every 2 to 4 hours, and report any changes. Remember that a fever can increase metabolic oxygen demands. Therefore, use an antipyretic, cooling blankets, or tepid sponge baths to help reduce the patient's fever.

Because the inflammatory process of pancreatitis can extend to the pericardial sac, causing pericarditis and possibly cardiac tamponade, auscultate the heart for S_3 and S_4 heart sounds and pericardial friction rubs. Also, check for a widening pulse pressure. During the acute period, implement cardiac monitoring, as directed. Evaluate electrocardiogram (ECG) waveforms for arrhythmias. If the patient has a pulmonary artery catheter, monitor hemodynamic values. Auscultate the patient's breath sounds at least every 4 hours to check for signs of heart failure, such as crackles.

Remember, a urine output of less than 30 ml per hour indicates that blood is being shunted away from the kidneys. Such shunting is a compensatory mechanism that occurs when cardiac output is impaired.

Respiratory function

Assess the patient for signs of hypoxemia, including changes in his LOC. Report any changes immediately. Assess his respiratory status every

Recognizing Cullen's sign and Grey Turner's sign

Cullen's sign appears as faint, irregularly formed hemorrhagic patches on the skin around the umbilicus. The discoloration progresses from blue-black to greenish brown to yellow, and then disappears. Cullen's sign results from the movement of blood from the retroperitoneal pancreatic tissue to the subcutaneous tissue of the umbilical region. This sign typically appears 1 to 2 days after the onset of severe abdominal pain characteristic of acute hemorrhagic pancreatitis.

Grey Turner's sign is an ecchymotic discoloration of the bilateral flank areas of the abdomen that spreads forward to the iliac fossae. Typically, this sign appears within 6 to 24 hours after the onset of a retroperitoneal hemorrhage from acute pancreatitis.

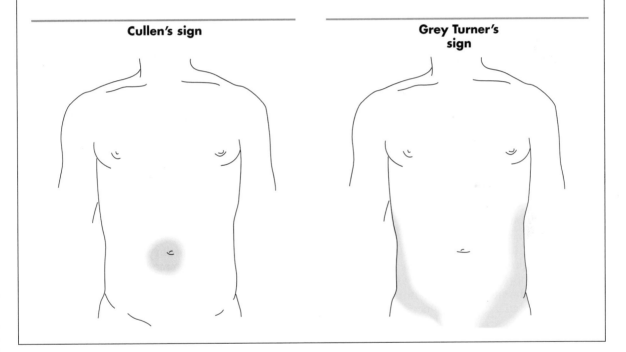

Cullen's sign

Grey Turner's sign

2 to 4 hours. Watch for signs of dyspnea and increased use of accessory muscles. Auscultate the lungs for decreased breath sounds and for crackles and wheezes, which may result from fluid overload and pulmonary edema.

Monitor the patient's ABG studies for signs of hypoxemia, such as a decreased partial pressure of oxygen. Continuously monitor his oxygen saturation level using pulse oximetry or ABG studies, as indicated. And give supplemental oxygen at the prescribed flow rate. If the patient's respiratory status declines, anticipate endotracheal intubation and mechanical ventilation.

If you administer meperidine for pain relief, monitor the patient for respiratory depression. Notify the physician immediately if it occurs.

Reposition the patient frequently, and elevate the head of the bed to maximize ventilation and to prevent pooling of respiratory secretions. Anticipate the need for a chest X-ray to check for a pleural effusion, infiltrates, or atelectasis.

Comfort measures
Make pain control a priority because the hyperventilation that accompanies pain commonly

leads to respiratory alkalosis, further complicating the patient's status. Closely monitor the patient's pain, being especially alert for any sudden increases.

Typically, a patient remains on bed rest for the first 3 to 5 days to decrease his metabolic rate and the production of pancreatic enzymes. Position your patient upright in bed, with his knees and spine flexed to relieve tension on the abdominal muscles. Maintain a calm environment and minimize distractions. Use alternative pain-control methods, such as relaxation, deep breathing, imagery, and distraction. And provide emotional support to allay anxiety and fear, which may increase the release of enzymes and, thus, pain.

Administer the prescribed dosage of meperidine, usually 75 to 100 mg every 3 to 4 hours. Assess the patient to determine the effectiveness of the analgesic. If pain persists, anticipate the need for a nerve block.

Nutrition

While the patient is taking nothing by mouth, administer I.V. fluids, as prescribed. Also, administer TPN or jejunal tube feedings, as prescribed. If your patient is receiving TPN, regularly monitor his blood glucose levels because of the high dextrose content of the solution. Obtain fingerstick blood glucose measurements as appropriate, usually every 6 hours. Anticipate the need for exogenous insulin to control the patient's blood glucose level.

When caring for the patient's TPN catheter, solutions, and insertion site, use strict aseptic technique. Keep in mind that the high dextrose, amino acid, and fat content of TPN provide a medium for the proliferation of microorganisms.

After the acute attack subsides, the patient's diet will be advanced to liquids and then to solid foods. Monitor his response and be alert for recurring signs and symptoms of pancreatitis.

If a patient with severe, acute pancreatitis experiences damage to the islet cells, he may need exogenous insulin and additional diet therapy. Enlist the aid of a dietitian to help plan meals and determine calorie needs.

As ordered, administer prescribed pancreatic enzyme replacements, such as pancreatin or pancrelipase, to correct your patient's enzyme deficit and to aid digestion.

Patient teaching

By teaching your patient with pancreatitis how to promote a healthy lifestyle, you can help prevent complications and recurrences. During the acute stage, focus your teaching on the disease process, treatments, and procedures. After the patient's condition stabilizes, focus your teaching on strategies to promote health.

Teach your patient about the relationship between pancreatitis and the factors that trigger exacerbations. Review the signs and symptoms of a recurrence and explain when he should notify his physician. Also, teach him about the hazards of continued alcohol intake, if appropriate. Refer him to Alcoholics Anonymous or other community resources.

Arrange for a consultation with a dietitian. Give your patient written instructions for a low-fat, high-protein, high-carbohydrate diet. Emphasize the need to avoid spices, caffeine, and nicotine.

Teach your patient about enzyme replacement therapy, if appropriate. Advise him to take the enzymes immediately after meals. Explain that he should swallow the pill whole and not disrupt the protective coating with hot foods or liquids. Remind him not to take these enzymes with antacids because antacids negate their effect.

If the patient needs insulin therapy, teach him and his family about insulin administration and blood glucose monitoring. Discuss appropriate meal and snack planning, blood glucose monitoring techniques, and the signs, symptoms, and treatment of hypoglycemia. Have the patient demonstrate the proper way to prepare and inject insulin. And make sure your patient's caregiver understands glucagon administration.

If your patient has had surgery, provide postoperative teaching. If he's being discharged with a surgical drain in place, obtain a home care referral for care of the drain site.

Pancreatitis and cirrhosis

In cirrhosis, a chronic liver disorder, liver cells are destroyed and replaced with fibrotic tissue. This results in obstructed hepatic blood flow, changes in liver structure, and a loss of liver function.

Because the pancreas and the liver are in close proximity in the abdominal cavity, a problem with one organ easily affects the other. What's more, the pancreatic venous system drains into the portal vein, and the common bile duct and pancreatic duct empty at the ampulla of Vater. Thus, a problem with the drainage of one organ can adversely affect the other organ (see *How pancreatitis leads to biliary cirrhosis*, page 380).

Commonly, alcohol causes both cirrhosis and pancreatitis, especially chronic pancreatitis.

Pathophysiology

In cirrhosis, the liver parenchymal cells are progressively destroyed and replaced with fibrotic tissue. Although some regeneration occurs, scarring causes irregularities in the shape of the hepatic lobules. As the central sections of the lobules become twisted and constricted, vascular flow is impeded and portal hypertension results. Lymphatic flow through the liver is also impeded. And fatty infiltration occurs. After long periods of liver damage and regeneration, hepatic necrosis and atrophy occur. Scarring eventually progresses to the hepatic ducts.

Because of the portal congestion, only some of the toxins carried to the liver are metabolized. The rest are carried through the liver and into the circulatory system. Also, ammonia continues to be formed in the intestinal tract as bacteria break down amino acids. But when this ammonia reaches the liver, the failing organ can't convert the ammonia into glutamine to be eventually broken down into urea and excreted. As a result, levels of ammonia in the bloodstream build up, interfering with normal cerebral metabolism and function and eventually leading to hepatic encephalopathy.

Other complications also arise as the liver fails. Because almost all clotting factors are produced in the liver, a patient may develop life-threatening bleeding complications. Also, the liver can't metabolize carbohydrates, fats, or vitamins, so the body can't maintain normal glucose and vitamin levels, and cellular nutrition suffers.

Alcoholic cirrhosis, which results from chronic alcohol abuse, is the most common type of cirrhosis. Acetaldehyde, a toxic metabolite of alcohol, damages and kills liver cells. Fibrotic tissue replaces the liver cells, eventually impairing all liver functions.

Biliary cirrhosis results from decreased bile flow, usually caused by long-term biliary duct obstruction.

Cardiac cirrhosis—most common in patients with severe, chronic right ventricular heart failure—is characterized by decreased oxygenation of liver cells and cell death.

Typically, a patient with cirrhosis experiences signs and symptoms when hepatic insufficiency and portal hypertension develop. With hepatic insufficiency, the patient may experience changes in his vital signs, renal function, ABG studies, acid-base balance, coagulation, and drug metabolism. With portal hypertension, the patient may have splenomegaly and variceal bleeding and will probably develop ascites, an accumulation of almost pure plasma in the peritoneal cavity. Ascites develops because portal hypertension leads to hepatic capillary congestion, which causes plasma and plasma proteins to leak into the peritoneal cavity.

Regardless of whether the cirrhosis develops from pancreatitis—as in biliary cirrhosis—or both disorders develop because of another factor—such as alcohol abuse—serious, life-threatening complications can develop as the two disorders interact.

For instance, if a patient develops biliary cirrhosis because pancreatitis causes edema of the pancreatic head, he's more likely to develop profound jaundice and pruritis. Or if a patient has alcoholic cirrhosis and pancreatitis, the cirrhosis may result in coagulation defects because of the liver's impaired ability to produce clotting factors, and the pancreatitis may lead to hypercoagulability because of an increase in platelets, factor VIII, fibrinogen, and possibly factor V. The complications of the two disorders then combine to increase the patient's risk for portal vein thrombosis and consequently GI hemorrhage. Because of these potential interactions, you'll need to monitor your patient closely for complications.

PATHOPHYSIOLOGY

How pancreatitis leads to biliary cirrhosis

Normally, bile flows through the common hepatic duct from the liver and through the cystic duct from the gallbladder. Bile then flows through the common bile duct, which is formed by the common hepatic duct and the cystic duct, to the ampulla of Vater. Here, the common bile duct joins the pancreatic duct and empties bile into the duodenum. Because the pancreas, the pancreatic duct, and the hepatic ducts are in such close proximity and are anatomically linked, a problem with the pancreas, such as occurs in pancreatitis, may affect the flow of bile from the liver and cause biliary cirrhosis.

In chronic pancreatitis, structural changes develop, including pancreatic duct obstruction, dilation, and atrophy as well as pancreatic tissue fibrosis. And fibrotic pancreatic tissue can cause common bile duct strictures, which can lead to common bile duct obstruction. With prolonged common bile duct obstruction, hepatic duct pressure rises, causing bile to stagnate in the liver. As excess bile accumulates, liver cells die, and tissue necrosis, edema, and fibrosis develop. Hepatic cells respond by regenerating and forming fine nodules between the fibrotic bands of tissue, giving the liver the characteristic cobbly appearance of cirrhosis. As a result of cirrhosis, liver function may be seriously impaired.

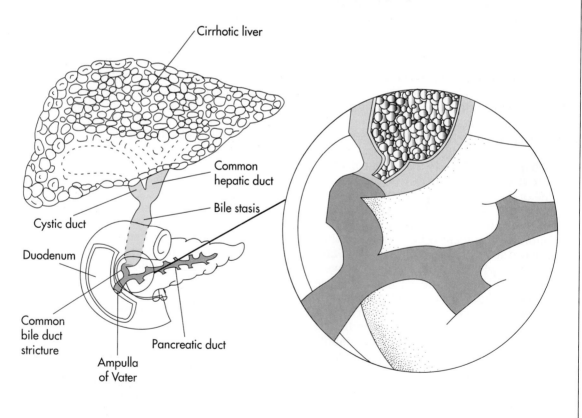

Adapting nursing care

Caring for a patient with pancreatitis and cirrhosis includes maintaining his fluid and electrolyte balance, promoting nutrition, monitoring his respiratory and cardiac function, preventing bleeding, making prescribed adjustments to his drug regimen, and monitoring his mental status. Before your patient is discharged, you'll need to teach him how to prevent complications at home (see *Teaching your patient with pancreatitis and cirrhosis*, page 382).

Fluid and electrolyte balance

For a patient with pancreatitis and cirrhosis, maintaining fluid balance is a nursing priority. Many patients with cirrhosis have ascites. And patients who also have pancreatitis may experience massive fluid shifts and losses, further exacerbating the fluid imbalance.

Typically, ascites in cirrhosis and acute pancreatitis is managed by restricting sodium and fluids and by administering a diuretic, such as spironolactone or furosemide. Limit diuresis to 2,000 ml per day to prevent rapid intravascular volume depletion and acute renal failure. Monitor the patient's intake and output closely, as often as every hour. If the patient is allowed nothing by mouth and has an NG tube attached to suction, be sure to include the drainage as part of his output. Administer I.V. fluids cautiously and use an infusion pump to control the infusion rate. Anticipate the need for albumin administration to improve plasma oncotic pressure and, consequently, vascular volume.

Measure abdominal girth at least every 4 hours. Mark the patient's abdomen with the first measurement to ensure that later measurements are accurate.

Carefully monitor the patient's serum electrolyte levels. Also, monitor him for signs and symptoms of electrolyte deficits or excesses. Anticipate the need for electrolyte replacement therapy.

Nutrition

Assess the patient's nutritional status. A common complication of cirrhosis, poor nutrition also occurs with pancreatitis, either from vomiting or from treatments, such as NG intubation.

Administer TPN, if indicated. Be sure to monitor the appropriate blood studies, including serum albumin and glucose levels. TPN should provide enough protein to compensate for the patient's catabolic state without causing an overload. If the patient's glucose levels are elevated, anticipate administering insulin.

When caring for a patient who's receiving TPN, use strict aseptic technique. Remember, he may already have leukopenia from an enlarged, overactive spleen and an altered immune function. Monitor his body temperature every 4 hours and institute measures to prevent infection, which can further exacerbate his fragile condition.

When the patient's diet advances to solid foods, anticipate a low-sodium, protein-restricted diet. Enlist the aid of a dietitian to teach the patient about food restrictions, appropriate food choices, and meal planning. Monitor the patient's weight daily and obtain calorie counts, as indicated.

Respiratory and cardiac function

Fluid buildup increases pressure on the diaphragm and interferes with lung expansion, making the patient work harder to breathe. This further increases the workload of the heart, which is already attempting to compensate for fluid shifts and fluid losses. Position the patient with the head of the bed elevated to ease the work of breathing and maximize lung expansion. Also, assist with measures to increase respiratory function, such as coughing, deep breathing, and incentive spirometry.

Monitor the patient's oxygen saturation levels, using pulse oximetry and ABG test results. Administer supplemental oxygen, as ordered.

Auscultate the patient's heart and lung sounds for abnormalities. Institute continuous cardiac monitoring, as indicated, and evaluate ECG waveforms for arrhythmias, which may result from electrolyte imbalances, and signs of ischemia.

Anticipate the need for pulmonary artery catheter insertion. Assess hemodynamic measurements every 2 hours or as needed. And note any changes, paying particular attention to trends.

Teaching your patient with pancreatitis and cirrhosis

Before going home, your patient needs to learn how to prevent recurrences of pancreatitis and minimize the effects of cirrhosis. Be sure you cover these points when you teach him and his family:

- Explain the disease processes and the relationship between cirrhosis and pancreatitis as well as the underlying causes and contributing factors.
- Describe the prescribed treatment plan and explain how the patient can incorporate it into his lifestyle. Explain that adhering to the plan can help prevent further attacks and thus avoid the need for surgery.
- Advise the patient to eat moderate-protein, high-carbohydrate foods; to plan small, frequent meals; and to take his prescribed enzymes with food. Tell the patient to avoid crash dieting and binge eating.
- Caution the patient to avoid alcohol, caffeine, nicotine, spicy foods, high-fat foods, foods that produce gas, and carbonated beverages.
- Advise the patient to try to avoid stress as much as possible.
- Teach your patient about his prescribed medications, such as a diuretic, electrolyte and enzyme replacements, and lactulose. Make sure he knows the name, dosage, and possible adverse effects of each.
- Teach the patient to check with his physician before taking nonprescription drugs, such as analgesics and cough remedies.
- Teach your patient to weigh himself and to measure his abdominal girth daily. Advise him to record these measurements.
- Tell your patient to notify his physician if he develops severe epigastric pain that's relieved by sitting, epigastric pain that radiates to the back, nausea and vomiting, or a loss of weight. He should also report dark urine, clay-colored stool, or greasy, foul-smelling stool.
- Discuss alternative pain-relief measures, such as relaxation techniques and guided imagery.
- Emphasize the need for follow-up laboratory testing, such as liver function studies, serum amylase and lipase levels, serum electrolyte levels, and coagulation studies.
- If appropriate, refer the patient to a community-based support group that will help him stop drinking alcohol.

Bleeding

Varices caused by cirrhosis and portal vein thrombosis caused by pancreatitis can lead to increased portal hypertension and predispose the patient to variceal rupture and life-threatening hemorrhage. Plus, changes in coagulation factors and platelets and the decreased absorption of vitamin K increase the patient's risk of bleeding. Therefore, you should try to protect your patient from injury and bleeding. Pad the side rails and, if possible, avoid invasive procedures.

Assess any drainage or excretions for frank or occult bleeding. Watch for petechiae, bruising, and oozing from injection and I.V. sites. Closely monitor the patient's coagulation test results, including his platelet levels. Anticipate the need for transfusion of blood and blood products, such as packed RBCs, fresh frozen plasma, and coagulation factors. And administer vitamin K, as prescribed.

Drug therapy

Cirrhosis decreases the metabolism of some drugs, so you should expect the patient's drug regimen to be adjusted. Meperidine, for instance, used for pain control in acute pancreatitis, is normally eliminated by the liver. In a patient with cirrhosis, however, meperidine metabolism is decreased. Thus, if a physician prescribes this drug, the prescription should be for smaller doses and longer intervals between doses to prevent toxic levels of the drug's metabolites.

Mental status

In pancreatitis, electrolyte and acid-base disturbances, hypoglycemia, hypoxia, anemia, hypotension, hemorrhage, and infection can affect the patient's mental status. These changes, together with the increased ammonia levels cause by cirrhosis, heighten the risk of encephalopathy.

Closely monitor the patient's LOC. Watch for such signs of decreasing LOC as disorientation, lethargy, somnolence, and difficulty awakening. Also note fluctuations in the patient's rate of response, memory, attention, and ability to concentrate.

To control ammonia levels, a physician may order neomycin and lactulose. Neomycin, a broad-spectrum antibiotic, destroys normal intestinal flora that convert urea to ammonia, thus decreasing protein breakdown and ammonia production. Lactulose creates an acidic environment in the intestine, converting nonionized ammonia to ionized ammonia, which can't be absorbed.

Complications

A patient with pancreatitis and cirrhosis may develop complications, such as jaundice, GI hemorrhage, and shock.

Jaundice

Also called icterus, jaundice results from an excessive accumulation of bilirubin (the yellow pigment of bile) in the blood. As you know, when the spleen destroys old RBCs, hemoglobin is released and converted to bilirubin. This non-water-soluble, unconjugated bilirubin travels to the liver, where it's converted to a water-soluble, conjugated form and secreted in bile. Bile then flows through the common bile duct to the intestines and is excreted from the body. When the conversion of unconjugated bilirubin to conjugated bilirubin is impaired or when normal bile flow is impaired, excessive amounts of bilirubin accumulate in the blood, producing the characteristic yellow pallor of jaundice.

In cirrhosis, jaundice results from the liver's inability to conjugate bilirubin. As a result, unconjugated bilirubin accumulates in the blood. And because unconjugated bilirubin is not water soluble, it can't be excreted in the urine.

In acute pancreatitis, bile production remains normal. But if the common bile duct becomes obstructed because of pancreatic pseudocysts or swelling of the pancreatic head, conjugated bilirubin accumulates in the blood. Because conjugated bilirubin is water soluble, however, some of it is excreted in urine.

A patient who has cirrhosis and pancreatitis is at risk for developing severe jaundice from elevated blood levels of both unconjugated and conjugated bilirubin.

Confirming the complication
Jaundice occurs when the serum bilirubin level exceeds 3.0 mg/dl. Typically, the patient develops a yellowing of the sclera, skin, and mucous membranes; pruritus; light clay-colored stools; tea-colored or mahogany-colored urine; and leukocytosis.

Nursing interventions
A patient with pancreatitis and cirrhosis who develops jaundice risks skin problems, such as skin breakdown and pruritis. The risk is increased because of the ascites resulting from both disorders and the increased peripheral edema resulting from cirrhosis.

Monitor the patient's skin routinely for signs of breakdown. Keep in mind that breaks in the skin can easily become infected because of the patient's compromised immune status. Encourage him to keep his fingernails short and his hands clean to decrease the risk of excoriation and infection.

Turn the patient frequently and regularly inspect bony prominences to detect early signs of skin breakdown. If the skin does break down, institute wound care measures, as prescribed.

To decrease itching, bathe the skin with cool water and apply lotion twice a day or as needed to prevent dryness. Also, advise the patient to wear cool, light, nonrestrictive clothing. As necessary, intervene to maintain a normal body temperature. And keep the environment cool.

Suggest that the patient use a soft cloth to pat his skin gently instead of scratching it. You may also try using diversionary activities to decrease the patient's awareness of itching.

Besides providing skin care, monitor your patient's serum bilirubin level regularly.

Before discharge, reinforce all care instructions. Be sure to review skin care and comfort measures to help prevent skin breakdown and control itching.

Gastrointestinal hemorrhage
A patient with cirrhosis may develop coagulopathies because clotting factors I (fibrinogen),

Determining the degree of blood loss

Your patient's signs and symptoms can help you determine how much blood he has lost. A mild blood loss is up to 20% of total blood volume, a moderate loss is 20% to 40%, and a severe loss is more than 40% of total blood volume.

Mild blood loss
- Slight tachycardia
- Normal supine blood pressure
- Systolic blood pressure decrease of more than 10 mm Hg with postural changes
- Pulse increase of more than 20 beats per minute with postural changes
- Capillary refill of more than 3 seconds
- Urine output of more than 30 ml/hr
- Cool, pale skin on arms and legs
- Anxiety

Moderate blood loss
- Rapid, thready pulse
- Supine hypotension
- Urine output of 10 to 30 ml/hr
- Severe thirst
- Cool skin on the trunk
- Restlessness, confusion, or irritability

Severe blood loss
- Marked tachycardia
- Marked hypotension
- Weak or absent peripheral pulses
- Urine output of less than 10 ml/hr
- Cold, mottled, or cyanotic skin
- Unconsciousness

II (prothrombin), V (proaccelerin), VII (proconvertin), IX (plasma thromboplastin component), and X (Stuart factor); fibrinolytic factor; and antithrombin III are synthesized in the liver. As a result, prothrombin time (PT) and activated partial thromboplastin time (APTT) are prolonged.

A patient with pancreatitis may develop hypercoagulability because of increased platelets, fibrinogen, factor VIII, and possibly factor V.

This hypercoagulable state increases his risk for disseminated intravascular coagulation, massive hemorrhage, and thrombus formation. Susceptibility to thrombus formation and localized pancreatic tissue inflammation increase the risk for portal vein, superior mesenteric, or splenic vein thrombosis. The patient may then develop portal hypertension from venous congestion in the liver and the gastric, mesenteric, and colonic varices.

If the patient has both cirrhosis—which leads to varices and coagulopathies—and pancreatitis, the risk of variceal rupture and massive GI hemorrage greatly increases.

Confirming the complication
You may detect blood loss from the GI tract in several ways. You may observe bright, bloody vomitus from fresh bleeding or coffee-ground vomitus from blood that has been in prolonged contact with gastric juices. Blood also may pass through the rectum. Melena is foul-smelling, tarry stool that results from the degradation of blood by stomach acids or intestinal bacteria. Maroon, black, or bright red blood also can pass through the rectum.

In some cases, GI bleeding can only be detected by testing the stool with a chemical reagent (guaiac). However, because GI drainage can test positive up to 10 days after a bleeding episode, the guaiac test isn't a reliable way to detect active bleeding.

Hematemesis and melena indicate acute upper GI tract bleeding. Bright red blood from the rectum usually indicates acute lower GI tract bleeding. The patient's other signs and symptoms depend on the degree of blood loss (see *Determining the degree of blood loss*).

Laboratory findings that indicate GI bleeding include decreased hemoglobin levels and hematocrit, a decreased RBC count, and increased blood urea nitrogen (BUN) levels. Panendoscopy may be performed to view the source of bleeding directly and to treat bleeding varices.

Nursing interventions
RAPID RESPONSE ▶ If your patient develops GI bleeding, you'll need to intervene quickly and efficiently to prevent hypovolemic shock from massive fluid loss and to stabilize his hemodynamic status.

- As soon as you suspect GI bleeding, notify the physician.
- Assess the patient's vital signs for indications of hypovolemic shock, such as hypotension and a weak, rapid pulse.
- Unless the patient is syncopal, frankly hypotensive, or severely tachycardic when supine, evaluate his orthostatic vital signs. Promptly report a systolic blood pressure decrease of 10 mm Hg or more or a pulse increase of 20 beats per minute or more.
- If the patient doesn't have an NG tube in place, assist with the insertion of one. The tube can be used to assess the severity of upper GI tract bleeding, maintain gastric decompression, and prevent vomiting. Perform gastric lavage, if indicated.
- Monitor the patient's platelet count, PT, APTT, hematocrit, and his hemoglobin, electrolyte, glucose, BUN, and creatinine levels. Obtain a urinalysis, a chest X-ray, and a 12-lead ECG, as indicated.
- Obtain blood for typing and crossmatching, as ordered. Ensure that several units of packed RBCs are available for transfusion.
- Establish and maintain I.V. access with a large-bore catheter to administer fluids and blood products. As appropriate, administer packed RBCs, fresh frozen plasma, platelets, or other blood components as well as volume expanders, such as plasma protein fraction or albumin. Monitor the patient's response.
- If bleeding results from esophageal varices, anticipate giving vasopressin by intermittent or continuous infusion. Also, anticipate the use of sclerotherapy or esophageal tamponade.
- If indicated, insert an indwelling urinary catheter and monitor the patient's urine output. Notify the physician if it drops below 30 ml per hour. Maintain accurate intake and output records, making sure you include emesis and stool.
- Administer oxygen by nasal cannula or mask, if indicated. Monitor the patient's oxygen saturation levels and ABG results for signs of hypoxemia. If breathing becomes severely compromised, prepare for endotracheal intubation and mechanical ventilation. ◄

Remember, a patient who undergoes emergency care for a GI hemorrhage is likely to be extremely frightened and upset. Be sure to provide comfort measures and emotional support (see *Hemorrhage: Allaying your patient's fears*, page 386).

Shock

If your patient with pancreatitis and cirrhosis develops bleeding that goes untreated, or if he can't compensate for the blood volume loss, hemorrhagic shock develops. In hemorrhagic shock, venous return decreases, which causes a corresponding decrease in cardiac output. The lowered cardiac output leads to inadequate tissue perfusion.

A patient with pancreatitis may already be experiencing a decreased cardiac output from massive fluid loss and fluid shifts. In a patient who also has cirrhosis, this situation is compounded by fluid shifting that results from decreased albumin production and decreased plasma oncotic pressure. Vasoconstriction, a vascular response to decreased cardiac output and decreased right atrial pressures, causes shunting to the cerebral and cardiopulmonary systems. If the vasoconstriction continues, decreased blood flow to the kidneys may lead to medullary tubular dysfunction or acute tubular necrosis.

Vasoconstriction and decreased tissue perfusion result in cellular dysfunction. The cells attempt to extract oxygen from the available blood, but as shock progresses and less blood is available, the cells shift to anaerobic metabolism. Energy production decreases, and large quantities of lactic acid are formed. The reduced blood flow to the hepatic and renal systems impairs their ability to break down lactic acid or remove it from the blood. Impaired liver function further interferes with the removal of toxins. As lactic acid accumulates, metabolic acidosis develops.

Normally, the body compensates for blood loss by releasing aldosterone and antidiuretic hormone, which trigger a shift of fluid from extravascular spaces to intravascular spaces. However, in a patient with cirrhosis, this compensatory effect is suppressed. The result is

COMFORT MEASURES

Hemorrhage: Allaying your patient's fears

Your patient with pancreatitis and cirrhosis is probably already anxious about the effects of these two disorders. If gastrointestinal bleeding develops while he's in the hospital, he's likely to become even more anxious about his condition. Therefore, as you're providing emergency care for his bleeding, make sure you take steps to keep him as calm and comfortable as possible.

- Take time to explain all interventions to your patient, even as you respond swiftly to his emergency. Use terms that he can understand. Also, be careful not to express dismay or anxiety. Maintain a calm, confident, matter-of-fact attitude.
- Use active listening to encourage your patient to express his feelings and fears. Acknowledge his fear by saying something like, "I know it must be scary to see all this blood. But we can treat this problem. We'll replace your blood by giving you a blood transfusion and I.V. fluids." Make sure you explain the risks and benefits of receiving blood products. And make sure a signed consent form has been obtained.

- Inform your patient and his family about any necessary diagnostic tests, such as endoscopy, and monitoring procedures.
- Throughout the bleeding episode, assess your patient's complaints of pain. Teach him to use relaxation techniques and guided imagery to relieve pain and anxiety. Keep in mind that the acuity of his condition can make it harder to maintain pain control. Check with the physician about increasing the dosage of meperidine or switching to another analgesic.
- Explain to your patient that he'll be transferred to the intensive care unit. Prepare him and his family for the transfer. Explain that he'll need to be monitored closely and thus may need continuous cardiac, central venous pressure, or pulmonary artery catheter monitoring. Discuss the possibility of endotracheal intubation and mechanical ventilation, if needed.

---

sodium and water retention. The extreme fluid losses that occur with pancreatitis further increase the risk of impaired compensation.

Confirming the complication

If you can see the bleeding, quantify the volume of blood loss and determine if the patient is likely to develop shock. Then, perform a focused assessment and intervene quickly and appropriately. If you can't see the bleeding, you'll need to be alert for hemodynamic and other changes that indicate shock. The patient may exhibit signs and symptoms, such as hypotension; shallow, rapid respirations; and cold, clammy skin. You also may note orthostatic hypotension and syncope.

Blood loss decreases both the hemoglobin level and hematocrit. As blood flow to the liver decreases, waste products accumulate in the blood, causing the BUN level to rise. Urine output, a sensitive measure of tissue perfusion and blood flow, decreases as blood is shunted to the vital areas. As shock progresses, the patient's LOC decreases. If the bleeding is untreated or uncontrolled, he eventually slips into a coma.

Nursing interventions

RAPID RESPONSE ▶ If your patient goes into hemorrhagic shock, notify the physician at once. Then follow these guidelines:

- Place the patient in the supine position.
- Assist with the insertion of a central venous or pulmonary artery catheter.
- Monitor the patient's vital signs and hemodynamic measurements every 15 to 60 minutes, according to the depth of the shock and the rate of its progression.
- Administer I.V. fluids, blood, and blood products, as prescribed. Monitor the patient's urine output and check for signs of fluid overload, such as crackles, neck vein distention, and an S_3 heart sound.
- Be alert for signs and symptoms of disseminated intravascular coagulation, such as blood

oozing from several sites, repeated bleeding episodes, petechiae, ecchymoses, hematomas, prolonged PT and APTT, a decreased fibrinogen level, a decreased platelet count, or an elevated level of fibrin split products.

• If bleeding continues and the patient's condition remains unstable, prepare him for surgery. Any coagulopathies need to be corrected—for example, with plasma or vitamin K administration. Otherwise, the patient will bleed uncontrollably during surgery. Surgery aims to repair the bleeding sites, such as esophageal varices. A surgical procedure, such as shunting, may be performed later to decompress the liver. ◄

Pancreatitis and diabetes mellitus

The combination of the endocrine dysfunction of diabetes and the exocrine dysfunction of pancreatitis puts a diabetic patient who develops pancreatitis at increased risk for complications, especially poor glucose control. Pancreatitis can also diminish pancreatic insulin production, which may cause some patients to develop diabetes.

Pathophysiology

A patient with Type I (insulin-dependent) diabetes mellitus lacks effective endogenous insulin and therefore needs exogenous insulin to survive. A patient with Type II (non–insulin-dependent) diabetes mellitus has a moderate or severe lack of effective endogenous insulin. He also may have resistance to available insulin and thus be unable to use it effectively. In either case, a patient with Type II diabetes may require oral hypoglycemic drugs, exogenous insulin, or both.

Without insulin, insulin-dependent cells can't use glucose, so cellular starvation develops despite an elevated blood glucose level. As a compensatory mechanism, catabolic hormones are secreted in an attempt to meet cellular energy needs. As a result, hyperglycemia increases, and cellular starvation continues.

A patient with pancreatitis and diabetes is under acute stress that's exacerbated by the pain of pancreatitis. The body's response to this stress makes glucose control more difficult. A diabetic patient who continues to take an oral hypoglycemic drug or insulin may suddenly develop hypoglycemia, especially if he has a poor appetite or if he's allowed nothing by mouth because of the pancreatitis.

Adapting nursing care

Assess your patient's hydration status closely. The acute stress of pancreatitis and hospitalization can increase his blood glucose levels, predisposing him to dehydration. This compounds the fluid imbalance caused by pancreatitis. Check the patient's skin turgor and mucous membranes. Monitor his intake and output and daily weight. And assess him routinely for signs and symptoms of fluid volume deficit, such as orthostatic hypotension and tachycardia. Also, monitor his serum electrolyte levels closely and administer replacements, as prescribed.

When your patient with diabetes can take nothing by mouth during the acute stage of pancreatitis, he may develop a glucose imbalance. Anticipate significant changes in his medication requirements, and prepare to adjust his drug therapy, as prescribed. If your patient uses insulin, the dosage may need to be increased. If he takes an oral hypoglycemic drug, he'll probably need to switch to insulin therapy. His physician may prescribe sliding scale doses of regular insulin every 4 to 6 hours based on blood glucose levels. Obtain blood glucose levels using fingerstick and venipuncture specimens, as ordered.

Depending on the patient's condition, insulin may be administered subcutaneously or I.V. In acutely ill patients, the I.V. route is preferred because absorption and circulatory uptake of subcutaneous injections is unpredictable.

If you administer a continuous insulin infusion, use an infusion device. Before beginning the infusion, flush the tubing with about 50 ml of regular insulin in 0.9% normal saline solution to prevent the insulin from adhering to the plastic I.V. tubing during the infusion. Monitor the patient closely. Frequently assess him for signs and symptoms of hypoglycemia and hyperglycemia.

After the patient's condition improves and he resumes taking food by mouth, readjust his insulin dosage, as needed. Work with the patient and the dietitian to develop appropriate meal plans that maintain adequate blood glucose control and prevent a recurrence of pancreatitis.

Monitor the patient's pain because pain heightens the stress response and places him at risk for hyperglycemia. Administer meperidine, as prescribed, and evaluate the patient's response. To help control pain, also use nonpharmacologic measures, such as positioning, relaxation, and deep breathing. Maintain the function of an NG decompression tube to promote rest for the pancreas, thus reducing pancreatic stimulation. Minimize the nasal discomfort from the NG tube by lubricating the nare and securing the tube properly. Be alert for sudden complaints of increased abdominal or referred pain, which may signal a rupture of a pseudocyst or pancreatic abscess.

Teach your patient to manage his disorders by taking his medications, maintaining his diet, modifying his lifestyle, and preventing long-term complications, such as retinopathy, nephropathy, and peripheral neuropathy. Have him return your demonstrations of all self-care procedures. And obtain a home care referral for assessment, evaluation, and follow-up support to ensure compliance.

Complications

A patient who has pancreatitis and diabetes mellitus risks developing complications, including hypoglycemia, diabetic ketoacidosis (DKA), and hyperglycemic hyperosmolar nonketotic (HHNK) syndrome.

Hypoglycemia

Hypoglycemia occurs when the blood glucose level drops below 60 mg/dl. However, many patients don't develop symptoms until the level falls to 45 mg/dl. Others may have a hypoglycemic reaction even when their blood glucose level is normal because they experience a rapid drop—for example, from 250 mg/dl to 100 mg/dl.

In a patient with pancreatitis and diabetes, hypoglycemia can develop because of an excessive dose of an oral hypoglycemic drug or insulin, missed meals, or an increase in exercise without a corresponding increase in food intake. Hypoglycemia can occur suddenly and, if untreated, may become life-threatening.

A patient with pancreatitis may already have poor nutrition, and his nutritional status can deteriorate rapidly if he develops hypoglycemia and its associated nausea and vomiting. The risk of hypoglycemia increases if he continues taking his diabetic medication—especially if he's receiving nothing by mouth.

Confirming the complication

A random blood glucose test reveals if the patient is having an episode of hypoglycemia. If you need immediate results, you can use bedside glucose monitoring.

Nursing interventions

The key to nursing care is preventing hypoglycemia by closely monitoring blood glucose levels, assessing the patient for signs and symptoms, and adjusting drug dosages appropriately. If the patient has signs and symptoms of hypoglycemia and his blood glucose level is below 70 mg/dl or has dropped sharply, you'll need to intervene immediately.

RAPID RESPONSE ▶ If hypoglycemia develops, follow these guidelines:

- If the patient is conscious and able to take food by mouth, give him 15 grams of a rapidly absorbed carbohydrate. For example, give 4 ounces of orange juice, 6 to 8 Lifesavers, 2 tablespoons of raisins, or a soft drink containing sugar. Depending on the severity of the hypoglycemia, he may need 15 to 30 grams of a rapidly absorbed carbohydrate.
- If the patient is experiencing neuroglycopenic signs or symptoms (such as mental confusion, slurred speech, disorientation, or seizures) or if he's unconscious or can't take anything by mouth because of acute pancreatitis, administer 25 to 50 g of 50% dextrose solution I.V. or

0.5 to 1 mg of glucagon subcutaneously, as prescribed. Begin an infusion of 5% dextrose, as prescribed, and continue it until the patient is alert and able to take oral nourishment.

- Recheck his blood glucose level in 15 minutes. If it's still depressed, repeat your intervention, as directed. ◄

If your patient is receiving TPN or a tube feeding, make sure it's administered without interruption. Give hypoglycemic drugs, as prescribed, and continue to monitor blood glucose levels.

When the patient's condition is stable, monitor him for signs and symptoms of a relapse. If he's allowed to take food by mouth, provide additional, longer-lasting sources of carbohydrates—for example, 8 ounces of milk or half a sandwich. If he's not allowed anything by mouth, administer I.V. glucose, as prescribed. Continue to monitor his blood glucose levels and adjust his insulin dose accordingly.

Also, review the possible causes of the hypoglycemic event and teach the patient how to prevent a recurrence. Reinforce all instructions about glucose management. And tell the patient to notify his physician if he's unable to consume adequate amounts of food. If appropriate, obtain a home care referral for follow-up support to evaluate the patient's understanding and compliance with treatment.

Diabetic ketoacidosis

In a patient with Type I diabetes, DKA can result from an absolute or relative deficiency of effective insulin and an increase in insulin counterregulatory hormones—catecholamines, cortisol, glucagon, and growth hormone. As a result, hepatic glucose production increases, peripheral glucose use decreases, fat mobilization increases, and ketogenesis is stimulated.

The most common cause of DKA is an acute illness, such as pancreatitis, which requires the pancreas to produce more insulin. In severe pancreatitis, damage to the alpha cells increases glucagon secretion, and damage to the beta cells may interfere with insulin secretion.

Confirming the complication
The signs and symptoms of DKA usually begin within 12 to 24 hours of the insulin deficiency

---

Detecting diabetic ketoacidosis in a patient with pancreatitis

Signs and symptoms of pancreatitis occur mainly in the gastrointestinal (GI) system. Diabetic ketoacidosis (DKA) triggers similar GI signs and symptoms, but it also causes a variety of other signs and symptoms throughout the body. Thus, you'll need to carefully assess a diabetic patient who has pancreatitis to determine if he's developed DKA. Here are the signs and symptoms to look for:
- lethargy
- irritability
- changes in level of consciousness
- fruity breath odor
- dry mucous membranes
- Kussmaul's respirations
- cardiac arrhythmias
- tachycardia
- orthostatic hypotension
- polyphagia (early)
- polydipsia (early)
- anorexia (late)
- nausea and vomiting (late)
- abdominal pain (late)
- rapid weight loss
- polyuria
- ketonuria
- muscle fatigue
- weakness
- poor skin turgor
- flushed, dry skin.

---

and may continue for several days before the patient seeks medical attention. Eventually, as his LOC decreases and polyuria, polydipsia, lethargy, and weight loss become intolerable, he realizes he's in crisis (see *Detecting diabetic ketoacidosis in a patient with pancreatitis*).

DKA affects many body systems. If the patient doesn't receive treatment soon enough, he may experience cardiac arrhythmias and become comatose. Such life-threatening complications can make diagnosing the underlying cause—in this case, pancreatitis—difficult. Therefore, be alert for signs of pancreatitis, such as acute abdominal pain, nausea, and vomiting.

At first, a patient with DKA may be hungry because of the hyperglycemia. As dehydration sets in and DKA progresses, however, the patient experiences anorexia, nausea, vomiting, and abdominal pain. Profound dehydration may lead to constipation. When you examine the patient with DKA and pancreatitis, you may note abdominal tenderness and reduced bowel sounds or none at all.

The extreme dehydration and hypovolemia that result from DKA cause tachycardia, orthostatic hypotension, dry mucous membranes, poor skin turgor, and flushed, dry skin. The patient may complain of weakness and fatigue. As his condition declines, so does his LOC.

When electrolytes, including potassium, are lost along with fluids, the signs and symptoms of hypokalemia appear. Initially, the patient experiences fatigue and muscle weakness. Eventually, as potassium and magnesium levels drop, he experiences flaccid muscle paralysis and cardiac arrhythmias.

As the body attempts to rid itself of excess carbonic acid, you may detect Kussmaul's respirations and a fruity acetone odor on the patient's breath.

In a patient with DKA, blood glucose levels usually range between 300 and 800 mg/dl. As bicarbonate is lost through osmotic diuresis, blood bicarbonate levels drop to less than 15 mEq/L. Dehydration causes BUN, hematocrit, and urine specific gravity to rise. Blood osmolality may soar as high as 330 mOsm/L.

In a patient with pancreatitis and diabetes who develops DKA, the WBC count may be elevated. Blood phosphate levels may be low. As ketones accumulate in the blood, the pH drops to less than 7.3, and ketones appear in the urine.

Nursing interventions

To prevent DKA from developing, you'll need to monitor your patient's blood glucose level, watch him closely for signs and symptoms, and make sure he receives his insulin as prescribed.

RAPID RESPONSE ▶ If DKA develops, follow these guidelines:

- Assess your patient for signs of inadequate gas exchange, including skin color changes, tachycardia, dyspnea, and decreased respiratory effort. Check his oxygen saturation levels and administer supplemental oxygen as indicated. To determine the degree of acidosis, check his ABG results for changes in pH and carbon dioxide and bicarbonate levels.

- Check your patient's vital signs. Postural or sustained hypotension, especially with tachycardia, may indicate impending shock. Remember that shock can result from fluid shifts, which occur in response to volume depletion. This risk is increased by the fluid shifts and losses of pancreatitis.

- Assess your patient's fluid balance to ensure adequate hydration. A central venous line may be inserted to monitor fluid status or to guide fluid replacement therapy, so you can prevent heart failure, pulmonary edema, and other serious complications. Watch for indications of central venous overload, including jugular vein distention, S_3 heart sounds, tachycardia, increased CVP, dyspnea, and pulmonary crackles. Also, note if breath sounds are decreased or absent.

- Check your patient's serum electrolyte levels, including sodium, potassium, bicarbonate, magnesium, and phosphate levels. Evaluate his ECG tracings to detect arrhythmias from abnormally high or low potassium levels.

- Monitor the patient's neurologic status closely because changes can result from fluid and electrolyte shifts in the body. Acidosis and dehydration may affect the patient's ability to concentrate, follow instructions, or engage in conversation. These deficits may linger for up to 72 hours after a DKA crisis. Expect the patient's LOC to improve when his blood glucose levels improve.

- If your patient needs an insulin infusion, mix regular insulin in 0.9% normal saline solution. Because insulin adheres to the I.V. tubing, flush it with about 50 ml of the insulin solution to saturate it. Otherwise, your patient won't receive the full insulin dose for several hours. Administer the I.V. insulin, using an infusion pump to control the infusion rate.

- Monitor the patient's blood glucose levels hourly. When they fall to about 250 mg/dl, obtain an order to switch the I.V. fluid-replacement solution to one that will help avoid hypoglycemia—for example, 5% dextrose with

0.45% normal saline solution. As blood glucose levels fall, monitor your patient closely for signs and symptoms of hypoglycemia. Continue to infuse insulin I.V. until subcutaneous injections begin. Evaluate the patient's body weight, intake and output, urine specific gravity, and blood osmolality. Assess skin turgor and mucous membranes for improved hydration. Maintain I.V. fluid replacement therapy, as prescribed, and frequently check the I.V. site for signs of infiltration or infection. ◄

Intervene as needed to provide comfort and hygiene measures. Although your patient is dehydrated and thirsty, he may not be able to eat or drink anything until he's no longer vomiting, feeling nauseous, or having abdominal pain. Provide frequent oral care to moisten his dry lips and mucous membranes.

Provide thorough skin care to reduce the risk of skin breakdown from dehydration and poor tissue perfusion. Turn and reposition your patient every 2 hours. Use an emollient to keep his skin from becoming scaly, flaky, and vulnerable to breakdown. As you provide skin care, check your patient's skin turgor, color, temperature, and perfusion.

After the patient's condition has stabilized and before discharge, reinforce the need to maintain adequate blood glucose control to minimize the risk of complications. Reinforce sick-day rules and explain when to notify the physician (see *Reviewing sick-day rules*). Obtain a home care referral, if appropriate.

Hyperglycemic hyperosmolar nonketotic syndrome

This syndrome may appear in a patient who has already been diagnosed with Type II diabetes, or it may be the first indication that he has it. Precipitating factors for HHNK syndrome include invasive procedures, certain types of drug therapy, and an acute or chronic illness, such as pancreatitis.

In this syndrome, a patient can produce enough insulin to prevent ketosis and acidosis but not enough to prevent severe hyperglycemia, diuresis, and loss of extracellular fluid.

 GOING HOME

Reviewing sick-day rules

The goal of sick-day rules is to prevent serious complications, such as diabetic ketoacidosis or hyperglycemic hyperosmolar nonketotic syndrome, and hospitalization when a diabetic patient becomes ill. A patient with diabetes should already be familiar with these rules. But a patient with diabetes and pancreatitis who has experienced diabetic ketoacidosis will benefit from a review.

Teach your patient to do the following when he's sick:
• Continue to take his usual dose of insulin.
• Monitor his blood glucose level every 2 to 4 hours.
• Check his urine for ketones if his blood glucose level is over 240 mg/dl and he isn't feeling well.
• Call his physician if his blood glucose level is over 250 mg/dl for two or more readings, if he has a large number of ketones in his urine, or if he has a fever and is vomiting.
• Drink at least 8 ounces of calorie-free fluid, such as water, diet soda, or tea, every hour.
• Drink clear fluids if he's been vomiting. When his blood glucose level is between 250 and 300 mg/dl, he should drink calorie-free beverages. When his blood glucose level is between 180 and 250 mg/dl before a meal, he should consume easily tolerated foods and beverages; he should consume the same amount of carbohydrate he usually does to prevent hypoglycemia.
• Consume the following easily tolerated foods if he's unable to follow his normal meal plan. (Each serving provides 15 grams of carbohydrate.)
 ½ cup of unsweetened apple juice
 1 cup of beef broth
 ½ to ¾ cup of caffeine-free soda
 1 cup of Gatorade
 ½ cup of Cream of Wheat
 1 slice of dry toast
 3 Graham cracker squares
 6 saltine squares

Confirming the complication

The syndrome usually begins slowly, with the patient experiencing extreme thirst and excessive urination over a period of days or weeks. Other common signs and symptoms include weight loss, weakness, anorexia, nausea, vomiting, tachycardia, hypotension, orthostatic hypotension, dry skin and mucous membranes, and poor skin turgor. Many patients with HHNK syndrome show a progressive neurologic deterioration, including a decreased responsiveness, confusion, lethargy, seizures, focal deficits, paralysis, and hemiparesis or hemisensory loss.

Laboratory test findings help confirm the diagnosis of HHNK syndrome. The patient's blood glucose level may be greater than 1,000 mg/dl and as high as 2,000 mg/dl. He may have ketones in his urine. ABG measurements may show metabolic acidosis with a pH of 7.26. The patient's serum osmolality may be greater than 330 mOsm/kg, and the BUN level between 70 to 90 mg/dl. The serum sodium level is usually elevated, typically to 145 mEq/L. The patient's hemoglobin level is commonly elevated, typically to 18 g/dl, and the hematocrit may be as high as 54%.

Nursing interventions

To prevent HHNK from developing, the patient will need close monitoring of his blood glucose level and treatment for pancreatitis.

RAPID RESPONSE ▶ If HHNK develops, follow these guidelines:

- Administer I.V. fluid replacement therapy, as prescribed. As you do, assess your patient's vital signs, intake and output, breath sounds, skin turgor, and mucous membranes. A central venous line may be inserted to monitor fluid status or to guide fluid replacement therapy, so you can prevent heart failure, pulmonary edema, and other serious complications. Watch for evidence of central venous overload, including jugular vein distention, S_3 heart sounds, tachycardia, increased CVP, dyspnea, and pulmonary crackles.
- Monitor your patient's electrolyte levels, especially his potassium, sodium, phosphate, and magnesium levels. A physician may order potassium supplements, which can be added to the I.V. replacement fluids. If your patient is receiving extensive potassium replacement, monitor his ECG tracings for arrhythmias.
- Determine your patient's neurologic status and then check it hourly, especially if cerebral edema occurs. As appropriate, initiate

seizure precautions, such as padding the side rails and keeping an airway at the bedside. Ensure a patent airway and protect the patient from injury. Typically, phenytoin is used to treat seizures; however, it can worsen hyperglycemia.

- If your patient is vomiting, anticipate inserting an NG tube. Assess his bowel sounds and check for increased abdominal tenderness.
- If an I.V. insulin infusion is prescribed, mix regular insulin in 0.9% normal saline solution. Because insulin adheres to the I.V. tubing, flush the tubing with 50 ml of the insulin solution to saturate it. Otherwise, your patient won't receive the full dose for several hours. Administer the I.V. insulin solution using an infusion pump to control the infusion rate.
- Monitor the patient's blood glucose levels hourly. When they fall to about 250 mg/dl, obtain an order to switch the I.V. fluid-replacement solution to one that will help avoid hypoglycemia—for example, 5% dextrose with 0.45% normal saline solution. As blood glucose levels fall, monitor your patient closely for signs and symptoms of hypoglycemia. Continue to infuse insulin I.V. until subcutaneous injections begin. If your patient is confused, comatose, or unconscious, you'll need to address your early teaching to his family. During the acute phase, explain the need for fluid and electrolyte replacement, invasive lines, and frequent monitoring. ◀

After your patient's condition stabilizes, teach him about the causes of HHNK syndrome and strategies for preventing it. Ask the physician for acceptable blood glucose levels and teach the patient what they are. Reinforce information about the proper use of home glucose-monitoring equipment. Give full instructions to patients who take oral hypoglycemic drugs or insulin. If insulin has been prescribed, observe the patient's technique as he administers it to himself. Suggest ways he can improve his technique.

Stress the importance of following the prescribed diet and recognizing the signs and symptoms of hyperglycemia and hypoglycemia. Instruct your patient and his family about emergency care for both conditions.

Obtain a home care referral for follow-up support to continue diabetic teaching.

Suggested readings

Banerjee AK, Haggie SJ, Jones RB, Basran GS. Respiratory failure in acute pancreatitis. *Postgrad Med J.* 1995;71(836):327-330.

Bradley EL. *Acute pancreatitis: diagnosis and therapy.* New York, NY: Raven Press; 1994.

De Beaux AC, Plester C, Fearon KC. Flexible approach to nutritional support in severe acute pancreatitis. *Nutrition.* 1994;10(3):246-248; discussion 249.

Delcenserie R, Yzet T, Ducroix JP. Prophylactic antibiotics in treatment of severe acute alcoholic pancreatitis. *Pancreas.* 1996;13(2):198-201.

Moscati RM. Cholelithiasis, cholecystitis, and pancreatitis. *Emerg Med Clin North Am.* 1996;14(4):719-737.

Noone J. Acute pancreatitis: an Orem approach to nursing assessment and care. *Crit Care Nurs.* 1995;15(4):27-35.

Parillo JE, Bone RE. *Critical care medicine: principles of diagnosis and management.* St Louis, Mo: Mosby–Year Book, Inc; 1995.

Rakel R. *Conn's Current Therapy.* Philadelphia, Pa: WB Saunders Co; 1996.

Ranson JH. The current management of acute pancreatitis. *Adv Surg.* 1995;28(9):93-112.

Renkes J. GI endoscopy: managing the full scope of care. *Nursing.* 1993;23(6):50-55.

Thompson JM, McFarland GK, Hirsch JE, Tucker SM. *Mosby's clinical nursing.* 3rd ed. St Louis, Mo: Mosby–Year Book; 1993.

Urban N, Greenlee KK, Krumberger J, Winkelman C. *Guidelines for critical care nursing.* St Louis, Mo: Mosby–Year Book, Inc; 1995.

Wilmink T, Frick TW. Drug-induced pancreatitis. *Drug Saf.* 1996;14(6):406-423.

Zaloga GP. *Nutrition in critical care.* St Louis, Mo: Mosby–Year Book, Inc; 1994.

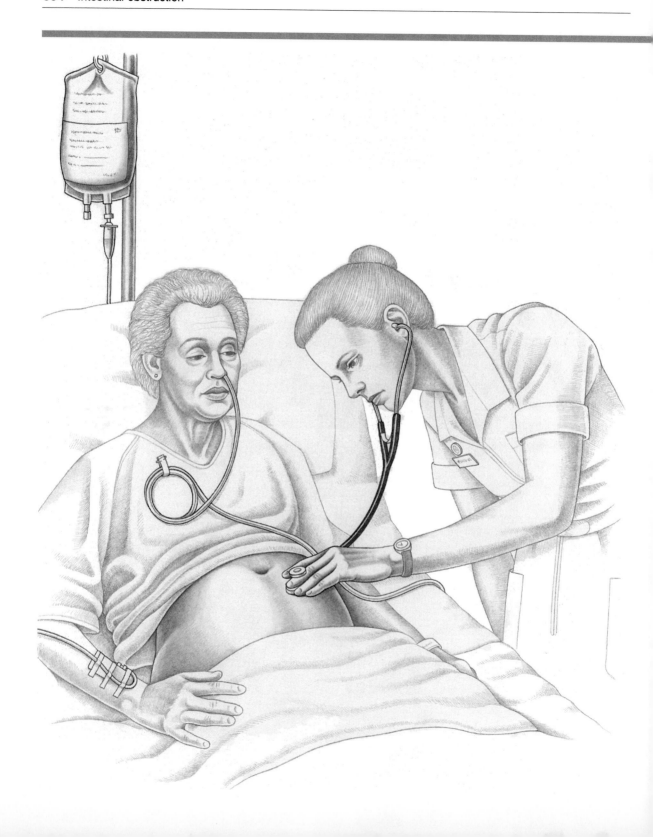

13

Intestinal Obstruction

Usually, abdominal pain means little more than passing indigestion. But sometimes it signals a more serious problem—an intestinal obstruction. Whether partial or complete, an intestinal obstruction can lead to a host of complications. And when a patient has an intestinal obstruction along with another disorder, such as a myocardial infarction (MI) or inflammatory bowel disease, she runs the risk of developing complications as serious as stress ulcers, intestinal infarction, fistulas, abscesses, peritonitis, and septic shock.

In some cases, an intestinal obstruction and its complications give you little time to spare.

To prevent serious problems and save the patient's life, you must act quickly.

Anatomy and physiology review

Between the stomach and the anus lie the small and large intestines, roughly 25 feet of gastrointestinal (GI) tract highly adapted to absorb nutrients from ingested foods and prepare remaining substances for elimination. Although each major section of the intestines serves a slightly different purpose, all are composed of the same four basic tissue layers: serosa, muscularis, submucosa, and mucosa.

In the serosa, layers of squamous cells secrete a thin film of serous fluid. Called the mesothelium, this smooth, slippery surface allows loops of intestine to slide past each other during body movements and peristalsis.

The muscularis actually contains two smooth-muscle layers, an outer layer of longitudinal fibers and an inner layer of circular fibers. The outer layer helps bend and twist the intestinal wall. The inner layer constricts the wall and narrows the lumen.

The submucosa contains connective tissue, nerves, blood vessels, lymph tissue, and many exocrine glands.

Just inside submucosa lies the mucosa, which has three layers:
- the lamina propria, which contains blood vessels, nerve endings, and lymphatic vessels
- a basement membrane
- the epithelium, which lines the lumen and helps with digestion.

Between the layers of the intestinal wall are two neural plexuses responsible for local and autonomic nerve stimulation. The myenteric plexus lies between the circular and longitudinal layers of the muscularis. The submucosal plexus lies between the circular layer of the muscularis and the submucosa. Distention stimulates these two neural networks, thus increasing peristalsis.

Small intestine

The small intestine is about 20 feet long and about 1 inch in diameter. It extends from the pyloric sphincter at the distal end of the stomach to the ileocecal valve at the beginning of the large intestine. Divided into three sections—the duodenum, jejunum, and ileum—the small intestine performs most of the chemical digestion and absorption of nutrients.

Most chemical digestion takes place in the duodenum, the first section of the small intestine. Brunner's glands secrete an alkaline mucus that helps neutralize acidic chyme as it leaves the stomach. Then digestive enzymes secreted by thousands of mucosal and submucosal glands break down carbohydrates, fats, and proteins in the duodenum. Hydrolytic enzymes from the pancreas and gallbladder enter the GI tract at the duodenum.

The jejunum, which is about 8 feet long, has thick walls and serves as the primary site of nutrient absorption. The ileum is longer and thinner than the jejunum. Its walls are narrower, and the villi are less numerous. Lymph clusters called Peyer's patches protect the mucosa of the ileum from foreign substances. By the time chyme reaches the ileum, it has been transformed into mostly water and food waste. In the small intestine, the mucosa and submucosa form tight folds called plicae circulares, which are covered with thousands of tiny projections called villi, each about 1 mm long. At the bases of the villi, intestinal glands open into the intervillous spaces.

Inside each villus is a central lymphatic vessel, called a lacteal, that absorbs lipids from passing chyme. Surrounding the lacteal is a network of tiny capillaries that absorb sugars and amino acids produced by carbohydrate and protein breakdown. Covering each villus is a layer of epithelial cells, called microvilli, that have a brushlike border. All these structures on the plicae circulares greatly increase the surface area available for the digestion and absorption of nutrients (see *Inside the intestines*).

Large intestine

Digestive products leave the small intestine through the ileocecal valve and enter the large intestine at the cecum in the right lower abdominal quadrant. Measuring 5 to 6 feet in length

ANATOMY REVIEW

Inside the intestines

The wall of the small and large intestines consists of four major layers: the serosa, muscularis (consisting of longitudinal and circular muscle sheaths), submucosa, and mucosa. In the jejunum, the submucosa and mucosa form the plicae circulares, which are covered with thousands of villi.

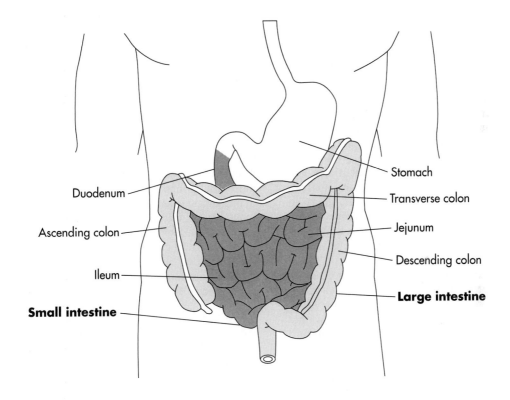

Duodenum

Ascending colon

Ileum

Small intestine

Stomach

Transverse colon

Jejunum

Descending colon

Large intestine

Layers of intestinal wall

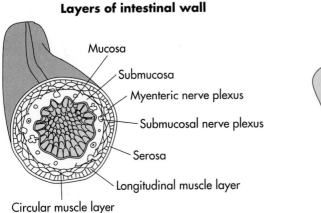

Mucosa

Submucosa

Myenteric nerve plexus

Submucosal nerve plexus

Serosa

Longitudinal muscle layer

Circular muscle layer

Plicae circulares

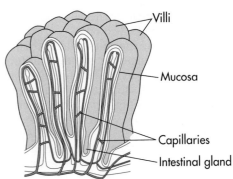

Villi

Mucosa

Capillaries

Intestinal gland

and about 2.5 inches in diameter, the large intestine extends up the right side of the abdomen, crosses just beneath the diaphragm, and extends down the left side to the rectum and anus. These three sections of large intestine are called the ascending colon, transverse colon, and descending colon, respectively.

The myenteric plexus regulates the large intestine's movements and secretions. Parasympathetic stimulation by the vagus nerve increases contractions from the cecum to the first portion of the transverse colon. Pelvic nerves stimulate the remaining portions of the colon, increasing its motility.

The large intestine looks looser and more saccular than the small intestine because of differences in the muscularis and mucosal layers. Although the mucosal layer of the large intestine has no plicae circulares or villi, it does continue the digestive process. Bacteria in the large intestine release additional nutrients from cellulose and other materials not fully digested in the small intestine, breaking down residual proteins into amino acids that the liver converts to urea. Columnar epithelial cells absorb water, electrolytes such as sodium and phosphate, and any remaining fats not absorbed by the ileum. Goblet cells secrete mucus that lubricates the mucosa so fecal matter can progress through the large intestine. And intestinal bacteria provide transport for some B vitamins and vitamin K needed for blood clotting.

In the large intestine, the longitudinal layer of the muscularis consists of three bands called taeniae coli. The circular layer of the muscularis forms outpouchings called haustra. Together, these structures give the large intestine its gathered appearance. Fat pads cling to the serosal surface of the ascending, transverse, and descending colons.

In the rectum, the muscularis forms the internal anal sphincter; the body wall forms a voluntary external anal sphincter. Sympathetic innervation keeps the internal anal sphincter contracted, and parasympathetic innervation stimulates it to relax when the rectum is full. Intrinsic nerve plexuses also relax the internal anal sphincter. Branches of the sacral division of the spinal cord innervate the external anal sphincter.

Pathophysiology

Normally, chyme flows smoothly through the intestinal tract, propelled by rhythmic peristaltic waves. The GI system, circulatory system, and nervous system all work together to digest food, absorb its nutrients, and expel its by-products from the body.

Sometimes, however, the process slows or stops because an obstruction develops in the small or large intestine. Anything that narrows or blocks the intestinal lumen (a mechanical cause) or interferes with peristalsis (a nonmechanical cause) can create an obstruction. An obstruction is more common in the small intestine. However, a complete obstruction in either intestine can lead to shock and death in a matter of hours if it's not successfully treated.

Postoperative adhesions that compress or kink areas of the intestine are the most common mechanical cause of obstructions. In children, intestinal obstructions usually result from a hernia. In people over age 65, the most common causes are tumors and diverticular disease. Colon cancer causes at least three out of four obstructions of the large intestine. Nonmechanical or paralytic causes include electrolyte disorders, medications that depress peristalsis, and neurologic deficits.

Not only can intestinal obstructions be classified by their cause but they can also be classified by onset, extent, location, type of lesion, and type of obstruction (see *Ways of classifying intestinal obstructions*).

Consequences of obstruction

When the intestinal lumen becomes partially or completely obstructed, digestive contents back up and begin forming a mass. Then gases and fluids begin to accumulate, distending the intestine. In an attempt to move the mass past a mechanical obstruction, peristaltic waves grow stronger, causing colicky, crampy abdominal pain. If the increased waves can't clear the obstruction, the proximal intestine continues to dilate, until the smooth muscle becomes atonic and peristalsis stops.

Ultimately, the effects of an intestinal obstruction depend largely on where it is, whether it's partial or complete, how much intraluminal

Ways of classifying intestinal obstructions

Usually, intestinal obstructions are classified by whether their cause is mechanical or nonmechanical. But obstructions can also be classified by onset, extent, location, type of lesion, and type of obstruction.

Classification	Description
Cause	
Mechanical	Physical obstruction resulting from a foreign body, a tumor, meconium (in cystic fibrosis), external compression, a hernia, abdominal adhesions, polyps, diverticular disease, volvulus, or intussusception
Nonmechanical or paralytic	Lack of peristalsis resulting from manipulation, anesthesia, peritoneal irritation (from bacteria or pancreatic enzymes), an electrolyte disturbance (such as hypokalemia, hypercalcemia, hypomagnesemia, hyperphosphatemia), gastrointestinal ischemia, neuromuscular disease (such as myasthenia gravis or multiple sclerosis), or intestinal infarction
Onset	
Acute	A single episode or periodic unrelated episodes, usually characterized by rapid onset of symptoms
Chronic	Repeated episodes of partial or complete obstruction related to an ongoing risk factor

Classification	Description
Extent	
Partial	Lumen partly open, causing slower passage of intestinal contents
Complete	Lumen occluded, causing intestinal contents to back up
Location	
High small intestine	Duodenum and upper jejunum
Low small intestine	Lower jejunum and ileum
Large intestine	Any portion of large intestine
Type of lesion	
Intrinsic, intraluminal, or mural	Lesion in lumen or intestinal wall
Extrinsic	Lesion outside intestine that exerts external pressure
Type of obstruction	
Simple	Lumen obstructed, blood flow to area intact
Strangulated	Blood flow to area compromised
Closed-loop	Section of intestine looped over itself and blocked on both ends

pressure it creates, and how much functional intestine is lost.

Gases that accumulate around the obstruction move into the bloodstream at increased rates, possibly altering the patient's acid-base balance. These effects vary with the location of the obstruction. If it's in the small intestine, carbon dioxide and nitrogen accumulate. As increased levels of carbon dioxide enter the patient's bloodstream, she may develop metabolic acidosis. If the obstruction is in the large intestine, bacteria continue to produce methane, but it can't escape. As a result, serum ammonia levels rise, and hyperammonemia may lead to alkalosis.

An obstruction also alters the patient's fluid and electrolyte balance. As the intestine distends, its wall grows edematous in response to increased intraluminal pressure. Capillary permeability rises, and massive amounts of fluid may shift out of the plasma and interstitial spaces into the distended intestine. Intraluminal pressure then exceeds the surrounding abdominal pressure, and trapped fluid leaks from the intestine into the peritoneum. If intraluminal pressure rises beyond the intestinal wall's ability to withstand it, the intestine can rupture.

Finally, because an intestinal obstruction prevents normal digestion and propulsion, the patient may develop a malabsorption syndrome.

Assessment findings

Primary signs and symptoms, those directly related to the obstruction, include abdominal pain, distention, altered bowel sounds, altered gastric drainage, and altered stool output. Secondary signs and symptoms, those that result from the effects of the obstructive process, include vomiting, malnutrition, hypotension, and fever (see *Locating an intestinal obstruction*).

Abdominal pain
An intestinal obstruction typically causes moderate to severe, crampy pain that comes and goes in a crescendo-decrescendo pattern. The pain commonly develops after the patient eats. An obstruction of the small intestine tends to produce more frequent pain than an obstruction of the large intestine.

Usually, increased pain with rebound tenderness suggests that the patient is at risk for an intestinal perforation. In some patients, however, as the distention grows, the pain decreases. Severe pain without periods of remission probably stems from a strangulated obstruction, a potentially life-threatening complication.

Distention
Every day the GI tract produces 7 to 10 liters of fluid to support its normal function. When an obstruction develops, this process of secretion doesn't stop. As a result, fluids from the stomach, pancreas, gallbladder, and small intestine accumulate behind the blockage. The results of this accumulation depend on the volume of retained secretions and the rate at which they accumulate.

Usually, if an obstruction develops in the upper small intestine—the duodenum, for example—the patient may vomit rather than develop abdominal distention. In the lower small intestine or the large intestine, however, accumulated fluids distend the patient's abdomen.

Eventually, the inflammatory process caused by the intestinal obstruction allows fluids to leak from the intestine into the peritoneum, raising the patient's risk of hypovolemia and peritonitis.

Drainage and stool
The color of vomitus or GI drainage can help reveal the location of the blockage. Clear vomitus comes from the stomach. Green vomitus comes from the duodenum or jejunum. Golden vomitus comes from below the bile duct. Feculent vomitus comes from the cecum. In a small-intestine obstruction, feculent vomitus is a poor prognostic sign. It suggests that stagnant intestinal drainage and ischemia have allowed an overgrowth of bacteria, which produces drainage that looks and smells like feces. If the patient has an intestinal strangulation or a tumor, a rectal exam may reveal bleeding.

Early on, an obstruction of the small intestine may not alter stool output. However, as it progresses, stool production may stop. Early in a large-intestine obstruction, a patient may have thin ribbonlike stools. Later (or with a more severe obstruction), the patient may produce small amounts of watery stool as increased peristalsis forces accumulated secretions around the blockage.

Bowel sounds and more
Expect to hear hyperactive bowel sounds proximal to the obstruction. If the intestine is blocked completely, you may hear pronounced, high-pitched, peristaltic rushes. You probably won't hear any bowel sounds over the obstruction. Distal to the obstruction, bowel sounds will be deceased or absent.

Also, the patient will likely be restless, hiccuping, and belching. She may complain of back

Locating an intestinal obstruction

The signs and symptoms of an intestinal obstruction vary, depending on its location. Use this table to help locate your patient's obstruction.

Characteristic	Upper small intestine	Lower small intestine	Large intestine
Location of pain	• Upper abdomen • Epigastrium	• Right upper quadrant	• Lower quadrants
Timing of pain	• Just after eating	• About 1 hour after eating	• Several hours after eating
Evidence of accumulated intestinal contents	• Vomiting	• Upper abdominal distention	• Lower abdominal distention
Evidence of malabsorption	• Reduced serum electrolyte levels • Reduced vitamin absorption	• Reduced serum electrolyte levels • Hypophosphatemia • Reduced vitamin absorption • Pernicious anemia from poor vitamin B_{12} absorption	• Fluid volume deficit • Hypophosphatemia • Pernicious anemia from poor vitamin B_{12} absorption
Drainage and stool	• Clear vomitus from stomach • Green vomitus from duodenum	• Green vomitus from jejunum • Golden vomitus from below entrance of bile duct into intestine • Feculent vomitus from cecum	• Abdominal gas, distention, and abnormal stools • Thin, ribbonlike stools with partial obstruction • Scant, watery stool with partial obstruction
Evidence of metabolic waste accumulation	• Acidosis from fatty acid conversion to carbon dioxide	• Acidosis from fatty acid conversion to carbon dioxide	• Alkalosis from hyperammonemia related to methane production
Other	• Hypovolemia that causes hypotension, low central venous pressure, and poor skin turgor	• Hypovolemia that causes hypotension, low central venous pressure, and poor skin turgor	• Coagulopathy from poor vitamin K absorption • Hypovolemia that causes hypotension, low central venous pressure, and poor skin turgor

pain and an inability to pass flatus or stool. If she's dehydrated, you'll detect decreased urine output, dry skin and mucous membranes, and hypotension.

As you assess your patient, keep in mind that complete obstructions usually produce more severe signs and symptoms and a more rapid onset of them than partial obstructions. Signs and symptoms also are more dramatic in obstructions that develop suddenly than in obstructions that develop more slowly.

Diagnostic tests

Together with an assessment of your patient's signs and symptoms, diagnostic testing can help confirm the likely location, cause, and severity of the obstruction.

Blood tests

A patient suspected of having an intestinal obstruction may have the following blood tests: complete blood count (CBC) with hematocrit,

Laboratory findings in intestinal obstructions

Location of obstruction	Abnormal finding	Reason for finding
Small intestine	Acidosis	Accumulated waste products of fatty acid breakdown
	Hypocalcemia	Decreased absorption in small intestine
	Hypokalemia	Decreased absorption in small intestine
	Hypomagnesemia	Decreased absorption in small intestine
Large intestine	Alkalosis	Accumulated methane
	Hyperammonemia	Accumulated methane
	Elevated blood urea nitrogen	Retained fecal matter leading to translocation of blood urea nitrogen
	Hypophosphatemia	Decreased absorption in large intestine
Small or large intestine	Elevated amylase	Peritonitis
	Hypernatremia	Fluid volume deficit caused by fluid shift from vascular to interstitial spaces
	Hyperosmolarity	Fluid volume deficit caused by fluid shift from vascular to interstitial spaces
	Prolonged prothrombin time	Malabsorption of vitamin K–dependent proteins leading to inadequate coagulation protein production and increased tendency to bleed
	Leukocytosis	Inflammation

serum electrolyte levels, blood urea nitrogen (BUN), serum amylase levels, serum osmolarity, and coagulation studies (see *Laboratory findings in intestinal obstructions*).

The CBC can help identify anemia, which may result from bleeding. Keep in mind, however, that hemoconcentration caused by dehydration can also raise the patient's hematocrit. The white blood cell (WBC) count may be increased because of inflammation. A simple obstruction causes a mild increase (10,000 to 15,000/mm^3), strangulation causes a moderate increase (15,000 to 25,000/mm^3), and mesenteric occlusion or perforation causes an extreme increase (more than 25,000/mm^3).

In a small-intestine obstruction, potassium, chloride, calcium, and magnesium levels may be decreased. Levels of other minerals, although not commonly measured, are also decreased in an obstruction of the lower small intestine. They include zinc, copper, iron, and folic acid. A loss of these minerals can cause poor wound healing and anemia. An obstruction of the lower small intestine or the large intestine interferes with vitamin K absorption, leading to poor production of coagulation proteins and possible coagulopathy.

A fluid volume deficit can result in hypernatremia, azotemia, and hyperosmolarity. And an obstruction of the large intestine causes hypophosphatemia. Elevated serum amylase levels suggest peritonitis.

Abdominal X-rays

Excess fluid and air cause intestinal distention that may be visible on an abdominal X-ray. If the patient has a perforated intestine, expect to see air under the diaphragm.

If the patient has a mechanical obstruction and a low risk of perforation, she may undergo a barium enema X-ray to pinpoint the location of the obstruction. A barium swallow X-ray is contraindicated because the barium will be retained behind the blockage.

Medical interventions

If an obstruction can be reversed without surgery or if a patient isn't a good surgical candidate, a physician will use conservative measures, such as decompressing the intestine, ordering dietary restrictions to rest the intestine, preventing or treating infection, reducing nausea and vomiting, and replacing fluids and electrolytes. If the obstruction can't be reversed with such measures, the patient may need surgery.

Decompression

For some patients, relieving the pressure behind a partial obstruction is enough to resolve the problem, or at least to resolve vomiting. Nasogastric (NG) or intestinal tubes can accomplish this task by draining GI fluids, thus reducing pressure and distention at and above the obstruction.

Typically, nonmechanical obstructions are treated with NG decompression. A Salem sump (double-lumen) or Levin (single-lumen) tube is attached to suction to drain the fluid.

For mechanical obstructions, a physician probably will choose a mercury-weighted intestinal tube. These tubes range from 6 to 10 feet in length and may have one, two, or three lumens. Each of these tubes has a balloon at the distal end that can be filled with mercury. Ideally, the mercury will be heavy enough to push the balloon through the obstructed area, even if peristalsis is weak or absent, thus allowing backed up fluids to drain.

Sometimes, an enema, rectal tube, sigmoidoscopy, or colonoscopy may be used to relieve a large mechanical obstruction.

Diet

A patient with an intestinal obstruction typically receives nothing by mouth, so the intestine can rest. If appropriate, she may be given ice chips to relieve her thirst and dry mouth. Some patients may need total parenteral nutrition to correct nutritional deficiencies, especially before and after surgery.

Drug therapy

Analgesics usually aren't prescribed because they tend to decrease peristalsis, worsening the obstruction. They also may mask abdominal pain, which indicates a complication, such as an intestinal rupture. For partial obstructions from nonmechanical causes, occasionally a physician may prescribe peristaltic stimulants such as cisapride, metoclopramide, or erythromycin.

The patient may receive an antibiotic to treat an infection. Also, she may be given an antiemetic, such as prochlorperazine, to relieve nausea and vomiting. Fluids and electrolytes may be given I.V. to help correct fluid and electrolyte imbalances.

Surgery

If an intestinal obstruction doesn't respond to conservative treatment, the intestine may perforate or rupture. A perforation is an erosion through the outside intestinal wall. A rupture is a break in the intestinal wall severe enough that intestinal contents can spill into the peritoneum. To prevent these complications, the patient may undergo surgery. Surgery is also used to remove large, immovable masses, such as tumors.

Whenever possible, a surgeon performs a resection with an end-to-end anastomosis. If the distal intestine is ischemic or the patient has extensive intestinal damage, however, she may need a temporary or permanent colostomy.

Nursing interventions

When caring for a patient with an intestinal obstruction, your priorities include promoting fluid and electrolyte balance, relieving discomfort, preventing complications, and teaching her about her condition and how to prevent its recurrence.

Promoting fluid and electrolyte balance

Remember that a patient who's vomiting or undergoing gastric decompression is at high risk for hypovolemia and fluid and electrolyte imbalance. That's because large amounts of gastric and intestinal fluid rich in sodium, potassium, chloride, and calcium may be lost. And the patient probably won't be allowed anything by mouth until her intestinal function improves.

This patient also has an increased risk of an acid-base imbalance because gastric fluid is highly acidic, and intestinal fluid is alkaline. Thus, a loss of acidic gastric fluid may predispose the patient to metabolic alkalosis, and a loss of alkaline intestinal fluid can raise her risk of metabolic acidosis.

Acid-base problems may also be related to intraluminal conditions. In small-intestine obstructions, the nonabsorbed lipids cause fatty acids to accumulate, resulting in acidosis. In large-intestine obstructions, bacteria produce methane, causing large amounts of ammonia to accumulate and resulting in alkalosis.

If the patient has trouble breathing because distended abdominal contents are pressing against her diaphragm, the risk of an acid-base imbalance increases further. The reason: When the lungs can't expand fully, oxygenation is reduced, and carbon dioxide is retained, raising the risk of respiratory acidosis.

To help prevent fluid, electrolyte, and acid-base problems, give I.V. fluids as prescribed. Be aware, however, that they can contribute to the patient's interstitial fluid leakage.

Be sure to monitor your patient's intake, output, and weight carefully. Include irrigation solution as part of the patient's input and decompression drainage as part of her output. Irrigate the tube every 2 hours, as ordered, to maintain patency. Irrigate with normal saline solution, which is isotonic. Water, if used frequently for irrigation, can increase electrolyte losses through osmosis. If you irrigate through an NG tube, check its position beforehand. To do so, attach a syringe to the end of the tube, and place a stethoscope on the patient's abdomen, over the left upper quadrant. Then inject 10 to 20 cc of air while auscultating for the sound of rushing air. Alternatively, you can attach a syringe to the end of the tube and aspirate for stomach contents. Assess the color, amount, and odor of the decompression drainage and check its pH.

If the patient's urine output drops below 30 ml per hour, notify the physician. Assess the patient for signs of dehydration, such as decreased skin turgor, dry mucous membranes, and lethargy. She also may complain of dry mouth, thirst, or weakness. Anticipate the need for central venous pressure (CVP) monitoring to evaluate her overall fluid status.

Remember that the patient's abdomen will grow as the volume of retained secretions increases, so measure her abdominal girth at least every 4 hours. Mark the spot where you took your original measurement, and take subsequent ones at the same spot.

To promote optimal lung expansion, keep the head of the bed elevated (if the patient's blood pressure can tolerate this position) and administer oxygen as indicated. Watch for signs of hypoxemia and hypoxia, such as dyspnea, cyanosis, and confusion. Monitor the patient's arterial blood gas (ABG) measurements and oxygen saturation levels. Be sure to reposition the patient frequently.

As indicated, obtain serum electrolyte levels and administer electrolyte replacement therapy to reverse deficits and reduce the risk of arrhythmias, seizures, or other complications. Be alert for signs and symptoms of electrolyte imbalance. And be especially careful when administering replacement therapy to avoid creating an imbalance in the opposite direction (see *Signs and symptoms of electrolyte imbalance*).

Providing comfort

After the decompression tube has been inserted, tape it securely in place. Wrap a piece of tape around the tube and pin the tape to the patient's gown, allowing enough slack for the patient to move her head comfortably. Apply water-soluble lubricant to her nares to prevent crusting and irritation. Maintain suction and check the tube's patency to be sure it's draining properly.

A patient with a decompression tube will probably complain that she's thirsty. Her thirst may result from fluid loss, fluid shifts, or the NG tube itself, which makes her breathe through her mouth. Of course, her thirst may also result from the fact that she's not allowed anything by mouth. Try giving her ice chips or hard candy, if appropriate, but remember to include the ice chips as intake. Also, have her rinse her mouth routinely and provide her with frequent mouth care.

Your patient also may complain of a sore throat. If she does, give her anesthetic lozenges, gargle solution, or saline rinses to relieve the discomfort.

If the tube becomes blocked, either because of drainage or because the lumen is pressed against the mucosal wall, gas and fluids can't drain, and your patient may complain of nausea and increased abdominal pain and distention. She may also begin to vomit. If this happens, irrigate the tube to clear it, and reposition the patient to move the lumen away from the mucosal wall. As excess gas and fluid decline, the distention will too, and the patient should become more comfortable. Check her bowel sounds frequently to make sure intestinal function returns.

Assess the patient's complaints of abdominal pain frequently. You probably won't be able to give her an analgesic, so use other comfort measures, such as distraction, massage, therapeutic touch, and relaxation therapy. Provide frequent explanations of her condition and offer reassurance. Also, note any increased pain or a change from cramping to constant pain or rebound tenderness. These developments may warn of an impending perforation.

If the patient is scheduled for surgery, take time to prepare her physically and mentally. If she'll have a colostomy after surgery, teach her about its purpose and the steps needed to care for it. Arrange a preoperative visit from an enterostomal therapist. And allow time for the patient to express her fears and concerns. Provide emotional support and guidance.

Signs and symptoms of electrolyte imbalance

By changing capillary and intestinal permeability, an intestinal obstruction raises the risk of electrolyte imbalances. Intestinal decompression may deplete electrolyte levels even more. To help spot the signs and symptoms of electrolyte imbalances common in patients with an intestinal obstruction, use this table.

Electrolyte imbalance	Signs and symptoms
Hypernatremia	• Disorientation, hallucinations • Seizures, possibly coma • Extreme thirst • Dry, sticky mucous membranes • Tachycardia and hypertension • Serum sodium level greater than 145 mEq/L
Hypokalemia	• Drowsiness, lethargy • Anorexia, nausea, vomiting • Leg cramps and muscle weakness • Hyporeflexia, paresthesia • Cardiac arrhythmias • Serum potassium level below 3.5 mEq/L
Hypocalcemia	• Confusion, mood changes, anxiety • Muscle cramps or tremors • Hyperactive deep tendon reflexes, paresthesia • Tetany • Positive Chvostek's and Trousseau's signs • Laryngeal spasm and bronchospasm • Seizures • Arrhythmias • Serum calcium level below 8.5 mg/dl (4.5 mEq/L)
Hypomagnesemia	• Memory loss, confusion, dizziness • Tremors • Tachycardia and hypotension • Arrhythmias • Anorexia, nausea • Tetany • Positive Babinski's reflex • Hyperactive deep tendon reflexes • Seizures, coma • Serum magnesium level below 1.5 mEq/L

Recognizing the signs and symptoms of intestinal rupture

An intestinal rupture can quickly become life-threatening, so monitor your patient closely for these warning signs and symptoms:
- local or diffuse abdominal pain
- rigid, boardlike abdomen
- increased abdominal distention
- rebound tenderness
- nausea, anorexia, and vomiting
- diminishing or absent bowel sounds
- fever
- elevated white blood cell count
- shallow respirations
- poor skin turgor from fever-related dehydration
- early signs and symptoms of shock, such as hypotension, tachycardia, tachypnea, oliguria, restlessness, and diaphoresis
- hiccups.

Preventing complications

Carefully monitor the patient for signs and symptoms that could warn of an intestinal perforation or rupture: fever, abdominal rigidity, rebound tenderness, and hypotension (see *Recognizing the signs and symptoms of intestinal rupture*). If not detected and reversed early, these complications can cause septic shock and death. Anticipate giving the prescribed antibiotics to prevent or treat peritonitis.

Patient teaching

If your patient has an increased risk of developing an intestinal obstruction, teach her to pay attention to her tolerance of specific foods, the frequency and consistency of her stool, and the fullness of her abdomen. Be sure to explain how the pain of an intestinal obstruction differs from the pain of other underlying conditions, such as a peptic ulcer. Also, teach the patient how to avoid future episodes of intestinal obstructions. For some patients, this may mean eating smaller, more frequent meals. For others, it may mean a regimen that includes laxatives and a high-fiber diet to prevent constipation.

If your patient had surgery to correct an intestinal obstruction, reinforce any postoperative instructions about wound care, diet, fluids, and exercise. If the patient has an ostomy, make sure you teach her how to care for it. Urge her to keep follow-up appointments. If appropriate, consult with her physician about obtaining a referral for home care.

Intestinal obstruction and myocardial infarction

An MI results from a coronary artery occlusion or spasm that blocks blood supply to the myocardium long enough for some myocardial cells to die. If a patient with an intestinal obstruction has an MI, she faces an increased risk of serious, possibly life-threatening complications. And a patient who has had an MI may face an increased risk of intestinal obstruction.

Pathophysiology

Having an MI creates great physiologic and emotional stress. In response to that stress, the body releases catecholamines and shunts blood away from nonessential tissues—including the GI tract—and toward the heart, lungs, and brain. This decreased GI blood supply can suppress peristalsis, which slows GI motility and may allow gas and fluids to stagnate in the intestine. In other words, by decreasing peristalsis, an MI can lead to a nonmechanical obstruction.

To make matters worse, the patient also risks an intestinal obstruction from the effects of drugs used to treat an MI. For example, sympathomimetics used to maintain blood pressure can compromise blood flow to the GI tract, thus increasing the risk of an obstruction. Other drugs can deplete potassium levels, which also can raise the risk of an obstruction.

Because of the tendency for an MI and its therapy to raise the risk of an intestinal obstruction, a patient who already has an intestinal obstruction before having an MI faces a greatly increased risk of serious complications.

Adapting nursing care

When caring for a patient with an MI and an intestinal obstruction, your priorities include balancing myocardial oxygen supply and demand, promoting cardiac function, maintaining nutrition and elimination, and contolling pain. Of course, you'll also need to teach your patient and her family about her condition.

Balancing myocardial oxygen supply and demand

An MI patient must minimize oxygen demand to aid myocardial function. As it happens, this strategy helps the GI tract as well by improving blood flow and peristalsis. Consequently, anything you can do to conserve the patient's energy and reduce her oxygen demand will help her avoid complications.

At first, an MI patient usually is placed on bed rest. However, prolonged bed rest can decrease peristalsis, which increases the risk of developing an intestinal obstruction or of complicating an existing obstruction. For a patient with an MI and an intestinal obstruction, the best option usually is to allow bed rest with a bedside commode for the first 24 hours. Reposition the patient frequently to promote movement and peristalsis. Help her with activities of daily living to minimize her energy expenditure and myocardial oxygen demand. Let her rest frequently, and always between activities, procedures, and treatments.

After this initial period, increase the patient's activity level gradually. Be sure to monitor her vital signs and other hemodynamic readings to track the effect of activity on her condition.

Nitrates, beta blockers, and calcium channel blockers also help reduce myocardial oxygen demand. Vasodilators and inotropic drugs help improve cardiac output, thus increasing oxygen supply. Patients with MIs usually receive an I.V. nitrate and, in some instances, an I.V. anticoagulant.

Give your patient supplemental oxygen through a nasal cannula, as indicated. Monitor her oxygen saturation levels using pulse oximetry and ABG studies. Be alert for restlessness and changes in the patient's level of consciousness (LOC), which may indicate hypoxemia.

Remember that fear and anxiety trigger the stress response, which increases myocardial oxygen demand and shunts blood away from the GI tract. So you'll want to take steps to keep the patient calm and relaxed. Use relaxation therapy and guided imagery to decrease her anxiety.

Help the patient and her family talk about their fears, feelings, and concerns. Explain the events going on around them and the rationales for treatments and procedures. Offer support and guidance. And encourage the use of positive coping strategies.

Promoting cardiac function

Throughout your care, monitor the patient's cardiac status and electrocardiogram (ECG) continuously. Assess her heart rate and rhythm. Track her vital signs, urine output, and peripheral pulses. Watch for a heart rate over 100 beats per minute, a urine output under 30 ml per hour, and pallor, cyanosis, and decreased peripheral pulses. These signs warn of a worsening hemodynamic status and require immediate intervention. Anticipate the insertion of a pulmonary artery catheter to assess the patient's hemodynamic status. Record readings every 2 to 4 hours, more frequently if indicated. And monitor the patient's cardiac enzyme levels to ensure that she isn't developing further myocardial ischemia or infarction.

If the patient experiences hypotension from her MI, she may receive a vasopressor, such as norepinephrine, to maintain her blood pressure. However, vasopressors can impair blood flow to the GI tract, thus decreasing peristalsis and increasing the risk of a nonmechanical obstruction. Give such a medication carefully and monitor the patient's cardiac and GI status closely.

If your patient receives thrombolytic therapy to lyse a clot in a coronary artery, monitor her coagulation studies closely for signs of bleeding. Also, note the color of the drainage from her decompression tube and test it for occult blood. Continuously assess her neurologic status for focal deficits and signs of increased

What you should know about drugs that enhance GI motility

Drug	Mechanism of action	Nursing considerations
Erythromycin	Irritates intestinal wall, which increases bowel motility.	• Give drug on an empty stomach. • Check for interactions with other drugs, such as digoxin, oral anticoagulants, theophylline, and corticosteroids. • Treat nausea and diarrhea, as necessary.
Metoclopramide	Increases sensitivity to acetylcholine, which increases upper gastrointestinal (GI) motility, relaxes pyloric sphincter and duodenal bulb, and accelerates gastric emptying and GI transit times.	• Give drug before meals and at bedtime. • Drug may cause sedation; institute safety precautions. • Be aware that some patients become jittery when taking this drug. • Monitor patient for mood changes. • Remember that drug decreases cimetidine's effect.
Cisapride	Enhances release of acetylcholine at myenteric plexus, which increases strength of esophageal peristalsis, increases lower esophageal sphincter pressure, and accelerates gastric emptying time.	• Give drug four times daily, 15 minutes before meals and at bedtime. • Monitor patient for arrhythmias. • Watch for potentiation with sedatives; institute safety precautions.

intracranial pressure. And take precautions to help the patient avoid bleeding and bruising, including putting pressure on needle puncture sites. If you observe signs of bleeding, notify her physician right away. Thrombolytic therapy or anticoagulant therapy may be stopped, and blood products may be administered to prevent life-threatening complications.

Remember, a patient with an intestinal obstruction faces an increased risk of fluid and electrolyte imbalances. And imbalances such as hypokalemia and hypocalcemia can adversely affect her already compromised cardiac function. So you'll want to monitor her ECG and her serum electrolyte levels routinely. If she develops an imbalance, expect to give electrolyte replacement therapy. But make sure she doesn't develop the opposite imbalance as a result of the therapy. Carefully monitor her intake, output, and daily weights.

Maintaining nutrition and elimination

During the acute phase, a patient with an intestinal obstruction and an MI takes nothing by mouth. When the obstruction resolves, she's usually allowed fluids. As her condition improves, her diet will be advanced based on her needs and ability to tolerate it. Typically, a patient will be placed on a low-cholesterol, low-fat, low-salt diet. She may tolerate small, frequent meals better than three large ones. Be sure to monitor her bowel sounds frequently. Also, assess her for increasing abdominal distention and note any complaints of nausea, vomiting, and increasing abdominal pain and pressure because they may indicate a recurring obstruction.

Make sure your patient is passing flatus and stool normally. If necessary, give her a stool softener to prevent straining. By changing her blood pressure and heart rate, straining (the Valsalva maneuver) can increase myocardial oxygen demand, possibly triggering ischemia, arrhythmias, pulmonary embolism, or even cardiac arrest.

If the patient's slowed GI motility results from circulatory insufficiency, she may receive a drug that increases motility by increasing the neurologic stimulus or irritating the intestine. As prescribed, administer metoclopramide or cisapride to induce neurologic stimulation of

DRUG ALERT

GI stimulants and MI drugs: Dangerous interactions

Gastrointestinal (GI) stimulants	Myocardial infarction (MI) drugs	Adverse effects	Nursing actions
• Cisapride	• Warfarin	• Increased coagulation times	• Monitor patient for signs and symptoms of bleeding. • Obtain baseline coagulation studies and monitor studies frequently. • Anticipate giving an H_2 blocker to minimize risk of GI bleeding. • Anticipate reducing warfarin dosage.
• Metoclopramide	• Digoxin	• Decreased digoxin absorption	• Monitor patient's serum digoxin levels to be sure they're in therapeutic range. • Assess patient's apical pulse rate and rhythm. • Anticipate increasing digoxin dosage to improve effectiveness. • If dosage is increased, monitor patient for signs and symptoms of digoxin toxicity.

peristalsis. Low-dose erythromycin can irritate the intestinal wall enough to enhance peristalsis as well. These drugs are ideal for patients with an MI-induced obstruction because they don't affect cardiovascular function (see *What you should know about drugs that enhance GI motility*). However, these drugs may interact with drugs used to treat an MI. Be alert for such interactions, especially when giving cisapride or metoclopramide (see *GI stimulants and MI drugs: Dangerous interactions*).

Controlling pain

Both an MI and an intestinal obstruction cause some degree of pain. Ask the patient to tell you right away if she feels increasing pain, so you can act fast to help prevent complications.

When monitoring your patient's pain, distinguish between chest pain and epigastric pain caused by an obstruction of the upper small intestine. Remember, chest pain probably indicates continuing myocardial ischemia. Look for nonverbal signals of chest pain, such as facial grimacing, rubbing the area, and guarding, and for changes in cardiopulmonary status, such as an elevated heart rate, respiratory rate, and blood pressure. Check too for increasing abdominal distention. And listen for changes in the patient's bowel sounds.

By reducing the patient's pain and apprehension, you can promote comfort and rest. And by decreasing sympathetic stimulation, you can reduce myocardial oxygen demand. Give oxygen, a nitrate, and morphine as prescribed to relieve chest pain. Also, if possible, position the patient with the head of the bed elevated to maximize lung expansion.

Keep in mind that opiate analgesics such as morphine may decrease peristalsis, further increasing the risk of an obstruction. If the patient already has an obstruction, morphine can raise the risk of complications, such as intestinal perforation. If morphine is prescribed, be sure to monitor the patient's bowel sounds and note any changes. Measure her abdominal girth every 4 hours. Be alert for complaints of increased nausea or vomiting. And monitor the drainage from the decompression tube, noting any increase in amount or change in color or consistency.

Because morphine also depresses a patient's respirations, monitor them carefully—especially if her abdominal contents are pressing upward on her diaphragm. Notify the physician if the patient's respiratory rate is consistently below 12 breaths per minute or consistently below her baseline rate. Assess the patient's oxygen saturation levels, using pulse oximetry. Anticipate the need for ABG measurements to check for acidosis or alkalosis.

Patient teaching

Initially, focus on simple, concrete explanations and directions. Tell the patient what's happening around her. In simple terms, explain the equipment being used, such as monitors, drainage tubes, and I.V. lines. Outline the procedures being performed, such as GI decompression. And tell her which medications she's receiving.

When the patient's condition stabilizes, teach her about her condition and any lifestyle changes she needs to make. Be sure she and her family understand her medication regimen and the reasons for any lifestyle changes. Reinforce the need for follow-up care. If appropriate, obtain a home care referral for continued assessment and education in the patient's home.

Complications

Common complications for patients with an intestinal obstruction and an MI include stress ulcers and intestinal infarction.

Stress ulcers

A stress ulcer is an erosion in the gastric or duodenal mucosa that results from prolonged physiologic or psychologic stress. Stress ulcers are common in patients with obstructions of the upper small intestine because acidic stomach contents tend to stagnate.

When cardiac output is compromised, as in an MI, the body shunts blood away from the GI tract and toward vital organs; the result can be GI mucosal ischemia and altered permeability. If a patient already has an intestinal obstruction, with its associated edema and altered membrane permeability, the ischemic mucosa may begin to erode (see *How an intestinal obstruction and an MI lead to stress ulcers*).

Confirming the complication

Typically, stress ulcers cause painless bleeding that you'll observe as hematemesis or melena

within 2 to 10 days. However, ulcers related to intestinal obstruction can be difficult to differentiate from a worsening obstruction, and they may be overshadowed by the patient's acute condition. Because these ulcers tend to be superficial, X-rays may not show them. An endoscopic examination may be the only sure way to confirm the problem.

Nursing interventions

In a patient with an MI and an intestinal obstruction, try to detect stress ulcers early and then respond quickly. First, be sure that the patient's blood has been typed and cross-matched and that blood or blood products are readily available. As you care for the patient, inspect all drainage from her decompression tube. Watch for red blood, which indicates frank bleeding, and for material that looks like coffee grounds, which indicates slow bleeding. Also, check the drainage for pH and for occult blood.

Be especially alert for bleeding if the patient is receiving a thrombolytic and anticoagulant therapy. Monitor her vital signs and hemodynamic measurements closely for changes that suggest bleeding and fluid loss.

If you see blood in the decompression-tube drainage, notify the physician right away. Anticipate the need for gastric lavage to help control the bleeding (see *When your patient needs gastric lavage*, page 412). Administer blood or blood products, as prescribed. And anticipate an order for an H_2 blocker, such as cimetidine or ranitidine. By blocking the action of histamine, these drugs reduce the production of hydrochloric acid and thereby increase the pH of the gastric contents. If the patient is receiving anticoagulant therapy, prepare to give an antidote, such as protamine sulfate (for heparin) or vitamin K (for warfarin), as prescribed. Continue to monitor the patient's vital signs and observe her for signs of hypovolemic shock, which can occur with prolonged or acute GI bleeding. Monitor the patient's intake and output. And frequently evaluate the results of her CBC, hemoglobin, hematocrit, and coagulation studies.

After the patient's condition stabilizes, continue taking steps to enhance her cardiac and GI function. Before discharge, reinforce all instructions about her medications and diet. Also, explain any activity restrictions. Review

PATHOPHYSIOLOGY

How an intestinal obstruction and an MI lead to stress ulcers

Gastric and duodenal stress ulcers typically stem from profound physiologic stress that decreases blood flow to the gastrointestinal mucosa. Either an intestinal obstruction or a myocardial infarction can cause such stress. This flowchart shows how the two disorders can combine to bring on stress ulcers.

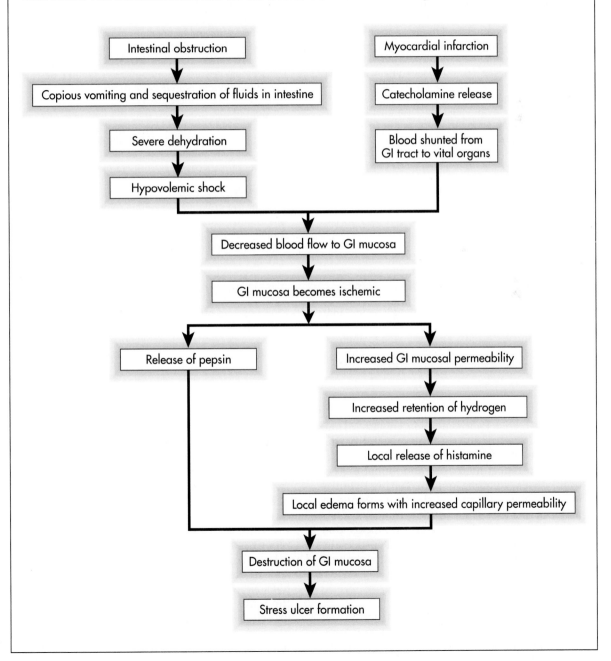

When your patient needs gastric lavage

If your patient with an intestinal obstruction and a myocardial infarction (MI) develops stress ulcers, they may bleed. That's because the thrombolytic and anticoagulant therapy used to treat the MI raises the risk of bleeding in the highly vascular gastrointestinal (GI) tract. If the patient's ulcers do bleed, you may need to assist with gastric lavage to help clear her stomach and small intestine of excess blood, clots, and corrosive gastric contents.

Before lavage
Find out which lavage fluid you'll be using. Most experts suggest using tap water rather than saline solution because it seems to break up clots better, and it's less expensive. For this patient, however, saline solution may be the better choice. That's because tap water can contribute to electrolyte imbalances, which a patient with an intestinal obstruction already has. Plus, electrolyte imbalances raise the risk of arrhythmias, which may be especially dangerous in an MI patient.

Find out what temperature the fluid should be. For this patient, you'll probably use a room-temperature or slightly cool solution that causes some vasoconstriction but doesn't lower the patient's core temperature.

Insert a nasogastric tube for lavage even if the patient has a tube in place for intestinal decompression. In most cases, an intestinal decompression tube extends past the site of stress ulcers. Thus, if you'd use the decompression tube for

lavage, you'd miss the area that needs treatment and raise the risk that extra fluid will increase the pressure on the obstruction.

During lavage
Instill 50 to 100 ml of solution into the tube. Leave it there for 2 to 3 minutes, then use a piston syringe to slowly and carefully aspirate it.

Carefully record the amount of solution instilled and the amount aspirated. Inspect the aspirated fluid for clots and increased bleeding.

Repeat this procedure until the fluid is lightly tinged or colorless and free from clots. If the aspirated fluid isn't clear within 30 minutes, notify the physician. The patient is still bleeding and may require different medical or surgical interventions.

After lavage
Monitor the patient's vital signs, electrocardiogram, and hemodynamic measurements frequently for changes that suggest increasing hypoxemia and shock.

Give supplemental oxygen as ordered, and assess oxygen saturation levels continuously, using pulse oximetry. Also, continue giving I.V. fluids, such as lactated Ringer's or normal saline solution.

Be sure to obtain a complete blood count. And have the patient's blood typed and cross-matched in case she needs a transfusion.

Anticipate giving an H_2 blocker to inhibit gastric acid secretion.

---

with her the risk factors associated with MI and intestinal obstruction and the possibility that the stress ulcer will bleed again. Instruct the patient to report increased abdominal distention, nausea, vomiting, or pain. Tell her to notify her physician right away if she vomits blood or material that looks like coffee grounds or if her stools become black and tarry. Emphasize that stress ulcers can start bleeding again, especially if she goes home while taking an anticoagulant.

Intestinal infarction
If your patient has an intestinal obstruction and an MI, she faces an increased risk of an intestinal infarction because reduced blood flow to

the intestines can make them ischemic. When blood and oxygen demand exceed supply, toxic metabolites accumulate in the intestines. The ischemia then causes epithelial cells to detach from the basement membrane, and subepithelial tissue protrudes into the villi. Besides worsening the patient's obstruction, ischemia, inflammation, and swelling may result in bloody diarrhea, perforation, or peritonitis.

Usually, a patient with an MI has an increased risk of thrombus formation and embolism because of the underlying atherosclerosis. If a thrombus or embolus occludes the mesentery artery, it can cause intestinal ischemia and altered membrane permeability. Initially, intestinal motility increases. It then decreases or stops. The damaged mucosa can't produce enough mucus to protect itself. And fluids shift into the intestinal wall and peritoneum, causing hypovolemia and a further decrease in blood flow. In some cases, collateral circulation develops to circumvent chronically decreased blood flow. However, the blood supply may not be adequate after eating, when the demand for blood increases. As the arterial occlusion progresses, infarction may develop.

Confirming the complication

Patients with chronic mesentery artery insufficiency typically develop colicky abdominal pain after eating. These patients may lose weight because they limit food intake to control the pain.

In an acute occlusion, the patient may complain of severe, continuous pain and bloody diarrhea. Her abdomen will be rigid, eventually distended, and bowel sounds may be absent. You may be able to hear a bruit over a partially occluded artery. Shock, fever, peritonitis, leukocytosis, and tachycardia may develop.

An angiograph of the mesenteric artery, an abdominal X-ray, and the patient's signs and symptoms help confirm the complication.

Nursing interventions

In a patient with an intestinal obstruction and reduced cardiac output from an MI, you can prevent an intestinal infarction by lowering the risk of ischemia. Nitroglycerin or another nitrate derivative dilates both the coronary and mesenteric arteries, thus increasing blood flow.

Assess the patient's abdomen frequently for changes in bowel sounds, abdominal pain, fever, and fluid extravasation. Measure her abdominal girth every 4 hours, and monitor her intake and output closely.

Continue to monitor the patient's cardiac status for changes that suggest ischemia. Give supplemental oxygen as ordered, and monitor the patient's oxygen saturation levels using pulse oximetry and ABG studies. Evaluate her ECG and hemodynamic measurements, too.

If the patient develops an intestinal infarction, anticipate the need for surgery to remove necrotic tissue. Try to stabilize the patient's condition as much as possible before surgery. Intervene as needed to maintain tissue perfusion, decompress the bowel, correct fluid volume

deficits, control pain and ischemia, maintain hemodynamic stability, and optimize cardiac and respiratory function. Provide appropriate patient teaching before and after surgery. Also, provide emotional support and guidance to the patient and family.

Intestinal obstruction and inflammatory bowel disease

Chronic inflammation of the intestinal wall raises the risk of an intestinal obstruction. That's why patients who have Crohn's disease (regional enteritis) or ulcerative colitis are at risk.

Because of its characteristic pathophysiologic changes, Crohn's disease is more likely than ulcerative colitis to cause intestinal obstruction.

Pathophysiology

In Crohn's disease, chronic inflammation typically begins in the submucosa of the small intestine and extends into the mucosa and serosa. It also may affect the large intestine, primarily the ascending and transverse colon.

As a result of the chronic inflammation, fibrous granulomas form in the mucosal wall, eventually reducing the lumen size. The intestinal wall becomes thickened, nodules form, and ulcers may develop. All these changes increase the risk of intestinal obstruction. The more often the patient has flare-ups of the disorder, the more damage her intestine sustains, and the greater her risk of infectious complications.

Usually, an obstruction develops during a flare-up of the disease, when the intestinal wall undergoes acute inflammatory changes. However, some patients with Crohn's disease also have chronic partial obstructions from the continuing inflammation and mucosal thickening. Strictures may develop as a result of scar tissue formation.

In ulcerative colitis, inflammation affects the large intestine, primarily the rectum and sigmoid colon. The mucosa erodes and may ulcerate. Abscesses and necrosis also may develop. The muscularis becomes edematous and thickened, causing the intestinal lumen to narrow.

Adapting nursing care

When caring for a patient with chronic inflammatory bowel disease, you'll need to be alert for signs and symptoms of an intestinal obstruction. Monitor the patient's GI status frequently. Auscultate her bowel sounds. Measure her abdominal girth and evaluate her stool patterns. Also, note any increased pain, abdominal distention, nausea, vomiting, or diarrhea.

Typically, during flare-ups, the patient with Crohn's disease receives an anticholinergic, an antidiarrheal, and an antispasmodic drug to allow the intestine to rest. If she has an obstruction, however, withhold these drugs. Also, avoid opiod analgesics because they slow peristalsis and may mask the signs of complications or a worsening intestinal obstruction.

For a patient who has an intestinal obstruction and inflammatory bowel disease, you'll need to control infection, monitor nutritional status and electrolyte levels, and establish a diet. In some cases, you may need to prepare the patient for surgery.

Managing infection

To help quiet the inflammatory process, give sulfasalazine, a corticosteroid, and an immunosuppressive drug, as prescribed. Also, give the prescribed antibiotics prophylactically to patients who are at risk for infection or who have intestinal strictures that cause stasis and bacterial proliferation.

Most complications of intestinal obstruction and inflammatory bowel disease are related to infection. It develops because of inflammation, endothelial tissue damage, and the use of corticosteroids. Keep in mind that corticosteroids decrease the number of circulating lymphocytes, basophils, and eosinophils, thus altering the patient's immune response. If a patient develops an infection, her regimen should include drugs that kill gram-positive, gram-negative, and anaerobic organisms. A common

regimen includes penicillin, an aminoglycoside, and either clindamycin or metronidazole.

Monitoring nutritional status and electrolyte levels

Keep in mind that a patient with Crohn's disease faces an especially high risk of malabsorption and fluid and electrolyte imbalances. That's because if an obstruction develops, it's likely to be in the small intestine. Plus, decompression used to treat the obstruction suctions potentially large volumes of electrolyte-rich fluids. And Crohn's disease tends to produce profuse diarrhea, which also leads to a loss of electrolytes.

For all these reasons, you should monitor the patient's serum electrolyte levels closely and administer replacement therapy as prescribed. Monitor the patient's daily weights, intake and output, and caloric intake closely. Anticipate the need for total parenteral nutrition.

Establishing a diet

When the patient's condition improves and she can eat, tailor her diet to her condition and tolerance. Stay away from raw fruits and vegetables, fatty foods, and spicy foods because they tend to increase diarrhea and abdominal pain. Ask the patient if she knows of any specific foods that trigger symptoms of her disease. And ask a dietitian to help you with meal planing. Offer suggestions for foods high in calories, protein, and minerals.

A patient with Crohn's disease may benefit from supplementation with elemental formulas. Consisting of free amino acids, simple sugar, and little fat, these predigested formulas require no digestion, only absorption. She'll probably need vitamin B_{12} and folic acid supplements.

Keep in mind that constipation may become a problem if a patient with Crohn's disease develops intestinal strictures. Stool softeners or suppositories may be needed because you won't be able to combat the problem by increasing bulk in her diet.

Preparing for surgery

If the patient has ulcerative colitis and develops a complication, such as an intestinal perforation, anticipate surgery. A partial intestinal resection may be performed, but the more typical procedure is a total proctocolectomy. This involves removal of the anus, rectum, and colon and the creation of a permanent ileostomy with an ileorectal anastomosis and a Kock pouch.

Crohn's disease tends to recur even after surgery. Surgery for these patients usually focuses on sparing as much of the intestine as possible to prevent malabsorption problems. The surgeon will try to remove only 5 to 10 cm above and below the area of visible damage. A temporary colostomy or ileostomy is performed whenever possible.

Whether your patient has ulcerative colitis or Crohn's disease, prepare her physically and emotionally for surgery; that is, prepare her for both the change in intestinal function and the change in body image.

After surgery, monitor the patient closely and provide emotional support, guidance, and education about the cause and treatment of the disease. Teach her how to care for the incision and, if appropriate, the ostomy. Obtain a referral for home care, if appropriate, to help the patient make the transition from hospital to home.

Patient teaching

Remember that patients with inflammatory bowel disease typically experience flare-ups and remissions. These changes can be frustrating, leaving the patient anxious and, at times, feeling powerless. Throughout your care of the patient with inflammatory bowel disease and an intestinal obstruction, help her develop and use her coping skills, and encourage her to participate actively in her care. Also, take time to teach her about her disease, its treatment, and the measures used to reduce the risk of complications (see *Teaching a patient with Crohn's disease and an intestinal obstruction*, page 416).

Complications

Common complications for patients with an intestinal obstruction and inflammatory bowel disease include fistulas and abscesses, peritonitis, and septic shock.

Fistulas and abscesses

The chronic inflammation of inflammatory bowel disease eventually causes erosive and fibrous changes in the intestinal wall. These changes increase the patient's risk of fistulas. This is especially true of patients who also have an intestinal obstruction because the obstruction raises intraluminal pressure. Fissures can easily develop, possibly deepening to communicate with nearby structures, such as reproductive organs, the urinary tract, or the peritoneum. If intestinal contents leak into these other areas, infectious complications, such as an abscess, typically develop.

As you know, an abscess is an encapsulated area of infection that doesn't communicate with other areas. Because few antibiotics can penetrate the enclosed area, most abscesses need to be drained.

Confirming the complication

With any fistula or abscess, a patient will have signs of infection: a fever, tachycardia, and an elevated WBC count. If a fistula communicates with the reproductive tract, intestinal contents will drain from the patient's vagina. If it communicates with the urinary tract, intestinal contents will drain into the urine. Also, the patient will have signs and symptoms of a urinary tract infection.

Nursing interventions

Patients who have Crohn's disease, an intestinal obstruction, and a fistula or abscess typically develop fluid and electrolyte imbalances. They also run the risk of developing a systemic infection, so observe your patient for the signs and symptoms of such an infection. Check her vital signs, especially her temperature and pulse, and monitor her WBC count.

Also, make sure the patient maintains an adequate fluid intake. Assess her nutritional status, fluid and electrolyte status, and daily weight. Administer fluid and electrolyte replacements as necessary, and urge her to eat a high-calorie diet. If the patient can't consume enough calories, prepare her for parenteral nutrition. Remember that her nutritional requirements will increase if she develops a systemic infection.

Anticipate the use of percutaneous drains to allow external drainage. Monitor the quantity and quality of the drainage. Provide meticulous

GOING HOME

Teaching a patient with Crohn's disease and an intestinal obstruction

If your patient with Crohn's disease has had an intestinal obstruction, you'll need to provide thorough teaching before her discharge. If you can help her minimize flare-ups of her Crohn's disease, you may just help her avoid another obstruction.

Start your teaching by explaining what's happening in her intestine. Keep it simple and make sure you explain how her symptoms relate to the disease process. Doing so will help decrease her anxiety, and it may help her detect early complications.

Then, go over the patient's drug regimen. For each drug, explain the purpose, dosage, and adverse effects. If she's taking a corticosteroid, warn her not to suddenly stop taking it because serious adverse effects can develop.

Next, teach her how to maintain nutrition and prevent complications.

Maintaining nutrition

- Encourage the patient to eat a high-calorie, high-protein diet. If her Crohn's disease flares up, tell her to avoid foods that make her symptoms worse—such as fresh fruits, vegetables, spicy foods, and fatty foods. Work with the patient, her family, and a dietitian to devise a personalized nutrition plan.
- Recommend the use of protein and calorie supplements, and encourage the use of multivitamin and mineral supplements.
- Urge the patient to drink about 3 liters of fluid a day to maintain hydration.
- Suggest that she drink a commercial electrolyte solution (such as a sports drink) if she begins to develop increasing intestinal irritation.
- Teach the patient and her caregiver how to perform parenteral nutrition therapy, if prescribed.

Find out whether the patient will receive it around the clock or intermittently.

- If the patient will receive continuous parenteral nutrition, instruct her to check her blood glucose levels every 6 hours. If she will receive intermittent therapy, tell her to check her blood glucose levels before, during, and after the therapy.
- Make sure the patient and her family know how to care for the catheter site properly.
- Tell the patient to take her temperature every day and to inspect the catheter insertion site for redness, swelling, warmth, and drainage. Urge her to report these changes to her physician right away.

Preventing complications

- Recommend that the patient keep a diary of her stool pattern and that she note any related medications she uses, such as stool softeners or suppositories.
- Tell her to call her physician if she hasn't had a bowel movement in 2 days. And warn her not to use bulk fiber laxatives, especially if she has an intestinal stricture.
- Tell the patient to be alert for pain, increased distention, nausea, vomiting, and diarrhea.
- Advise the patient to notify her physician if she vomits bright red blood or material that looks like coffee grounds or if her stools become tarry or red.
- Review the signs and symptoms of infection, and tell the patient to notify her physician if they develop.
- Remind the patient that her compliance with therapy is crucial. Urge her to keep all follow-up appointments.
- Suggest a referral for home care to make sure the patient receives the care she needs.

---

skin care for the drain insertion site and check for signs of skin breakdown. Give parenteral antibiotics, as prescribed.

Prepare the patient for surgical repair of a fistula, if appropriate. After surgery, provide the appropriate incision care.

Before discharge, reinforce all aspects of the patient's regimen. Teach her to care for the

wound, if appropriate. Review the signs and symptoms of infection and tell her to notify her physician if they develop. Urge the patient to take her temperature every day. If she takes a corticosteroid, explain that she has an increased risk of infection. And because corticosteroid use may suppress her inflammatory response, explain that she may experience fever or chills if or when a severe infection first develops.

Finally, anticipate a referral for home care to provide follow-up evaluation and education about the disease and wound-care measures.

Peritonitis

Patients who have an intestinal obstruction and inflammatory bowel disease face an increased risk of intestinal perforation from the increased intraluminal pressure and erosion of the intestinal wall. If the intestine perforates or a fistula forms, intestinal contents can leak into the peritoneum, causing peritonitis. To make matters worse, patients with inflammatory bowel disease commonly take corticosteroids, which increase the risk of infection.

Bacterial peritonitis commonly involves such organisms as *Escherichia coli*, alpha-hemolytic and beta-hemolytic streptococci, *Staphylococcus aureus*, enterococci, and gram-negative rods. These organisms enter the peritoneal cavity through a break in the GI tract, possibly from a mucosal erosion or a change in mucosal permeability.

Chemical peritonitis also results from a break in the mucosa that allows GI contents to spill into the peritoneum. Once the bacteria and GI fluids enter the peritoneum, they spread easily through the abdominal cavity. An inflammatory reaction occurs, changing the permeability of the peritoneal membrane. This change causes water and electrolytes to shift rapidly into the abdominal cavity. In response to this inflammatory process, blood is shunted to the area to combat the infection. The result is further distention with additional fluid and gas accumulation in an already obstructed intestine.

Many times, a patient has both bacterial and chemical peritonitis.

Confirming the complication

A patient with peritonitis typically complains of continuous abdominal pain. At first, she may have a rigid abdomen. Then, she may experience a less painful period, in which rebound tenderness develops and profound fluid shifting and hypovolemia occur. The patient may try to relieve the pain by lying supine with her knees flexed. She may complain of weakness, malaise, nausea, vomiting, and diarrhea. She

also may have a fever, tachycardia, hypotension, and shallow respirations.

In the early stages of peritonitis, you'll hear hyperactive bowel sounds. Later, as the condition progresses and causes paralytic ileus, you won't hear any bowel sounds.

In a patient with the typical signs and symptoms, elevated serum amylase levels usually confirm the diagnosis of peritonitis. The patient's WBC count may be increased, and her serum protein levels may be decreased. In some cases, a physician may perform peritoneal aspiration and culture and sensitivity testing to identify blood, bacteria, pus, bile, or amylase in the peritoneal fluid.

Nursing interventions

Patients with peritonitis need immediate antibiotic therapy and massive amounts of I.V. fluids, electrolytes, and blood or blood products to correct hypovolemia, electrolyte imbalances, and anemia. Throughout the patient's care, monitor her vital signs, hemodynamic measurements, and fluid and electrolyte status. Also, check her WBC count for changes. If she has a CVP catheter attached to a monitoring device, check the values for signs of continuing hypovolemia. Maintain her CVP between 2 and 6 mm Hg (or 5 to 12 cm H_2O), as ordered.

Promote ventilation by placing the patient in the semi-Fowler or high Fowler position. These positions help shift fluid to the lower abdomen, removing pressure from the diaphragm and allowing the patient to breath more effectively. Give supplemental oxygen and monitor the patient's oxygen saturation using pulse oximetry. Note the rate, depth, and character of her respirations.

Maintain NG or nasointestinal decompression to relieve the obstruction and decrease the distention. Monitor the amount, color, and odor of the drainage. Irrigate the tube as needed to maintain patency. Make sure the patient receives nothing by mouth. And anticipate the need for total parenteral nutrition.

To alleviate severe pain and anxiety, administer a narcotic analgesic and a sedative, as prescribed.

When peritonitis appears to result from a perforation caused by an intestinal obstruction, emergency surgery is usually performed. Prepare the patient for surgery and provide supportive care. If the patient isn't a surgical candidate and other interventions haven't been effective, the physician may perform peritoneal lavage using rapid dialysis exchanges and antibiotics.

When the patient's condition has stabilized, explain what happened and what she can do to prevent a recurrence. Reinforce all aspects of the treatment plan to control the inflammatory bowel disease.

Septic shock

A patient with an intestinal obstruction and inflammatory bowel disease is at high risk for systemic infection that may progress swiftly to septic shock—a systemic inflammatory reaction that results when the infecting organism is broken down by WBCs and releases endotoxins. These endotoxins release chemical mediators that cause massive vasodilation, selective vasoconstriction, and increased capillary permeability. As a result, the patient suffers dramatic fluid shifts, hypovolemia, and hypotension that's unresponsive to fluid resuscitation.

An intestinal obstruction can lead to septic shock in a few ways. For one, increased intraluminal pressure and altered mucosal permeability may allow bacteria to translocate across the intestinal wall and into the bloodstream. For another, microorganisms can enter the bloodstream when mucosal erosion results in draining fistulas, abscesses, or peritonitis. Also, patients with inflammatory bowel disease commonly take a corticosteroid, which can increase the risk of infection and mask its signs and symptoms. This tendency may delay treatment for perforation or peritonitis, thus increasing the risk of septic shock.

Septic shock eventually causes decreased tissue perfusion and cellular hypoxia. Without adequate nutrition and oxygenation, cells die, and tissues and organs become dysfunctional. Because prolonged septic shock can be fatal, you'll need to monitor your patient carefully for its signs and symptoms—and be prepared to intervene swiftly.

Confirming the complication

Typically, a patient with early septic shock has a high fever, hypertension with bounding peripheral pulses, tachycardia, tachypnea, and flushed, warm skin. As the condition progresses, the patient becomes hypotensive, and her respiratory rate slows. Her peripheral pulses may become weak and thready. Now, she may look pale and have cool, clammy skin. You may hear crackles and wheezes in her lungs. Her urine output will decrease as will her LOC. She may grow confused, lethargic, or drowsy.

The patient's WBC count and erythrocyte sedimentation rate probably will be elevated. If renal dysfunction has developed, her BUN, creatinine, potassium, and sodium levels also may be elevated. Her ABGs probably will reveal metabolic acidosis, with a bicarbonate level below 22 mEq/L and a pH below 7.35. A blood culture may identify the pathogen.

Nursing interventions

RAPID RESPONSE ▶ When your patient is in septic shock, you'll focus on enhancing tissue perfusion, promoting gas exchange, and restoring body temperature.

- Every 15 minutes, monitor the patient's vital signs.
- Monitor the patient's urine output and assess her intake and output hourly.
- Assist with the insertion of a pulmonary artery catheter or central venous line and check the values hourly. Also, monitor other hemodynamic values, such as systemic vascular resistance, as indicated.
- Administer I.V. fluids, such as colloids and crystalloids, blood or blood products, and electrolytes, as prescribed.
- Give a vasopressor and inotropic drug, as prescribed, to increase blood pressure and cardiac output.
- Monitor ABG results for hypoxemia and acidosis.
- Provide supplemental oxygen and assess oxygen saturation continuously, using pulse oximetry.
- Without causing the patient discomfort, elevate the head of the bed to improve chest expansion.
- If the patient develops respiratory distress or cardiopulmonary arrest, assist with endotracheal intubation and mechanical ventilation.

- Administer an I.V. antibiotic, as prescribed.
- Monitor the patient's CBC results, including the WBC count, hemoglobin, and hematocrit.
- Administer an antipyretic, as prescribed, to reduce fever. Use a hypothermia blanket or tepid sponge baths to lower the patient's body temperature.
- Monitor the patient for restlessness, confusion, and a decreased LOC, which may indicate decreased cerebral perfusion. ◄

Septic shock is more likely to be a surgical emergency in a patient with an intestinal obstruction than in other patients. That's because the patient's intestine continues to feed the infection until the break in the intestinal wall is repaired. During surgery, the patient probably will receive intraperitoneal antibiotics and systemic therapy.

Prepare your patient for surgery and monitor her closely afterward. Assess her cardiac and respiratory status. Check her vital signs and hemodynamic measurements frequently. Also, give supplemental oxygen and monitor her oxygen saturation levels, using pulse oximetry. Monitor her ABG results, CBC, and electrolyte levels.

Observe the patient's abdomen closely after surgery. Auscultate her bowel sounds and be alert for distention. Maintain decompression drainage as ordered and anticipate advancing the diet as the patient's bowel function returns.

Throughout the patient's care and before discharge, reinforce all instructions. Review the need to control the inflammatory bowel disease. And urge the patient to monitor herself closely for signs and symptoms of obstruction and infection. Finally, obtain a referral for home care, if appropriate.

Suggested readings

Abrams JH, Cerra FB. *Essentials of surgical critical care.* St Louis, Mo: Quality Medical Publishing; 1993.

Cerrato PL. New acute MI guidelines. *RN.* 1997; 60(1):25-26.

Cumbie B, Clement S. Action stat: bowel obstruction. *Nursing.* 1996;26(1):33.

Ferrin M. Restoring electrolyte balance: magnesium. *RN.* 1996;59(5):31-34.

Huether SE, McCance KL. *Understanding pathophysiology.* St Louis, Mo: Mosby–Year Book, Inc; 1996.

Isselbacher K, Braunwald E, Wilson J, Martin J, Fauci A, Kasper D. *Harrison's principles of internal medicine.* 13th ed. New York, NY: McGraw-Hill, Inc; 1994

Kirtin CA. Assessing for ascites. *Nursing.* 1996; 26(4):53.

Pagana KD, Pagana TJ. *Mosby's diagnostic and laboratory test reference.* 3rd ed. St Louis, Mo: Mosby–Year Book, Inc; 1997.

Parrillo JE, Bone RC. *Critical care medicine: principles of diagnosis and management.* St Louis, Mo: Mosby–Year Book, Inc; 1995.

Price SA, Wilson LM. *Pathophysiology: clinical concepts of disease processes.* 5th ed. St Louis, Mo: Mosby–Year Book, Inc; 1997.

Rakel R. *Conn's Current Therapy.* Philadelphia, Pa: WB Saunders Co; 1996.

Urban N, Greenlee KK, Krumberger J, Winkelman C. *Guidelines for critical care nursing.* St Louis, Mo: Mosby–Year Book, Inc; 1995.

White VM. Hyperkalemia. *Am J Nurs.* 1997; 97(6):35.

Zaloga GP. *Nutrition in critical care,* St Louis, Mo: Mosby–Year Book, Inc; 1994.

Index

---

i indicates an illustration; t indicates a table.

---

i indicates an illustration; t indicates a table.

R